OXFORD MEDICAL PUBLICATIONS

Paediatric Dermatology

Oxford Specialist Handbooks published and forthcoming

General Oxford Specialist Handbooks
Addiction Medicine
Applied Medicine and Surgery in Dentistry
Day Case Surgery
Infection in the Immunocompromised Host
Perioperative Medicine, 2e
Pharmaceutical Medicine
Postoperative Complications, 2e
Renal Transplantation
Retrieval Medicine

Oxford Specialist Handbooks in Anaesthesia
Anaesthesia for Emergency Care
Global Anaesthesia
Neuroanaesthesia
Obstetric Anaesthesia, 2e
Paediatric Anaesthesia, 2e
Regional Anaesthesia, Stimulation and Ultrasound Techniques
Thoracic Anaesthesia
Vascular Anaesthesia

Oxford Specialist Handbooks in Cardiology
Adult Congenital Heart Disease, 2e
Cardiac Catheterization and Coronary Intervention
Cardiovascular Computed Tomography, 2e
Cardiovascular Imaging
Cardiovascular Magnetic Resonance
Echocardiography, 2e
Fetal Cardiology, 2e
Heart Disease in Pregnancy
Heart Failure, 2e
Hypertension
Inherited Cardiac Disease
Nuclear Cardiology
Pacemakers and ICDs, 2e
Pulmonary Hypertension
Valvular Heart Disease

Oxford Specialist Handbooks in Critical Care
Advanced Respiratory Critical Care
Cardiothoracic Critical Care

Oxford Specialist Handbooks in End of Life Care
Dementia
Heart Failure
Kidney Disease
Respiratory Disease

Oxford Specialist Handbooks in Infectious Disease
Infectious Disease Epidemiology

Oxford Specialist Handbooks in Neurology
Parkinson's Disease and Other Movement Disorders, 2e
Stroke Medicine, 2e

Oxford Specialist Handbooks in Oncology
Practical Management of Complex Cancer Pain

Oxford Specialist Handbooks in Paediatrics
Community Paediatrics
Manual of Childhood Infections, 4e
Paediatric Dermatology 2e
Paediatric Endocrinology and Diabetes
Paediatric Gastroenterology, Hepatology, and Nutrition, 2e
Paediatric Intensive Care
Paediatric Nephrology, 3e
Paediatric Neurology, 3e
Paediatric Palliative Medicine, 2e
Paediatric Radiology
Paediatric Respiratory Medicine
Paediatric Rheumatology

Oxford Specialist Handbooks in Pain Medicine
Spinal Interventions in Pain Management

Oxford Specialist Handbooks in Psychiatry
Addiction Medicine, 2e
Forensic Psychiatry
Medical Psychotherapy

Oxford Specialist Handbooks in Radiology
Head and Neck Imaging
Interventional Radiology
Musculoskeletal Imaging
Thoracic Imaging

Oxford Specialist Handbooks in Surgery
Burns
Cardiothoracic Surgery, 2e
Colorectal Surgery
Current Surgical Guidelines
Gastric and Oesophageal Surgery
Hand Surgery, 2e
Oral and Maxillofacial Surgery, 2e
Otolaryngology and Head and Neck Surgery
Plastic and Reconstructive Surgery
Surgical Oncology
Urological Surgery
Vascular Surgery, 2e

Oxford Specialist Handbooks in Paediatrics

Paediatric Dermatology

SECOND EDITION

EDITED BY

Sue Lewis-Jones

Consultant Dermatologist,
Department of Dermatology, Ninewells Hospital and Medical School, Dundee, UK

Ruth Murphy

Consultant Dermatologist and Paediatric Dermatologist,
Department of Dermatology, Royal Hallamshire Hospital, Sheffield, UK

OXFORD
UNIVERSITY PRESS

OXFORD
UNIVERSITY PRESS

Great Clarendon Street, Oxford, OX2 6DP,
United Kingdom

Oxford University Press is a department of the University of Oxford. It furthers the University's objective of excellence in research, scholarship, and education by publishing worldwide. Oxford is a registered trade mark of Oxford University Press in the UK and in certain other countries

First Edition published in 2010
Second Edition published in 2020

Published in the United States of America by Oxford University Press
198 Madison Avenue, New York, NY 10016, United States of America

British Library Cataloguing in Publication Data

Data available

Library of Congress Control Number: 2019942870

ISBN 978–0–19–882130–4

Dedication

To the founders of the British Society for Paediatric Dermatology, especially Professor Julian Verbov, Professor John Harper, Dr David Atherton, and other members of the founding committee.

Acknowledgements

We are grateful to our numerous colleagues for their hard work, patience, and helpful support in producing this book, especially the first edition authors and the British Society for Paediatric Dermatology (BSPD). We would like to thank all the children and their parents who have made this book possible by allowing us to use their images. Our thanks also go to the medical photography departments at Ninewells Hospital, Perth Royal Infirmary, Addenbrookes Hospital, and colleagues too numerous to mention who have helped to provide other suitable photographs.

Foreword

Skin disease in children is extremely common but paediatric dermatologists are scarce. In practice most paediatric skin disease is managed by general practitioners, paediatricians, emergency physicians, and increasingly physicians' assistants, nurses, health visitors, and pharmacists. Recognizing this, members of the British Society for Paediatric Dermatology (BSPD) chose to make their specialty more accessible to other professionals by producing this useful handbook. Ten years on from the first edition, the need is greater than ever as many dermatology consultant posts remain vacant, skin clinics are moving to the community, and patients are increasingly 'skin aware' and wanting expert advice.

A key attraction of this book is its practical, problem-based format. The enquiring doctor just needs to observe what colour or shape the skin condition is, where it is on the body, or how it feels, to find the right information. This meant that contributors had to think creatively as well as thoroughly researching their topic. Sue Lewis-Jones and Ruth Murphy, both past presidents of the BSPD, have done a sterling job in cajoling and supporting their authors to contribute and to update their sections.

The authors are all enthusiasts for paediatric dermatology. Many have subspecialty expertise ranging from common disorders such as eczema to the more niche genodermatoses. But the message throughout is restrained and focused: not 'this is what we know' but 'this is what you need to know'. It comprises the condensed wisdom of dedicated paediatric dermatologists motivated to reach out and share their skills with all those caring for children with skin disease.

Professor Celia Moss
Consultant Dermatologist
Birmingham Children's Hospital
and University of Birmingham, UK

Contents

Section 4 Rashes

Section 5 Textural skin changes

Section 6 Discolouration of the skin

Section 7 Rashes in rheumatology and transplant patients

Contributors

Paula Beattie
Consultant Dermatologist, Department of Dermatology, Royal Hospital for Sick Children, Glasgow, UK
Chapter 16

Sarah Bridges
Consultant Paediatrician, Musgrove Park Hospital, Taunton and Somerset NHS Trust, UK
Chapter 24

Nigel Burrows
Consultant Dermatologist, Department of Dermatology, Cambridge University Hospitals NHS Foundation Trust, Cambridge, UK
Chapter 29

Sheila Clark
Consultant Dermatologist, The Leeds Teaching Hospital and Mid Yorkshire Hospitals NHS Trust, Leeds and Wakefield, UK
Chapters 18, 21

Tim Clayton
Consultant Paediatric Dermatologist, Central Manchester University Hospitals NHS Foundation Trust, Manchester, UK
Chapter 7

David de Berker
Consultant Dermatologist, Department of Dermatology, Bristol Royal Infirmary, Bristol, UK
Chapter 15

Carsten Flohr
Chair in Dermatology and Population Health Science and Consultant Dermatologist, St John's Institute of Dermatology, St Thomas, Hospital, London, UK
Chapter 17

Richard Goodwin
Consultant Dermatologist, Department of Dermatology, Royal Gwent Hospital, Newport, UK
Chapters 1, 2, 3

Helen Goodyear
Consultant Paediatrician and Associate Postgraduate Dean, University Hospitals of Birmingham and Health Education England, West Midlands, UK
Chapter 25

Gordon Hale
Specialist Registrar, Royal Hallamshire Hospital, Sheffield Teaching Hospitals NHS Trust, UK
Chapters 4, 14

Ross Hearn
Consultant Dermatologist, Department of Dermatology and Photobiology, Ninewells Hospital and Medical School, Dundee, UK
Chapter 23

Mary Judge
Consultant Dermatologist, Department of Dermatology, Salford Royal NHS Foundation Trust, Salford, UK
Chapter 27

Cameron Kennedy
Consultant Dermatologist, Departments of Dermatology, Bristol Royal Infirmary, and Paediatric Dermatology, Bristol Royal Hospital for Children, Bristol, UK
Chapters 5, 28

Thomas King
Specialist Registrar, Royal Hallamshire Hospital, Sheffield Teaching Hospitals NHS Trust, UK
Chapters 11, 12, 30

Veronica Kinsler
Consultant Paediatric Dermatologist and Academic Lead Clinician, Paediatric Dermatology, University College London Hospitals NHS Foundation Trust, London, UK
Chapter 34

Bisola Laguda
Consultant Paediatric Dermatologist, Department of Dermatology, Chelsea and Westminster Hospital NHS Foundation Trust, London, UK
Chapter 6

Susan Lewis-Jones
Hon Consultant Dermatologist, Department of Dermatology, Ninewells Hospital and Medical School, Dundee, UK
Chapters 9, 24, 26

Anna Martinez
Consultant Paediatric Dermatologist, Department of Dermatology, Great Ormond Street Hospital, London, UK
Chapter 38

Cassandra McDonald
EB Fellow, Great Ormond Street Hospital, London, UK
Chapter 38

Jemima Mellerio
Consultant Dermatologist, St John's Institute of Dermatology Guy's and St Thomas' NHS Foundation Trust, London, UK
Chapters 25, 38

Andrew Messenger
Consultant Dermatologist, Department of Dermatology, Royal Hallamshire Hospital, Sheffield, UK
Chapter 14

Ruth Murphy
Consultant Dermatologist and Paediatric Dermatologist, Department of Dermatology, Royal Hallamshire Hospital, Sheffield, UK
Chapters 4, 10, 11, 12, 13, 30, 38

Siobhan Muthiah
Dermatology Specialist Registrar, Royal Victoria Infirmary, Newcastle Upon Tyne, UK
Chapter 22

Sivakumar Natarajan
Consultant Dermatologist, Department of Dermatology, Royal Victoria Infirmary, Newcastle upon Tyne, UK
Chapter 22

Malobi Ogboli
Consultant Dermatologist and Paediatric Dermatologist, Department of Dermatology, Sandwell and West Birmingham Hospitals NHS Trust, UK
Chapters 19, 20

Emma Ormerod
Dermatology Specialist Registrar, Department of Dermatology, Bristol Royal Infirmary, Bristol, UK
Chapter 15

David Rutkowski
Dermatology Specialist Registrar, Salford Royal Foundation Trust, Manchester, UK
Chapter 7

Muriel Sadlier
Dermatology Specialist Registrar, Our Lady's Children's Hospital Crumlin, Dublin, Ireland
Chapter 8

Graham Sharpe
Consultant Dermatologist, Clatterbridge Hospital, Wirral, UK
Chapters 32, 33, 35, 36, 37

Lindsay Shaw
Consultant Dermatologist and Paediatric Dermatologist, Department of Dermatology, University Hospitals Bristol NHS Foundation Trust, Bristol Royal Infirmary, Bristol, UK
Chapters 24, 31

Rosemarie Watson
Consultant Paediatric Dermatologist, Department of Dermatology, Our Lady's Children's Hospital Crumlin, Dublin, Ireland
Chapter 8

Paul Yesudian
Consultant Dermatologist and Paediatric Dermatologist, The Grosvenor Hospital, Chester, UK
Chapters 32, 33, 35, 36, 37

Symbols and Abbreviations

➲	cross-reference
⚑	red flag
AA	alopecia areata
ACEI	angiotensin converting enzyme inhibitors
ACTH	adrenocorticotropic hormone
AE	atopic eczema
AGEP	acute generalized exanthematous pustulosis
APEC	asymmetric periflexural exanthem of childhood
AT	alopecia totalis
BAD	British Association of Dermatologists
BCG	bacillus Calmette-Guérin
BIE	bullous ichthyosiform erythroderma
BNF	British National Formulary
BSACI	British Society for Allergy and Clinical Immunology
CAH	congenital adrenal hyperplasia
CALM	café-au-lait macule
CAVLM	capillary–arteriovenolymphatic malformation
CAVM	cerebral arteriovenous malformation
CCE	cornified cell envelope
CIE	congenital ichthyosiform erythroderma
CINCA	chronic infantile neurologic cutaneous and articular syndrome
CLVM	capillary–lymphatic–venous malformation
CM	capillary malformations
CMN	congenital melanocytic naevus
CMTC	cutis marmorata telangiectatica congenita
CMV	cytomegalovirus
CNS	central nervous system
CRMO	chronic recurrent multifocal osteomyelitis
CRP	C-reactive protein
CSU	chronic spontaneous urticaria
CU	chronic urticaria
CVM	congenital vascular malformation
DA	dermatitis artefacta
DEJ	dermoepidermal junction
DIC	disseminated intravascular coagulation
DLSO	distal lateral subungual onychomycosis
DRESS	drug rash with eosinophilia and systemic symptoms
EB	epidermolysis bullosa
EM	erythema multiforme
EMLA®	Eutectic Mixture of Local Anaesthetics
FBC	full blood count
FCAS	familial cold autoinflammatory syndromes
FDA	Food and Drug Administration
FFP	fresh frozen plasma
FG	faltering growth
FSH	follicle-stimulating hormone
FTU	fingertip unit
GA	granuloma annulare
GH	growth hormone
GVHD	graft versus host disease
HDU	high dependency unit
HPA	hypothalamic-pituitary-adrenal
HPV	human papilloma virus
HSV	herpes simplex virus
HUVS	hypocomplementaemic urticarial vasculitis
ICU	intensive care unit
IH	infantile haemangioma
ILVEN	inflammatory linear verrucous epidermal naevus
IM	intramuscular
ISSVA	International Society for the Study of Vascular Anomalies
IU	intrauterine
IV	intravenous
KOH	potassium hydroxide

KTS	Klippel–Trenaunay syndrome
LBW	low birth weight
LC	Langerhans cells
LCH	Langerhans cell histiocytosis
LE	lupus erythematosus
LH	luteinizing hormone
LI	lamellar ichthyosis
MEN	multiple endocrine neoplasia
MMR	measles, mumps, rubella
MSH	melanocyte-stimulating hormone
NAI	non-accidental injury
NICH	non-involuting congenital haemangioma
NICU	neonatal intensive care unit
NOMID	neonatal onset multisystem inflammatory disease
OD	once daily
OTC	over the counter
PASH	pyoderma gangrenosum, acne, suppurative hidradenitis
PCOS	polycystic ovary syndrome
PCR	polymerase chain reaction
PLE	polymorphic light eruption
PROS	progressive overgrowth syndrome
PWS	port-wine stain
QOL	quality of life
RAS	recurrent aphthous stomatitis
RCT	randomized controlled trial
RICH	rapidly involuting congenital haemangioma
SCID	severe combined immunodeficiency
SLE	systemic lupus erythematosus
SPF	sun protection factor
SWS	Sturge–Weber syndrome
TA	tufted angioma
TB	tuberculosis
TCS	topical corticosteroids
TEN	toxic epidermal necrolysis
TNF	tumour necrosis factor
UAS	Urticaria Activity Score
UV	ultraviolet
VA	vascular anomalies
VM	venous malformations
VZV	varicella-zoster virus
WHO	World Health Organization
XLRI	X-linked recessive ichthyosis
XP	xeroderma pigmentosum
YAG	yttrium aluminium garnet

Glossary

Abscess* collection of acute inflammatory cells (polymorphs).
Acantholysis* loss of intercellular keratinocyte adhesions predisposing to clefting or blister formation at various layers in epidermis.
Acanthosis* increase in epidermal thickness.
Alopecia absence of hair in normally hairy site.
Anetoderma localized skin laxity causing either depressions or out pouching of the skin due to loss of elastic tissue.
Anhidrosis absence of sweating.
Anonychia absence of nails.
Apoptosis* individual cell death resulting in condensation of nucleus (pyknosis).
Atrophy term used for loss of tissue from any layer of skin or subcutis or all, causing thinning of the skin.
Autoinflammatory syndrome a clinical syndrome caused by an exaggerated response of the innate immune system resulting in spontaneous episodes of inflammation affecting multiple organs.
Blister fluid-filled lesion that may be serous or blood-filled.
Bulla large blister, may be unilocular or multilocular.
Closed comedo (whitehead) plug of keratin or sebum within skin pore and covered by epithelium.
Collagenoma a connective tissue naevus derived from too much collagen.
Comedone (pl. nes) (blackhead) plug of keratin or sebum distending the skin pore.
Crusting dried serous exudate.
Dyschromatosis altered, abnormal discolouration of the skin, often with several shades of colour.
Ecchymosis extravasation of blood cells into the skin (bruise) > 2mm in diameter.
Elastolysis* disintegration of the dermal elastin.
Elastoma a connective tissue naevus characterized by overgrowth of elastic fibres.
Enanthem superficial mucosal lesions usually associated with infection.
Epidermis the outer layer of the skin.
Erosion superficial loss of epidermis (leaves no scarring).
Erythema redness of the skin (may be difficult to assess in dark skin where it may manifest as increased pigmentation).
Erythroderma erythema covering all or most of the body.
Escutcheon (shield-shaped) hair growing upwards and outwards rather than downwards, e.g. male pattern of pubic hair in a female.
Exanthem skin rash, usually associated with infection.
Excoriation scratch mark causing loss of skin tissue.
Exfoliation separation of outer keratin layer of skin in scales or sheets.
Exocytosis* presence of inflammatory cells within spongiotic epidermis.
Fibroma benign tumour composed of fibrous or connective tissue.
Fissure splitting of the skin.

Follicular associated with opening of hair follicle (skin pore).
Granuloma* collection of chronic inflammatory cells in dermis and/or subcutis.
Hamartoma* local overgrowth of tissue of one or more cell types.
Hyper/hypo/depigmentation increased/reduced/complete loss of pigment.
Hypercornification increase of the horny (cornified) layer.
Hyperhidrosis increased sweating.
Hyperkeratosis increased horny (cornified) layer.
Hyperplasia excessive formation of cells.
Hypertrichosis increased body hair in non-male pattern.
Hypohidrosis decreased sweating.
Ichthyosis dry skin, usually refers to inherited dry skin conditions.
Keratoderma thickening of horny layer of skin.
Leukonychia white nails (or white patches on nails).
Lichenification exaggeration of the normal skin creases due to protective thickening of the epidermis (usually from chronic rubbing).
Lipoatrophy localized loss of fat tissue resulting in overlying skin depression.
Lipoma benign overgrowth of fat cells, causing subcutaneous swellings.
Macule flat, non-palpable area of change in skin colouration.
Maculopapular erythematous (red) rash consisting of macules and papules, e.g. measles.
Milium a tiny keratin-filled cyst.
Monomorphic all lesions are similar, e.g. molluscum contagiosum.
Morbilliform measles-like, i.e. widespread, blotchy macular red rash with tiny papules within.
Naevus* a 'nest' of cells of same histological type.
Nikolsky's sign deemed positive when, on lateral pressure, the superficial skin layers slip free from the underlying tissue extending or producing a blister.
Nodule larger palpable lesion >5mm size (approximately, varies in different textbooks).
Onycholysis lifting of nail from nail bed.
Panniculitis inflammation of the subcutaneous fat tissue presenting as painful skin lumps.
Papule small raised palpable lesion <5mm size (approximately, varies in different textbooks).
Parakeratosis* abnormal retention of nuclei within stratum corneum.
Paronychia inflammation of nail fold and loss of cuticle.
Patch flat area of skin change, usually considered larger than 2cm in diameter.
Pathergy lesions arising in sites of minor trauma seen particularly in Beçhet's disease and pyoderma gangrenosum.
Perifollicular around margin of follicular opening.
Periungual around nail.
Petechia (pl. iae) tiny haemorrhagic dot (1–2mm).
Phlebolith calcification within vein, hard and nodular.
Pica compulsion to eat non-food items such as fabric, coal, hair, etc.
Pityriasis fine branny scaling.
Plaque raised area of skin rash, usually >2cm, e.g. psoriasis.

Poikiloderma areas of skin showing mixture of altered pigmentation, telangiectasia, and atrophy.
Polymorphic rash several different types of lesions present, e.g. acne has papules, comedones (blackheads), pustules, and cysts.
Progeria various rare inherited conditions resulting in premature ageing (cutaneous and systemic).
Pruritus itching without a visible rash.
Purpura area of skin haemorrhage 5mm or more in diameter (exact size varies between texts) often used to describe bruising.
Pustule small blister containing neutrophils (or other leukocytes).
Pyoderma any purulent skin disease.
Rhagades fissuring or splitting of the skin.
Scales adherent keratinocytes (from stratum corneum).
Sclerosis induration of subcutaneous tissue, which may include the epidermis.
Serpiginous snake-like linear lesions.
Spongiosis* intercellular oedema within epidermis that makes prickles stand out.
Striae linear marks, ridge, or groove on the skin surface.
Subungual below the nail.
Target lesion three or more concentric rings of alternating pale and red skin, usually with central erythema or purpura.
Telangiectasia small capillaries visible below skin.
Tinea ringworm. Latin names used to designate body site affected, e.g. for ringworm of scalp (*T.capitis*), hand (*T.manuum*), foot (*T.pedis*), body (*T. corporis*), groin (*T.cruris*), face (*T.faciei*), nails (*T.unguium*).
Ulcer loss of epidermis and dermis (or deeper).
Ungual pertaining to the nails.
Vacuolation* degenerative change in epidermal basal cells in which intracellular vacuoles occur.
Varioliform lesions resembling smallpox.
Verrucous rough, irregular surface resembling a viral wart.
Vesicle small blister.
Weal or wheal transient raised pale area of oedema, usually surrounded by red flare.
Xanthoma (pl. ta) yellowish lipid-filled papules, nodules, or plaques.
Xerosis mildly dry skin often associated with eczema.

* Denotes histological terminology

Section 1

Basics of dermatology

Chapter 1

Structure and function of the skin

Structure and function of the skin

The skin is comprised of three layers (Fig. 1.1):

- The epidermis.
- The dermoepidermal junction.
- The dermis.

The epidermis has digitate (finger-like) folds known as *rete pegs*, which project down into the dermis. Similarly the dermis projects upwards as *dermal papillae*. This helps to protect the integrity of the skin from mechanical frictional shearing forces.

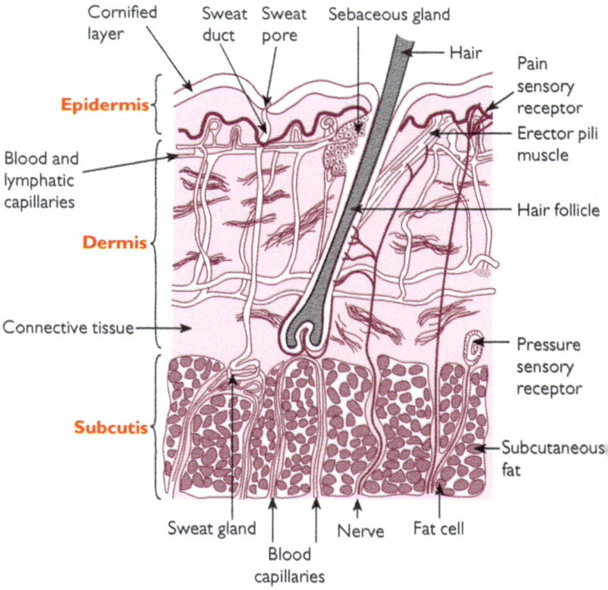

Fig. 1.1 The structure of the skin.

Adapted with permission from Warrell D.A. *et al.* (Eds.) (2004). *Oxford Textbook of Medicine*, Fourth Edition. Oxford, UK: Oxford University Press

The epidermis

- See Fig. 1.2.

The epidermis is immensely complex and comprised of several layers of keratinocytes with different functions and structure interspersed with melanocytes and occasional Merkel cells.

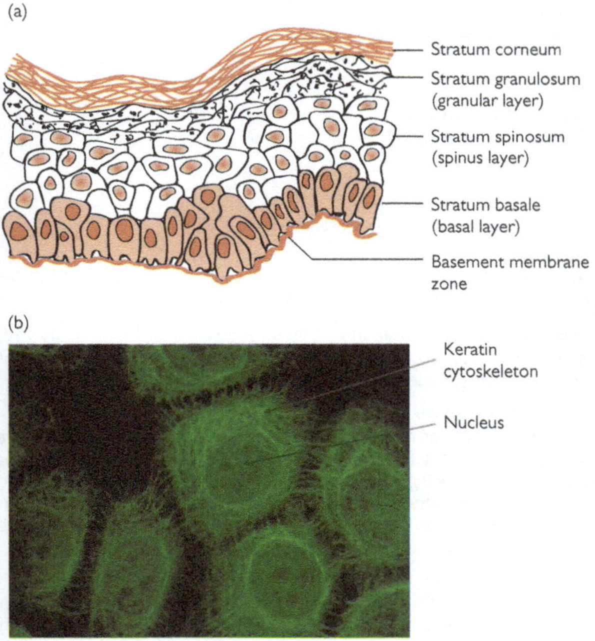

Fig. 1.2 (a) The epidermis. (b) Keratinocytes in culture showing cytoskeleton of keratin.

Reproduced courtesy of Birgitte Lane, Chief Scientist, Skin Research Institute of Singapore, Singapore

Cells found in the epidermis

- *Keratinocytes*—the main cells of the epidermis that change their shape and function over 28 days as they migrate to the surface to form the cornified cell envelope, and are eventually shed. Keratin filaments containing paired keratin proteins form fibrils by interlinking heterodimers. This provides a rigid cell cytoskeleton. The pairs differ within each layer of epidermis and with the type of epithelium. Intercellular adhesion is achieved by complex bodies known as desmosomes and at the dermoepidermal junction by hemidesmosomes. Gap junctions allow intercellular communication.
- *Langerhans cells*—dendritic antigen-presenting cells forming part of the immune surveillance system of the skin, conveying antigen to T lymphocytes.
- *Melanocytes*—dendritic cells interspersed between the basal keratinocytes containing melanin pigment (within melanosomes), which overlie the nucleus and act as a protective cap against ultraviolet damage.

- ***Merkel cells***—mechanoreceptors, function poorly understood.
- ***Sweat ducts and pilosebaceous orifice***—pass through the epidermis to open out on to the skin surface.
- ***Bare nerve endings***.

Layers of the epidermis

There are four main layers of the epidermis:
- Basal layer.
- Spinous layer.
- Granular layer.
- Stratum corneum (cornified cell envelope, CCE).

Basal layer

Attached to the dermoepidermal junction by hemidesmosomes. Active cell division occurs to replenish cells lost from CCE.

Spinous layer (stratum spinosum)

Lipid biosynthesis occurs in upper cell layer (and granular layer) with formation of lamellar granules (membrane-coating granules).

Granular layer (stratum granulosum)

Keratohyalin granules contain proteins such as profilaggrin (filament aggregating protein) that aids terminal cell-differentiation by keratin filament aggregation and flattening of the cell. Other granules contain involucrin, which acts together with other envelope precursors such as loricrin, plakins, and transglutaminases (and others) with degradation of corneodesmosomes and construction of a durable, flexible cell envelope forming the CCE.

Cornified cell envelope (CCE) (stratum corneum)

Outermost layer of flat (dead) corneocytes with impermeable cell envelope surrounded by lipid layer of ceramides, free sterols, and free fatty acids. The function of the CCE is to act as a semi-permeable barrier to reduce cellular water loss and prevent entry of noxious substances such as irritants, allergens, and micro-organisms.

The dermoepidermal junction (DEJ)

This region lies between the epidermis and dermis, incorporating the plasma membrane of the basal keratinocytes, melanocytes, and Merkel cells (Fig. 1.3), and the basement membrane which is composed of three main layers:
- Lamina lucida.
- Lamina densa.
- Lamina fibroreticularis.

Structural abnormalities in and antibodies against various components are found, respectively, in genetic and acquired blistering, dry, scaly skin diseases.

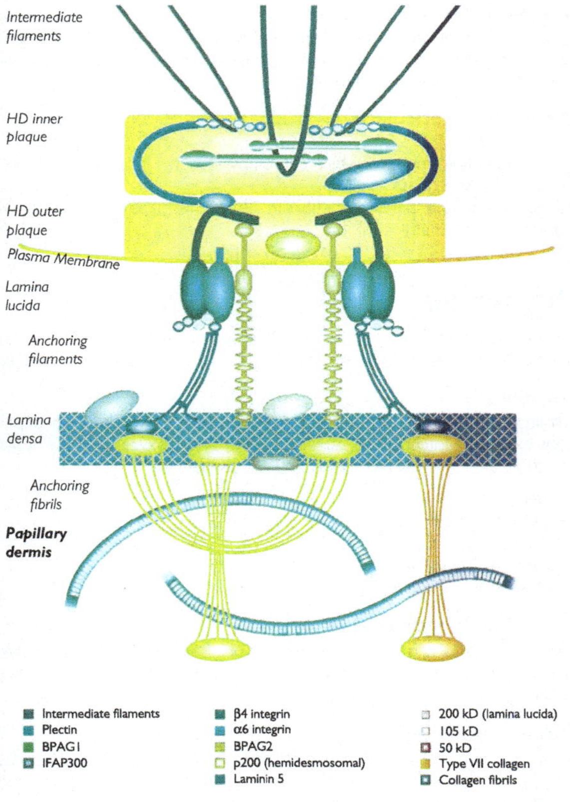

Fig. 1.3 The dermoepidermal junction.

Reproduced with permission from Pulkkinen L. and Uitto J. (1998) Hemidesmosomal variants of epidermolysis bullosa. Mutations in the alpha6beta4 integrin and the 180-kD bullous pemphigoid antigen/type XVII collagen genes. *Exp Dermatol*. 7(2–3):46–64

Lamina lucida

Appears as a clear zone on electron microscopy lying below the basement cells and above the lamina densa.

- *Anchoring filaments:* perpendicular fine filaments that traverse the lamina lucida from the plasma basement membrane into the lamina densa. Particularly concentrated around the hemidesmosomes.
- *Hemidesmosomes:* complex structures that attach basal cells to the basement membrane.

Lamina densa

Appears as an electron-dense zone below and parallel to the lamina lucida. Anchoring filaments pass upwards to connect with basal cells, while anchoring fibrils help to anchor it to the upper dermis.

Lamina fibroreticularis

This contains:

- *Anchoring fibrils:* many of which curve upwards in a loop to insert twice into the lamina densa.
- *Elastic microfibrils:* particularly fibrillin. Usually as bundles interlacing with dermal elastin bundles.

The dermis

The dermis lies below the DEJ and is attached to it by anchoring fibrils formed from collagen VII. Within the dermis lie many important structures:

Vasculature

Forming deep and superficial reticulate capillary networks with papillary loops extending into dermal papillae, which supply oxygen and nutrients to the whole skin (the epidermis has no blood vessels).

Functions

- Metabolite transport.
- Thermoregulatory.
- Aiding wound repair.
- Part of immunosurveillance system.

Dermal connective tissue

Consisting mainly of collagen and elastin fibrils contained in a mucopolysaccharide ground substance. This provides structure, texture, and elasticity for the skin and protects specialized organs.

Cutaneous nerves

Follow same pattern as vasculature with deep and superficial plexuses. Autonomic supply to sweat and sebaceous glands and arrector pili muscle.

There are various nerve receptors:

- *Pencillate free nerve endings*—'paint brush' shape, extensive network common in papillary dermis, around hair papillae and intraepidermal layer for precise touch, pain, itch, and temperature.
- *Pacinian corpuscles*—'onion' shaped and layered pressure and vibration receptors found mainly in subcutis and around arterio-venous anastomoses, especially palms and soles (some on genitals and nipples).
- *Meissner corpuscles*—papillary shape found individually in dermal papillae of volar skin (hands, feet, and fingertips) for touch.
- *Merkel cells*—slow-acting mechanoreceptors.

Nerve endings are abundant in non-hairy erogenous zones of nipple and genitalia.

Sweat glands

For disorders, see ➲ Disorders of sweating, pp. 11–13.

- *Eccrine glands*—located all over the body but greatest concentration on palms and soles. Secretory coil lies deep in reticular dermis and duct opens directly on the skin surface. Sympathetic (cholinergic) fibres cause secretion of mainly water and electrolytes essential in maintaining body temperature control. Full control is not complete until age 2–3y.
- *Apocrine glands*—large, coiled, tubular glands deep in the dermis of scalp, face, axillae, nipples, and anogenital areas. Duct opens directly into infundibulum of hair follicle. Secretion occurs by loss of apical projection directly into lumen (holocrine secretion) mediated mainly by alpha adrenergic stimuli caused by powerful emotions or pain but not heat. Function is uncertain (Fig. 1.4).

Pilosebaceous unit

Name given to a hair and its related structures, the sebaceous gland, and the arrector pili muscle. Types of hair:

- *Lanugo*—fetal hair, found in newborn. Fine, non-medullated, with little pigment. Replaced by intermediate and then terminal scalp hair by 2y.
- *Terminal*—long, coarse, and medullated, usually pigmented.
- *Vellus*—short, fine, soft, non-medullated hairs.

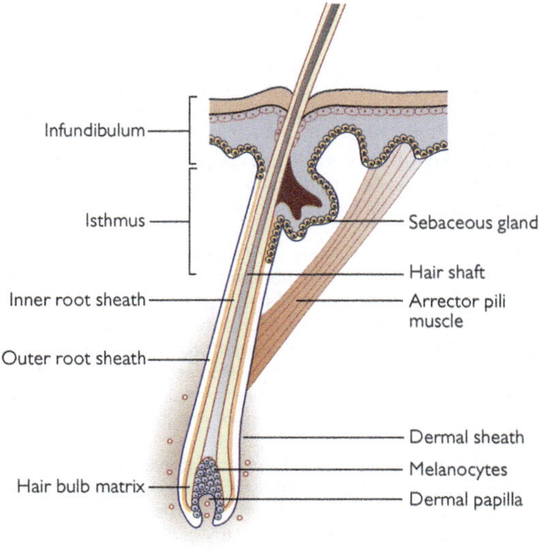

Fig. 1.4 Diagram of anagen hair follicle.

Reproduced with permission from Burns T. *et al.*, (Eds.) (2016). *Rook's Textbook of Dermatology*, Tenth Edition. Oxford, UK: Wiley Blackwell

Fully formed terminal hair has a central medulla, cortex, and cuticle surrounded by varying thickness of inner and outer root sheaths (site dependent).

- *Hair bulb*—contains the dermal papilla (hair germinal cells) and lies in the subcutaneous tissue. Its size determines the hair thickness.
- *Sebaceous gland*—secretes sebum into duct that opens into the hair follicle at the infundibulum (which is lined by stratified squamous epithelium). Most numerous on face, scalp, and upper chest. Specialized glands are found on lips and buccal mucosa (Fordyce spots), eyelids (Meibomian and Zeis), glans penis, prepuce (Tyson's), and nipple (Montgomery's tubercles).
- *Arrector pili muscle*—composed of smooth muscle, attaches to the outer root sheath at the isthmus. Contraction causes hair erection. Adrenergic and cholinergic innervation.
- *Apocrine sweat glands*—also open into the infundibulum.

Functions of the skin

The skin is a highly complex structure with multiple functions. It may be modified in different body sites. The following is a simplified outline:

- *Barrier function*—the stratum corneum acts as waterproof covering, retains moisture, prevents entry of harmful substances including bacteria and allergens, and limits mechanical damage.
- *Percutaneous absorption*—the majority of substances applied to the skin will be absorbed to some degree and this is increased by occlusion with dressings or in areas of thinner skin (e.g. face, axillae, and genital area). Tape stripping or frictional trauma thins the epidermis and increases absorption.
- *Thermoregulatory*—the extensive and complex vasculature can undergo constriction to retain heat or dilatation to lose heat.
- *Sweating*—reduces heat by water loss and helps to maintain electrolyte balance.
- *Sensory function*—to detect pain, light touch, itch, thermal, pressure, and vibratory changes via a three-dimensional network of afferent (sensory) and efferent (autonomic) nerve fibres. Loss of sensation and pain can lead to neuropathic changes (e.g. in diabetes or leprosy).
- *Immunosurveillance*—the skin has a major protective immune function and is part of the body's defence against infection and malignancy. Keratinocytes and Langerhans cells within the epidermis can act as antigen-presenting cells to the T lymphocytes found mainly in the dermis.
- *Synthesis of vitamin D*—under influence of ultraviolet light (sunlight).
- *Production of keratins*—to form cytoskeleton of keratinocytes, giving structure and helping to protect against mechanical damage.
- *Formation of extracellular lipids* (particularly ceramides)—vital to the function and integrity of the stratum corneum.
- *Formation of specialized structures*—hair, nails, sweat glands, sebaceous glands. All have their own particular function.
- *Sexual*—the appearance of skin, hair, and nails plays a major role in sexual attraction and is specially modified in areas such as the anogenital area, axillae, and breasts.

In different body sites, the skin is modified for specific functions, e.g.
- ***Palms and soles***—protective epidermal thickening with absence of hair.
- ***Nipples***—modified for lactation and contain specialized Montgomery tubercles.
- ***Nails***—provide protection and act as tools for manipulation.
- ***Scalp hair and eyebrows***—for heat retention and sexual characteristics.
- ***Secondary sexual hair***—at puberty, growth of specialized axillary and pubic hair, and increased beard and moustache hair in the male.

Disorders of sweating

There are two types of sweat glands: eccrine and apocrine (➲ see Sweat glands, p. 9).

Disorders of the eccrine glands

Abnormalities of sweating are common and may be inherited or acquired. Main problems are:
- Decreased sweating—hypohidrosis.
- Increased sweating—hyperhidrosis.

Rarely there may be problems with:
- Coloured sweat—from drugs such as isoniazid or infection.
- Unusual smell—some metabolic disorders.

Causes of hypohydrosis

Several genetic disorders are linked to poor sweating, which often presents in infancy as febrile convulsions. The best known is *hypohidrotic ectodermal dysplasia:* X-linked is commonest but autosomal dominant and recessive forms occur. Main features are:
- Sparse fair hair.
- Peg-like (tiger) teeth.
- Poor sweating.
- Erythroderma and scaling at birth.
- Characteristic facies, with frontal bossing, saddle nose with depressed ridge, large lower lips.
- Significant mortality from hyperthermia and infection.

Its management requires a multidisciplinary approach.

Causes of hyperhidrosis

It may be primary (idiopathic) or secondary, and diffuse or localized. Several problems arise (Box 1.1).

Presentations of hyperhidrosis in children

Primary type (constitutional)

Commonest type: usually localized hand and foot sweating, often with malodour; sometimes axillae. Red palms, often cold and dripping sweat (autonomic effect). Feet often develop pitted keratolysis (Fig. 1.5) caused by several different Gram-positive filamentous organisms including *Micrococcus, Dermabacter, Janibacter, Kytococcus*, and *Propionibacterium* species. Hyperhidrosis causes markedly impaired quality of life.

Box 1.1 Problems associated with hyperhidrosis

- Social (peer rejection), embarrassment, and loss of confidence.
- *Feet:* malodour, skin maceration, pitted keratolysis, bromhidrosis, increased risk of contact dermatitis to foot wear, worsening of pre-existent skin disease, e.g. juvenile plantar dermatosis (forefoot eczema; ➲ see Fig. 12.7) or epidermolysis bullosa (➲ see Genetic causes of blisters, pp. 387–390).
- *Hands*: difficulty writing and holding pens, ruins paper and clothes, etc.
- *Axillae:* malodour and damage to clothes.

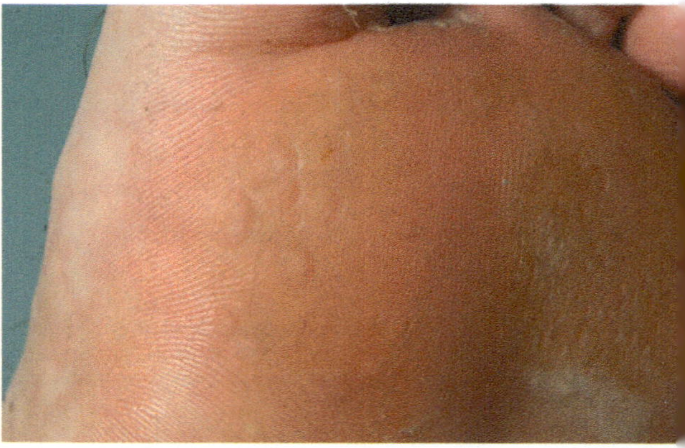

Fig. 1.5 Pitted keratolysis of the sole.

Reproduced courtesy of Susan Lewis-Jones, Hon Consultant Dermatologist, Ninewells Hospital and Medical School, Dundee, UK

Treatment

- ***Local hygiene measures:*** cotton socks, leather (non-patent) shoes, cork insoles.
- ***Numerous topical agents***: for example, topical aluminium chloride solutions (Driclor® or Anhydrol Forte® over-the-counter (OTC)) apply at night (2 weeks then weekly or bi-weekly—irritant); several topical antibiotics (e.g. erythromycin, clindamycin, benzoyl peroxide).
- ***Iontophoresis:*** with either tap water or, more effectively, anticholinergic agents (e.g. glycopyrronium preparations).
- ***Systemic drugs:*** oxybutynin or propiverine hydrochloride can be helpful in teenagers. Avoid anticholinergics if possible.
- ***Injection:*** botulinum toxin is proving helpful for axillary hyperhidrosis in teenagers but is a second-line therapy; sympathetic blocks; both require specialist training.
- ***Local axillary surgery:*** local denervation or destruction, avoid in children
- ***Surgical sympathectomy:*** a last resort, avoid in children.

Secondary types

Generalized

- ***Various emotional stimuli*** and following vomiting.
- ***Systemic diseases*** (e.g. hyperthyroidism, acromegaly, diabetes mellitus, Cushing's syndrome).
- ***Drug overdose:*** salicylism; alcohol or neonatal heroin withdrawal.
- ***Increased catecholamine secretion*** from shock, hypoglycaemia.
- ***Causes of fever*** (e.g. tuberculosis, brucellosis, malaria).
- ***Neurological:*** brain tumours, encephalitis; cerebral hypoxia.

Localized

- Some diseases listed previously may cause localized sweating of palms and soles (e.g. neurological tumours, endocrine disease).
- Local eccrine tumours (very rare).
- Gustatory sweating of cheeks (malar areas)—Frey's or auriculotemporal syndrome. Causes red patch on cheeks following eating.

Rare genetic syndromes with hyperhidrosis include nail-patella, dyskeratosis congenita, Papillon–Lefèvre, Charcot–Marie–Tooth, and others.

Apocrine disorders

Usually in adults—very uncommon in children.

- ***Tumours:*** such as apocrine hidrocystoma (cystadenoma) or syringocystadenoma papilliferum (usually in conjunction with sebaceous tumours).
- ***Hidradenitis suppurativa:*** recurrent abscesses, boils, and keloid scarring in anogenital, axillary, and submammary areas (➲ see Chapter 11).

Chapter 2

The dermatological consultation

Introduction

It is vital to take a good history, which in many cases will provide the diagnosis. This chapter describes what should take place in a dermatologica[l] consultation and includes some basic investigations.

Taking a dermatological history

History of rash or lesion

A carefully taken dermatological history is essential, providing the diagnosis in most cases. Include a knowledge of the following:

- *Length of time* of evolution of a rash or lesion, its duration, and its relation to preceding medical events (e.g. pyrexia, new medication). Is there any fluctuation? If episodic: how long does it last; how long do individual lesions last? Is there any history of similar rash or lesions?
- *Character*: colour; size; shape; edges (well- or poorly defined). Is it flat, raised, papular, nodular? Are there any blisters, crusts, or scales? Has there been a change in character (e.g. in colour, shape, or size of lesions)? Is the texture soft/hard, smooth/rough, regular/irregular?
- *Pattern*: is there a recognizable pattern of lesions or distribution of rash (➲ see Chapter 4)?
- *Body site(s)*: where it started; does it move around (e.g. in urticaria lesions move within 24h) or does it recur in the same place (e.g. herpes simplex, fixed drug reaction)? Is it always located in a particular distribution, e.g. peripherally or centrally or on limbs (extensor or flexural) or scalp, face, etc.?
- *Symptoms*: note presence or absence of itching? Is anyone else in family itching (e.g. scabies), is it worse at night (e.g. scabies)? Itching alone without skin signs is known as pruritus (➲ see Itching, pp. 262–4). Is there any soreness, burning, or pain?
- *Seasonal variation*: or reaction to light, cold, trauma, etc.
- *Relieving or provoking factors*: including treatment, stress, and exercise?
- *Previous skin problems and response to therapies*.

General health and development

Should usually include a full paediatric history:

- Birth and feeding history, dietary intake, and growth (particularly relevant in young children), vaccination programme.
- General development and milestones, including progress at school.
- Other medical complaints including recurrent infections.
- Birthmarks, natal teeth, clefting, accessory lesions, pits, or other unusual features.
- Abnormalities of hair, nails, teeth, sweating, sight, or hearing.

Detailed drug history

Extremely important. List all drugs, including over the counter (OTC), herbal, alternative/complementary therapies and topicals, particularly in the last 6 weeks. Is there any temporal relationship to the rash? Most drug rashes start within 3 weeks of starting drug (➲ see Chapter 23).

Allergies

To drugs (including local anaesthetics; topical medicaments), foods, cosmetics, jewellery (e.g. nickel), rubber products, animals, sunlight, and plants. Note type of allergy (i.e. immediate or delayed), and any associated symptoms such as rash, vomiting, or other gastrointestinal symptoms, wheezing, or difficulty breathing or swallowing, loss of consciousness, or cardiovascular collapse (➲ see Chapter 21, Anaphylaxis, pp. 311–13).

Treatments

Record:

- *Past and present*: including length of use and any OTC or alternative/complementary therapies, topical and systemic drugs, phototherapy, laser, etc.
- *Success of treatments*: any adverse reactions; adherence (compliance) with therapies.

Family history

Ask about skin diseases, especially atopy (eczema, asthma, hay fever), psoriasis, acne, autoimmunity. In family tree—check for consanguinity, miscarriages/still births, especially where 'genetic' diseases are suspected. Has anyone else had a similar problem in the past? If urticaria is suspected (➲ see Chapter 21) ask if there is thyroid disease in the family.

Social history

Who lives at home? In a separated family, is there medication at both homes? Any severe stress (bereavement, teasing, domestic violence)? Any pets, or contact with animals outside the home (e.g. grandparents, childminders, etc.)? Any school problems? List hobbies and sports.

Quality of life (QoL) measurement

Very important to consider this in children with skin diseases. Research suggests that skin diseases affect children (and families) across all aspects of their lives. The visible nature of skin disease makes concealment from peers difficult, and having eczema or urticaria, for example, is worse than having many other chronic diseases such as asthma or diabetes.

QoL effects include:

- Questions about disease/teasing/bullying, which may cause loss of confidence.
- Mood changes including depression, withdrawn or aggressive behaviour, which often result in school problems and school avoidance.
- Symptoms such as itching or pain affect sleep, causing tiredness and loss of concentration, particularly in atopic eczema (➲ see Chapter 17).
- Restriction of activities such as games or sports and swimming.
- Embarrassment from having to wear concealing clothes, make-up, or wigs, or getting undressed with others.
- Difficulties on holidays or at friends' houses.
- Restriction of diets or avoidance of pets.
- Difficulty with treatments.

Impairment in health-related QoL occurs from the combination of physical, psychological, or social malfunction. Factors influencing this include age, gender, ethnicity, social class, education, life experience, and cognitive ability. In those with impaired cognition or in young children, information is obtained by proxy from parent(s) or carer(s) and may be biased.

How to measure QoL in clinic

QoL assessment is an important part of clinical assessment and may reveal some surprising evidence. It can be done by:

- Informally asking a child (or parent/carer) how much the skin problem is bothering them; does it affect their confidence or sleep, etc.?
- Using a visual analogue scale, the result of which may be expressed as a % of the whole.
- QoL questionnaires. There are specific dermatological quality of life scales available (free for clinical assessment) from http://www.dermatology.org.uk/ (click on quality of life).
    - The Children's Dermatology Life Quality Index* (CDLQI©) for children of school age with any skin disease.
    - The Infants' Dermatitis Quality of Life index* (IDQoL©) for atopic eczema.
    - The Dermatitis Family Index* (DFI©)—impact of atopic eczema on the family.
    - The Family Dermatology Quality of Life Index (FDLQI©)—a measure of the impact of a patient's skin disease on adult family members.
    - Cardiff Acne Disability Index (CADI©).

Examining the skin

Skin examination

This should be done in a good light, with a magnifying lens for close examination. The whole skin should be inspected (Box 2.1). Look at distribution and pattern of rash or lesions and try to characterize the rash/lesion

Box 2.1 Things to consider when examining a child

- The child (and parents) must be at their ease.
- The room should be child friendly and warm.
- Get down to their level—if necessary, on the floor.
- Use toys to distract (or to 'look' at child for you!).
- Use a nurse, play therapist, or parent to help with a very apprehensive child or if child requires holding to keep still.
- Tell parents and children what you wish to do. Don't ask a toddler for permission to examine; they will usually say no, but do explain what you are doing—demonstrating on a toy can be helpful.
- If necessary, examine the upper body first and allow them to dress again before looking at the lower part. Respect modesty of all ages but especially teenagers.

* **Declaration of interest:** Dr Sue Lewis-Jones (editor) owns co-copyright to the questionnaires marked with *.

according to type (➲ see Chapter 4). Always check the hands and feet (and genitalia if relevant or scabies is suspected). If hand dermatitis is present, also check the feet for signs of athlete's foot (➲ see Chapter 22). Examine mouth, ears, and eyes, teeth, hair, and nails, especially if genetic disorders are suspected.

General examination

Should include growth charts for height and weight. Head circumference in certain circumstances, e.g. suspected neurofibromatosis (➲ see Localized forms of brown pigmentation, pp. 491–4). Look for faltering growth (➲ see Chapter 6), obesity, unusual body habitus, skeletal problems, or dysmorphic facial features.

Dermoscopy (dermatoscopy)

A hand-held oil-immersion lens or polarized, magnified light, used for aiding differential diagnosis of pigmented or vascular skin lesions, e.g. melanocytic naevi (moles, ➲ see Chapter 34) but also increasingly for hair disorders and even inflammatory skin changes. Requires some specialist training but is non-invasive and can be very helpful to demonstrate scabies mites or nits non-invasively (Fig. 2.1) or view nail fold telangiectasia in connective tissue disease.

Wood's light

UVA black light (wavelength 365nm), used for examination (in the dark) of white macules, e.g. in tuberous sclerosis complex (ash-leaf macules) or vitiligo (➲ see White skin (hypomelanosis), pp. 480–6). Different colours of fluorescence may be seen, e.g. yellow or green in some dermatophyte infections (ringworm; Fig. 2.2) or a salmon pink in erythrasma (➲ see p.167).

Photography

Be aware of guidelines on the taking and storage of medical photographs on personal or hand-held devices. Obtain informed consent and take good photographs of any lesions, especially dermoscopy images of any melanocytic lesion (mole) that requires monitoring (➲ see Chapter 34), rashes that are unusual or undiagnosed, and especially for suspected child abuse.[1]

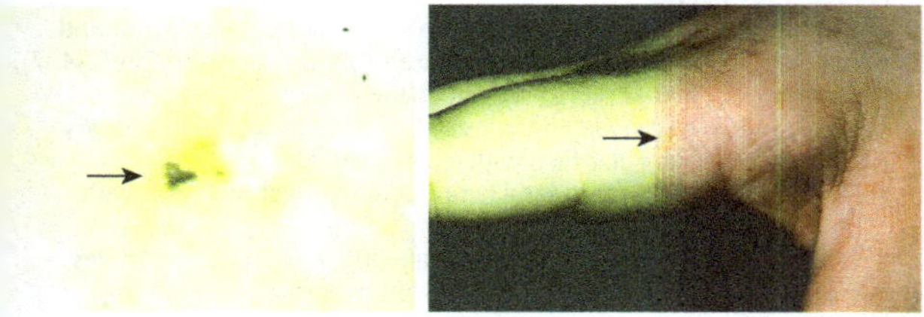

Fig. 2.1 Dermoscopy showing scabies mites in burrows.

Reproduced courtesy of Susan Lewis-Jones, Hon Consultant Dermatologist, Ninewells Hospital and Medical School, Dundee, UK

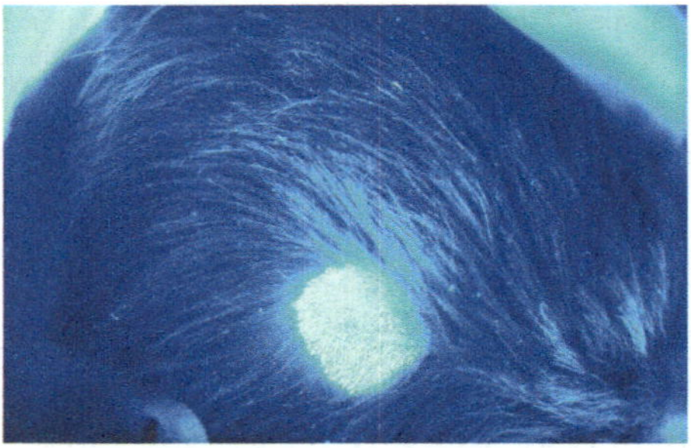

Fig. 2.2 Wood's light and ringworm of scalp.

Reproduced courtesy of Susan Lewis-Jones, Hon Consultant Dermatologist, Ninewells Hospital and Medical School, Dundee, UK

Height, habitus, and skin changes

Abnormally tall

- *Marfan's syndrome*: multiple skeletal abnormalities including tall, thin body habitus; long fingers (arachnodactyly); joint hypermobility; pectus excavatum or carinatum; increased arm span to height ratio; scoliosis. Also, upward dislocation of lens, dilatation of the aorta (aortic aneurism—frequently fatal). Skin changes are minimal (e.g. striae and may have bluish sclera).
- *Acromegaly*: large hands, feet, and head. May be associated with acne vulgaris and increased sweating.

Abnormally small stature

- *Atopic eczema*: (approximately 10%) usually severe cases (➲ see Chapter 17) often found with asthma and oral corticosteroids. Very rarely from topical corticosteroids.
- *Faltering growth*: various vitamin deficiencies (➲ see Chapters 32 and 33). May also be associated with erythroderma and immunodeficiency (➲ see also Chapter 6).
- *Genetic diseases*: numerous, e.g. Bloom's, Cockayne's and Rothmund–Thomson syndromes (➲ see Exaggerated sunburn reaction, pp. 234–7), and all types of acrogeria (➲ see Fat changes, pp. 452–3).
- *Turner's syndrome (gonadal dysgenesis)*: females 45, XO, with primary amenorrhoea. Triangular face with micrognathia.
  - *Newborn*: transient peripheral lymphoedema; webbed neck with redundant skin folds.
  - *Older*: low-set hairline; sometimes café-au-lait macules and moles.
- *Russell–Silver syndrome*: dwarfism, limb anomalies, café-au-lait macules.
- *Xeroderma pigmentosum*: extreme photosensitivity, skin tumours, and premature ageing—various types (➲ see Chapter 16, Exaggerated sunburn reaction, pp. 234–7).

Skin problems associated with exceptional obesity

- *Frictional dermatitis*: particularly inner thighs from rubbing.
- *Pigmentation*: particularly acanthosis nigricans (➲ see Fig. 33.6).
- *Generalized hypertrichosis and hirsutism* (➲ see Fig. 14.14).
- *Intertrigo*: redness and itching in moist flexures—often with secondary candidiasis. Commoner in diabetics (➲ see Diabetes mellitus, pp. 60–2).
- *Striae*: stretch marks; common in puberty (adolescent striae) (➲ see Fig. 29.6).

Skin problems associated with excessive weight loss

- *Anorexia nervosa*: dry skin with downy hypertrichosis but also scalp loss (telogen effluvium); pili torti; pigmentary changes—often carotenaemia (➲ see Introduction, Yellow or orange colouration, p. 520); acrocyanosis; periungual erythema; brittle nails.
- *Loose skin*: redundant folds.
- *Associated vitamin deficiencies*, e.g. pellagra—darkening of skin pigment, photosensitivity (➲ see Vitamin deficiencies, p. 494).

Dermatological procedures: skin surgery

Skin biopsy

Used for diagnosis of skin rashes or to remove a lesion. This must be done by a practitioner suitably trained in skin surgery and trained in dealing with children. The child and parent(s)/carer must have fully consented and be informed about the procedure and its possible risks (bleeding, infection, and unsightly scar or keloid formation are the commonest). Young babies can often be biopsied under local anaesthesia, perhaps with a sedative, provided they are appropriately swaddled and held. Otherwise most procedures in young children will require general anaesthesia. All tissue samples removed should be sent for histopathological examination.

Local anaesthesia

Always ask about allergy prior to use. Consider a short-acting topical anaesthetic preparation first, e.g. EMLA® cream (Eutectic Mixture of Local Anaesthetics 2.5% lignocaine, 2.5% prilocaine), LMX4® (4% lidocaine), or Ametop (4% tetracaine) under film occlusion, followed by infiltration of the biopsy site with a suitable local anaesthetic. As a rule, adrenaline should be avoided in young children (Box 2.2).

Note: EMLA® should not be used in premature babies or neonates up to 3 months of age because of the risk of methemoglobinemia.

Types of biopsy procedure

Incisional ellipse biopsy

Used for diagnosis of skin rashes or large tumours to help aid management plan†.

Punch biopsy

An alternative to ellipse biopsy. Various sizes of disposable punches (usually 3–5mm) are available. Useful for tissue diagnosis (e.g. tumour)†.

†*All require wound closure with suturing.*

Box 2.2 Tips for reducing pain in children

Reducing fear

- Prepare beforehand: explain procedure, use play therapist if possible.
- Use child-friendly surroundings, with their music, a story, or parent's 'phone.
- Keep instrument tray out of sight.
- Let a parent stay (provided they can cope) or use a nurse to distract.

Reducing the pain of injection

- Use topical anaesthetic for an adequate time first.
- Use narrow 30-gauge needle.
- Prewarm local anaesthetic to body temperature.
- Rubbing and gently pinching skin at same time as injection helps.
- Prior use of ice or ethyl chloride spray helps to numb area.
- Give injection very slowly.

Excisional ellipse biopsy

Used for excision of whole lesion or tumour. This results in a scar approximately three times as long as the lesion[†].

Sutures

There are two main types:

- Absorbable (e.g. Vicryl™, PDS™).
- Non-absorbable (e.g. synthetic nylon such as Ethilon™, or polypropylene such as Prolene™).

Size depends on type of wound and body site. The higher the number the finer the suture. Generally 4/0 gauge is suitable for the body and limbs and 5/0 or 6/0 for the face. For simple excisions use an interrupted suture method and avoid tension across the wound.

Not requiring wound closure

Curettage and cautery

A small razor-sharp ring curette pares away surface skin layers for superficial removal (e.g. of warts, pyogenic granulomas). The raw area is cauterized with electrocautery or hyfrecation or chemical cautery with aluminium chloride hexahydrate solution.

Hyfrecation

Hyfrecation is a form of cold electrocautery. This is a radiofrequency-based treatment that heats and destroys tissue. Local anaesthetic may or may not be required prior to treatment depending on the site and condition being treated. Can be used to treat telangiectatic vessels, comedones, small skin tags, and to stop bleeding.

Shave biopsy

Shaving across base of lesion to leave flat area flush with skin surface (e.g. pedunculated skin tags. Bleeding can be stopped by pressure or a cautery technique).

[†]*All require wound closure with suturing.*

Skin snip

A useful technique of cutting a piece from the free edge of peeling skin in some blistering conditions such as staphylococcal scalded skin syndrome (➲ see Neonatal erythroderma, p. 87). It is painless so does not require anaesthesia and does not scar. Histopathological examination will determine the depth of blistering and aid diagnosis. Check with pathologist first because not all are familiar with this technique. A special transport medium may be required.

Electrolysis

Can be used to remove hair that will not respond to laser epilation. Can be painful and occasionally causes postinflammatory pigmentary changes and scarring.

Histopathological examination

Interpretation of skin biopsy specimens requires a histopathologist with a specialist knowledge of cutaneous pathology, particularly for pigmented (melanocytic) lesions, which may be erroneously interpreted as malignant by the unwary. The request form should contain sufficient clinical details to aid interpretation of histopathological features. In cases of diagnostic uncertainty, it is often wise to have a discussion with the pathologist to aid interpretation of the biopsy specimen (Box 2.3).

Box 2.3 Some commonly used histological terms

- For further information, ➲ see Glossary, p. xv.
- *Abscess*—collection of acute inflammatory cells (polymorphs).
- *Acantholysis*—loss of intercellular keratinocyte adhesions predisposing to clefting or blister formation at various layers in epidermis.
- *Acanthosis*—increase in epidermal thickness.
- *Apoptosis*—individual cell death resulting in condensation of nucleus (*pyknosis*).
- *Exocytosis*—presence of inflammatory cells within spongiotic epidermis.
- *Granuloma*—collection of chronic inflammatory cells in dermis and/or subcutis.
- *Hamartoma*—local overgrowth of tissue of one or more cell types.
- *Naevus*—nest of cells of same histological type.
- *Parakeratosis*—abnormal retention of nuclei within stratum corneum.
- *Spongiosis*—intercellular oedema within epidermis that makes prickles stand out.
- *Vacuolation*—degenerative change in epidermal basal cells in which intracellular vacuoles occur.

Note: this is merely a brief description of commonly used basic surgical techniques. For further information readers are referred to appropriate texts on skin surgery.

Other dermatological investigations

Skin scrapes

Essential where tinea (ringworm) is suspected—note that this can rarely occur in neonates. Any red scaly rash should be scraped if the diagnosis is uncertain, especially red scaly faces. Swab skin first with an alcoholic wipe to eradicate bacteria, which can contaminate culture plates. In young children where use of a scalpel blade might be dangerous, try a plastic knife or similar object; or alternatively, a cervical brush or toothbrush can be used to obtain samples (including scalp) to directly impregnate into culture plate

Hair samples

Hair plucking or cutting (➲ see Investigations, pp. 196–7). Used mainly for microscopical examination. However, in tinea capitis (scalp ringworm) the hairs may be loose and easily plucked for culture.

Direct microscopy

Useful for hair shaft abnormalities, staging of hair papillae to determine growth cycle, examination of skin scrapings with potassium hydroxide (KOH) for tinea (ringworm) or scabies mites and nits (head lice, which cause pediculosis capitis, Fig. 2.3).

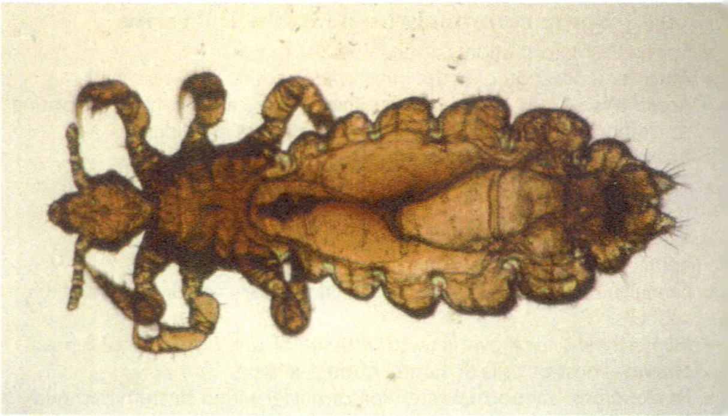

Fig. 2.3 Head louse (*Pediculus capitis*) on microscopy.

Reproduced from CDC/Dr. Dennis Juranek. ID#: 19067, https://phil.cdc.gov/Details.aspx?pid=19067

Patch testing

Used where delayed type IV contact allergy (contact eczema/dermatitis) to substances in contact with the skin is suspected, e.g. rubber (Figs. 2.4 and 2.5), perfume, sticking plaster, or metal (usually nickel). A standard battery of common allergens and any other suspected substances are placed under small metal discs (Finn chambers) pre-mounted on hypoallergenic tape. These are placed on normal areas of skin over the back, held in place with occlusive hypoallergenic tape for 48h before removing for readings with repeat readings at 96h (reading times may vary in different centres). Reactions are deemed positive (Fig. 2.6) when the area tested shows a

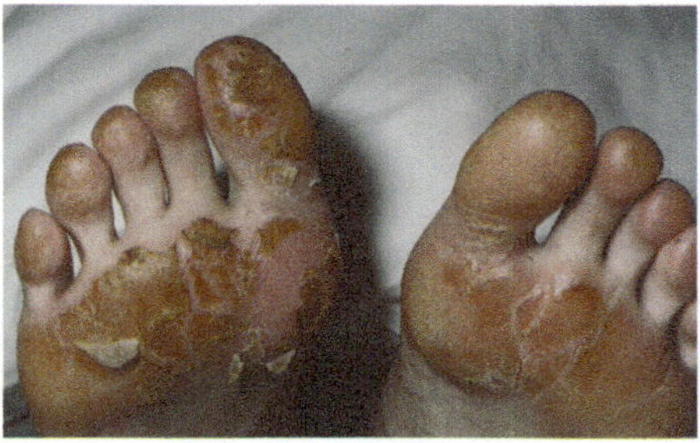

Fig. 2.4 Severe contact allergy to shoes. Note sparing of toe-webs not in direct contact with the sole.

Reproduced courtesy of Susan Lewis-Jones, Hon Consultant Dermatologist, Ninewells Hospital and Medical School, Dundee, UK

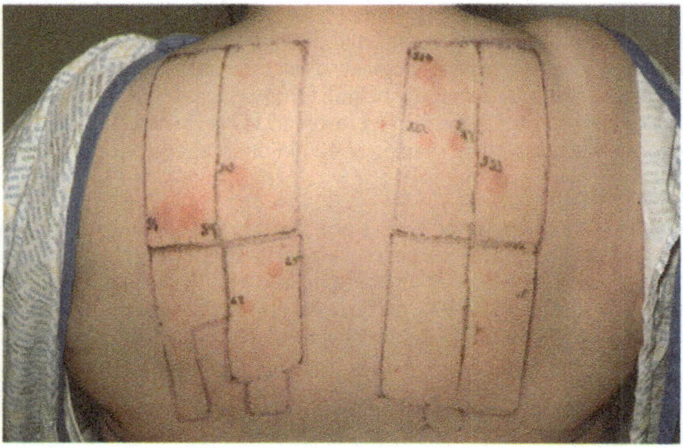

Fig. 2.5 Positive patch test results.

Reproduced courtesy of Susan Lewis-Jones, Hon Consultant Dermatologist, Ninewells Hospital and Medical School, Dundee, UK

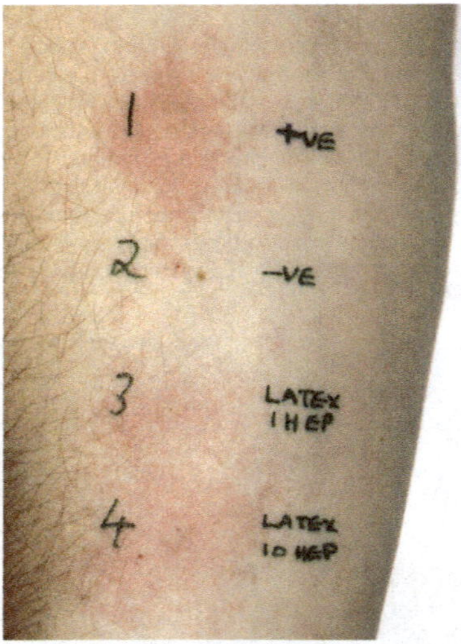

Fig. 2.6 Prick testing showing positive wheal and flare reaction to latex and positive histamine control.

Reproduced courtesy of Graham Lowe, Ninewells Hospital, Dundee, UK

reaction from erythema (redness) through to frank eczema or even vesicles or bullae (blisters) and are graded from 1+ to 3+ depending on severity. However, irritant reactions are common and interpretation requires specialist dermatological training, so it is only available in secondary care specialist dermatology centres in the United Kingdom. It is difficult to do in very young children and is normally reserved for those older than 6/7y.
Note: patch testing is not usually helpful for investigation of urticaria and related allergies (➲ see Chapter 21). However, some immediate type I allergic reactions can be tested by reading at 40min or so after occlusion.

Prick testing

This tests for immediate or type 1 allergy and is used to test for allergies such as latex allergy, acute urticaria caused by food allergy, or airborne allergens (pollens, pet dander, etc.) especially when associated with atopic eczema (➲ see Chapter 17). It requires specialist training and availability of resuscitation equipment and training because of the risk of anaphylaxis.

References

1. British Association of Dermatologists, *UK Guidance on the use of Mobile Photographic Devices in Dermatology*, http://www.bad.org.uk/shared/get-file.ashx?itemtype=document&id=5776

Chapter 3

Dermatological treatments

Introduction

Topical therapies: all substances applied to the skin are absorbed to some extent and it is important to remember that children have thinner skin and a greater body surface area to weight ratio compared to adults so care should be exercised, especially in premature babies, when applying a product over the whole body (e.g. topical corticosteroids).

Treatments are available as creams, ointments, gels, pastes, lotions, paints, sprays, mousses, scalp preparations, soaks, and impregnated tapes.

Available topical therapies

Acne treatments

- ➲ See Chapter 18.

Anaesthetic agents

- ➲ See Chapter 2.

Anti-inflammatory treatments

- Corticosteroids
- Calcineurin inhibitors
- Zinc
- Non-steroid anti-inflammatory medication

Antimicrobials

- Antibacterial
- Antifungal
- Antiviral
- Antiseptic

Antiperspirants

- Aluminium chloride hexahydrate

Antipruritics (anti-itch)

- Calamine
- Crotamiton
- Doxepin (may cause drowsiness)
- Antihistamines (may cause allergic contact dermatitis)

Barrier preparations

Hydrating agents

- Emollients
- Urea
- Lactic acid

Treatments for psoriasis

- Tar
- Dithranol
- Vitamin D analogues
- Salicylic acid
- Vitamin A analogues

Preparations for warts

- Salicylic acid, which softens keratin. Available in various strengths. Avoid in children age less than 1y (due to possible systemic absorption and acidosis) and preparations greater than 12.5–26% in children (weaker preparations of 2–5% can be used to descale scalps).
- 4% glutaraldehyde soaks.
- Podophyllin preparations (caution—highly neurotoxic if taken orally).

Sunscreens

- Physical blocks containing titanium dioxide.
- Chemical sunscreens—a huge number are available and may sometimes cause allergic sensitization.

Bases

Bases act as carriers for active ingredients and may alter drug bioavailability. Different forms of skin treatments are available, dependent upon the base used.

Cream

Useful on wet or delicate sites. Water-based and contain preservative chemicals to prevent colonizing microbes. In general, the 'thinner' the cream, the higher the water and preservative content. Preservatives can irritate or sting inflamed or sensitive skin and occasionally cause allergic contact dermatitis.

Ointment

Grease-based, so better hydration for dry and/or inflamed skin (e.g. eczema). Contain fewer preservative chemicals and are therefore less irritant but messy to use and may cause folliculitis, particularly under occlusive dressings.

Lotions

Used predominantly for the scalp. Usually in an alcohol base which can cause stinging or irritation.

Gels

Useful for the scalp, especially if there is marked inflammation, weeping, or erosions when alcohol-based lotions can cause significant local discomfort or irritation

Note: some gels are also alcohol-based.

Others

- Foams and mousses mainly available as scalp preparations.
- Soaking solutions (e.g. potassium permanganate soaks 1/10,000, pale pink colour) to clean infected dermatoses or ulcerated areas.
- Paints (e.g. for fungal nail problems).

Tape

Steroid impregnated tape is useful where additional occlusion is advantageous (e.g. for fissuring on feet or fingers).

Anti-inflammatory treatments

Topical corticosteroids (TCS)

Used to treat actively inflamed itchy skin, particularly eczema (Box 3.1) and some autoimmune skin diseases (➲ see First line treatment, p. 255).

Three major properties:

- *Anti-inflammatory and immunosuppressive.*
- *Vasoconstriction*: a test of which is used to determine the potency of a particular TCS formulation.
- *Reduce cell turnover*: long-term use, especially of very potent TCS may lead to reduced collagen production by fibroblasts causing skin thinning (epidermal and dermal atrophy), that may be reversible in the early stages but with continued use, striae can occur.

Note: TCS use causes considerable anxiety among parents because of side effects and undertreatment is common. 'Thinning' of the skin is rarely seen with judicious use. It is important to explain this verbally to parents and emphasize it with written explanation.

Available topical corticosteroid preparations

TCS are available in four different potencies and many formulations.
Appropriate steroid quantities: there are no hard and fast rules about the amount of TCS that is safe to use but 'fingertip units' (FTUs) (Fig. 3.1) are currently the best method (Box 3.2).

Two FTUs weigh approximately 1g.

Box 3.1 Topical corticosteroid recommendations for atopic eczema

Explain that:

- The benefits of TCS outweigh the risks when applied correctly.
- TCS should only be applied to areas of active atopic eczema (or eczema that has been active in the past 48h).

Do not use:

- Potent TCS on the face or neck.
- Potent TCS in children under 12 months without specialist dermatological supervision.
- Very potent preparations without specialist dermatological advice.
- Prescribe TCS for application only once or twice daily.
- Where more than one TCS is appropriate within a potency class, prescribe the drug with the lowest acquisition cost, taking into account pack size and frequency of application.

For full recommendations on TCS usage for atopic eczema, see NICE guidelines.[1]

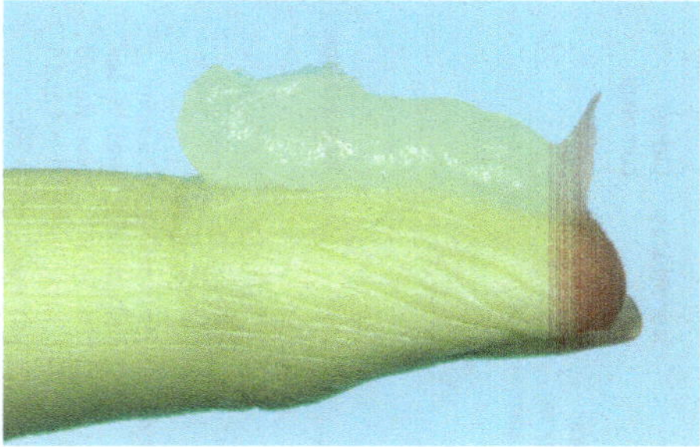

Fig. 3.1 Fingertip unit.

Reproduced courtesy of Susan Lewis-Jones, Hon Consultant Dermatologist, Ninewells Hospital and Medical School, Dundee, UK

Box 3.2 Fingertip unit usage

- *1 FTU* = the quantity of steroid squeezed from a standard (5mm nozzle) tube in a line from the distal crease to the tip of the index finger.
- *1 FTU* should be used to treat an area of skin equivalent to twice the flat area of that same adult hand with the fingers together.

Source: data from Long C.C. *et al.* (1998). A practical guide to topical therapy in children. *Br J Dermatol.* 138(2):293–6. https://doi.org/10.1046/j.1365-2133.1998.02077.x

Potency: TCS are divided in to four groups depending on potency: mild, moderate, potent, and super potent (Table 3.1).

Note: potency is not the same as strength. Strength is measured in percentages and this does not compare with potency (e.g. 0.1% betamethasone valerate is potent compared with 1% hydrocortisone, which is of weak potency).

Additives: TCS preparations combined with other active ingredients are available. These include antiseptics, antibiotics, antifungals, antipruritic, and keratolytic agents (Table 3.2).

Table 3.1 Approximate guide to appropriate quantities of topical steroids

Age of child	Area of skin (FTU application)				
	Head and neck	Upper limb	Trunk anterior	Trunk lower posterior	Limb
3–6 months	1	1	1	1.5	1.5
1–2y	1.5	1.5	2	3	2
3–5y	1.5	2	3	3.5	3
6–10y	2	2.5	3.5	5	4

Adapted with permission from Long C.C. *et al.* (1998). A practical guide to topical therapy in children. *Br J Dermatol.* 138(2):293–6. https://doi.org/10.1046/j.1365-2133.1998.02077.x

Table 3.2 Topical corticosteroid preparations

Steroid potency	Plain steroid	Steroid + antiseptic	Steroid + antibiotic	Steroid + antifungal	Steroid + other	Steroid scalp prep	Other/ comment
Mild	Hydrocortisone *Hydrocortisone* *Efcortelan*®	*Vioform HC*® (clioquinol) *Timodine*® (benzalkonium chloride)	*Fucidin H*® (fusidic acid)	*Canestan HC Daktacort*® (miconazole) *Econacort*® (econazole) *Nystaform HC*® (nystatin) *Timodine*® (nystatin)	*Alphaderm*® (urea) *Calmurid HC*® (urea) *Eurax HC*® (crotamiton)		
Moderate	Clobetasone butyrate *Eumovate*®		*Trimovate*® (oxytetracycline)	*Trimovate*® (nystatin)			
	Flurandrenolone *Haelan*®						Tape available
Potent	Alclometasone dipropionate *Modrasone*®						
	Betamethasone *Betnovate*® *Diprosone*®		*Fucibet*® (fusidic acid)	*Lotriderm*® (clotrimazole)	*Diprosalic*® (salicylic acid)	*Betnovate scalp lotion*® *Betacap*® *Bettamousse*® *Diprosalic*® (salicylic acid)	Dilutions available for plain steroid (1 in 4 and 1 in 10)

Steroid potency	Plain steroid	Steroid + antiseptic	Steroid + antibiotic	Steroid + antifungal	Steroid + other	Steroid scalp prep	Other/ comment
	Fluocinolone acetonide *Synalar*®	*Synalar C*® (clioquinol)	*Synalar N*® (neomycin)			*Synalar gel*®	Dilutions available for plain steroid (1 in 4 and 1 in 10)
	Fluocinonide (*Metosyn*®)						
	Fluticasone (*Cutivate*®)						
	Hydrocortisone butyrate (*Locoid*®)						
	Mometasone furoate (*Elocon*®)					*Elocon*® *scalp lotion*	
	Triamcinolone acetonide		*Aureocort*® (tetracycline)	*Tri-Adcortyl*® (nystatin)			
Super potent	Clobetasol Propionate (*Dermovate*®)						

Topical corticosteroid combination products

TCS can be used short term (up to 2 weeks) in combination with antibacterial agents where skin infection is associated with significant eczematization or inflammation (e.g. eczematized scabies, impetiginized eczema). Avoid using where viral infection is suspected to be the predominant problem (e.g. herpetic or varicella infection).

Which steroid to use?

It is important to be aware that occasionally contact sensitization to either a topical steroid or an excipient in the cream or ointment may occur. If reactions are suspected referral to a dermatologist for contact allergy (patch) testing (➲ see Patch testing, pp. 25–6) is appropriate. Remember that creams are more likely to produce contact reactions (both irritant and allergic) than ointments.

Which corticosteroid is most appropriate to use will depend on:

- Body site
- Severity of inflammation
- Previous steroid usage and response
- Age

Site

- Certain (delicate) body sites such as face, neck, flexures, and genital areas are more prone to thinning with repeated use of TCS, particularly potent and super potent preparations and these should not generally be prescribed for children without specialist dermatological advice (Box 3.3).
- Whenever possible use weak preparations in these sites but if potent TCS are required for severe inflammation then use should be limited to a few days except under specialist dermatological supervision (e.g. for genital conditions such as lichen sclerosis, lichen planus or ulcerative bullous disorders where inflammation is severe and/or may lead to scarring, atrophy, or ulceration).
- Avoid anything other than mild TCS in the periocular area. Eyelid skin is very thin and TCS easily absorbed, increasing the risk of atrophy, cataract, and glaucoma.
- At hair-bearing sites such as scalp, lotions, or mousses are often easier to use but if inflammation is severe, a gel or ointment may be least irritant.
- Around and on the nail bed, lotion application may be helpful, sometimes with occlusion (➲ see Anti-inflammatory treatments, pp. 30–6).

Severity of inflammation

- ***For mild inflammation***: use a mild TCS, taking note that emollient therapy alone may be sufficient (e.g. mild atopic eczema).
- ***For moderate inflammation***: use a moderate potency TCS and reduce the potency as symptoms and inflammation settle.
- ***For severe inflammation***: short-term use of a potent TCS (only up to 7 days without dermatological advice) is appropriate for rapid relief of symptoms to improve patient morale, sleep, and treatment adherence. Reduce frequency and/or potency as inflammation settles.

Box 3.3 Before deciding on appropriate potency of topical corticosteroid ensure that:

- The diagnosis is correct and steroid therapy is appropriate.
- Other therapies appropriate to the condition being treated are optimized (e.g. emollients in atopic eczema).
- The condition being treated is not complicated by infection (e.g. candidiasis in the nappy area; *Staph. aureus* or herpes simplex virus associated with eczema).

Age

- *In young infants and children*, avoid potent steroids if possible (Box 3.3).
- *At puberty* the risk of stretch marks/striae increases significantly. Take extra care using potent TCS at sites prone to growth-related striae (see Dermal atrophy, p. 445).

Frequency of topical corticosteroid use

- Most TCS are recommended once or twice daily. However as inflammation settles, frequency of use can be reduced.
- Intermittent use of potent TCS reduces the risk of local and systemic side effects.

Duration of use depends on:

- Condition being treated.
- Severity of inflammation.
- Degree of lichenification/thickening of the skin.
- Adherence to therapy.
- Site—avoid longer-term use at delicate sites.

- *For moderate or severe inflammation* and skin barrier impairment (dry skin): ointment preparations are preferable to cream preparations, which often cause stinging and irritation due to preservative content.
- *For very severe inflammation*: super potent TCS are appropriate for conditions unresponsive to less potent steroid therapy (e.g. lichen sclerosis, morphoea). They are safer for sites where the epidermis is very thick (e.g. palms and soles). *They should not be used in children without specialist dermatological supervision.*
- TCS potency may need to be increased if a condition fails to settle. *However*, before doing so ensure that:
  - There is appropriate use of other therapies for the condition being treated (e.g. emollients in eczema, antimicrobial agents for infection).
  - There is appropriate adherence to previous treatments used.
  - Quantity used is appropriate—FTU quantities help.
  - The diagnosis is correct. You may be missing other conditions such as scabies in eczematized skin or contact allergy.
- *For acute inflammatory conditions*: 1–2 weeks is usually appropriate.
- *For chronic conditions*: a longer course may be necessary (1–3 months or more) particularly if considerable lichenification from chronic scratching. Reduce potency and frequency of use as soon as possible.
- *In inflamed areas of eczema continue use of a TCS for 2 days after the redness has disappeared to prevent a flare* (see NICE Guideline CG057).[1]

Topical corticosteroid under occlusion

Using TCS under occlusion (e.g. with local dressings, bandages or stockingette garments) increases skin absorption increasing the risk of topical and systemic side effects (equivalent to using a more potent preparation). Occlusion is useful in sites where TCS is often washed or rubbed off and it reduces the frequency of steroid application.

Can be used to treat:

- Localized areas of chronic dermatitis to switch off scratching.
- Inflammatory nail diseases.
- To flatten hypertrophic scars.
- To treat painful fissures (e.g. on digits or feet).

A steroid impregnated tape preparation is available on prescription.

Note: TCS used over a wide area under stockingette bandages or garments for longer than a week increases the risk of systemic absorption and hypothalamic-pituitary-adrenal (HPA) axis suppression.

Other topical immunosuppressants

Calcineurin inhibitors

These block the cytokine reaction triggered by inflammatory T cells. Two different preparations are currently available:

- Pimecrolimus (Elidel®)—1% cream.
- Tacrolimus (Protopic®)—0.03% and 0.1% ointment.

A National Eczema Society UK written information sheet is available (https://www.eczema.org).

Use of calcineurin inhibitors

- Licensed from 2y and above (0.1% tacrolimus is licensed from 12y) in atopic eczema.
- Use in quantities similar to TCS.
- All sites (best for face and neck)—no atrophy.
- Twice daily reducing to once daily with improvement.
- Discontinue if eczema clears (tacrolimus is now licensed for twice-weekly use for 12 months for long-term prevention of eczema flares).
- Give advice on sun avoidance and sun protection.
- Provide appropriate vitamin D supplementation if advising sun avoidance (➲ see Chapter 16).

Do not use:

- On infected skin.
- Under occlusion.
- Four weeks either side of vaccination.
- In pregnancy and lactation.
- In patients receiving phototherapy.
- In immunosuppressed individuals or with history of skin cancer.

Side effects

Short term

- Stinging, soreness, burning.
- Acne and folliculitis.

- Skin sensitivity to heat/cold.
- Skin infection—particularly viral (e.g. herpes simplex virus, HSV).

Long term

Not clearly known. These treatments do not affect DNA directly but may impair immunosurveillance.

- Possible cancer risk—skin and systemic (lymphoma). A small number of cases of postmarketing malignancies have been reported both at the site of application and elsewhere.

Current NICE recommendations for calcineurin inhibitor use

- Not recommended for mild atopic dermatitis or as first-line treatment for any severity of eczema.
- Both are recommended (pimecrolimus for face only) for moderate or severe atopic dermatitis where there is a serious risk of adverse effects from TCS use.
- Treatment should only be initiated by physicians with a special interest/ experience in dermatology.[1]

Zinc

Zinc has anti-inflammatory and antiseptic properties. It is found in barrier preparations and in some zinc impregnated bandages.

Topical treatments for psoriasis

Coal tar

Coal tar has anti-inflammatory and antiscaling properties. Crude coal tar is available in paraffin base (coal tar BP). Cleaner proprietary preparations are more practicable for home use. Tar baths, shampoos, and impregnated bandages are also available. Side effects include unpleasant smell, irritation, folliculitis, and contact allergy. Tar preparations can be useful in some forms of eczema.

Dithranol

Dithranol decreases the rate of keratinocyte differentiation thus reducing epidermal thickening and scaling. It is available as a paste (sometimes mixed with other active ingredients such as salicylic acid), ointment, and cream. It can be used:

- Short contact—washed off after 10–60min.
- Long contact—wash off if irritation occurs.

Varying concentrations are available. Start with the lowest concentration and increase to a higher concentration every 3 days if tolerated. *To reduce burning, apply to a small test area first with each new concentration prior to more widespread use.*

Side effects

- Burn-like skin irritation that can be severe.
- Staining—skin, hair, nails, and fabrics, fades over 1–2 weeks (except on fabrics). Apply with gloves taking care to avoid surrounding normal skin.

Do not use on:
- Pustular psoriasis.
- Delicate sites—face, genitals, flexures, or in skin folds.
- Inflamed, broken, blistered, raw, or oozing areas of skin.
- Infants and young children.
- Pregnant females.

Vitamin D analogues

Calcipotriol, calcitriol, and tacalcitol are available to treat plaque psoriasis; but only calcipotriol is licensed under 12y (from 6y).
- They do not stain unlike tar and dithranol but local irritation is not uncommon so they should be used with caution on face, genitals, and flexures (see manufacturers' recommendations).
- Occasional aggravation of psoriasis can occur.
- Hypercalcaemia may occur if used excessively.

Avoid in generalized pustular or erythrodermic psoriasis because of irritation and enhanced risk of hypercalcaemia.

Keratolytic agents

These are useful for descaling especially of the scalp, hands, and feet. They may be combined with other products such as tar.

Keratolytic agents

These soften keratin and are used as anti-wart agents and to soften and descale hard, thickened skin (hyperkeratosis) on scalp, palms, and soles. Salicylic acid is most commonly used, but urea preparations can also be helpful (➲ see Hydrating agents, p. 28).

Salicylic acid

- Available in a number of proprietary and hospital manufactured preparations as pastes, ointments, and lotions, often combined with other topical treatments (e.g. corticosteroid, zinc, or tar).
- Local skin irritation can occur.
- In young children, if used over wide areas or where the skin barrier is significantly impaired, systemic absorption can occur with the risk of salicylate toxicity.
- It should be avoided in infants under 2y and used with caution and in small amounts only in those under 6y.

Emollients

Indicated for all dry and scaling skin disorders to hydrate, smooth, and soothe the skin. Choice depends on the severity of the condition, site, and patient preference. Apply in direction of hair growth to minimize follicular irritation and smooth in to facilitate absorption (rubbing hinders absorption).

Emollient preparations with antimicrobial agents are available. These are only appropriate if infection is present or is a frequent complication as antimicrobial may cause irritation and less commonly contact allergic reactions.

Emollient preparations available

- Creams
- Ointments
- Lotions
- Bath oils
- Shower gels
- Vaporized spray

Commonly used plain cream and ointment preparations in approximate order of thickness

Greasy/thick

- Emulsifying ointment
- Hydromol® ointment
- Epaderm® ointment
- 50/50 mix of emulsifying ointment and liquid paraffin
- 50/50 mix of liquid paraffin and white soft paraffin
- Diprobase® ointment
- Creamy paraffin

Creamy/light

- Unguentum Merck®
- Oilatum® cream
- Doublebase® cream
- Hydromol® cream
- Cetraben® cream
- Ultrabase® cream
- Neutrogena® dermatological cream
- Aveeno® cream
- Balneum Plus® cream
- E45® cream
- Aqueous cream
- Dermol 500® lotion

Notes: Creams contain preservative chemicals that may cause contact irritation. If this occurs, change to an ointment preparation.

Unless infection is a problem, avoid preparations with antimicrobials as contact irritation/stinging may occur.

Quantity of emollient to be used per week

For most conditions, emollients should be applied all over the body to prevent skin dryness, not just to actively involved areas especially in atopic eczema. It is essential to ensure that appropriate quantities are prescribed regularly to ensure adequate benefit and treatment adherence. Suggested approximate amounts per week[2]:

- Infant—¼ large 500g tub
- Small child—½ large 500g tub
- Older child—1 large 500g tub

Side effects of emollients

- *Local irritation*—more common with lotions and creams, and those preparations with antiseptics. Aqueous cream is cheap and therefore commonly used but is irritant in almost half of patients so should be avoided as a leave on emollient.

- *Contact allergy*—most commonly to added fragrances, preservatives, antimicrobials, and sunscreens (excipients) in creams.
- *Follicular occlusion/folliculitis*—more likely to occur with greasier emollients especially if used under occlusion or in hot weather.
- *Systemic allergy*—e.g. to products applied to which the subject is allergic, e.g. soya or nut containing products (very rare).

Other hydrating agents

Urea

The stratum corneum contains natural water-retaining substances, including urea that can therefore be used to treat dry skin conditions and keratosis pilaris. Urea is found in various emollients and occasionally used with other topical agents such as TCS to enhance penetration. Can be used in high concentrations (such as 40%) to soften and remove nails provided that the surrounding skin is protected (avoid under 2y).

Sunscreens

Sunscreens are used to protect skin from burning and ageing and in photoaggravated and photo-induced skin diseases (➲ see Chapter 16) to prevent/reduce flares. Preparations contain substances that protect the skin against UVB (ultraviolet radiation with wavelength between 280 and 320nm) that can cause sunburn, and UVA (ultraviolet radiation with wavelength between 320 and 400 nm) that penetrates the skin more deeply and causes long-term skin ageing. Sunscreens are available as creams, lotions, gels, and sprays.

The sun protection factor (SPF) gives guidance on the degree of protection offered against UVB (SPF 30 is usually recommended but higher SPFs of 50 may be required on occasion). It indicates the multiple time of protection against burning compared with unprotected skin.

The star rating (maximum 5 stars) gives guidance on the degree of protection against UVA, 5 stars is recommended (British Association of Dermatologists (BAD) guidelines).

Unfortunately, the thickness of application used to provide guidance ratings is often far greater than quantities applied in everyday life.

No sunscreen blocks completely—clothes provide the best protection.

The active ingredients in sunscreens include:

- *Physical blocks*—opaque materials that reflect light (e.g. titanium dioxide and zinc oxide).
- *Chemical blocks*—organic chemical compounds that absorb light (e.g. oxybenzone and cinnamates).

For optimum photoprotection, sunscreens should be applied liberally and frequently (2-hourly) and after bathing or swimming.

Side effects include:

- *Local irritation.*
- *Contact allergic dermatitis*—to active ingredients (more commonly chemical blocks), fragrances, or preservatives.

Adverse reactions to topical treatments

The likelihood of an adverse reaction increases with the severity of skin condition being treated.

Adverse reactions may include:

- *Irritant contact reaction*—more likely to occur with products containing higher quantities of excipient additives/preservatives and therefore more frequent with creams than ointments. As the skin barrier improves creams are better tolerated. On areas of broken skin due to excoriation, erosion, etc., alcohol-containing preparations can cause significant stinging (e.g. in lotion preparations). Switching to an ointment-based preparation can help.
- *Allergic contact reaction*—can occur due to added fragrances, preservatives, antimicrobials, or more rarely TCS. Reactions to dressings and bandages may also occur (e.g. due to colophony in Elastoplast/ adhesive dressings, or latex in bandages). *Investigation:* detected by patch tests (➲ see Chapter 2).
- *Other local side effects*
  - *Atrophy, striae, and telangiectasia*—TCS.
  - *Infection risk*—topical immunosuppressants.
  - *Folliculitis*—tar and emollients.
  - *Burn-like reaction*—dithranol.
  - *Caustic burns*—from inappropriate dilutions (e.g. potassium permanganate solution, salicylic acid preparations).
  - *Temporary skin staining*—dithranol, potassium permanganate.
  - *Pressure effects*—of inappropriate/incorrect bandaging.
- *Systemic side effects*
  - *HPA axis suppression* after significant or long-term use of potent TCS that may affect growth (rare).
  - *Anaphylaxis* (e.g. to latex in sensitized individuals).
  - *Salicylism* from topical salicylates (do not use under 2y and use only small amounts under 6y).
  - *Increased absorption* of any drug may occur in prems and neonates and those with erythroderma (≥90% generalized redness).
- ➲ See also Chapter 23.

Other modalities of treatment

Medicated dressings and bandages

These are occlusive and used for protection, support, to aid healing, or for treatment such as hydration of the skin. A wide variety is available:

- *Dry bandages*—with or without elastication, gauzes, tubular bandages, garment type occlusive dressings.
- *Wet-wrap dressings and garments* (Fig. 3.2).
- *Non-adhesive dressings*—numerous types.
- *Impregnated bandages*—usually with zinc oxide paste and other excipients such as tar, ichthammol or antimicrobial agent (Fig. 3.3).

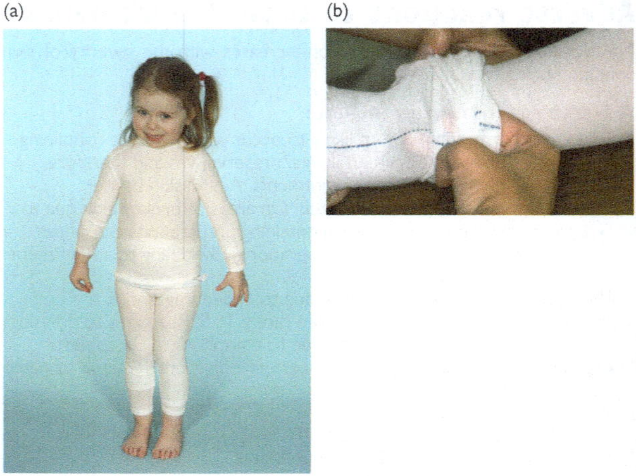

Fig. 3.2 (a) Wet-wrap therapy with two layers of garments or (b) tubular bandages, the first layer being damp with a dry layer on top.

Reproduced courtesy of NHS Tayside Clinical Photography, Dundee,UK

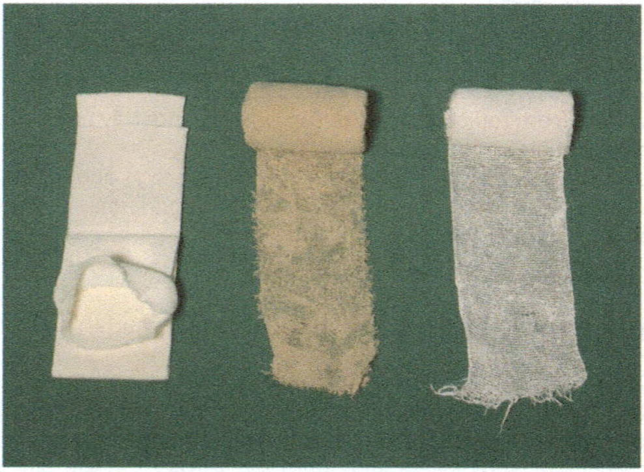

Fig. 3.3 Medicated bandages (dressings) with zinc oxide paste; on the left is a tubular bandage; the central bandage also contains ichthammol.

Reproduced courtesy of NHS Tayside Clinical Photography, Dundee, UK

Use:

- For localized dermatoses where secondary lichenification has occurred due to chronic scratching (e.g. eczema, to switch off the itch–scratch cycle).
- When local trauma (intentional or non-intentional) is exacerbating or inducing a skin condition.
- To reduce the need for frequent treatment applications.
- To improve compliance.
- To increase the efficacy of topical therapy.
- For the compressive effect (e.g. to improve venous return).

Correct usage requires appropriate training and they should be avoided if skin infection is suspected or in those with a risk of vascular compromise.

Medicated bandages may contain:

- Zinc
- Tar
- Calamine
- Ichthammol (anti-inflammatory)
- Corticosteroid
- Alginates

Their usage often requires secondary tubular or other bandage on top to hold them in place. Frequency of use will depend on the condition and site. Usually changed daily but can be left on for longer depending on type.

Side effects include:

- Local skin irritation including folliculitis.
- Contact allergy—to the bandage material or impregnated medication.
- Vascular compromise—if applied too tightly or in patients with impaired circulation.

For a full description of all available dressings, see the *British National Formulary for Children.*[2]

Botox® injection

Injection of botulinum toxin into the skin to reduce hyperhidrosis (➲ see Disorders of sweating, pp. 11–13). It is expensive and only available in some NHS units but often very effective. Theoretically, it can cause temporary localized weakness. The effect initially lasts a few months but is progressively longer lasting with each administration. Not licensed for use under 16y.

Cosmetic camouflage

Important aspect of care for facial conditions in particular. The British Red Cross runs a free service in the United Kingdom and some other countries with referral through the local dermatology department in most cases. Various tinted creams are available on NHS prescription to help camouflage conditions such as acne or port-wine stains. Camouflage is often used alongside laser treatment until such time as benefit occurs.

Electrolysis

Electrolysis is a method of permanent hair removal, mostly superseded by laser techniques. An electrical thin metal probe is slid into the hair follicle avoiding puncture of the skin to deliver a charge causing local damage to the hair follicle. Treatment can be painful and time-consuming. There is a risk of scarring, postinflammatory pigmentary change, and secondary infection.

Iontophoresis

A non-invasive method of propelling a charged substance transdermally, using a small electrical charge and a liquid such as tap water, with or without an active agent such as an anticholinergic drug. The charge alters permeability of the skin to the active ingredient. Main use is for treatment of hyperhidrosis (➲ see Disorders of sweating, pp. 11–13) but benefit is only temporary and maintenance treatment is required (e.g. every 6 weeks). Only available in some hospitals but if successful, home machines (using tap water) can be purchased. Treatment is contraindicated in pregnancy and for those with metal orthopaedic implants or a pacemaker.

Intralesional injections

Most commonly using corticosteroids to treat keloid scars or alopecia areata. May cause local atrophy that usually recovers with time.

Dermojet

High pressure spray injection as alternative to using needles, mainly used for intralesional corticosteroids.

Tattooing

Can be used for absent eyebrows, nipples, etc. NHS availability is patchy.

Wigs

In cases of extensive hair loss certain wigs can be partially funded by the NHS but there is considerable regional variation and in some areas only consultant dermatologists may prescribe.

Laser treatment

A variety of lasers are used to treat skin conditions and all require specialist training and knowledge. Most young children require general anaesthesia although older children may cope with local anaesthesia. The effectiveness of therapy is often highly variable and it is important not to raise the child and parents' expectations too much. They must also be informed of any potential side effects (pain, scarring, hyper/hypopigmentation, recurrence of lesions).

Some lasers are used for several different functions and there are too many on the market to comment on them all. The following are currently found to be useful:

- Argon pumped tunable dye laser for vascular lesions (e.g. port-wine stains).
- Flashlamp excitable dye (pulse dye) has less side effects and is currently the best for superficial vascular lesions.
- Carbon dioxide for resurfacing or removing small tumours.
- Q-switched yttrium aluminium garnet (YAG) for some pigmented lesions such as lentigines and naevus of Ota.
- Alexandrite and Q-switched ruby lasers used for pigmented lesions and tattoo removal.
- Hair removal lasers are only useful for dark hair and the effect is not permanent—regular treatment every few weeks is usually required.

Phototherapy

Phototherapy can be used to treat many skin diseases including psoriasis, eczema, acne vulgaris, vitiligo, and cutaneous T-cell lymphomas. However, it is not used in very young children because of practical difficulties and *even in older children it should be used with caution because of the potential for increased risk of skin cancer in later life.*

It encompasses a wide range of treatments using various wavelengths of ultraviolet light in the UVA to UVB spectrum (290–400nm). The most widely available are:

- Narrow wave band UVB or TL-01 (311nm)—currently the most often used.
- Broad band UVB (290–320nm)—used less often now.
- UVA (320–400nm); UVA-1 (>340nm) is not available in many centres.
- PUVA (Psoralens—photosensitizing drugs with **UVA** light) is rarely used in children (due to the increased risk of skin cancer in later life), except in those with skin type III–VI to treat vitiligo.

UVB phototherapy is often used in combination with topical treatments such as emollients, TCS, tar preparations (Goeckerman regime) or dithranol (Ingram regimen).

Phototherapy should only be initiated and undertaken in specialist centres with staff trained in its use. Records should be kept of the number of treatments given and the total joules used.

Photodynamic therapy

The use of a phototoxic agent in combination with a source of light to destroy abnormal areas of skin such as skin cancers. Rarely used in children.

Systemic therapies

Many systemic therapies are used in dermatology and are mentioned in specific sections throughout this book. Many are not licensed for use in children and should be used with caution.

The majority fall into the following categories:

- Antibiotics and other antimicrobial agents including antivirals and antifungals; for infections or as acne treatment.
- Anti-inflammatory agents.
- Antihistamines—mainly for urticaria and to combat itch.
- Antimalarials such as hydroxychloroquine for systemic lupus erythematosus (SLE).
- Agents to reduce hyperhidrosis (teenagers mainly), e.g. oxybutynin.
- Immunosuppressive therapy—including methotrexate, ciclosporin, azathioprine, mycophenolate mofetil (all mainly for eczema and psoriasis, less commonly SLE or other autoimmune disorders). Systemic corticosteroid therapy can be given orally or as pulsed IV methyl prednisolone (e.g. in severe autoimmune disease).
- Sulphones such as dapsone (used mainly for immunobullous disorders).
- Retinoids, such as isotretinoin (for severe acne) and acitretin (for severe psoriasis and ichthyosis). These are both teratogenic and must be avoided in pregnancy.

- Biological agents—monoclonal antibody therapies, initially directed against antitumour necrosis factor-alpha but now also against an expanding number of other molecular targets involved in inflammatory pathways. Etanercept, adalimumab, and ustekinumab are now licensed to treat psoriasis in children. The first licensed therapy for atopic eczema, dupilumab, an interleukin 4 receptor antagonist, is now also available.
- Apremilast, a phosphodiesterase inhibitor, is now licensed for the treatment of psoriasis in adults. It does not require blood monitoring.
- Intravenous gamma globulin for replacement in immunodeficiency syndromes. It has also been used in Kawasaki disease, dermatomyositis, and toxic epidermal necrolysis and others.

Further guidance

Alopecia UK: (0800 101 7025); www.alopecia.org.uk.
National Alopecia Areata Foundation: www.naaf.org

References

1. NICE, *Atopic Eczema in Under 12s: Diagnosis and Management*, https:www.nice.org.uk/guidance/cg57
2. Long, C.C., Mills, C.M., and Finlay, A.Y. (1998). A practical guide to topical therapy in children. *Br J Dermatol* **138**(2):293–6.

Chapter 4

Patterns, shapes, and distribution in skin disease

Introduction

The pattern and shape of individual lesions and how they are distributed on the body is crucial in helping to form a diagnosis. It is important to ask about the evolution of a rash when taking the history (➲ see Taking a dermatological history, pp. 16–8) since the presenting features may have disappeared at the time of examination and many skin diseases fluctuate and vary with time. Some of the classic patterns in this chapter are described in greater detail elsewhere, in particular diseases found in different body sites are described in Section 3. However, it is important to remember that these descriptions are only a guideline and atypical presentations occasionally occur with most diseases.

Terminology: patterns and distribution

Acral—restricted or localized preferentially to the peripheries of hands, feet, and sometimes face, nose, and ears (Fig. 4.2), e.g. hand, foot, and mouth disease (Fig. 4.1), Stevens–Johnson syndrome, chilblains (Box 4.1).

Annular—ring-shaped with central clearance (Fig. 4.3; Box 4.2), e.g. granuloma annulare, tinea corporis (ringworm; ➲ see Fig. 22.8).

Arcuate (circinate)—arch shaped, incomplete ring shape (Fig. 4.4), e.g. elastosis perforans serpiginosum seen in connective tissue disorders such as Marfan's syndrome, Wilson's disease, Down syndrome, penicillamine therapy; urticaria (➲ see Chapter 21); partially healed tinea infections (➲ see Chapter 22, Fungal infections of the skin, pp. 330–1), or psoriasis.

Blaschko's lines—embryonic epidermal cell migration lines. Linear (limbs) or whorled lesions (trunk) representing genetic mosaicism, e.g. incontinentia pigmenti (Figs. 4.5 and 4.6).

Bullous—blistered (➲ see Chapter 25).

Clustered/grouped—e.g. insect bites (➲ see Fig. 19.4).

Extensor:

- Red scaly rash on elbows, knees, lumbar area and scalp is seen in psoriasis (➲ see Psoriasis—clinical variants, p. 322).
- Blisters with urticated rash on knees, elbows, buttocks, and scalp is seen in dermatitis herpetiformis (➲ see Fig. 25.9).
- Red papules on legs and buttocks, elbows, and sometimes cheeks is seen in Gianotti–Crosti (➲ see Figs. 19.2 and 19.3; see also Papular acrodermatitis of childhood, pp. 282–3).
- Purpuric rash on buttock and lower legs is seen in Henoch–Schönlein purpura (➲ see Fig. 31.4).

Digitate—finger-shaped. Sometimes seen in Mycosis fungoides (➲ see pp. 340).

Discoid—circular area of rash, e.g. in discoid eczema (➲ see Fig. 17.12).

Flexural—mainly confined to body creases (groin, axillae, submammary), e.g. seborrhoeic eczema, intertrigo, flexural psoriasis (➲ see Fig. 11.3; see also Box 11.1).

Follicular—centred around hair follicles, e.g. keratosis pilaris (➲ see Chapter 12).

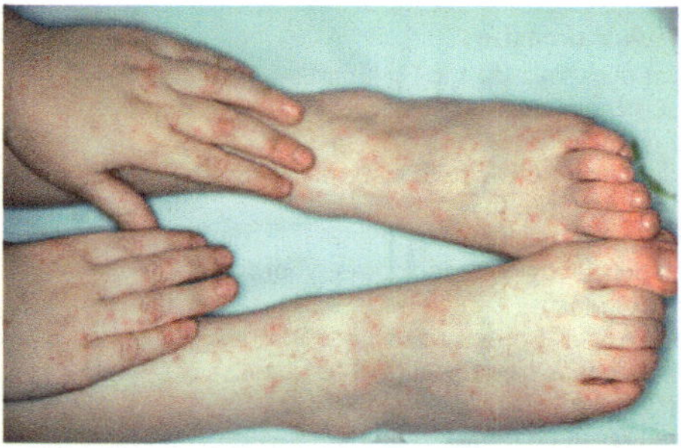

Fig. 4.1 Acral rash—hand, foot, and mouth disease.

Reproduced courtesy of Susan Lewis-Jones, Hon Consultant Dermatologist, Ninewells Hospital and Medical School, Dundee, UK

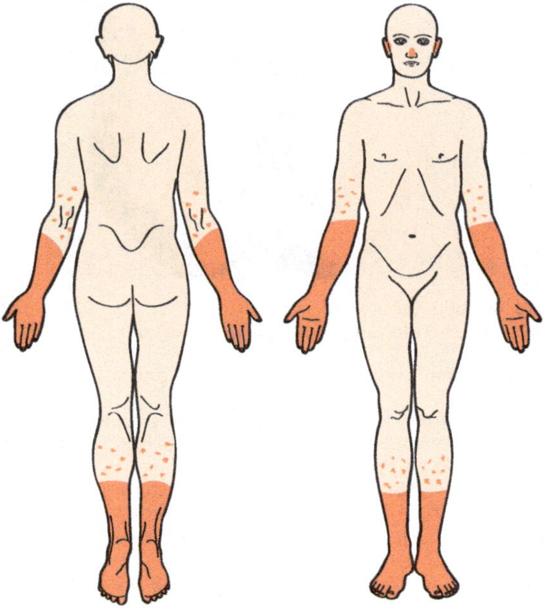

Fig. 4.2 Distribution in acral rash.

Box 4.1 Acral rashes

- Cryoglobulinaemia (➲ see Fig. 38.3).
- Chilblains (perniosis) (➲ see Fig. 31.9).
- Erythema multiforme.
- Fixed drug eruptions—tend to be acral (➲ see Chapter 23).
- Hand foot and mouth disease (Fig. 4.1).
- Infantile acral pustulosis.
- Papular-purpuric gloves and socks syndrome.
- Purpura fulminans (➲ see Fig. 31.7).
- Scabies (may also present as an eczematous rash on the trunk).
- Stevens–Johnson syndrome (➲ see Chapter 22).

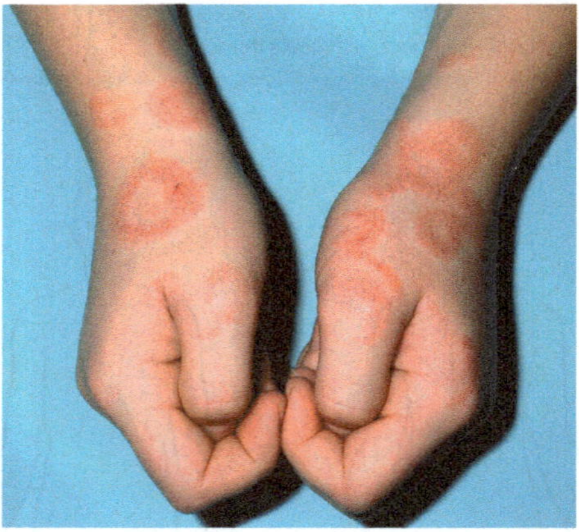

Fig. 4.3 Annular lesions on wrists.

Reproduced courtesy of NHS Tayside Clinical Photography, Dundee, UK

Guttate—raindrop pattern of small lesions, e.g. guttate psoriasis (➲ see Fig. 22.3).

Herpetic/herpetiform—blisters tightly clustered or grouped together as in herpes simplex *or* herpes zoster (Fig. 4.7; ➲ see also Fig. 25.2); or dermatitis herpetiformis (➲ see Fig. 25.9).

Koebner (Köbner) phenomenon—rash or lesions occurring in site of injury, e.g. in psoriasis (Fig. 4.8), lichen planus, vitiligo, viral warts, and others.

Langer's lines—distribution following normal skin creases (Fig. 4.9), e.g. pityriasis rosea (➲ see Fig. 22.7).

Linear—in straight lines, e.g. linear warty epidermal naevus (Fig. 4.10; and Box 4.3).

Note: some limb lesions in the distribution of Langer's lines and Blaschko's lines occur in a linear pattern (➲ see Fig. 25.13).

Box 4.2 Annular red rashes

Common

- Granuloma annulare (often skin coloured) (➲ see Fig. 28.3).
- Healing psoriasis (clears centrally first, may become arcuate).
- Urticaria (➲ see Chapter 21).
- Discoid eczema (➲ see Chapter 17).
- Resolving haemangioma (➲ see Chapter 8).
- Erythema multiforme.

Less common

- Tinea* (ringworm) (➲ see Fig. 22.8).
- Necrobiosis lipoidica diabeticorum (➲ see Fig. 5.2).
- Erythema annulare centrifugum (➲ see Chapter 22).
- Erythema chronicum migrans (➲ see Fig. 22.12).
- Tuberculoid leprosy (➲ see Chapter 22).
- Neonatal lupus erythematosus (➲ see Fig. 7.2).

Very rare in children

- Annular sarcoid.
- Annular lichen planus.
- Annular syphilis.
- Erythema marginatum (in rheumatic fever).
- Familial annular erythema.
- Ichthyosis linearis circumflexa (Netherton syndrome)—double edges with scaling.

**Note*: most annular lesions in UK children are not due to ringworm—but are usually discoid eczema, psoriasis, urticaria, or granuloma annulare.

Oval—many lesions are oval (e.g. moles or café-au-lait macules) but in some rashes, such as pityriasis rosea, the majority of lesions are typically oval.

Photosensitive—sun exposed sites such as face (with periorbital sparing) 'V'—of neck, dorsal hands (➲ see Fig. 16.1).

Polymorphic (also multiform)—lesions of different shapes and sizes, e.g. in polymorphic light eruption or erythema multiforme (where not all lesions are target shaped).

Reticulate (livedo)—lace pattern, net-like, or branching pattern, e.g. oral lichen planus, erythema ab igne, livedo reticularis (Fig. 4.11) (seen in vasculitis).

Seborrhoeic distribution—flexures of neck, axillae, and groin; perinasal and eyebrows; central chest and central upper back; scaling of scalp, e.g. seborrhoeic eczema (➲ see Fig. 17.13), Langerhans cell histiocytosis.

Targetoid—multiple target lesions, often of various sizes resembling a target with central red area surrounded by rings of alternating red and white (Fig. 4.12), e.g. Bullous erythema multiforme (➲ see p. 191).

Segmental or zosteriform—localized to a dermatome (see Box 4.4), e.g. herpes zoster, facial port-wine stains (Fig. 4.13).

Serpiginous—snake-like, wavy lines (Fig. 4.14; Box 4.5), e.g. in cutaneous larva migrans (➲ see pp. 167–9).

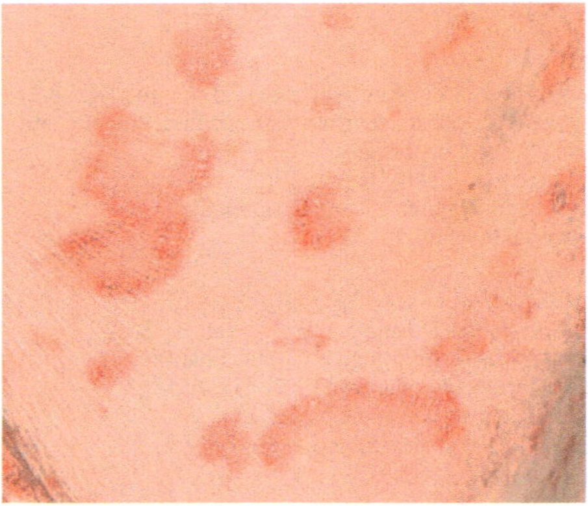

Fig. 4.4 Arcuate lesions in healing psoriasis.

Reproduced courtesy of Susan Lewis-Jones, Hon Consultant Dermatologist, Ninewells Hospital and Medical School, Dundee, UK

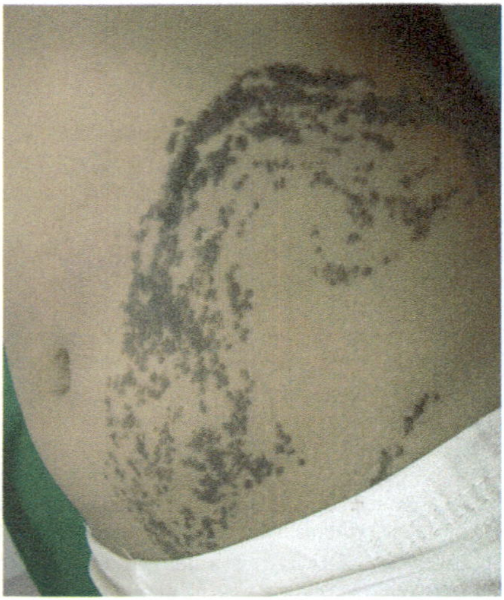

Fig. 4.5 Pigmented epidermal naevus following the typical whorled pattern of Blaschko's lines.

Reproduced courtesy of Patrick Yesudian, Consultant Dermatologist, Chennai, India

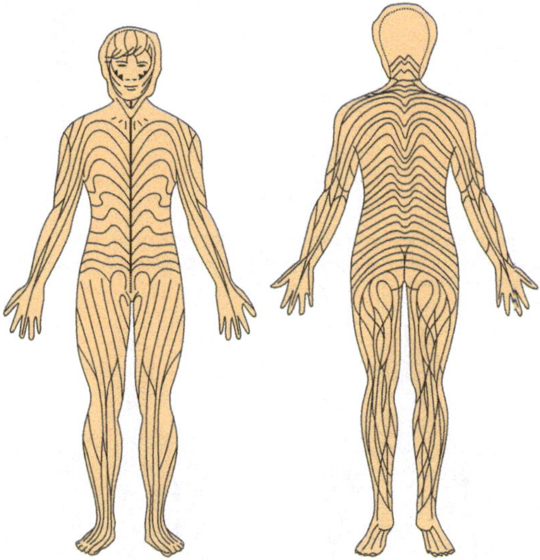

Fig. 4.6 Blaschko's lines are linear and whorled and are thought to follow embryonic migration lines. The abnormal areas represent a form of cutaneous genetic mosaicism.

Reproduced from Blashko A. (1901). *Die Nervenverteil ung in der Haut in Ihrer Bezeihung Zu Den Erkrankungen der Haut*. Vienna, Leipzig: Braumuklller

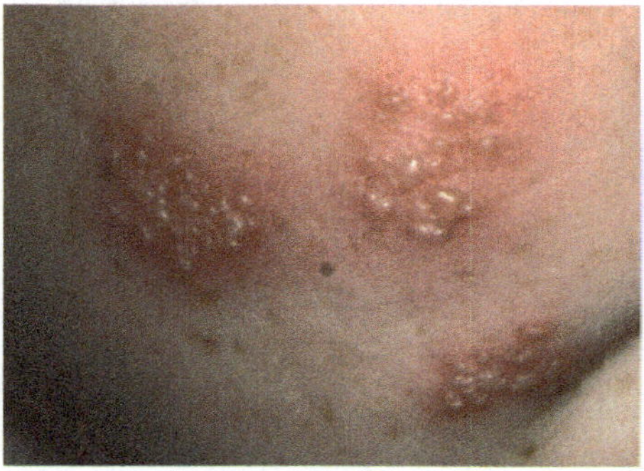

Fig. 4.7 Herpetiform group of blisters.

Reproduced courtesy of Susan Lewis-Jones, Hon Consultant Dermatologist, Ninewells Hospital and Medical School, Dundee, UK

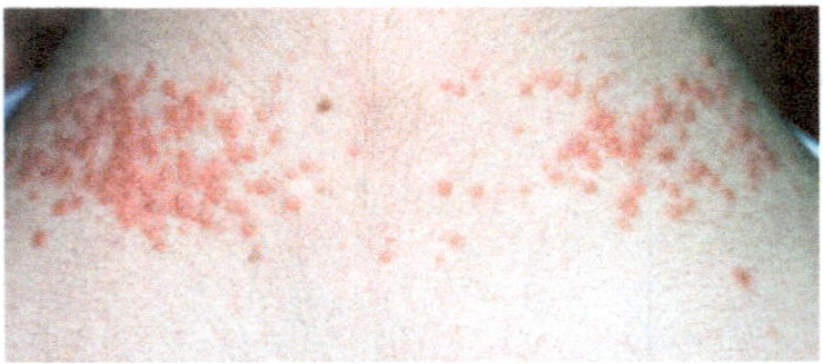

Fig. 4.8 Koebnerized lesions of psoriasis following sunburn on neck.

Reproduced courtesy of Susan Lewis-Jones, Hon Consultant Dermatologist, Ninewells Hospital and Medical School, Dundee, UK

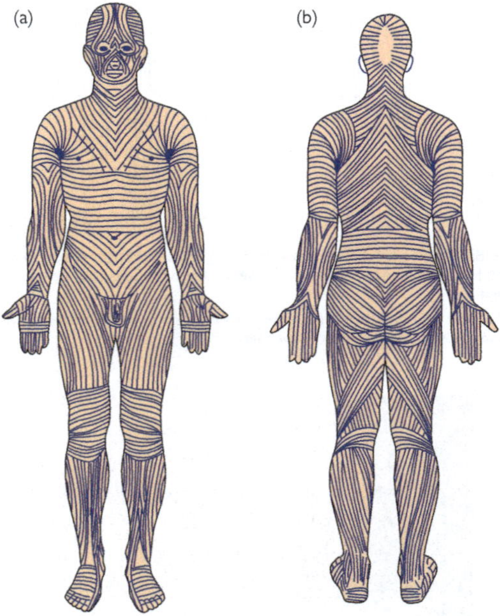

Fig. 4.9 Langer's lines.

Reproduced with permission from Dorland W. A. M (2007). *Dorland's Illustrated Medical Dictionary*, 31st Edition. Philadelphia, USA: Saunders an imprint of Elsevier

Shield-shaped—'V' of chest and upper back e.g. acne vulgaris (➲ see Fig. 18.1). Photosensitivity often fits this pattern but can affect any exposed site (➲ see Chapter 16).

T-shirt and shorts distribution—e.g. pityriasis rosea, lesions distributed in 'fir-tree' pattern on trunk (➲ see Fig. 22.7).

Box 4.3 Rashes/lesions occurring in a linear pattern

- Blaschko's lines are linear on limbs.
- Dermatitis artefacta (➲ see Chapter 24).
- Koebnerized lesions (e.g. psoriasis, warts).
- Jellyfish stings—may leave linear or bizarrely shaped pigmentation.
- Lesions in Langer's lines on the limbs.
- Lichen striatus (➲ see Fig. 17.5).
- Linea alba and linea nigra.
- Linear psoriasis.
- Linear lichen planus.
- Linear eczema.
- Inflammatory linear verrucous epidermal naevus (ILVEN).
- Linear blisters of phytophotodermatitis (➲ see Chapter 16).
- Linear epidermal naevus (Fig. 4.10).
- Plantar warts may present in a linear pattern.

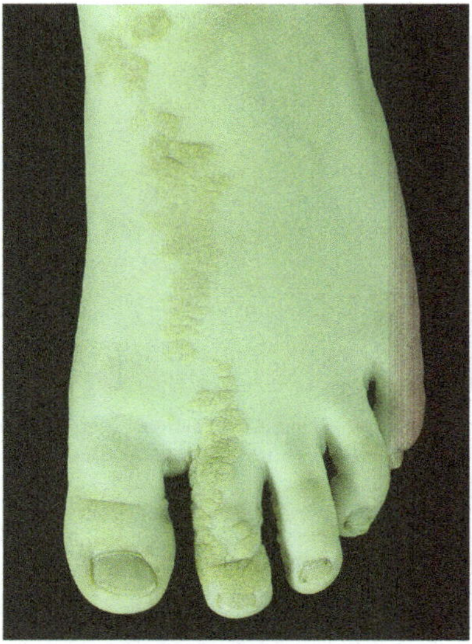

Fig. 4.10 Linear warty epidermal naevus. These particular lesions follow Blashko's lines which are linear in some areas on the limbs.

Reproduced courtesy of NHS Tayside Clinical Photography, Dundee, UK

T-shirt only distribution—pityriasis versicolor (➲ see Fig. 11.1).

Whorled—swirls of lesions representing cutaneous mosaicism (see Blaschko's lines, Fig. 4.6), e.g. epidermal naevi (Fig. 4.5) or incontinentia pigmenti (➲ see p. 389).

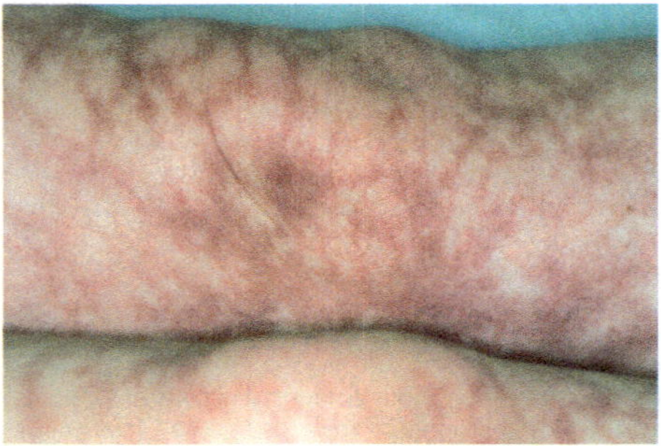

Fig. 4.11 Livedo (lace-like) pattern of rash—in systemic lupus erythematosus.
Reproduced courtesy of Susan Lewis-Jones, Hon Consultant Dermatologist, Ninewells Hospital and Medical School, Dundee, UK

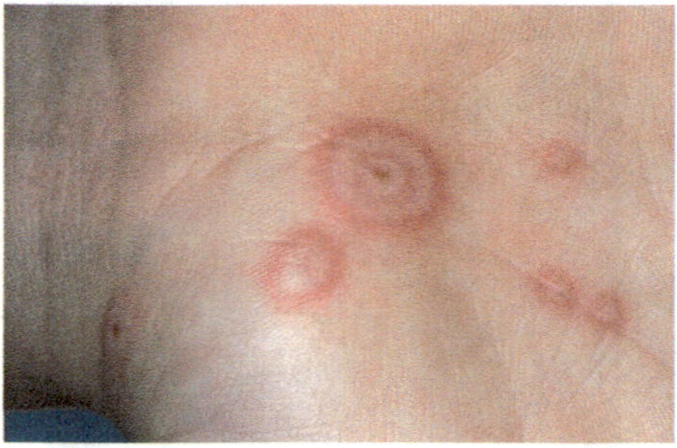

Fig. 4.12 Close-up of target lesion and early blistering in erythema multiforme.
Reproduced courtesy of Susan Lewis-Jones, Hon Consultant Dermatologist, Ninewells Hospital and Medical School, Dundee, UK

Box 4.4 Segmental/zosteriform

Common:
- Port-wine stains (Fig. 4.13).
- Herpes zoster infections (➲ see Fig. 25.5).

Rare:
- Becker's naevus (➲ see Fig. 33.2).
- Café-au-lait macules in McCune-Albright syndrome.
- Cutis marmorata telangiectatica congenita (➲ see Fig. 8.20).
- Segmental vitiligo (➲ see Vitiligo, pp. 480–1).
- Naevus depigmentosus (➲ see White skin (hypomelanosis), pp. 480–6).

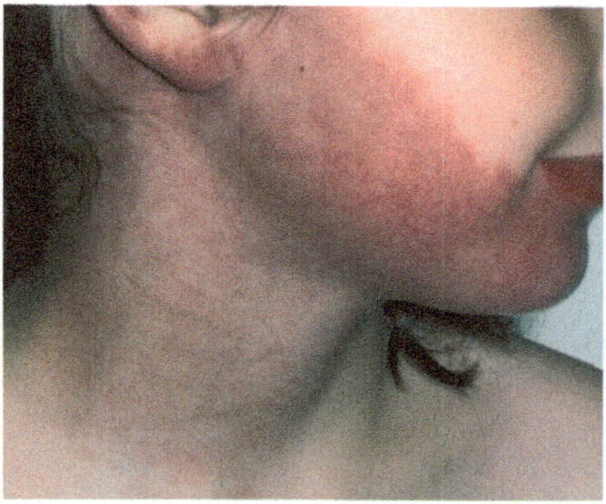

Fig. 4.13 Segmental/zosteriform rash. Facial port-wine stain in V3 distribution.
Reproduced courtesy of Susan Lewis-Jones, Hon Consultant Dermatologist, Ninewells Hospital and Medical School, Dundee, UK

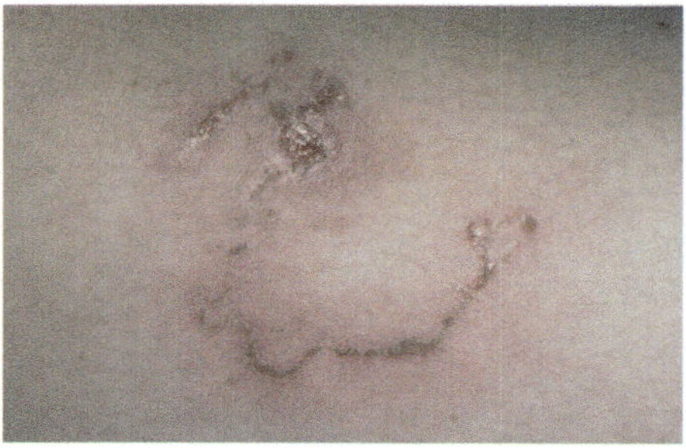

Fig. 4.14 Serpiginous lesions of larva migrans.
Reproduced courtesy of Susan Lewis-Jones, Hon Consultant Dermatologist, Ninewells Hospital and Medical School, Dundee, UK

Box 4.5 Serpiginous (snake-like) and arcuate rashes

- Tinea infections or psoriasis–during clearance.
- Cutaneous larva migrans (various hookworm larvae) (Fig. 4.14).
- Elastosis perforans serpiginosa (➲ see Chapter 20).
- Larva currens (nematode—*Strongyloides* spp).
- Urticaria (➲ see Chapter 21).

Chapter 5

Endocrine dysfunction and the skin

Introduction

Skin changes may occur as part of many endocrine disorders, and can provide diagnostic clues towards the underlying diagnosis. Occasionally the skin changes may be the presenting feature. The following categories of endocrine disorders are considered:

- Diabetes mellitus.
- Disorders of thyroid function.
- Disorders of adrenal function.
- Pituitary dysfunction.
- Disorders of sex hormones.
- Polyglandular syndromes.
- Multiple endocrine neoplasia syndromes.

Diabetes mellitus

Childhood diabetes mellitus has a prevalence of approximately 1 in 500, with the majority of cases being insulin dependent (type 1 diabetes), although recent studies suggest a 20% increase in type 2 diabetes and it is thought to be widely underreported. The most common cutaneous features of diabetes are listed in Box 5.1.

Insulin injection site reactions

- *Lipoatrophy*—commoner in females and children. Often commences as reddened areas due to inflammation of the fat.
- *Lipohypertrophy*—localized soft tissue hypertrophy (like lipomas). Rotation of injection sites may help to prevent this.
- *Allergic reactions*—redness and swelling (minutes to hours later).

Box 5.1 Skin changes in diabetic children

Bacterial infections: furunculosis (boils), cellulitis, erysipelas.
Candidal infections: intertrigo, vulvovaginitis, balanitis, angular cheilitis, oral candidiasis, paronychia.
Diabetic dermopathy: (rare) small brown papules, may scar. No treatment is required.
Granuloma annulare (GA): several forms. Usually seen as raised ringed lesions (➲ see Fig. 28.3) in non-diabetics. GA in diabetics may be more extensive. Lesions are either flat purplish circles or more florid plaques (Fig. 5.1).
Injection site reactions: lipoatrophy, lipohypertrophy, allergic reactions, localized abscesses.
Necrobiosis lipoidica diabeticorum: well-defined yellow/brown/orange plaques with atrophic centres, usually located over the shins (Fig. 5.2). Active lesions can be treated with potent topical corticosteroids or intralesional corticosteroids.
Waxy skin thickening (cheiroarthropathy) with limited joint mobility (especially of the hands).
Xanthomas: Fig 5.3 (➲ see also Fig. 37.2).

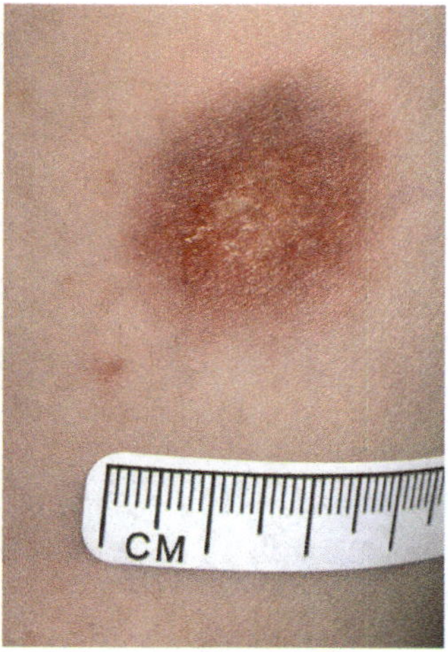

Fig. 5.1 Granuloma annulare in a diabetic girl showing circular raised plaque.
Reproduced courtesy of Susan Lewis-Jones, Hon Consultant Dermatologist, Ninewells Hospital and Medical School, Dundee, UK

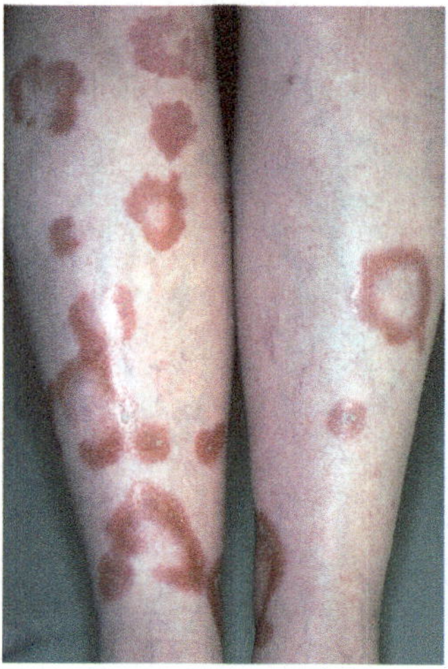

Fig. 5.2 Necrobiosis lipoidica diabeticorum: typical purplish shiny annular areas on shins.
Reproduced courtesy of Susan Lewis-Jones, Hon Consultant Dermatologist, Ninewells Hospital and Medical School, Dundee, UK

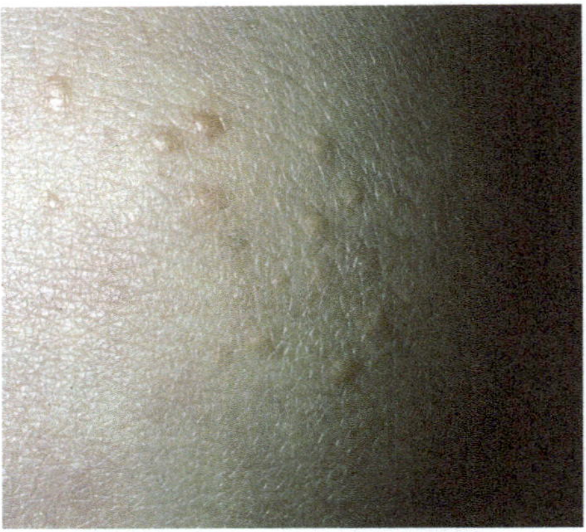

Fig. 5.3 Eruptive xanthomas.

Reproduced courtesy of Cameron Kennedy, Consultant Dermatologist, Departments of Dermatology, Bristol Royal Infirmary and Paediatric Dermatology, Bristol Royal Hospital for Children, Bristol, UK

- *Localized abscesses*—usually *Staphylococcus aureus* or *Streptococcus pyogenes*, but there may be unusual pathogens; pus should be cultured.
- *Generalized purpuric reactions* to insulin (very rare).

Disorders of thyroid function

Hyperthyroidism

The commonest cause in children is autoimmune disease (Graves' disease or Hashimoto's thyroiditis). With the exception of pretibial myxoedema, most skin changes in hyperthyroidism are a direct result of excess circulating thyroid hormones (see Box 5.2). Autoimmune thyroid disease may also be associated with other autoimmune skin diseases such as vitiligo.

Management: normalization of circulating thyroid hormone levels will cause resolution of most cutaneous signs.

Pretibial myxoedema: very rare in children and only seen in Graves' disease when circulating autoantibodies stimulate production of glycosaminoglycans by fibroblasts. This leads to the formation of firm, non-pitting skin-coloured or purple nodules and plaques, usually over the shins. Later lesions may have an orange peel-like surface.

Box 5.2 Cutaneous signs of hyperthyroidism

- Moist skin.
- Palmar erythema.
- Flushed appearance.
- Thinning of scalp hair (uncommon).
- Onycholysis and other nail changes.

Box 5.3 Cutaneous signs of acquired hypothyroidism

- Cool, dry skin.
- Yellow-tinged pallor (due to anaemia/carotenaemia).
- Myxoedema (non-pitting thickening) of tongue and skin, especially face, hands, and feet.
- Thinning of scalp hair.
- Loss of lateral third of eyebrows.
- Hypertrichosis of back.

Treatment: it is very unsatisfactory as the disease is driven by autoantibodies. Potent topical corticosteroids or intralesional corticosteroids can be tried in combination with compression bandaging.

Hypothyroidism

May be congenital, or acquired at any stage of childhood.

- *Congenital hypothyroidism*
  - Incidence of approximately one in 4000 births; it is tested for as part of neonatal screening programmes, so untreated congenital hypothyroidism is rare in the Western world.
  - Untreated infants develop characteristic signs of poor muscle tone, umbilical hernia, poor feeding, excessive sleeping, constipation, prolonged neonatal jaundice, and hypothermia.
  - Cutaneous features: these include cool dry skin, jaundice, periorbital puffiness, cutis marmorata (➲ see Fig. 31.8), pallor (secondary to anaemia), which may be followed by generalized thickening of the skin and tongue through excess glycosaminoglycan production.
- *Acquired hypothyroidism*
  - Usually due to autoimmune thyroid disease in the Western world.
  - Generally presents with non-cutaneous symptoms such as lethargy, constipation, developmental delay, hypertrichosis, goitre, and cold intolerance.
  - Cutaneous signs are given in Box 5.3.

Management: the cutaneous features of hypothyroidism are reversible upon restoration of euthyroidism with thyroxine therapy.

Disorders of adrenal function

Cushing's syndrome

This results from chronic glucocorticoid excess, which may be exogenous or endogenous in origin.

Endogenous causes include tumours of the adrenal cortex, and adrenocorticotropic hormone (ACTH)-secreting pituitary adenomas. The clinical features in children are similar to those in adults, although growing children with Cushing's syndrome may have short stature. A characteristic distribution of fat, typified by central adiposity, buffalo hump, and moon face may be present.

The following skin signs may be seen:

- Purple striae.
- Skin fragility.
- Plethoric facies.
- Easy bruising.
- Hypertrichosis.

- Acneiform rash on face and upper trunk—comedones will be absent unless true acne (➲ see Chapter 18) is also present.

In Cushing's disease (which is specifically due to ACTH-secreting pituitary adenoma), there may also be Addisonian-like hyperpigmentation (➲ see Addison's disease, p. 64).

Addison's disease

- ➲ See also Metabolic/endocrine, p. 495.

Primary adrenocortical insufficiency (hypoadrenalism) causes excess ACTH and melanocyte-stimulating hormone secretion by pituitary gland. It is very rare in children.

Cutaneous signs: increased pigmentation of skin, hair, and mucosae, best seen in the palmar creases and buccal mucosae.

Presentation: either acute Addisonian crisis, or chronic ill health and pigmentation.

Cause: most are due to autoimmune destruction of the adrenal cortex; rarer causes include adrenal infarction, tuberculosis (TB), and genetic disorders.

Pituitary dysfunction

- ➲ See also Cushing's syndrome, pp. 63–4.

Hypopituitarism

- Global reduction in secretion of pituitary hormones.
- Commonest cause in childhood is craniopharyngioma.

Presentation: failure of growth and pubertal development, or symptoms of diabetes insipidus.

Cutaneous changes: not prominent except for reduced or absent pubic hair, pallor, and dryness.

Gigantism/acromegaly

- *Gigantism*: growth hormone (GH) excess occurring before epiphyseal closure.
- *Acromegaly*: GH excess occurring after epiphyseal closure.

Cutaneous features: include hyperhidrosis, increased sebum production, skin tags, hyperpigmentation, acanthosis nigricans (➲ see Fig. 33.6), and cutis verticis gyrata of the scalp (➲ see Cutis verticis gyrata, p. 450).

Cause: usually GH-secreting pituitary adenoma.

Disorders of sex hormones

Androgens and the skin

Androgen levels rise with puberty in both sexes and are responsible for the development of pubic and axillary hair, oily skin (seborrhoea), acne, and body odour.

- *In females*: androgens are secreted by maturing adrenal glands (adrenarche).

- *In males*: higher levels result from combined secretion by adrenal glands and testes causing a general coarsening of skin texture, increased hair growth on face and chest, and genital enlargement.

In later life (occasionally late teens), androgens can drive androgenetic alopecia in both sexes.

Androgen excess

Prepubertal

Children present with penile enlargement or clitoromegaly, accelerated growth, deepening voice, pubic and facial hair, seborrhoea, and acne.

Postpubertal

- *Females*—present with hirsutism, acne, and irregular periods. More severe cases may also have a deepening voice, clitoromegaly, and male pattern alopecia.
- *Males*—androgen excess often not clinically apparent.

Cause: adrenal disease (adrenal tumour, congenital adrenal hyperplasia), gonadal tumours, hyperprolactinaemia, or obesity (enhanced peripheral conversion of androstenedione to testosterone, which may occur as part of the polycystic ovary syndrome; ➲ see Chapter 18, Associations with other disorders, p. 267).

Androgen deficiency: see ➲ Hypogonadism, p. 65.

Oestrogens and the skin

Oestrogen excess

Cutaneous signs: spider naevi, palmar erythema, chloasma, and pigmentation of the nipples and linea alba. Oestrogen excess in males produces breast enlargement with puffiness and pigmentation of the areolae.

Causes: usually pregnancy or with combined oral contraceptive use. Rarely oestrogen-producing tumours of the adrenal glands or testes.

Note: oestrogen-secreting tumours may also secrete androgens (see earlier), giving rise to a mixed clinical picture.

Oestrogen deficiency: see ➲ Hypogonadism, p. 65.

Hypogonadism

- *Prepubertal*: failure of development of some secondary sexual characteristics, such as breast development and menstruation in females, and genital enlargement in males. However, pubic and axillary hair will develop under the influence of adrenal androgens, although typically in a female pattern in hypogonadal males.
- *Postpubertal*: oligo- or amenorrhoea in females, and impotence and reduced requirement for shaving in males.

Cause: primary gonadal failure (e.g. Klinefelter syndrome, Turner's syndrome) or inadequate pituitary gonadotrophin release (e.g. prolactinoma, hypopituitarism).

Precocious puberty

This is defined as the appearance of secondary sexual characteristics before the age of 8y in a female and 9y in a male.

- *Cutaneous signs*: pubic and axillary hair, acne, facial hair.

Note: if pubic/axillary hair and acne are the only positive signs of precocious puberty, then this is usually the result of premature adrenarche.

Causes: may be constitutional, head trauma, hydrocephalus, central nervous system (CNS) tumour/infection, severe hypothyroidism, Addison's disease, adrenal tumours, ovarian tumours, testicular tumours, McCune–Albright syndrome, congenital adrenal hyperplasia.

Polyglandular autoimmune syndrome type 1 (PGAS1)

PGAS1

Autoimmune polyendocrinopathy-candidiasis-ectodermal dystrophy syndrome. The three most common manifestations are:

- Chronic mucocutaneous candidiasis, earliest manifestation typically before age 5.
- Hypoparathyroidism.
- Addison's disease.

Less common manifestations: vitiligo and alopecia areata. A variety of endocrine (hypogonadism, diabetes mellitus, thyroid disease) and non-endocrine (pernicious anaemia, hepatitis, nephritis) disorders may also occur.

Cause: rare, autosomal recessive inheritance due to mutations of the autoimmune regulator gene (*AIRE*).

PGAS2 and *PGAS3* are distinct syndromes occurring in adults.

Multiple endocrine neoplasia syndromes

Three autosomal dominant, multiple endocrine neoplasia syndromes are described.

MEN1

Parathyroid hyperplasia, pituitary and pancreatic tumours.

Cutaneous features: facial angiofibromas (similar to tuberous sclerosis complex, ➲ see pp. 483–4) may be seen.

MEN2a

Medullary thyroid carcinoma, phaeochromocytoma, and parathyroid hyperplasia.

Cutaneous features: sometimes lichen amyloidosis (very itchy papules coalescing to form dark plaques, often rippled in appearance) on upper back.

MEN2b

Medullary thyroid carcinoma, phaeochromocytoma, Marfanoid body habitus (tall, thin, with elongated limbs and digits).

Cutaneous features: multiple mucosal neuromas (small non-pigmented papules) causing a bumpy thickening of lips, eyelids, tongue, and mouth from birth or first few years of life.

Chapter 6

Faltering growth and the skin

Introduction

Definition: Faltering growth (previously termed failure to thrive) is a descriptive term and not a specific diagnosis. Most would accept the definition of weight measurement falling by two major percentiles when plotted on an appropriate growth chart for children of the same age, sex and ethnicity. It may be associated with several cutaneous manifestations.

Pathophysiology

Normal growth in term infants

The average birth weight in the United Kingdom is 3.3kg (Table 6.1). Weight drops as much as 10% in the first few days of life. However, birth weight should be regained within 2 weeks, with breastfed babies regaining weight a little later than bottlefed babies (➲ see Fig. 6.1 for an example growth chart).

Normal growth in premature babies

When plotting growth charts for premature babies, a 'corrected age' should be calculated by subtracting the number of weeks of prematurity from 40 weeks (term). When catch-up growth is attained, normal growth charts can be used (i.e. approx. 18 months for weight and 40 months for height).

Table 6.1 Average increase in weight in children

Age	Average daily weight gain (g)
0–3 months	26–31g
3–6 months	17–18g
6–9 months	12–13g
9–12 months	9g
1–3y	7–9g
4–6y	6g

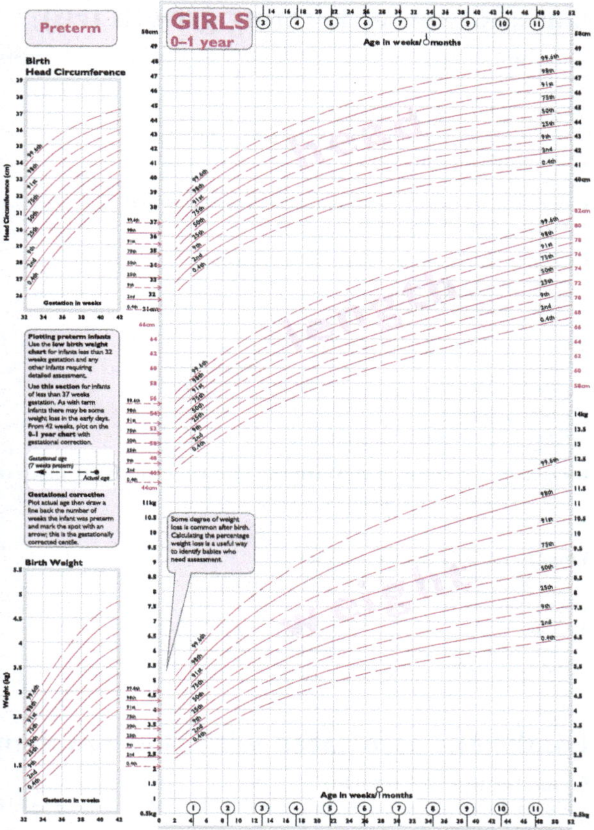

Fig. 6.1 Growth chart (0–1 girls).

Chart developed by RCPCH, WHO, and Department of Health. Reproduced with permission of Royal College of Paediatrics and Child Health

Classification of faltering growth (FG)

There are a number of mechanisms by which this may occur. The following give examples of each:

Reduced intake of nutrients

- Feeding difficulties such as in gastro-oesophageal reflux.
- Cows' milk protein allergy.
- Neglect and withholding of food.
- Anorexia, mechanical, and coordination problems with swallowing.
- Kwashiorkor or marasmus.

Inability to digest or absorb nutrients

- Pancreatic insufficiency.
- Small intestinal disease.

Excessive loss of nutrients

- Vomiting.
- Protein-losing enteropathy.
- Chronic diarrhoea.
- Renal failure/renal tubular acidosis.

Increased nutrient requirements due to underlying disease

- Chronic cardiac or respiratory failure.
- Chronic infection.

Unable to fully utilize nutrients

- Metabolic disorder such as biotin deficiency.
- Zinc deficiency.
- Cystic fibrosis.
- Hypohidrotic ectodermal dysplasia.
- Chromosomal/genetic abnormality.

Conditions associated with skin problems

Neonates (up to 1 month)

- Congenital or acquired infections such as CMV, HIV, *Treponema pallidum* (➲ see Chapter 7).
- Netherton syndrome (Fig. 6.2; ➲ see also Structural abnormalities of hair shaft, pp. 199–200, and Fig. 27.6).
- Immunodeficiency:
  - Severe combined immunodeficiency (SCID).
  - Omenn syndrome.
- Junctional/dystrophic epidermolysis bullosa (EB) (Figs. 6.3, 6.4) (➲ see Chapter 25).
- Severe atopic dermatitis with associated gastrointestinal problems (gastro-oesophageal reflux, cows' milk allergy) (➲ see Chapter 17).
- CINCA (chronic infantile neurologic cutaneous and articular syndrome) (➲ see Chapter 21).

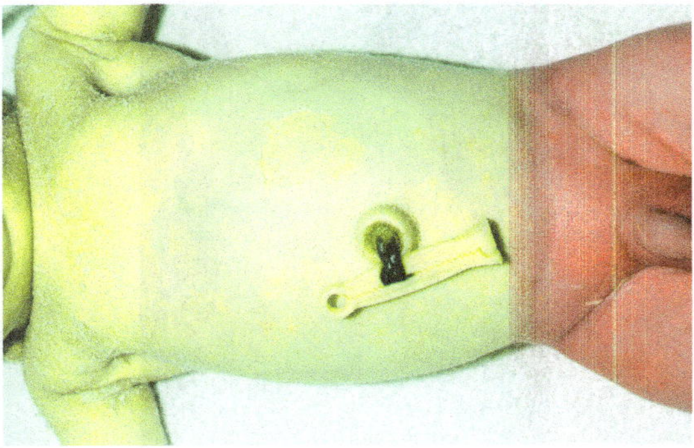

Fig. 6.2 Baby with Netherton syndrome.

Reproduced courtesy of Bisola Laguda, Chelsea and Westminster Hospital NHS Foundation Trust, London, UK

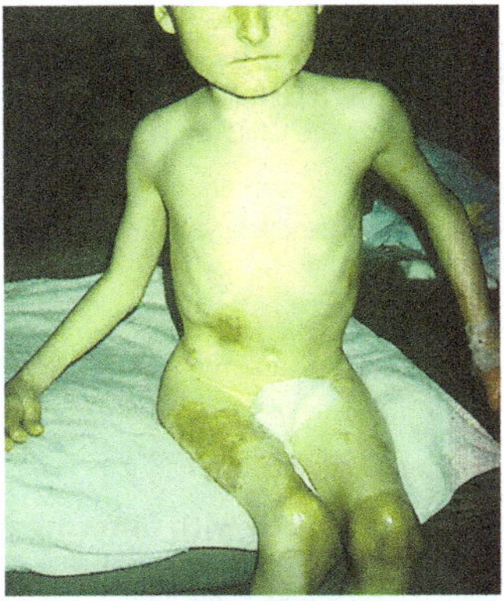

Fig. 6.3 A markedly underweight child with dystrophic epidermolysis bullosa before insertion of a gastrostomy.

Reproduced courtesy of Bisola Laguda, Chelsea and Westminster Hospital NHS Foundation Trust, London, UK

Infancy (up to 2y)

All of those listed for neonates plus:

- Severe ichthyosis (➲ see Chapter 25).
- Cystic fibrosis.
- Metabolic conditions—thyroid/adrenal disorders.
- Acrodermatitis enteropathica—zinc deficiency (➲ see Fig. 7.4 and Fig. 13.4).

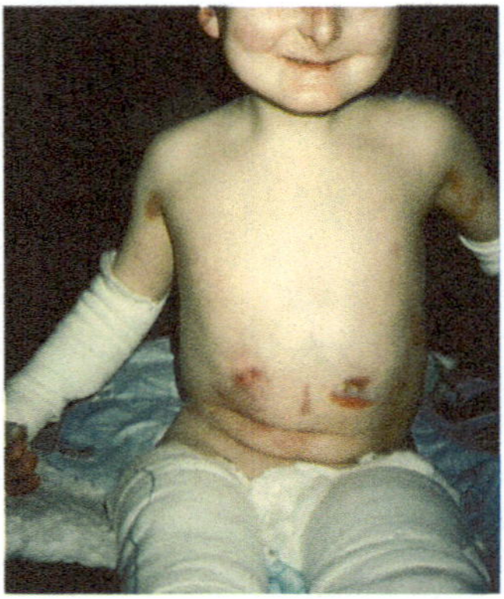

Fig. 6.4 Button gastrostomy still in use. Child showing weight gain.
Reproduced courtesy of Bisola Laguda, Chelsea and Westminster Hospital NHS Foundation Trust, London, UK

- Chronic infection—such as HIV.
- Langerhans cell histiocytosis (LCH) (➲ see Fig. 13.5).
- Drugs—corticosteroids (➲ see Chapter 3).

Children (2y and over)

All of those listed for neonates and infancy plus:

- Inflammatory bowel disease.
- In-born errors of metabolism.
- Mucopolysaccharidoses.
- Chronic inflammatory illness—autoimmune/rheumatological conditions (➲ see Chapter 38).
- Chronic renal disease.
- Degenerative neurological conditions.

Rare skin disorders associated with faltering growth (FG) to consider

- Costello and cardiofaciocutaneous syndrome.
- Hutchinson–Gilford progeria (➲ see Chapter 29, Fat changes, pp. 452–3).
- Menkes disease (X-linked recessive disorder of copper metabolism, FG, kinky hair, neurological deterioration).
- SAVI (stimulator of interferon genes—associated vasculopathy with onset in infancy).
- Infantile systemic hyalinosis.
- Congenital disorders of glycosylation.

Clinical evaluation

An accurate history is vital. FG may be related to a specific underlying condition or psychological disorder, or may be a combination of the two.

History

Take a detailed history of:

- Diet (dietetic input may be necessary).
- Family history and antenatal history including drugs.
- Recurrent infections.
- Diarrhoea and or vomiting.
- Respiratory distress.
- Chronic cough.

Examination

- Height, weight, head circumference (especially in a child under 1y).
  - Useful to have several weight measurements—consult child's NHS handheld information booklet (red book).
  - May also be useful to obtain parental heights.
- General appearance—does the child look unwell?
  - Decreased skin turgor.
  - Wasting.
  - Oedema.
  - Hepatosplenomegaly.
  - Lymphadenopathy.
  - Rash or skin changes (erythroderma, scaling, hypo or hyperpigmentation, blistering).
  - Hair colour and textural changes.
  - Alopecia.
  - Signs of vitamin deficiency.

Initial investigations

- If infection is suspected then take appropriate microbiology samples (e.g. skin swabs, throat swabs, blood for microscopy and culture).
- TORCH or HIV serology may be required.
- Full blood count.
- Electrolytes.
- Liver function tests, calcium, and phosphate.
- Thyroid function tests.
- Urinalysis.
- Skin biopsy if indicated.

Other specific tests: as required, e.g. in erythroderma (➲ see Chapter 22).

Classification

Dependent on whether onset was at, or soon after birth, or acquired later. Congenital presentation is indicative of a developmental or inherited disorder. The cutaneous appearance is helpful for diagnosis (Table 6.2).

Table 6.2 Causes of faltering growth with skin manifestations

Clinical condition	Dermatological features	Specific tests
Acrodermatitis enteropathica	Papulosquamous scaly erythematous rash with perioral, perirectal and acral involvement; alopecia	Serum zinc level
CINCA (➲ see Chapter 21)	Persistent migratory urticarial skin rash	Mutations of *CIAS1* gene
Cystic fibrosis (CF)	Generalized erythema, scaly papules, exfoliative dermatitis	Sweat test, mutations of the *CFTR* gene
Epidermolysis bullosa (EB) (➲ see Chapter 25)	Generalized blistering; in dystrophic EB, blisters heal with dystrophic scarring—milia formation	Shave skin biopsy for electron microscopy and immunofluorescence. DNA mutation analysis
Langerhans cell histiocytosis (➲ see Fig. 13.5)	Seborrhoeic dermatitis-like rash; yellow brown papules associated with scaling and crusting, often purpura	Skin biopsy with S100 and CD1a immunohistochemistry stain
Netherton syndrome (➲ see Fig. 6.2 and Chapters 14, 27)	Erythroderma, alopecia, or short hair, ichthyosis linearis circumflexa (older children)	Skin biopsy shows absent LEKTI stain. Hair microscopy for bamboo hair (➲ see Structural abnormalities of hair shaft, pp. 199–200). Mutation in *Spink 5* gene
Omenn syndrome	Erythroderma desquamation, alopecia, often visible adenopathy	T-cell subsets showing increased numbers of activated T cells, full blood count (FBC)—eosinophilia, *RAG-1*, *RAG-2* mutational analysis
Hyperhidrotic ectodermal dysplasia (➲ see Chapter 1)	At birth, affected males show marked scaling, eczema, periorbital hyperpigmentation, sparse fine blonde hair or alopecia, dental abnormalities, diminished sweating	DNA-based molecular genetic diagnosis

Management

Dependent on the diagnosis:

- For the acutely ill child hospital admission is usually necessary (Fig. 6.5) and requires the involvement of a paediatrically trained physician.
- A multidisciplinary approach may be required and include specialities such as immunology, gastroenterology, and genetics.
- The basic management of FG is to achieve weight gain by ensuring adequate nutritional/calorific intake (Fig. 6.3).
- Tailoring treatment to diagnosis can be:
    - *Curative*—e.g. zinc replacement for acrodermatitis enteropathica.
    - *Highly effective*—e.g. topical corticosteroid therapy for atopic dermatitis.

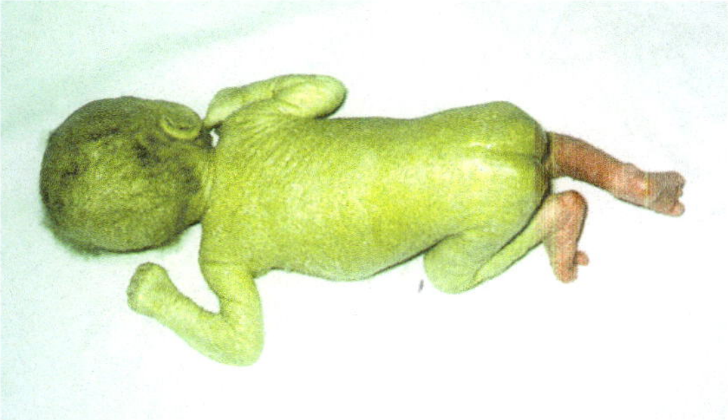

Fig. 6.5 Ichthyosiform erythroderma as a manifestation of a nutritional/metabolic abnormality. Child was admitted for investigation.

Reproduced courtesy of Bisola Laguda, Chelsea and Westminster Hospital NHS Foundation Trust, London, UK

- *Limited symptomatic*—e.g. genetic disorders like Netherton syndrome (Fig. 6.2; ➲ see also Chapters 14, 17, and 25).
- *Lifesaving* for FG conditions like SCID or Omenn syndrome when bone marrow transplant may be necessary in the long term.

FG in low- and middle-income countries

Can be as a result of inadequate nutritional intake, e.g. kwashiorkor (protein–energy malnutrition), which is the most common. It is often as a result of prolonged breastfeeding and improves on mixed feeding.

Kwashiorkor

Cutaneous features develop over a few days:

- Initially skin lesions are erythematous becoming purple to reddish brown, with marked skin peeling and sloughing. Fissuring (splitting) of drier, darker areas causes paler patches—'crazy pavement dermatosis'. There can also be patchy hyper- and hypopigmentary discolouration and peripheral oedema in severe cases.
- *Hair* becomes dry and brittle, may change colour and have lighter coloured banding known as the 'flag sign'. Examine older siblings for this.
- *Nail* plates are thin and soft and may be fissured or ridged.

Marasmus

Cutaneous features—the skin is dry and scaly with muscle wasting and loss of subcutaneous fat. There is also desquamation.

Hair—falls out easily with areas of alopecia.

Nails—grow slowly and are brittle.

Section 2

Neonatal

Chapter 7

Neonatal skin problems

Introduction

The skin of a newborn infant is different from adult skin. It is 40–60% thinner and topical agents are easily absorbed, sometimes resulting in toxicity (Table 7.1). It is prone to injury from seemingly innocuous trauma such as skin stripping from removal of adhesive dressings potentiating secondary infection and/or scarring. These properties are particularly marked in preterm infants and in children who suffer from a blistering skin eruption, known as epidermolysis bullosa (EB) (➲ see Figs. 6.4, 6.5, 25.10–12; see also Chapter 25, Genetic causes of blisters, pp. 387–90).

In any newborn with blistering: always ask for an urgent dermatological opinion.

Table 7.1 Risks of transcutaneous absorption of topical products in newborn babies, infants, and children

Compound	Toxicity
Aniline (dye used in laundry)	Methemoglobinemia
Pentachlorophenol (laundry disinfectant)	Tachycardia, sweating, hepatomegaly, metabolic acidosis
Hexachlorophene (topical antiseptic)	Vascular encephalopathy
Resorcinol (topical antiseptic)	Methemoglobinemia
Boric acid (baby powder)	Vomiting, diarrhoea, erythroderma, seizures
Lindane (scabicide)	Neurotoxicity
Salicylic acid	Metabolic acidosis
Isopropyl alcohol under occlusion	Haemorrhagic skin necrosis
Urea (exfoliating, emollient)	Uraemia
Povidone-iodine (topical antiseptic)	Hypothyroidism, goitre
Neomycin	Neural deafness
Corticosteroid	Cutaneous atrophy, adrenal suppression
Benzocaine (topical antiseptic)	Methemoglobinemia
Prilocaine (topical anaesthetic)	Methemoglobinemia
Methylene blue (dye)	Methemoglobinemia

Reproduced with permission from Fernandes J. D. et *al.* Children and newborn skin care and prevention. *An Bras Dermatol.* 86(1):102–10. Copyright © 2011. http://dx.doi.org/10.1590/S0365-05962011000100014

Physiology of neonatal skin

Key physiological considerations in newborn skin include:

- Increased evaporation of water from the surface of the skin resulting in electrolyte disturbance, particularly hypernatraemic dehydration.

- Diminished thermoregulatory capability, due to increased water and heat loss, lack of subcutaneous fat, and poor autonomic control of cutaneous vasculature.
- Increased transcutaneous absorption, which may result in systemic toxicity from topical agents.
- Reduced skin surface area to body mass ratio, providing further increased risk for systemic toxicity from topical treatments.
- Barrier function of skin is reduced in preterm infants below 34 weeks' gestation, resulting in increased risk of infection.

Care of premature skin

The goals of skin care for premature infants should be to:
- Prevent physical injury to the skin.
- Minimize insensible water loss.
- Maintain thermostability.
- Prevent infection.

Significant absorption of substances applied to the skin occurs in neonates (Table 7.1). Not all emollients are safe to use. For suitable emollients see Box 7.1.

Box 7.1 Emollients suitable for neonates and premature babies

Preservative-free paraffin-based emollients are best:
- 50% white soft paraffin or 50% liquid paraffin.
- Emulsifying ointment.

Transient benign neonatal dermatoses

Physiological desquamation

Occurs in most newborn infants. Premature infants do not show desquamation until 2–3 weeks of life. Postmature babies are often born with cracked peeling skin. If it persists beyond 1 week, consider other diagnoses (e.g. ichthyosis; ➲ see Chapter 27).

Milia

Very common, occurring mainly on the face as tiny papules (inclusion cysts) which resolve spontaneously. May also occur as a result of damage to the skin in certain syndromes including EB.

Epstein's pearls

Also known as oral mucosal cysts of the newborn. They occur as a result of epithelial tissues that become trapped during fusion of the palate. They appear as smooth yellowish papules, around 1–2mm in size, and are most commonly seen on the palate. Also found on alveolar ridges, they usually resolve spontaneously by 5 months.

Miliaria

Obstruction of the sweat glands resulting in superficial trapping of sweat under the skin surface (not follicular), producing small fragile, clear droplets (miliaria crystallina). Miliaria rubra usually present as 1–3mm red papules on head, neck, and trunk, favouring intertriginous or occluded areas. It is common in overheated or febrile infants. Responds to reducing ambient temperature and reduction of fever.

Transient neonatal pustulosis

Usually occurs at birth as very small pustules, eventually resolving to leave hyperpigmented macules with a collarette of scale that may last months. More common in Fitzpatrick skin type 6. Differential diagnosis includes erythema toxicum neonatorum, miliaria, candidiasis, and impetigo. No treatment is necessary.

Benign cephalic pustulosis (neonatal acne)

Neonatal non-follicular pustulosis typically appears within the first 5–21 days, presenting with erythematous papules, and pustules on the face, neck, and scalp. There are no comedones, unlike true acne.
Cause: possible association with *Malassezia* species. Self-limiting but responds to topical ketoconazole (➲ see Chapter 18).

Erythema toxicum neonatorum

Very common, mostly seen in full-term infants with onset between 24 and 48h of life (up to 10 days, rarely longer) as 1–3mm yellow papules or pustules, with surrounding erythematous flare (Fig. 7.1) sparing the palms and soles. Pustules are filled with eosinophils. Differential diagnosis includes herpes simplex, impetigo, and neonatal pustular melanosis (➲ see Pustular rashes in neonates and infants, pp. 298–9). No treatment is necessary.

Other rashes in the newborn

Neonatal lupus erythematosus (LE)

Rare rash which commonly involves the head, especially around the eyes (owl eyes; Fig. 7.2) but any area may be affected. It generally starts as red macules and evolves into annular red scaly plaques (Fig. 7.3). It usually resolves spontaneously, sometimes with mild atrophy. Mothers are Ro (or sometimes La) antibody positive. Forty-five per cent (45%) of infants are at risk of heart block that may require a pacemaker but both skin changes and heart disease are only seen in 10%.

Zinc deficiency and acrodermatitis enteropathica

Rare, but important to recognize. Well-demarcated erythematous patches and plaques with flaccid bullae around mouth, eyes and ears, napkin area, and distal extremities. Associated with diarrhoea and other features, including hair loss. May be a primary inherited disease or secondary to intrauterine growth retardation or faltering growth (e.g. amino-acid disorders, or low zinc in breast milk; ➲ see Table 6.2 and Fig. 13.4). For other skin problems associated with faltering growth, ➲ see Classification of FG and Conditions association with skin problems, pp. 70–2.

(a)

(b)

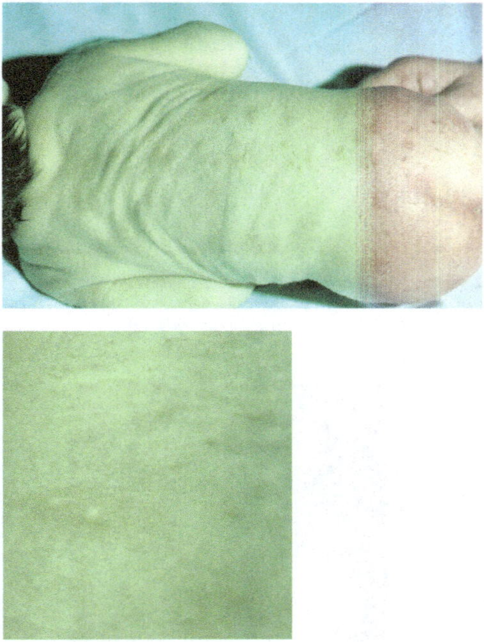

Fig. 7.1 (a) Toxic erythema of newborn with small pustules and areas of erythema—the so-called flea-bitten appearance; (b) a close-up of erythema pustules.

Reproduced courtesy of Susan Lewis-Jones, Hon Consultant Dermatologist, Ninewells Hospital and Medical School, Dundee, UK

Subcutaneous fat necrosis of the newborn

Red/purplish firm, subcutaneous nodules appearing within the first weeks of life. There is a higher incidence in premature infants and it may follow hypothermia (➲ see Thickening of fat layer, p. 453). Commonest over the buttocks, thighs, and back, and nodules may ulcerate or become calcified with time. Hypercalcaemia can occur, therefore monitor calcium levels until 1 month after lesions have abated.

Birthmarks

These are collections of cells of one or more of the skin elements: epidermis, melanocytes, blood vessels, lymphatics, dermis, connective tissue, and smooth muscle (Box 7.2). They are usually present at birth or present within the first few months of age. They may be:

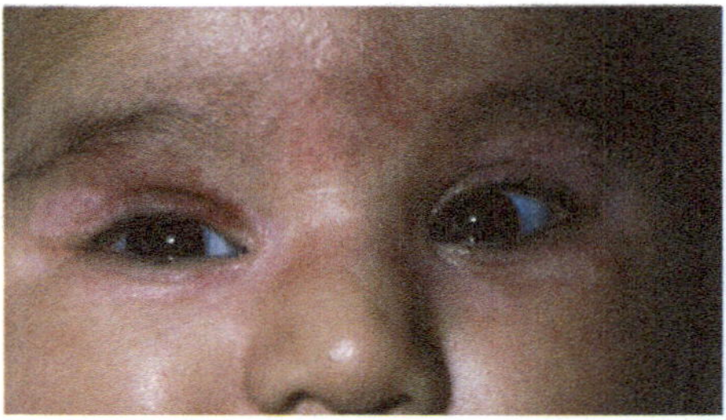

Fig. 7.2 Neonatal lupus erythematosus around the eyes (owl eyes).
Reproduced courtesy of Rosemarie Watson, Consultant Paediatric Dermatologist, Department of Dermatology, Our Lady's Children's Hospital Crumlin, Dublin, Ireland

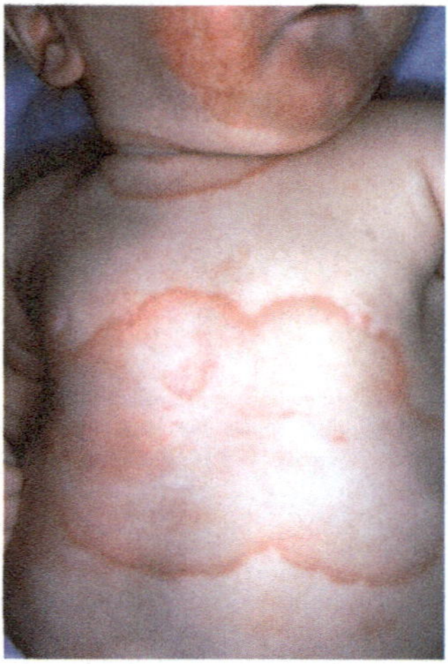

Fig. 7.3 Neonatal lupus erythematosus showing annular lesions on chest.
Reproduced courtesy of Susan Lewis-Jones, Hon Consultant Dermatologist, Ninewells Hospital and Medical School, Dundee, UK

- Vascular (➲ see Chapter 8).
- Pigmented/coloured (➲ see Chapters 31–37).
- Epidermal (➲ see Chapters 28 and 29).
- Connective tissue (➲ see Chapters 28 and 29).

Box 7.2 Common 'birth' marks

Flat red (➲ see Chapter 8)
- Salmon patches (midline telangiectatic naevi).
- Port-wine stains (usually lateral, not midline).
- Haemangiomas—often small flat lesions at birth, rapid growth thereafter in first 7 months, and then regress (50% resolve by 5y, 90% by 9y, although some skin marks/scars often remain).

Brown (➲ see Chapters 33 and 34)
- Café-au-lait macules (coffee-coloured).
- Melanocytic naevi (congenital moles).

Blue (➲ see Chapter 35)
- Mongolian blue spot (Fig. 7.5 and ➲ Fig. 24.2).
- Blue naevi.

Orange/skin-coloured (➲ see Chapters 32 and 37)
- Sebaceous naevus—usually on scalp (➲ see Fig. 14.5).
- Epidermal naevus—may be pale brown.
- Connective tissue naevus—usually skin-coloured or white.

White (➲ see Chapter 32)
- Ash-leaf macules (tuberous sclerosis complex)— ➲ see Fig. 32.4.

Primary irritant napkin dermatitis

This is extremely common, although incidence is falling due mainly to the introduction of disposable nappies (➲ see Nappy rash, pp. 176–83). Its main causative factors are prolonged contact with faeces, urine, and chemical irritants, friction, excessive hydration, increased temperature, and infection, particularly candida.

Clinical appearance

Shiny, confluent erythema on the buttocks, perineum abdomen, and thighs (➲ see Figs. 13.1 and 13.2).

Differential diagnosis

- *Candidal nappy rash*—affects skin folds, bright red scaly patches with satellite lesions/pustules (➲ see Fig. 13.3).
- *Seborrhoeic dermatitis*—greasy yellowy well-demarcated patches typically found in the groin and intertriginous areas (➲ see Fig. 17.13).
- *Bullous impetigo*—large flaccid bullae with erosions (➲ see Fig. 13.8).
- *Psoriasis*—rare, sharply demarcated plaques (➲ see Fig.11.3).
- *Acrodermatitis enteropathica* (➲ see Zinc deficiency, pp. 179–82)—facial rash (Fig. 7.4). Consider in atypical or recalcitrant nappy rash (➲ see Fig. 13.4).
- *Langerhans cell histiocytosis* (➲ see Langerhans cell histiocytosis, pp. 182–3)—this rare neoplastic condition may present with intractable nappy rash.

Note: atopic dermatitis typically spares the nappy area.

Management

Reduce contact with urine and faeces, change nappy more frequently. Clean skin gently with water and apply barrier preparations. For resistant cases, a topical anticandidal drug combined with 1% hydrocortisone ointment can be applied. Avoid topical preparations containing antiseptics and other sensitizers such as talc.

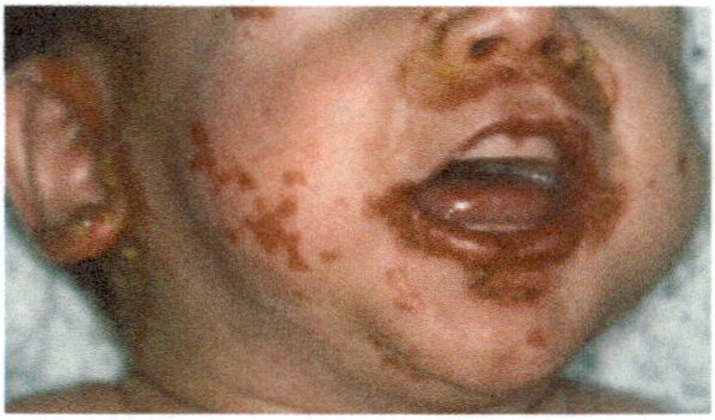

Fig. 7.4 Zinc deficiency in low birth weight newborn showing well-demarcated perioral and perinasal red/brown rash. A similar rash is seen on the buttocks (➲ see Fig. 13.4).

Reproduced courtesy of Dr Shevaun Mendelssohn.

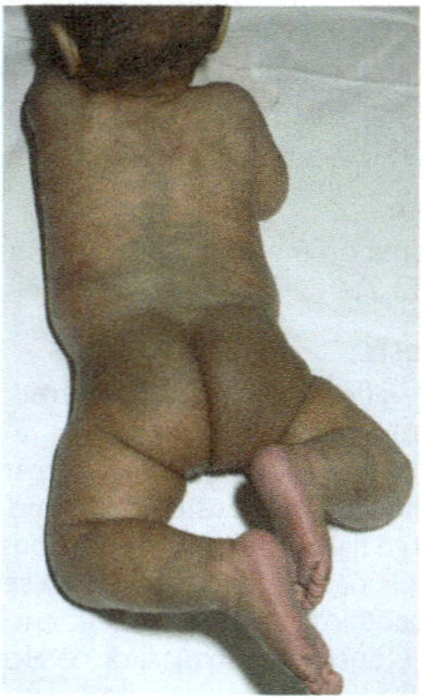

Fig. 7.5 Mongolian blue spot in typical site over back and buttocks.

Reproduced courtesy of Susan Lewis-Jones, Hon Consultant Dermatologist, Ninewells Hospital and Medical School, Dundee, UK

Neonatal erythroderma

If >90% of the body surface area is involved, this is potentially life-threatening with a high mortality rate. Always ask for an urgent **dermatological** opinion (see Erythroderma, faltering growth, and recurrent infection, p. 346).

Causes include:

- *Inflammatory*—atopic dermatitis, psoriasis, seborrhoeic dermatitis.
- *Infectious*—neonatal candidiasis, congenital syphilis. Staphylococcal scalded skin syndrome (Fig. 7.6) may be preceded by neonatal impetigo.
- *Inherited*—the ichthyoses, in particular congenital ichthyosiform erythroderma (see Fig. 27.4), lamellar ichthyosis (see Fig. 27.5), bullous ichthyosiform erythroderma (see Fig. 27.6), and Netherton syndrome (see Fig. 6.2 and Fig. 27.7).
- *Immunological*—any immunodeficiency syndrome, Omenn syndrome (see Table 6.2), and graft-versus-host disease (see Chapter 39).
- *Drug reaction*—very rare in neonates. Hypersensitivity to a drug can cause a wide spectrum of clinical features, including morbilliform rash, acute generalized pustular dermatosis (AGEP), drug rash with eosinophilia and systemic symptoms (DRESS), or Stevens–Johnson syndrome/toxic epidermal necrolysis (SJS/TEN; see Chapter 23). A detailed timeline of any new treatment prescribed to the mother in the last trimester of pregnancy and to the neonate in the first month of life should be established.

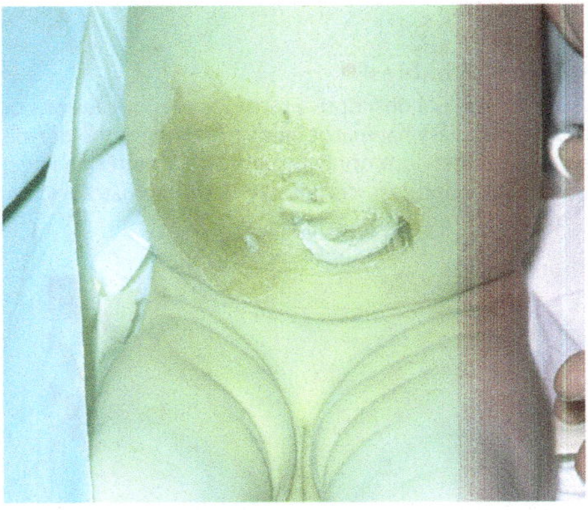

Fig. 7.6 Early staphylococcal scalded skin syndrome. Periumbilical raw area of impetigo with superficial peeling and extensive erythema spreading over trunk and proximal limbs.

Reproduced courtesy of Susan Lewis-Jones, Hon Consultant Dermatologist, Ninewells Hospital and Medical School, Dundee, UK

Management

- Control temperature.
- Monitor fluid input/output.
- Monitor electrolytes.
- Nutritional supplementation.
- Emollients.
- Screen for sepsis.

Collodion baby

Collodion babies are encased in thickened, shiny, variably erythematous skin that resembles cellophane. It is usually shed within 2–3 weeks but most cases have an underlying genetic ichthyosis (➲ see Fig. 27.8, and Collodion baby, p. 413). Seek a dermatological opinion.

Congenital infection

Usually presents in the neonatal period and many have associated characteristic skin rashes, including blueberry muffin baby (Box 7.3). Prognosis is usually worse if infection occurs in first trimester:

- Herpes simplex.
- *Cytomegalovirus (CMV)*.
- Rubella.
- Syphilis.
- Varicella.
- *Candida*.

Blueberry muffin babies

Blueberry muffin baby is a descriptive term for purpuric lesions occurring as a result of extramedullary haematopoiesis occurring in the dermis (Fig. 7.7). The clinical lesions most commonly result from intrauterine infections, such as rubella and CMV, and less commonly with haematological malignancy (Box 7.3).

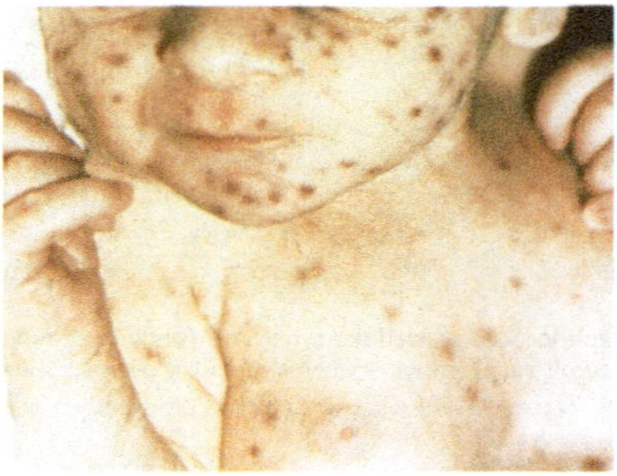

Fig. 7.7 Blueberry muffin lesions in a child with leukaemia.

Reproduced courtesy of Cameron Kennedy, Consultant Dermatologist, Departments of Dermatology, Bristol Royal Infirmary, and Paediatric Dermatology, Bristol Royal Hospital for Children, Bristol, UK

Box 7.3 Blueberry muffin lesions are seen in:
- CMV infections.
- Syphilis.
- Congenital toxoplasmosis.
- HIV.
- Rubella.
- Malignancies such as leukaemia.

Herpes simplex

This has a high morbidity including death. May show localized or disseminated vesicles, erosions, or even deep atrophic ulcers.

Cytomegalovirus (CMV)

Presents with systemic upset, jaundice, hepatosplenomegaly, microcephaly, and intrauterine growth retardation. Skin lesions consist of petechiae, purpura, and vesicles.

Rubella

Twenty to fifty per cent (20–50%) have skin rashes, usually blueberry muffin (Fig. 7.7). Later changes include cutis marmorata (➲ see Chapter 31, Fig. 31.8, and Causes of purple patches other than purpura, p. 474) and hyperpigmentation. Associated abnormalities include cataracts, deafness, growth retardation, and microcephaly.

Syphilis

Often born without symptoms but manifests within first 2 months, although snuffles and perioral rhagades are seen. Findings include maculopapular, vesiculobullous (only seen in early syphilis before aged 2y), and papulosquamous lesions. Generalized desquamation may occur. Look for hepatosplenomegaly and lymphadenopathy.

Varicella-zoster virus (VZV)

Follows intrauterine (IU) chicken pox from maternal infection:
- In early IU first and second trimester, congenital varicella syndrome occurs. There may be cutaneous loss, CNS, ocular, GIT, and skeletal defects. The skin shows varying degrees of cropped or widespread vesicles that can follow a zoster-like distribution and lead to deep scarring.
- In late IU (5–2 days prior to delivery) neonatal varicella occurs. It lacks the congenital defects but a widespread vesicopustular rash can occur.

Treatment: with VZV immune globulin and intensive care unit (ICU) care, which has reduced mortality risk to around 7%.

Candida

Congenital candidiasis may present with oral lesions, erythema, and pustules, particularly in the skin creases, palms, and soles. Usually acquired by maternal transmission during birth. Rarely may become systemic—preterm, low birth weight, or immunosuppressed babies are at particular risk.

Treatment: depends on disease extent. Prompt treatment with parenteral anticandidal agents (usually amphotericin B) is vital for systemic forms.

Tumours in the newborn

(➲ See Fibromatoses, p. 450.)

Errors during fetal embryogenesis can result in several developmental anomalies that are first recognized in the newborn. They include various tumours including:

- ***Preauricular cysts***—abnormality of first branchial cleft, more common in girls, and may be associated with hearing loss. May also have clefting.
- ***Accessory tragus***—may be multiple and can be associated with other branchial arch defects such as Goldenhar syndrome.
- ***Wattles***—branchial arch remnants, sometimes containing cartilage. Usually found on the anterior neck and not to be confused with a skin tag (Fig. 7.8).
- ***Dermoid cysts***—soft small tumours of 1–4cm diameter found on the forehead and anywhere on the face or scalp. They are not usually detected until childhood. Although small and superficial they can extend intracranially, therefore CT/MRI should be performed prior to excision (➲ see Fig. 28.1).
- ***Thyroglossal cysts***—small 1–3cm, soft, midline neck tumours. They are a common developmental abnormality of the anterior neck.
- ***Aplasia cutis congenita***—these present as a focal absence of skin on the scalp with an absence of hair growth typically along the midline (➲ see Fig. 14.6).
- Vascular lesions (➲ see Chapter 8).

Malignant tumours: These are very rare but include melanoma, various cutaneous sarcomas, and systemic malignancies such as leukaemia cutis or secondary deposits (➲ see Fig. 28.7). **If in doubt, refer to a dermatologist for a skin biopsy** (➲ see Malignant skin tumours, p. 435).

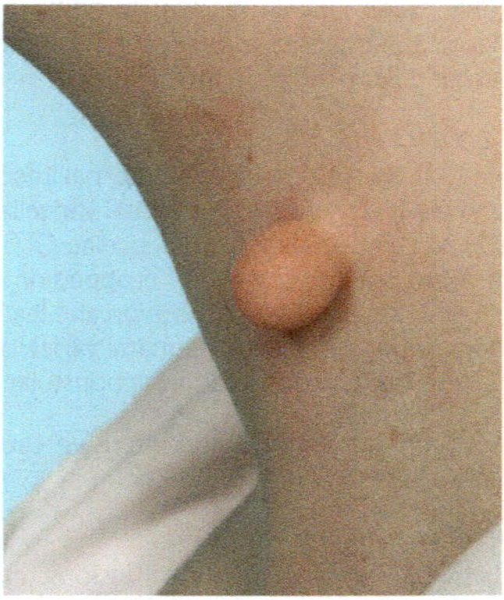

Fig. 7.8 Wattle on neck—branchial arch remnant.

Reproduced courtesy of NHS Tayside Clinical Photography, Dundee, UK

Vascular birthmarks

Introduction

Vascular birthmarks are common. Most are small and harmless and require no additional investigations or treatment. It is important to be aware of the minority which are associated with severe disfigurement, compression of vital organs, functional disability, associated structural abnormalities, or visceral involvement. Improvement in the classification of these lesions, combined with a multidisciplinary approach has revolutionized management. Advances in our understanding of the genetic basis of vasculogenesis is leading to improved therapies, the ultimate goal is to prevent life-threatening complications, improve quality of life, and to minimize disfigurement.

Classification

Correct diagnosis is important due to differences in morbidity, treatment, and prognosis. The 2018 International Society for the Study of Vascular Anomalies (ISSVA) classification divides vascular birthmarks into two main groups; lesions with a proliferative component ('vascular tumours') and those that are relatively static ('vascular malformations'). See Fig. 8.1.

Vascular tumours

Characterized by endothelial hyperplasia.

Vascular malformations

Are caused by faults in construction of vascular pathways during embryogenesis. They are congenital structural lesions composed of anomalous dilated vessels with abnormal walls lined by normal endothelium without hyperplasia. They occur in 0.3–0.5% of the population with an equal sex distribution. Although present at birth, they may not become clinically apparent until much later. Untreated, they persist throughout life and grow proportionately to the patient. Trauma, infection, hormonal changes, puberty, intervention, and thrombosis may cause rapid enlargement. These are divided into four groups:

- *Simple malformations* which involve only one type of vessel (i.e. capillaries, lymphatics, or veins) with the exception of arteriovenous malformations which include capillaries, arteries, and veins.
- *Combined* (defined as two or more vascular malformations found in one lesion).
- *Malformations associated with other anomalies*.
- *Malformations of major named vessels*.

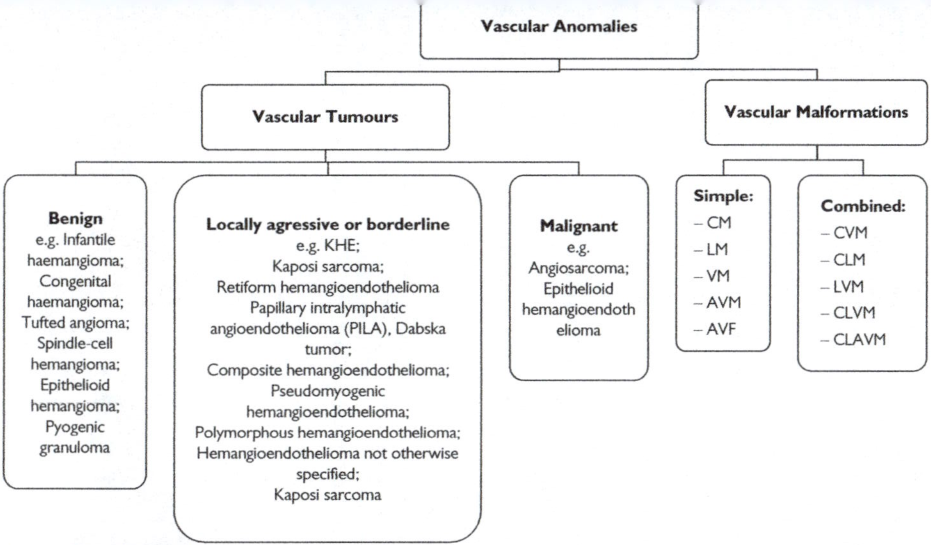

Fig. 8.1 Classification of vascular anomalies.

Key: C = capillary; A = artery; V = venous; M = malformation; F = fistula; KHE = kaposiform haemangioendothelioma

Adapted with permission from ISSVA Classification of Vascular Anomalies © 2018 International Society for the Study of Vascular Anomalies Available at https://www.issva.org/UserFiles/file/Classifications-2014-Final.pdf

Vascular tumours

Infantile haemangiomas (IH)

IH are the most common tumour of infancy affecting 4–10% of infants. They are characterized by a benign proliferation of endothelial cells. While the exact pathogenesis of IH is unknown local tissue hypoxia is thought to play a pivotal role. Most are sporadic, however up to 1/3 of patients report a family history of IH suggesting genetic factors may also contribute to their development. They are more common in Caucasian, female (4:1), low birth weight and preterm babies, with increased maternal age, multi-gestation pregnancies, and pregnancies complicated by pre-eclampsia, placental abnormalities, gestational diabetes, and maternal hypertension.

Classification of infantile haemangiomas

Based on location:
- Superficial (bright red) 50–60%. Old terminology—strawberry capillary haemangiomas (Fig. 8.2).
- Deep (blue or skin coloured) 10%. Old terminology—cavernous haemangiomas (Fig. 8.3).
- Combined 25–30% (Fig. 8.4).

Based on morphology, extent, and distribution:
- Focal (the majority).
- Multifocal.
- Segmental (increased risk of complications and other vascular and non-vascular anomalies) (Fig. 8.5).
- Indeterminate.

Clinical features

Most appear postnatally usually before 4 weeks of age. Subtle precursor lesions are present at birth in up to half of cases (i.e. a hypopigmented or pale red macule or patch +/– telangiectasia; Fig. 8.6). Around 80% are solitary; 60% occur on the head and neck; 25% on trunk; and 15% on the

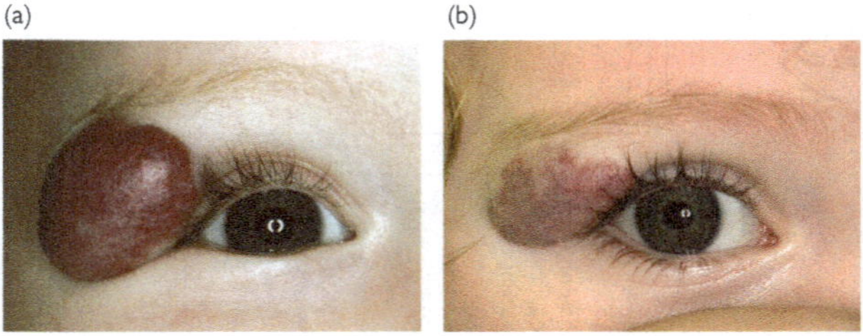

Fig. 8.2 (a) Periocular haemangioma. Bright red colour indicates proliferative phase. Ophthalmic review showed no visual axis obstruction. (b) Much reduced after 3 months on propranolol.

Reproduced courtesy of Rosemarie Watson, Consultant Paediatric Dermatologist, Department of Dermatology, Our Lady's Children's Hospital Crumlin, Dublin, Ireland

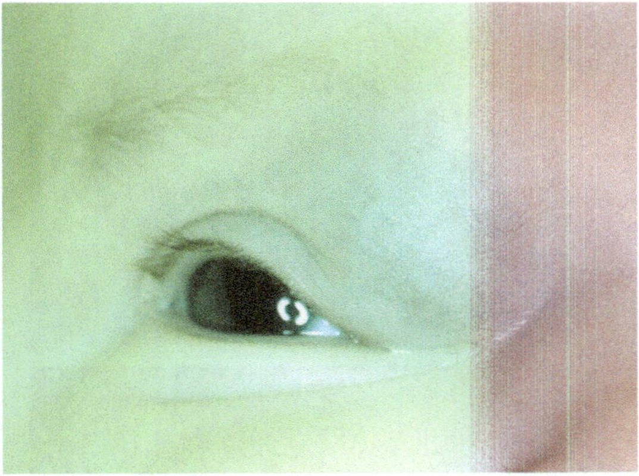

Fig. 8.3 Deep haemangioma indicated by blue colouration. Risk of astigmatism due to compression of the globe. Ophthalmological follow-up, imaging to assess extent of lesion and close monitoring required.

Reproduced courtesy of Rosemarie Watson, Consultant Paediatric Dermatologist, Department of Dermatology, Our Lady's Children's Hospital Crumlin, Dublin, Ireland

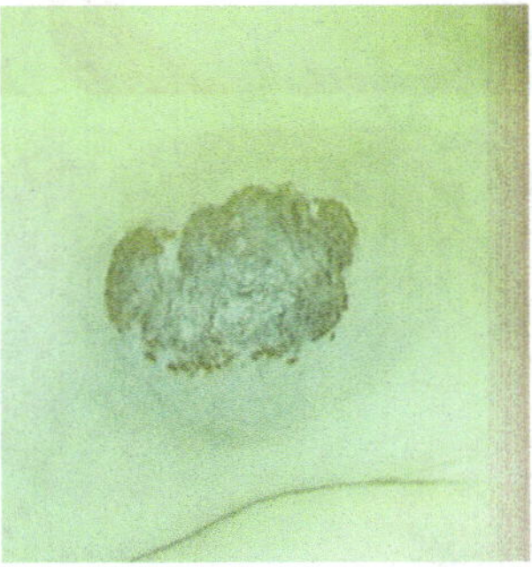

Fig. 8.4 Combined superficial (red) and deep (blue) haemangioma on chest, non-critical location, however consider treatment as can interfere with breast bud development.

Reproduced courtesy of Rosemarie Watson, Consultant Paediatric Dermatologist, Department of Dermatology, Our Lady's Children's Hospital Crumlin, Dublin, Ireland

extremities. They are non-blanching and firm to rubbery on palpation. There are three phases in the natural history:

- ***Proliferative phase***: initial growth phase lasting 3–9 months. Most rapid growth occurs between 5.5 and 7.5 weeks of age, suggesting the optimal timing for referral for IH that may require systemic treatment is ~4 weeks of age.

(a) (b) (c)

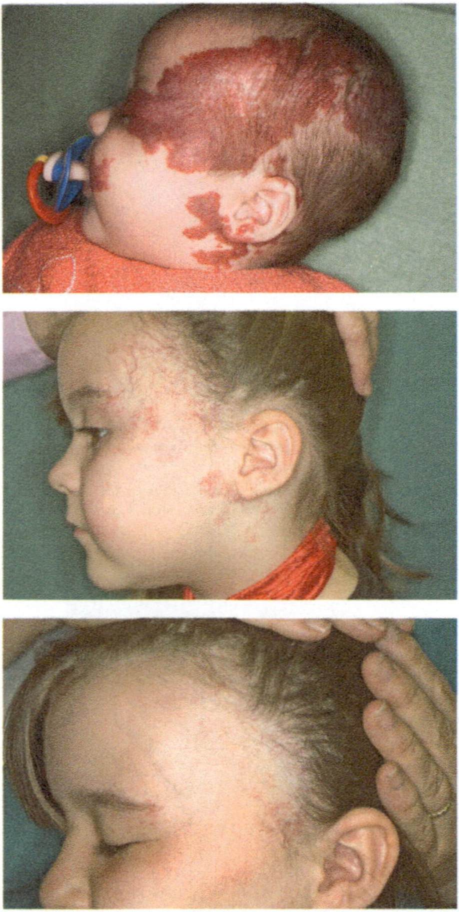

Fig. 8.5 Segmental haemangioma; negative screening for PHACES. (a) Proliferative phase; (b) persistent telangiectasias age 6; (c) cosmetic result post-laser treatment, few residual telangiectasias.

Reproduced courtesy of Rosemarie Watson, Consultant Paediatric Dermatologist, Department of Dermatology, Our Lady's Children's Hospital Crumlin, Dublin, Ireland

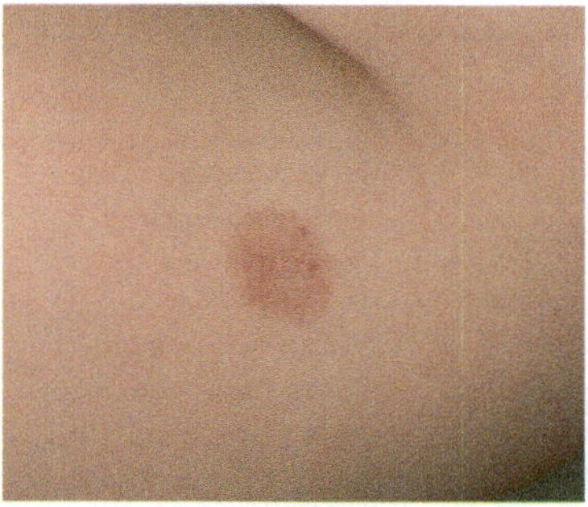

Fig. 8.6 Precursor lesion: superficial haemangioma. Pale red telangiectatic patch on left upper thigh present at birth.

Reproduced courtesy of Rosemarie Watson, Consultant Paediatric Dermatologist, Department of Dermatology, Our Lady's Children's Hospital Crumlin, Dublin, Ireland

- *Stabilization phase*: 80% IH have reached their maximum growth by 5 months; (a small proportion have a prolonged growth phase that may last 1–2y).
- *Involution phase*: slow. Most have completed involution by 4y. A central grey/white colour may herald this phase. Around 30% leave entirely normal skin after involution. Residual telangiectasia, atrophy, and dermal scarring can occur especially if there has been ulceration or if the superficial component had a steep or abrupt border. Large lesions may leave redundant lax skin and those affecting the lip, nasal tip, eyelid, or ear often have fibro-fatty thickening which may require surgical correction.

Diagnosis

Based on clinical examination. Imaging (ultrasonography/MRI) is rarely indicated unless there is diagnostic uncertainty, to determine the extent and relationship to adjacent structures (e.g. periorbital extension), or to rule out associated structural abnormalities or visceral involvement. Suspect visceral involvement in patients with multifocal lesions (>5) or if there is jaundice, stridor, dyspnoea, or bloody stools. Biopsy if suspicious of malignancy (e.g. sarcoma). Haemangiomas stain positive with GLUT-1.

Complications

- See Table 8.1.

Ulceration occurs in 15%; usually during the proliferative phase and results in scarring. Heralded by early grey-white discolouration. Further complicated by infection, bleeding, and pain (Fig. 8.7).

Risk factors for ulceration: large, segmental, and mixed subtypes. Lesions on flexures, lower lip, or anogenital area. Prematurity, low birth weight, and female infants.

Other complications: compression of underlying structures/vital organs, functional abnormality, associated structural abnormalities or visceral lesions, high-output cardiac failure (rare), disfigurement.

Table 8.1 Haemangiomas: when to worry

Location	Association
Periocular (Figs. 8.2 and 8.3)	Ocular abnormalities (amblyopia, astigmatism, ptosis, proptosis, strabismus)
Beard (Fig. 8.8)	Airway haemangioma
Lip/mucosal Philtrum (blocking nares)	Feeding difficulties Breathing difficulties
Multiple >/= 5 (Fig. 8.7)	Visceral haemangiomas
Very large haemangiomas	Cardiac failure, coagulopathy
Segmental cervicofacial haemangiomas (Fig. 8.8)	PHACES syndrome
Lumbosacral, perineal, and segmental leg	LUMBAR syndrome * PELVIS syndrome ** SACRAL syndrome ***
Parotid	Conductive hearing loss
Hepatic	Hypothyroidism
Hands or feet	Functional impairment

* LUMBAR: Lower body haemangioma and other cutaneous defects, Urogenital anomalies, ulceration, Myelopathy, Bony deformities, Anorectal malformations, arterial anomalies, Renal anomalies.

** PELVIS: Perineal haemangioma, External genital malformations, Lipomyelomeningocele, Vesicorenal abnormalities, Imperforate anus, Skin tag.

*** SACRAL: Spinal dysraphism, Anogenital, Cutaneous Renal, and urologic anomalies, associated with an Angioma of Lumbosacral localization.

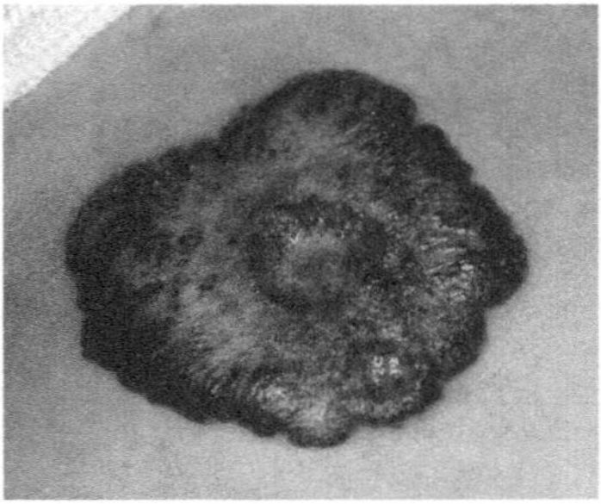

Fig. 8.7 Large proliferating haemangioma on the back with central ulceration. Grey surface colour may indicate impending further extension of ulceration.

Reproduced courtesy of Rosemarie Watson, Consultant Paediatric Dermatologist, Department of Dermatology, Our Lady's Children's Hospital Crumlin, Dublin, Ireland

PHACE(S) syndrome

Posterior Fossa defects, Haemangioma (segmental, cervicofacial), Arterial anomalies, Cardiac anomalies, and coarctation of the aorta, Eye abnormalities (e.g. microphthalmia), Sternal clefting, or supraumbilical median raphe (Figs. 8.8, 8.9). Investigations: segmental facial IH with echocardiogram, MRI and MR angiogram of head and neck, and ophthalmology assessment*.

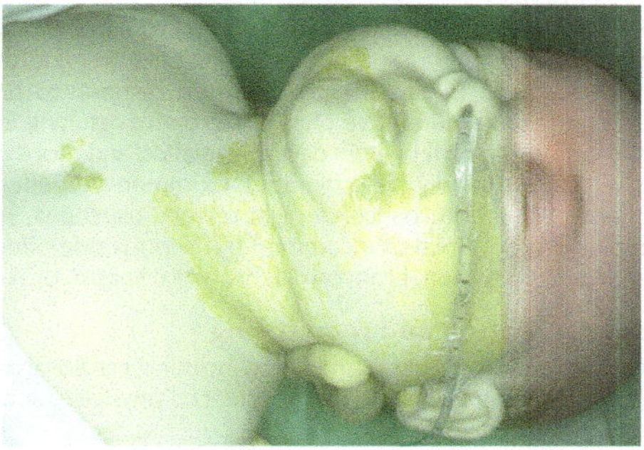

Fig. 8.8 Beard haemangioma with subglottic and sternal clefting (PHACES syndrome).

Reproduced courtesy of Rosemarie Watson, Consultant Paediatric Dermatologist, Department of Dermatology, Our Lady's Children's Hospital Crumlin, Dublin, Ireland

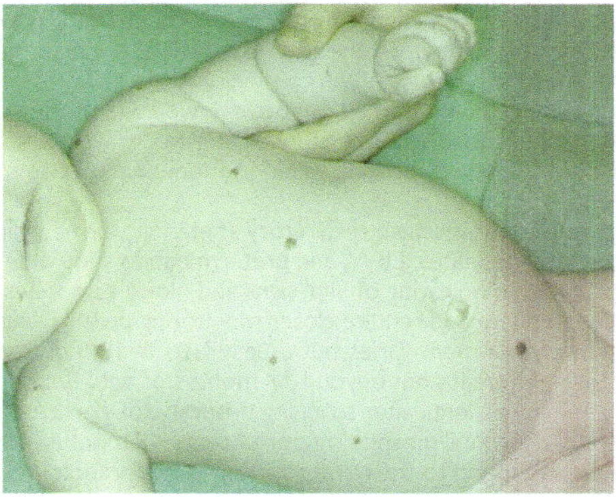

Fig. 8.9 Diffuse haemangiomatosis. More than five lesions warrants investigation for haemangiomas involving internal organs.

Reproduced courtesy of Rosemarie Watson, Consultant Paediatric Dermatologist, Department of Dermatology, Our Lady's Children's Hospital Crumlin, Dublin, Ireland

*Most children affected have only 1–2 extracutaneous manifestations.

Treatment of haemangiomas

The vast majority of IH are of little clinical significance and parents should be reassured regarding the natural benign course. However, approximately 15% result in complications such as disfigurement or visual field/airway obstruction and require therapeutic intervention.

First-line treatment

Oral β-blockers have revolutionized the treatment of IH. The non-selective β-adrenergic receptor blocking agent propranolol is first-line therapy for IH requiring treatment. Most patients (98%) will respond to propranolol when given during the proliferative phase of growth, resulting in softening and reduced colour of the IH within days of initiation and more rapid involution (Fig. 8.11). It is usually well-tolerated. Common side effects include cold peripheries, sleep disturbance, or night terrors, diarrhoea, vomiting or constipation, and bronchiolitis. Uncommon but serious side effects include hypoglycaemia, hypotension, bradycardia, bronchial spasm, or A-V block.

Propranolol initiation and monitoring

1. Comprehensive history and examination including cardiovascular and respiratory examination by an experienced physician, abdominal examination for hepatomegaly.
2. Rule out any contraindications to propranolol†.
3. Routine pretreatment electrocardiogram (ECG)/echocardiogram is not necessary unless there are specific clinical indications.
4. Recommended starting dose is 1mg/kg/day in divided doses, increase to 2–3mg/kg/day after 24h**.
5. Parents should be advised on strategies to avoid hypoglycaemia by scheduled feedings and administration of the medication, as well as withholding treatment when the baby is unwell or during periods of prolonged fasting.
6. Patients with uncomplicated IH can be reviewed 2–3 months after starting to adjust dose according to weight gain.
7. Clinical photography is recommended to monitor response to treatment.
8. Patients with cardiovascular, respiratory, metabolic, or neurological comorbidities, neonates, LBW, and preterm babies should be admitted for appropriate monitoring of vital signs and blood sugar levels during the initiation phase and require closer monitoring during treatment.

The duration of treatment varies but usually lasts 6–12 months. Most patients do not need treatment beyond 17 months of age. Rebound growth occurs in ~14% of patients after stopping propranolol, particularly in those with a deep or segmental morphology, or patients <9 months of age. These patients usually respond to the reintroduction of propranolol.

†**Absolute contraindications:** Hypoglycaemic episodes, second or third degree heart-block, hypersensitivity to propranolol. **Relative contraindications:** Frequent wheeze, heart rate/blood pressure outside normal range (treat in conjunction with paediatrician), severe coarctation of the aorta.

** Dose and monitoring are modified in PHACES.

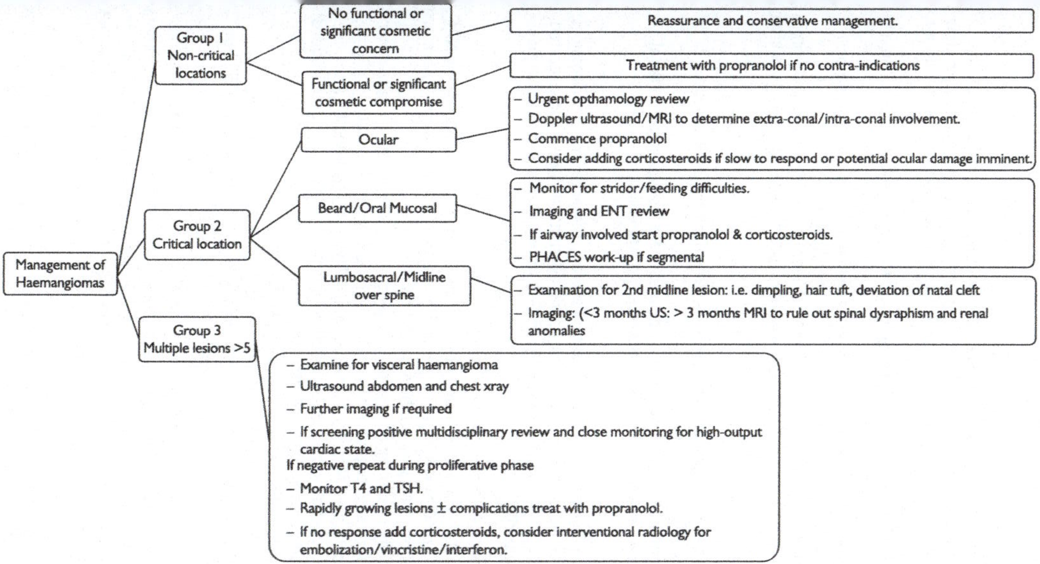

Fig. 8.10 Management of haemangiomas.

Reproduced courtesy of Rosemarie Watson, Consultant Paediatric Dermatologist, Department of Dermatology, Our Lady's Children's Hospital Crumlin, Dublin, Ireland

Other treatment modalities

- *Systemic corticosteroids*
  - See Fig. 8.10.
  - Administered during proliferative phase.
  - 2–3mg/kg/day for 4–6 weeks, until proliferative phase complete.
  - Used alone, one-third experience shrinkage and one-third stabilization.
  - Can be used in combination with propranolol when a rapid response is essential.
- ***Topical β-blockers***: off-label timolol maleate 0.5% gel BD/TDS for small (<5mm) superficial lesions.
- ***Superpotent topical steroids/intralesional steroids*** can be used alone or in combination with topical timolol for small lesions.
- ***Pulsed dye laser*** has been used to treat small or ulcerated haemangiomas but is used more frequently to treat residual redness/telangiectasia after involution is complete.

Surgery

- Reduced need for surgery since widespread use of β-blockers but occasionally still required.
- Indications include pedunculated or persistent lesions, selected facial lesions, unsightly scarring, or thickening postinvolution.

Other

- Arterial embolization, compression therapy for large limb IH. Dressings, topical antibiotics, barrier creams, and adequate analgesia for ulcerated lesions. Ophthalmology/ENT/plastic surgery, psychological input may be required.

Congenital haemangiomas

Rare GLUT-1 negative haemangiomas due to somatic mutations in *GNAQ*, *GNA11*, or GNA14. Lesions present and fully formed at birth. There are three subtypes based on their natural history:

1. Rapidly involuting congenital haemangioma (RICH): rapid improvement in first few months of life (usually regress fully by 14 months as compared to several years for IH). May be surrounded by a characteristic rim of pallor. Ulceration common. Serious complications include potential life-threatening bleeding from ulcerated RICH, coagulopathy, high-output heart failure (Fig. 8.12).
2. Non-involuting congenital haemangioma (NICH): no involution at 1y.
3. Partially involuting congenital haemangioma: presents like a RICH but fails to completely involute and persists as a NICH-like lesion.

Other tumours and swellings mimicking haemangiomas

These can include pyogenic granuloma, kaposiform haemangioendothelioma (KHE), tufted angioma (TA) (Fig. 8.13‡), haemangiopericytoma, fibrosarcoma, rhabdomyosarcoma, nasal gliomas, encephalocoele, glomuvenous tumours (➲ see also Chapter 28).

‡Kasabach–Merritt phenomenon is a life-threatening coagulopathy associated with KHE and TA characterized by profound thrombocytopaenia due to platelet trapping within the tumour and consumption of blood coagulation factors. These tumours require treatment with antiplatelet agents, vincristine, or sirolimus with a good response in majority. Small lesions may be amenable to excision.

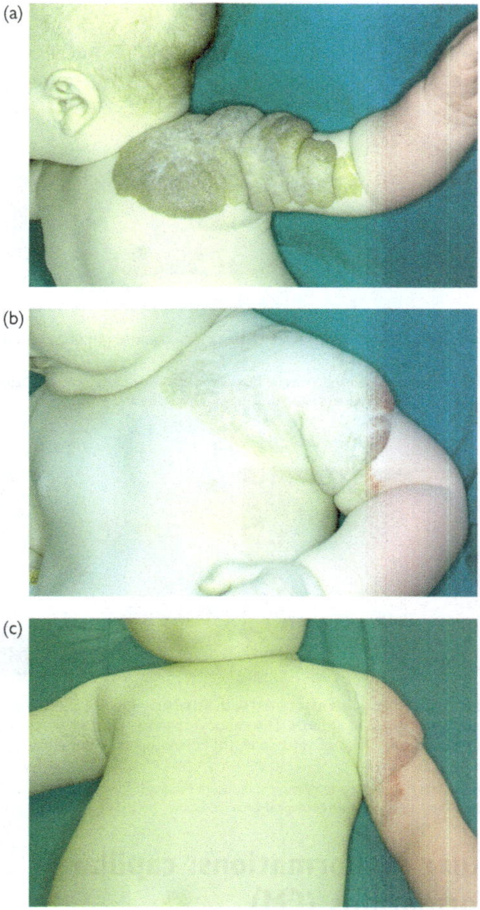

Fig. 8.11 (a) Large bulky haemangioma at risk of ulceration in the creases at age 2 months. (b) Significant resolution after 4 months on propranolol (c) Dramatic resolution 6.5 months on propranolol.

Reproduced courtesy of Rosemarie Watson, Consultant Paediatric Dermatologist, Department of Dermatology, Our Lady's Children's Hospital Crumlin, Dublin, Ireland

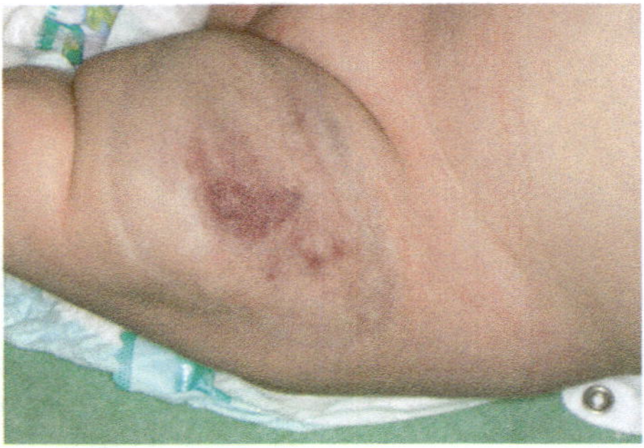

Fig. 8.12 Rapidly involuting congenital haemangioma; note rim of pallor surrounding lesion.

Reproduced courtesy of Rosemarie Watson, Consultant Paediatric Dermatologist, Department of Dermatology, Our Lady's Children's Hospital Crumlin, Dublin, Ireland

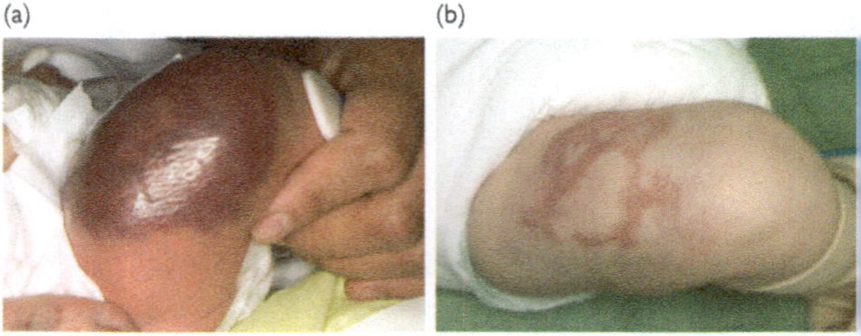

Fig. 8.13 (a) Tufted angioma associated with Kasabach–Merritt phenomenon. Born at 31 weeks, lesion present at birth. Thrombocytopaenia. Treated with compression, prednisolone, and five cycles of vincristine. (b) Follow-up at 1y demonstrating resolution with atrophy.

Reproduced courtesy of Rosemarie Watson, Consultant Paediatric Dermatologist, Department of Dermatology, Our Lady's Children's Hospital Crumlin, Dublin, Ireland

Vascular malformations: capillary malformations (CM)

Salmon patch

- See Fig. 8.14.
- Very common, present in ~80% of infants.
- Synonyms: stork bite, angel's kiss, naevus simplex.
- Faint pink patches on nape of neck, eyelids, glabella, blanching on pressure—more obvious during crying or febrile illness.
- Minor dermal capillary ectasias that tend to fade after 1–3y (nape of neck more persistent).

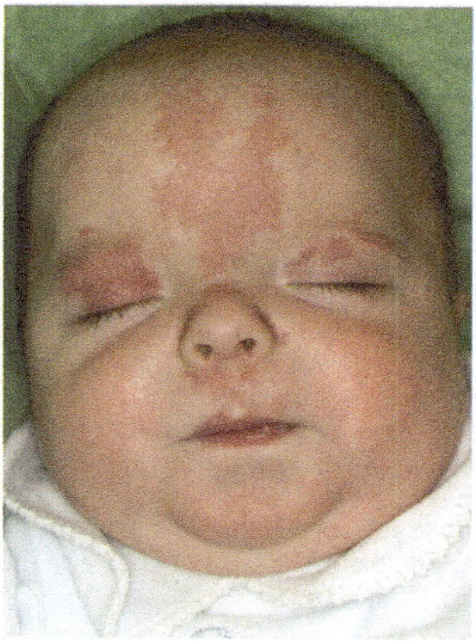

Fig. 8.14 Salmon patch, pink ill-defined patches crossing the midline. Persistent mid-facial lesions may be associated with macrocephaly.

Reproduced courtesy of Rosemarie Watson, Consultant Paediatric Dermatologist, Department of Dermatology, Our Lady's Children's Hospital Crumlin, Dublin, Ireland

Port-wine stain (PWS)

Usually sporadic, slow-flow permanent CM due to somatic GNAQ mutation. One in 300 newborns. Equal sex incidence. Characterized by groups of ectatic malformed tortuous dilated vessels in the upper dermis. May be associated with other VAs, structural anomalies, or syndromes.

Clinical features

- See Fig. 8.15.
- Usually noted at birth as a pink to red well-defined macular area.
- Facial PWSs may darken and thicken with time with or without blebs, hyperkeratotic areas, or soft tissue overgrowth.
- Often located on the face, sharp midline cut-off, often segmental.
- Clinical diagnosis.

Note: early facial haemangiomas may mimic a PWS in neonates.

Treatment

- Pulsed dye laser is the gold standard—coagulation of vessels.
  - Multiple treatments (6–12 average) required and may recur after treatment.
  - 80% achieve a 50% lightening; 10% achieve 90% clearing; 20–30% fail to lighten.
  - Best response is seen in smaller facial lesions (<20% facial surface area) and those in the V1 dermatome. Children respond better than adults.
  - Least responsive are crown of cheek and distal extremities.
- Cosmetic camouflage.

Syndromes associated with capillary malformations

Sturge–Weber syndrome (SWS)

- Sporadic congenital neurocutaneous disorder characterized by a triad of features:
  - Facial PWS
  - Ipsilateral leptomeningeal/brain vascular malformation
  - Ipsilateral ocular abnormalities
- Due to somatic activating mutation in GNAQ.
- Occurs in 1 in 20,000 to 50,000 births; equal sex distribution.
- Strongest predictor of SWS is distribution of PWS based on vascular embryological development of the face and not the distribution of the trigeminal nerve as previously thought.
- Children with PWS on upper face (any part of forehead) have up to 16% risk of developing SWS. Risk is increased if large areas, middle, or both sides of the face are involved.
- The commonest extracutaneous manifestations are seizures by age 2y (>70%), intellectual impairment (50%), hemiplegia (30%), and ipsilateral glaucoma (15–25%).

Screening for SWS:

- Ophthalmology assessment.
- Role for routine imaging controversial as age at which MRI can reliably exclude SWS unknown.
- If PWS extensive/high-risk (hemi-facial/bilateral), consider early neurology referral and MRI with gadolinium.
- Parents should receive education regarding neurological red flags, seizure symptoms, and early seizure management. Early diagnosis is important as prophylactic aspirin may reduce number of seizures and stroke-like episodes.

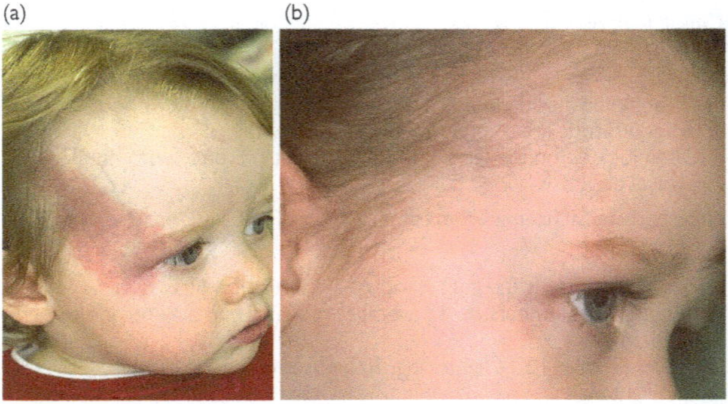

Fig. 8.15 (a) Port-wine stain forehead. No other features to suggest Sturge–Weber syndrome but requires long-term ophthalmology follow-up because of glaucoma risk with eyelid involvement (b) Excellent clearing after three pulsed dye laser treatments.

Reproduced courtesy of Rosemarie Watson, Consultant Paediatric Dermatologist, Department of Dermatology, Our Lady's Children's Hospital Crumlin, Dublin, Ireland

Fig. 8.16 Small capillary malformation with subtle rim of pallor on cheek. *RASA1* positive. Brother and father have multiple similar lesions. No internal abnormalities or history of stroke in this family. Lifelong monitoring required because of significant risk internal arteriovenous malformations.

Reproduced courtesy of Rosemarie Watson, Consultant Paediatric Dermatologist, Department of Dermatology, Our Lady's Children's Hospital Crumlin, Dublin, Ireland

Capillary malformation—arteriovenous malformation (CM-AVM) syndrome

- Multiple atypical pale pink, red, or brown CM with surrounding white halo develop in childhood and increase in number over time (Fig. 8.16).
- Autosomal dominant inheritance, mutations in *RASA1* and *EPHB4* identified in familial and sporadic cases.
- Associated limb > brain/spine > head and neck fast-flow AVMs in 30% patients.

Other syndromes associated with CM

Several complex combined syndromes are described. Many are associated with tissue overgrowth resulting in disability and deformity. These include: Klippel–Trenaunay syndrome (KTS), Parkes–Weber syndrome, Cobb syndrome, Proteus syndrome, CLOVES syndrome, Beckwith–Wiedemann syndrome, Von Hippel–Lindau syndrome, and phakomatosis pigmentovascularis.

Vascular malformations: venous malformations (VM)

VMs are slow-flow vascular malformations composed of ectatic venous channels within the dermis. Usually sporadic and solitary. Common, accounting for 2/3 of all congenital vascular malformations (1 in 5000). They may affect skin, mucous membranes, vessels, bone, joints, and viscera. Associated with somatic activating mutations in *PIK3CA* and *TEK* genes.

Clinical features

- Blue or purple, soft spongy, easily compressible swelling (Fig. 8.17). A hyperkeratotic verrucous variant is also described.
- Swells with exertion, in dependant positions or with venous pressure alteration (e.g. Valsalva manoeuvre).
- Though present at birth, may not become clinically apparent until much later. Puberty is often a time of expansion.
- Hard nodules—phleboliths (hard due to calcification) are diagnostic when present.
- Differential diagnosis includes deep haemangioma, lymphatic malformation, glomuvenous malformation§.
- Head and neck lesions often more extensive than initially thought.

Investigations: MRI may be used to measure the extent and depth.

Complications:

- Pain, phleboliths, thrombophlebitis, hyperhidrosis over lesions, disfigurement, compression of vital organs, haemarthrosis, limb girth/length discrepancy, skeletal distortion, localized intravascular coagulation.

Treatment:

- Multidisciplinary approach.
- Pain management important: non-steroidal anti-inflammatory drugs (NSAIDs), paracetamol, aspirin/anticoagulation, address neuropathic pain.
- Compression.
- Sclerotherapy can relieve symptoms and reduce lesion size.
- Nd:YAG laser, surgical excision, or a combination.
- Low molecular weight heparin if fibrinogen low/recurrent thrombosis.
- Possible role for treatment with inhibitors of the mTOR or AKT pathway (e.g. sirolimus) but further studies needed.

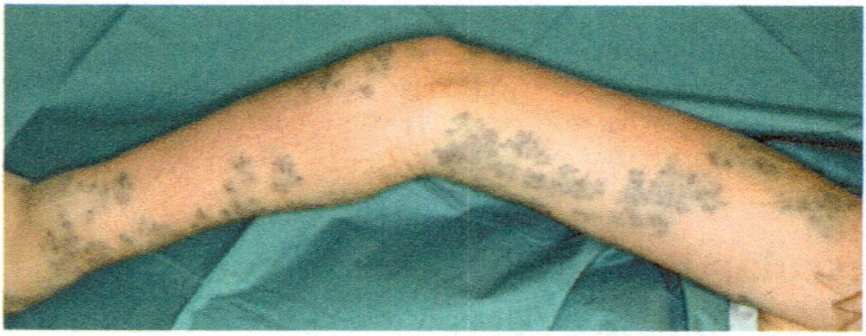

Fig. 8.17 Venous malformation. Blue spongy compressible swellings. Phleboliths palpable. Compression therapy helped discomfort.

Reproduced courtesy of Rosemarie Watson, Consultant Paediatric Dermatologist, Department of Dermatology, Our Lady's Children's Hospital Crumlin, Dublin, Ireland

§ Glomuvenous malformations present as distinctive blue-purple painful papules and nodules with a 'pebbly' surface (Fig. 8.18). They are firm and less compressible than typical VMs. Associated with glomulin gene mutation.

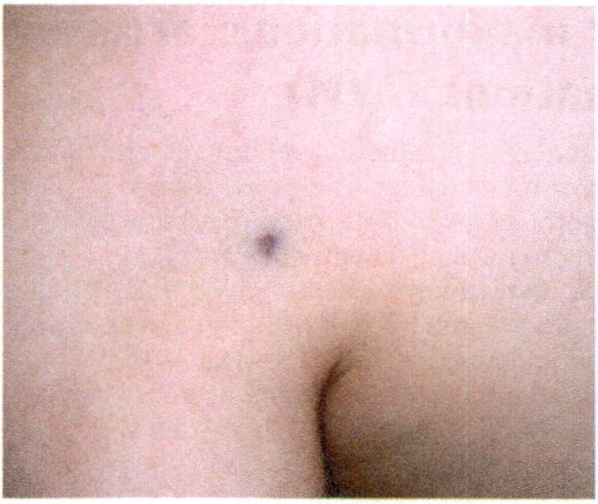

Fig. 8.18 Glomuvenous malformation may be difficult to differentiate from blue rubber bleb naevus syndrome. Family history can be positive in either. Histology will distinguish the two.

Reproduced courtesy of Rosemarie Watson, Consultant Paediatric Dermatologist, Department of Dermatology, Our Lady's Children's Hospital Crumlin, Dublin, Ireland

Associated syndromes

Blue rubber bleb naevus syndrome (Bean syndrome)

- Sporadic condition due to somatic mutation in receptor tyrosine kinase (*TEK/TIE2*) gene, with numerous mucocutaneous and gastrointestinal VM.
- Multiple dome-shaped dark blue, compressible papules and nodules, generally asymptomatic but may be tender and often recur after excision.
- *Differential*—multiple glomus tumours, diffuse neonatal haemangiomatosis, Anderson–Fabry disease.
- *Associations*—intestine is most common internal organ involved, resulting in abdominal pain and bleeding. Check for anaemia and coagulopathy. Other viscera frequently involved.
- Some promising reports of response to treatment with sirolimus.

Maffucci syndrome

- Spindle cell haemangioendotheliomas that mimic VMs especially on hands and feet.
- Phalangeal and long-bone enchondromas, fractures.
- Transformation to chondrosarcoma (15–20%).

Servelle-Martorell syndrome

- Rare, limb VM associated with limb hypoplasia.

Fibro-adipose vascular anomaly (FAVA)

- Recently described solid intramuscular and extrafascial fibrofatty and slow-flow venous vascular malformation.
- May present with pain and contracture of limb (usually lower limb).

Vascular malformations: arteriovenous malformations (AVM)

- Structurally abnormal arterial and venous vessels connected directly to one another without an intervening capillary bed.
- Permits dangerous flow of high-pressure arterial blood into thin-walled vessels which can result in bleeds/stroke.
- Most sporadic; familial form associated with *RASA1* mutations.
- Somatic mutations in the RAS—MAPK signalling pathway recently implicated in the development of sporadic AVMs.
- Disease associations include hereditary haemorrhagic telangiectasia and syndromes with *PTEN* mutations (i.e. Cowden's).

Clinical features

- See Fig. 8.19.
- Fifty per cent (50%) clinically apparent at birth.
- Most common locations include intracranial, head and neck (70%), cheeks, and ears.

Schobinger staging system

- Stage I (quiescent): asymptomatic macular stain. May resemble PWS.
- Stage II (expansion):
  - Enlargement may be triggered by puberty, trauma, infection, and some therapeutic interventions.
  - Warm red/purple subcutaneous lesions with tortuous tense veins, pulsation, thrill, bruit +/– pseudosarcomatous change.
- Stage III (destruction):
  - Dystrophic changes, ulceration, intermittent bleeding, pain, bony invasion.
- Stage IV: (decompensation):
  - Cardiac failure.

Management

- Diagnosis is primarily clinical.
- Ultrasonography and colour Doppler evaluation can confirm the diagnosis and MRI/MRA evaluates extent.
- Therapeutic interventions can be very challenging.
- Recurrence is high if nidus is not removed. Multidisciplinary approach required.
- Angiography is indicated prior to embolization followed by resection when possible in symptomatic lesions.
- Personalized medical treatments targeting the RAS—MAPK pathway with drugs such as the *BRAF* inhibitor vemurafenib under investigation.

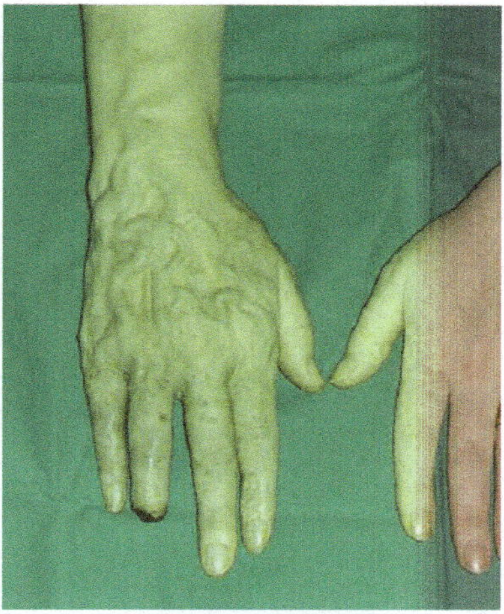

Fig. 8.19 Arteriovenous malformation with steel phenomenon resulting in ischaemia and gangrene.

Reproduced courtesy of Rosemarie Watson, Consultant Paediatric Dermatologist, Department of Dermatology, Our Lady's Children's Hospital Crumlin, Dublin, Ireland

Other vascular birthmarks

Telangiectasia

- Tiny, visible, superficial dilated dermal vessels (0.1–1mm). May blanch but do not fade with time.
- May be punctuate, stellate, or linear.
- May be isolated, dermatomal, or associated with a syndrome.

Causes in childhood include:

- Telangiectatic haemangioma (likely an aborted IH).
- Generalized essential telangiectasias.
- Unilateral naevoid telangiectasia.
- Telangiectatic vascular malformation.

Hereditary haemorrhagic telangiectasia (Osler–Weber–Rendu)

Rare autosomal dominant disorder characterized by mucocutaneous telangiectasia with a tendency to bleed. Epistaxis is a common presenting feature. Anaemia develops secondary to mucosal bleeds. Other viscera especially the lung may be affected by fast-flow lesions (AVMs).

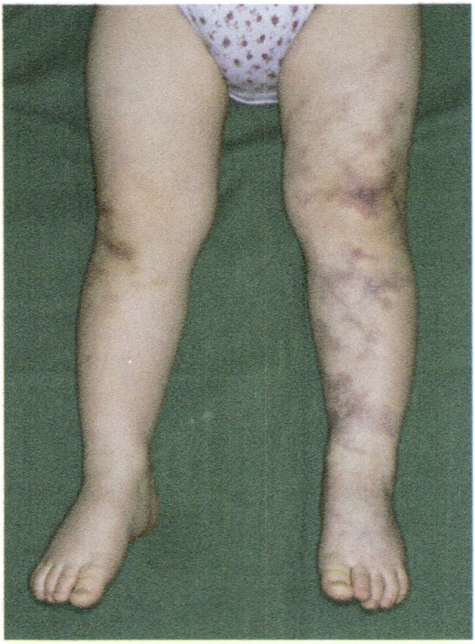

Fig. 8.20 Cutis marmorata telangiectasia congenita. Distinctive reticulated vascular anomaly. Check head and limb circumference.

Reproduced courtesy of Rosemarie Watson, Consultant Paediatric Dermatologist, Department of Dermatology, Our Lady's Children's Hospital Crumlin, Dublin, Ireland

Cutis marmorata telangiectasia congenita (CMTC)

A rare sporadic distinctive red/purple reticulated vascular anomaly ± atrophy, ulceration, venous dilation.

- Localized, segmental, generalized. Congenital, persistent, enhanced by crying, exercise, cold (Fig. 8.20)

Differential diagnosis: physiological cutis marmorata (➲ see Fig. 31.8), neonatal lupus, and antiphospholipid syndrome.

- Most frequently isolated but may be associated with limb hypoplasia, craniofacial, neurological, or other abnormalities.

Vascular malformations: lymphatic malformations (LM)

This is a diverse group of developmental anomalies of the lymphatic system caused by abnormal formation of lymphatic vessels resulting in cysts of varying size filled with lymphatic fluid or lymphoedema.

Primary lymphoedema results in tissue swelling due to an interruption in the lymphatic channel which normally returns interstitial fluid to the thoracic duct, then the bloodstream (Fig. 8.21).

- It may be isolated or associated with structural abnormalities (spina bifida) or syndromes including Turner's syndrome, Noonan syndrome, and Trisomy 21 (Fig. 8.22).
- Several causative mutations have been identified the commonest of which is VEGFR3.

Secondary lymphoedema is the most common lymphatic abnormality seen and may be associated with infection or surgical intervention (more frequent in adults).

Management of lymphoedema

- Meticulous attention to hygiene to prevent cellulitis.
- Compression therapy and manual lymphatic drainage.
- Prophylactic penicillin if recurrent cellulitis.

Primary localized lymphatic malformations

Macrocystic lymphangioma (cystic hygroma)

Occurs in 1 in 12,000 births; equal sex incidence.

Clinical features

- See Fig. 8.23.
- Usually visible at birth, 80% by 2y.
- Most often neck and axilla. Often diagnosed by prenatal ultrasound.
- Single or multiloculated fluid-filled cavities present as soft translucent swellings under normal skin.
- Size may vary from millimetres to several centimetres. May be painful or tender.
- Skin to blueish colour. Readily transilluminates on examination.
- May suddenly enlarge and become tender following secondary infection (upper respiratory infection or poor dental hygiene), or minor trauma with intralesional bleeding.

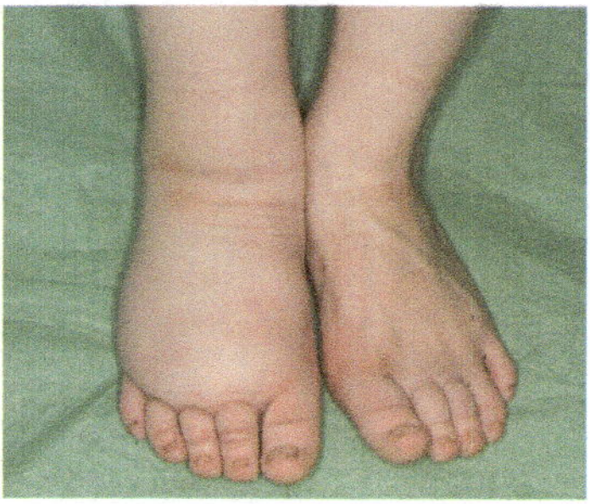

Fig. 8.21 Unilateral lymphoedema. Improved with compression and manual lymphatic drainage.

Reproduced courtesy of Rosemarie Watson, Consultant Paediatric Dermatologist, Department of Dermatology, Our Lady's Children's Hospital Crumlin, Dublin, Ireland

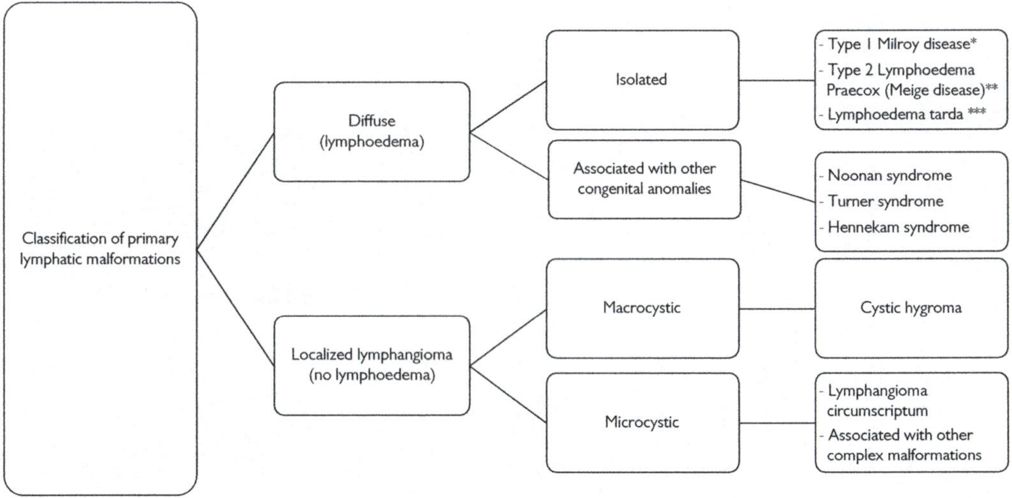

* Rare, congenital, positive family history
** Represents 80% patients with primary lymphoedema. Presents from adolescence to age 35
*** Presents over age 35

Fig. 8.22 Classification of lymphatic malformations.

Reproduced courtesy of Rosemarie Watson, Consultant Paediatric Dermatologist, Department of Dermatology, Our Lady's Children's Hospital Crumlin, Dublin, Ireland

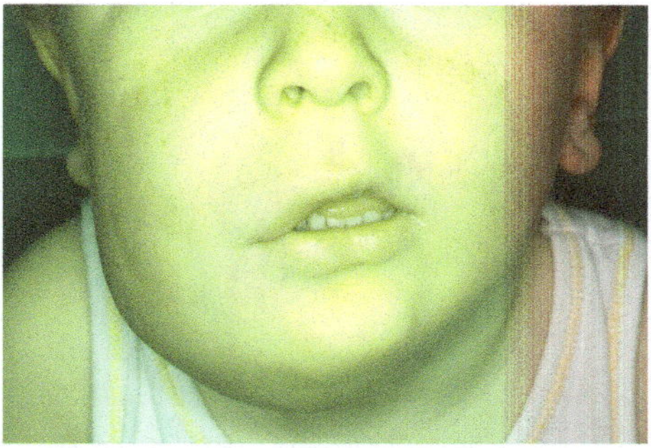

Fig. 8.23 Combined macro- and microcystic lymphatic malformation. Present at birth, now age 5. MRI demonstrated multiloculated cysts of varying size. Partial response to sclerotherapy with alcohol.

Reproduced courtesy of Rosemarie Watson, Consultant Paediatric Dermatologist, Department of Dermatology, Our Lady's Children's Hospital Crumlin, Dublin, Ireland

Complications

Compression of neighbouring structures, infection, skeletal overgrowth, large lesions, may impede vaginal delivery.

Management

- Ultrasonography/MRI useful to confirm diagnosis, delineate extent.
- Consider C-section delivery, maintain vital functions, treat infection.
- Aspiration and injection of sclerosants. Surgical excision.

Microcystic (lymphangioma circumscriptum)

Small cysts caused by dilated lymph channels and vesicles.

Clinical features

- See Fig. 8.24.
- Present at birth but may not become evident until complications such as infection or bleeding arise.
- Persistent crops of irregular groups of thin-walled vessels or hyperkeratotic papules. Recurrent oozing of clear fluid is common.
- May also present as verrucous lesions with superficial black dots.
- Mixed microcystic/macrocystic forms also can occur.

Complications

Bleeding, secondary infection, ulceration, and rarely squamous cell carcinoma.

Treatment

- Imaging (ultrasound and MRI) is used to confirm diagnosis and determine extent of the lesion.
- No current definitive gold standard treatments—the cysts are not usually amenable to sclerosants although there are reports of success

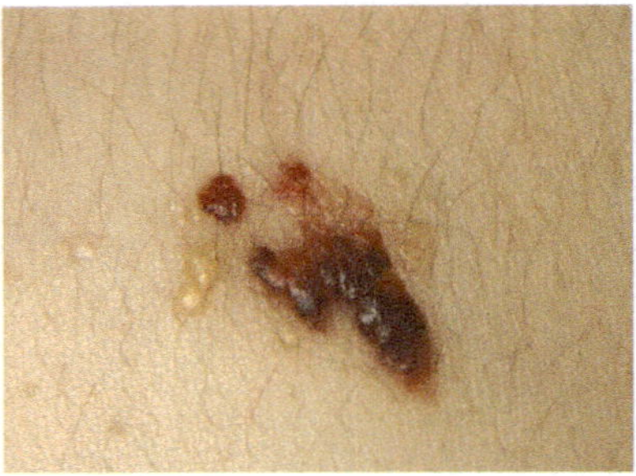

Fig. 8.24 Lymphangioma circumscriptum—microcystic lymphatic malformation. Note clear and haemorrhagic vesicles. May have deep involvement.

Reproduced courtesy of Rosemarie Watson, Consultant Paediatric Dermatologist, Department of Dermatology, Our Lady's Children's Hospital Crumlin, Dublin, Ireland

with bleomycin and other sclerosants. Ablative laser therapy (or localized surgery) is occasionally helpful in superficial lesions but recurrence is frequent.

- Topical sirolimus, oral sirolimus, or sildenafil reported as beneficial but further studies are needed.

Generalized lymphatic anomaly (previously known as lymphangiomatosis)

- Rare progressive congenital disorder of lymphatic channels.
- May present with fetal hydrops or faltering growth in infancy.
- Affects different tissues and organs including intestines and bone (Gorham-Stout vanishing bone disease).
- May be complicated by chylous pleural effusions and ascites, hypoalbuminaemia, hypogammaglobulinaemia, lymphopenia, coagulopathy.
- Prognosis guarded.

Treatment (guided by symptoms): sclerotherapy, surgical debulking. For large congenital vascular malformations, sirolimus is emerging as an effective treatment option but requires careful monitoring.

Complex combined vascular malformations with overgrowth

Complex combined vascular malformations may have a combination of components of capillary (C), lymphatic (L), venous (V), and arterial (A) vessels. Clinical examination and imaging will usually identify these components.

May be associated with localized or asymmetric tissue overgrowth. A myriad of heterogenous overgrowth phenotypes occur due to somatic *PIK3CA* activating mutations, classified under the umbrella term of *PIK3CA*-related overgrowth spectrum (PROS) disorders. Examples include:

Klippel–Trenaunay syndrome

- See Fig. 8.25.
- Sporadic, severe combined capillary–lymphatic–venous malformation (CLVM) with limb overgrowth—slow flow.
- More common in males.
- Agenesis, aplasia, or duplication of anomalous deep veins with deformed, reduced, or absent valves. Persistent embryonic lateral marginal vein.
- Most commonly involves lower leg (95%), unilateral in 85%, associated with limb overgrowth, leg length discrepancy, venous varicosities.
- Complications include pain, infection, bleeding, ulceration, venous thrombosis, and thromboembolism, lymphoedema, localized intravascular coagulation, and protein-losing enteropathy.

Management

- Meticulous attention to hygiene to prevent cellulitis prophylactic penicillin (if recurrent episodes).

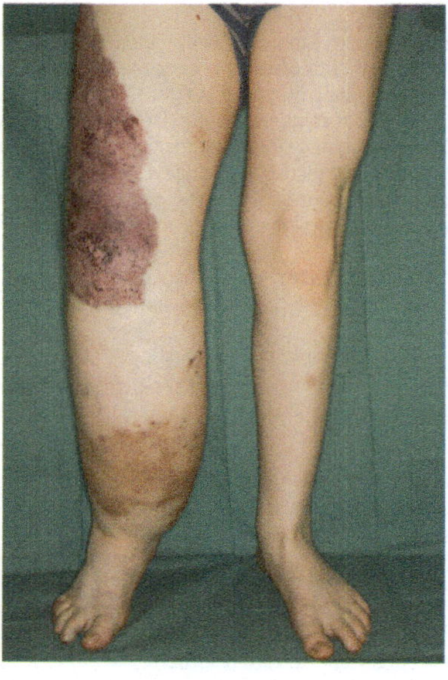

Fig. 8.25 Klippel–Trenaunay syndrome. Note geographic pattern capillary malformation with history of surface ooze and crusting and episodes of cellulitis. Marked limb hypertrophy and haemosiderin staining lower leg.

Reproduced courtesy of Rosemarie Watson, Consultant Paediatric Dermatologist, Department of Dermatology, Our Lady's Children's Hospital Crumlin, Dublin, Ireland

- Compression and manual lymphatic massage may improve oedema. Check a baseline coagulation screen in particular D-dimers and fibrinogen and repeat prior to any surgery because of potential increased risk of bleeding.
- ECHO examination may detect pulmonary hypertension secondary to thromboembolism.
- Surgical intervention to be undertaken with extreme caution only after imaging (including venography) and multidisciplinary review with input of interventional radiology.

Parkes–Weber syndrome

- High-flow combined cerebral arteriovenous malformation and capillary–arteriovenolymphatic malformation (CAVLM) with limb overgrowth.
- Usually lower leg.
- Bruit or thrill may be evident on examination.
- Distinguished from KTS by presence of AVM.
- *RASA1* mutation.

Multidisciplinary management: required and medical care should be directed to patient's needs.

Proteus syndrome[¶]

- Progressive overgrowth syndrome with multiple abnormalities that may be present from birth, but often only become apparent with age.
- Due to somatic activating mutation in AKT1, resulting in insulin receptor stimulation which leads to an increase in P13 kinase activity.
- CM, VM, LM, or combined slow-flow malformations occur in addition to epidermal naevi, connective tissue naevi, and lipomas.
- Asymmetrical enlargement of soft tissue and bone affects any area of the body, most often involves hands and feet especially digits (macrodactyly).
- There may be hemi-hypertrophy of one side of the body.
- Plantar collagenomas give a cerebriform appearance to the soles of the feet.
- Benign and malignant neoplasms may occur.
- Targeted treatment with AKT inhibitors is under investigation.

CLOVES syndrome

- See Fig. 8.26.

Due to somatic mutation in *PIK3CA* gene:

- Congenital Lipomatosis.
- Asymmetric Overgrowth.
- Lymphatic, capillary, Venous, and combined vascular malformations.
- Epidermal naevi.
- Skeletal abnormalities/scoliosis/sandal gap deformity of big toe.
- Associated with neurological abnormalities including hemimegalencephaly and seizure disorders.

[¶] Named after the Greek sea-god Proteus (a shape-changer) due to the highly variable manifestations of this disorder.

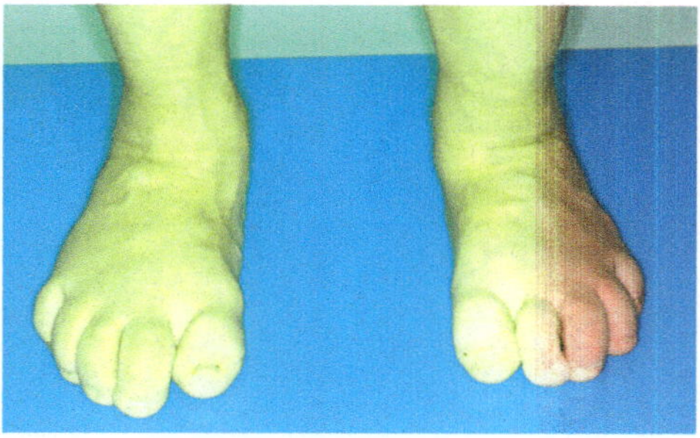

Fig. 8.26 CLOVES syndrome. Note overgrowth of toes, venous dilatation, and capillary malformation.

Reproduced courtesy of Rosemarie Watson, Consultant Paediatric Dermatologist, Department of Dermatology, Our Lady's Children's Hospital Crumlin, Dublin, Ireland

Risk for Wilms' tumour

An increased risk of Wilms' tumour (nephroblastoma) has been described in overgrowth syndromes, in particular Beckwith–Wiedemann syndrome. Further study is required to determine which overgrowth syndromes are at increased risk. Consideration should be given to screening for Wilms' tumour (i.e. 3-monthly renal ultrasound exams until age 8y) in children with overgrowth disorders.

Further reading

British Association of Dermatologists (BAD), *Propranolol for Haemangiomas of Infancy*, http://www.bad.org.uk/shared/get-file.ashx?id=177&itemtype=document

Kohout, M.P., Hansen, M., Pribaz, J.J., and Mulliken, J.B. (1998). Arteriovenous malformations of the head and neck: natural history and management. *Plast Reconstr Surg* 102:643–54.

Mulliken, J.B. (1997). Vascular anomalies. In: Aston S.J., Beasley, R.W., and Thorne C.H.M. (eds.) *Grabb and Smith's Plastic Surgery*, 5th edition, p. 201. Philadelphia, PA: Lippincott-Raven.

Solman, L., *et al.* (2018). Oral propranolol in the treatment of proliferating infantile haemangiomas: British Society for Paediatric Dermatology consensus guidelines. *Br J Dermatol* **179**:582–9.

Section 3

Diagnosis by body distribution

[illegible]

[illegible]

[illegible]

[illegible]

[illegible]

14 Hair and scalp disorders

15 Nail disorders

16 Photodermatology

Chapter 9

Skin problems of the face, nose, eyelids, and ears

Introduction

The face, and particularly the nose, are the most visual body sites and any skin disease in these areas can cause considerable distress and embarrassment with loss of confidence ('loss of face'). This should be considered when treatment decisions are made.

Most of the diseases listed in this chapter are described in more detail elsewhere in this book. For mouth, lips, and perioral problems, ➲ see Chapter 10.

Facial problems

Take note of any dysmorphic features that might point to underlying genetic disorders (e.g. coarse features, low set or abnormally shaped ears, low hairline, widely spaced eyes, small lower jaw, abnormally shaped nose, etc.).

Common

- *Acne*—a mixture of red inflamed papules, pustules, comedones (blackheads, whiteheads), scars and occasionally deep cysts (➲ see Chapter 18). Distribution is typically face, back, and chest.
- *Angioedema*—swelling of lips and or periorbital areas (Box 9.1); ➲ see also Fig. 21.2.
- *Allergic contact eczema*—often caused by makeup, may complicate atopic eczema (➲ see Chapters 2 (patch-testing) and 17).
- *Atopic eczema*—(➲ see Chapter 17) often starts on cheeks in infants and there may be excoriations, dryness, weeping, and crusting with associated cradle cap. Postinflammatory dyschromia (white and or dark patches) is common in chronic cases, often giving a rippled appearance on neck. In older children atopic eczema may localize around the eyes (airborne allergens) (➲ see Fig. 17.9). Lick eczema is common around the mouth (➲ see Fig. 10.1).
- *Bites*—from insects: usually small papules, sometimes blisters, or pustules in crops (➲ see Fig. 20.5), very itchy often with surrounding urticarial wheal (➲ see Chapters 19 (Fig. 19.4) and 25).
- *Blisters*—(➲ see Chapter 25), impetigo, herpes simplex virus, chickenpox (Fig. 9.1), sunburn (➲ see Chapter 16), drug rashes (➲ see Chapter 23), rarely acute contact dermatitis, e.g. hair dye.
- *Bruises*—➲ see Chapters 24 and 31.
- *Chickenpox*—often starts on the face as blisters (Fig. 9.1).
- *Freckles*—(ephelides) and *lentigines* (➲ see Chapter 33).
- *Infantile haemangiomas* (➲ see Chapter 8)
- *Keratosis pilaris*—rough texture due to tiny papules of follicular keratin plugs, usually cheeks (commonest upper, outer arms) often with some inflammation. Mild forms probably physiological but can be autosomal dominant trait. Often associated with atopic eczema and several rare genetic diseases. Rarely atrophic forms occur.
- *Molluscum contagiosum*—➲ see Fig. 19.1.
- *Photosensitive rashes*—(➲ see Fig 16.1) typically spare upper eyelids, below a fringe and around scalp margin, below chin.
- *Pityriasis alba*—(➲ see Chapter 32 and Fig. 32.3) hypopigmented slightly scaly, pale areas, common in eczema.

- *Port-wine stains (PWS)*—(➲ see Figs. 4.13 and 8.15a) commonest on face in distribution of the trigeminal nerve.
- *Psoriasis*—facial lesions commoner in children than adults. Well-demarcated fine red scaling especially around scalp margin, ears, and often around the eyes in children (Fig. 9.2).
- *Scars*—traumatic or following acne vulgaris.
- *Streptococcal infections*—e.g. scarlatina, which is becoming more common again (➲ see Chapter 22).
- *Viral rashes (exanthems)*—e.g. 'slapped cheeks' in erythema infectiosum (➲ see Chapter 22, Fig. 22.4).
- *Viral warts*—often filiform on the face (Fig. 9.5) and also flat planar warts (➲ see Chapter 29, Fig. 29.5).
- *Vitiligo*—whiteness, usually in a perioral or periorbital distribution (➲ see Chapter 32, Fig. 32.1).

Uncommon to rare

- *Arteriovenous shunts*—feel for warmth and a thrill.
- *Atrophoderma vermiculata*—rare atrophic keratosis pilaris (KP) causing worm-like superficial scars on cheeks.
- *Dermatomyositis*—purplish heliotrope rash on eyelids (➲ see Chapter 29, Fig. 29.11).
- *Erysipelas*—*Streptococcus pyogenes* (group A most common): acute redness and swelling of cheek(s) with sharply demarcated margins and a 'peau d'orange' surface.
  Treatment: oral or IV penicillin or erythromycin if penicillin allergy[1]
- *Gustatory sweating*—(auriculotemporal or von Frey's syndrome): redness of cheeks following eating. *Causes*: injury, surgery, CNS lesion, postinfective but often no obvious cause in children.
- *Kawasaki syndrome*—perioral redness and dryness (Fig. 9.4; see also ➲ Chapter 22).
- *Langerhans cell histiocytosis*—seborrhoeic eczema-like rash, often petechial on face and flexures (➲ see Chapter 13 and Fig. 13.5).

(a) (b)

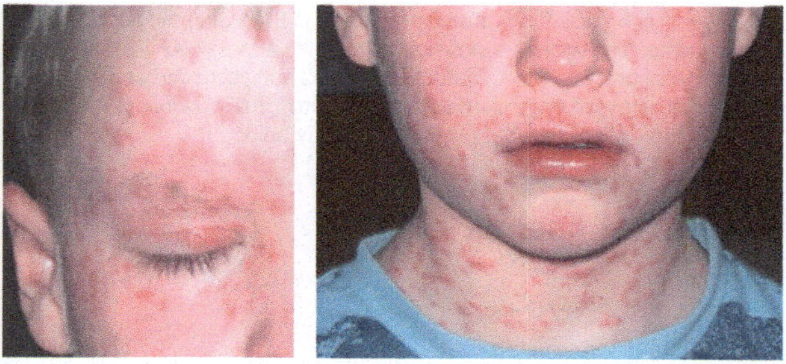

Fig. 9.1 Chickenpox face.

Reproduced courtesy of Susan Lewis-Jones, Hon Consultant Dermatologist, Ninewells Hospital and Medical School, Dundee, UK

- *Leishmaniasis*—slow/non-healing lesions (crusts, eschars, ulcers, nodules) following bites (➲ see Chapters 19, 26, 30, and Fig. 26.4a and b). Endemic and common in many countries but not United Kingdom. Ask about holidays abroad. Contact tropical disease unit for help.
- *Melasma*—teenage girls: brown pigmentation especially periorbital, cheeks, and nose (➲ see Chapter 33).
- *Naevus of Ota:* blue pigmentation usually forehead and around eye (➲ see Chapter 35).
- *Perioral dermatitis*—monomorphic non-itchy inflammatory papular rash, usually teenage girls (➲ see Chapter 20).
- *Poxvirus infections*—orf (or very rarely, cowpox) (➲ see Chapter 26, Fig. 26.8).
- *Progressive facial hemiatrophy*—a form of linear morphoea (➲ see Chapter 29).
- *Pyoderma faciale*—very rare: severe facial pustules, usually in girls and possibly related to acne (➲ see Chapter 18). Treatment is difficult.
- *Lupus pernio*—chronic violaceous plaques (usually of nose). Associated with respiratory sarcoidosis. Very rare—mainly seen in Afro-Caribbean teenagers or adults.
- *Seborrhoeic eczema*—nasolabial folds, glabellar area, and eyebrows (➲ see Chapter 17), in infants and teens (also think of Langerhans cell histiocytosis (➲ see Chapter 13) or HIV/AIDS if severe (➲ see Chapter 39).
- *Syndromal lentiginous syndromes*—e.g. perioral freckling in Peutz-Jegher syndrome (➲ see Fig. 33.5) and others (➲ see Chapter 33 and Fig. 33.4).
- *Syndromal vascular anomalies*—e.g. Sturge–Weber likely if extensive facial PWS in V1–3 (➲ see Chapter 8).
- *Systemic lupus erythematosus (SLE)*—typically butterfly erythema of cheeks and nose (➲ see Chapter 38 and Fig. 9.3). In neonatal LE a periocular rash is typical (➲ see Chapter 7, Fig. 7.2) and there may be annular lesions on trunk (➲ see Fig. 7.3). Localized discoid LE causes scarring and sometimes pigmentary changes but is very rare in children.
- *Syphilis and Yaws*—periorificial and mucous membrane lesions. Saddle nose in congenital syphilis (➲ see Chapters 7 and 22).
- *Tinea faciei* (T. faciale)—caused by dermatophyte infections: red scaling easily missed in this site and it has even been reported in neonates. Animal ringworm can cause florid pustular reactions (➲ see Chapter 20, Fig. 20.4).
- *Ulerythema ophryogenes*—uncommon atrophic variant of KP (see earlier under facial problems) with redness of cheeks and particularly eyebrows and gradual loss of eyebrow hair laterally. Autosomal dominant inheritance. *Treatment*: topical retinoid preparations may help.

Red facial rashes

Common

- High fever from any cause.
- Infective:
  - Slapped cheeks (erythema infectiosum or other viral exanthems—➲ see Chapter 22, Fig. 22.4), bacterial toxins, e.g. scarlet fever, staphylococcal scalded skin syndrome (➲ see Chapter 7, Fig. 7.6).
- Eczema (➲ see Chapter 17).

- Psoriasis (Fig. 9.2; ➲ see also Chapter 22).
- Sunburn.
- Photosensitivity (➲ see Chapter 16).
- Postinflammatory (e.g. following a skin disease such as eczema or psoriasis).
- Vascular (➲ see Chapter 8):
  - Salmon patches (➲ see Fig. 8.14).
  - PWS (➲ see Fig. 8.15a).

Uncommon to rare

- Erythroderma from any cause (➲ see Chapter 22).
- Systemic disease:
  - SLE (Fig. 9.3; ➲ see also Chapters 22 and 38).
  - Dermatomyositis (mainly eyelid; ➲ see Chapter 29, Fig. 29.11).
- Von Frey's syndrome (see section on Uncommon to rare, this chapter).
- Rosacea: redness, papules, and pustules (➲ see Chapter 20).
- Arteriovenous malformations—may resemble a PWS, but area feels warm and there may be a thrill (➲ see Chapter 8).
- Kawasaki's disease—(Fig. 9.4; ➲ see also Chapter 22).
- Dyes and metabolic diseases (➲ Chapter 36).
- Tinea faciei (ringworm) (➲ see Chapter 20, Fig. 20.4).
- Ulerythema ophryogenes—cheeks and eyebrows (see section on Uncommon to rare, this chapter).

Facial tumours and developmental problems

- ➲ See Chapter 28.
- ***Angiofibromas (adenoma sebaceum)***—seen in tuberous sclerosis complex (perinasal and chin areas, ➲ see Box 32.1).
- ***Dermoid cysts***—eyebrow area in infants and young children (➲ see Fig. 28.1).
- ***Dental sinus***—small red/purple nodule from chronic dental abscess which may discharge. Site: around jawline/chin.
- ***Dermatosis papulosa nigra***—small brown to black warty lesions (face and/or neck). Common in black skins. Autosomal dominant trait starting in teens.

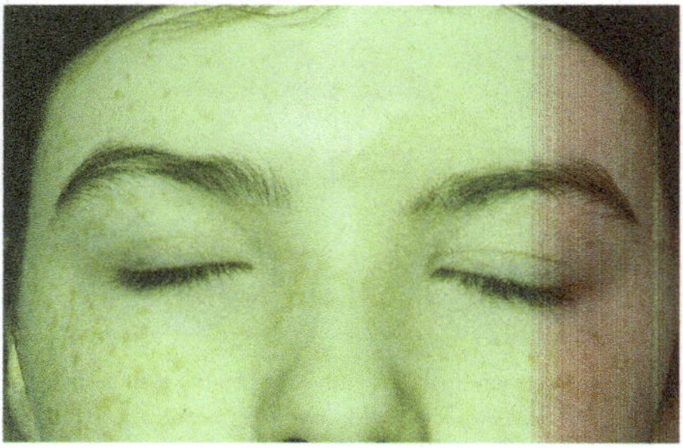

Fig. 9.2 Psoriasis of face.

Reproduced courtesy of Ross Hearn, Ninewells Hospital, Dundee, UK

- *Fibrous forehead plaques*—brown flat lesions seen in tuberous sclerosis complex (➲ see Chapter 32, Box 32.1).
- *Histiocytic lesions*—e.g. juvenile xanthogranuloma (➲ see The histiocytoses, pp. 287–8).
- *Infantile haemangiomas*—may enlarge rapidly. Particular danger sites: periorbital (may occlude sight); ➲ see Figs 8.2 and 8.3; Segmental facial lesions (risk of PHACES syndrome) (➲ see Chapter 8).
- *Malignant skin tumours*—melanoma, basal cell, and squamous cell cancers (very rare except in xeroderma pigmentosum, (➲ see Xeroderma pigmentosum, p. 235 and Chapters 28 and 34).
- *Milia*—in newborn (➲ see Chapter 7). Often cheeks, across nose, or periocular in older children (Fig. 9.6).
- *Moles*—various types (➲ see Chapter 34).
- *Molluscum contagiosum*—small umbilicated papules (Fig. 9.7, ➲ see also Chapter 19, Fig. 19.1).
- *Mycobacterium infections*—tuberculous lymph nodes on neck (scrofuloderma) (➲ see Chapter 22, Fig. 22.11).
- *Pilomatrixoma*—hard, calcifying whiteish tumours of hair follicle origin (➲ see Chapter 28, Fig. 28.15).
- *Preauricular pits and tags* (➲ see Chapters 7 and 28).
- *Pyogenic granuloma*—vascular pedunculated tumours, friable bleed easily (➲ see Chapter 28, Figs. 28.5 and 28.12).
- *Warts*—verrucae vulgaris, often filiform pattern (Fig. 9.5).
- *Xanthomas*—yellowish/skin coloured/reddish brown. Several types, juvenile xanthogranuloma (➲ see Figs. 28.11 and 37.3) is the more common (➲ see Chapters 5, 28, and 37).

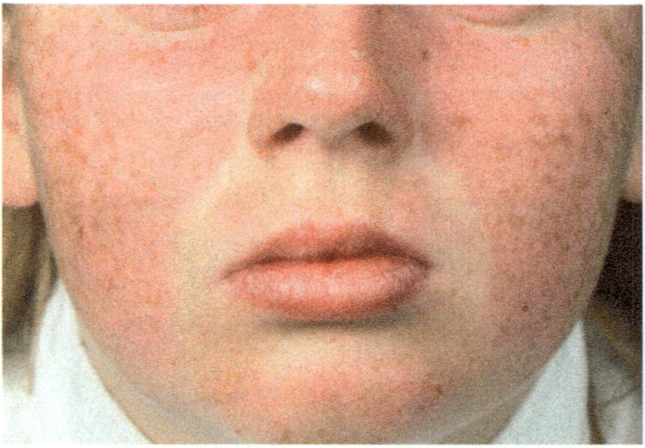

Fig. 9.3 Systemic lupus erythematosus with red butterfly rash on face.

Reproduced courtesy of Susan Lewis-Jones, Hon Consultant Dermatologist, Ninewells Hospital and Medical School, Dundee, UK

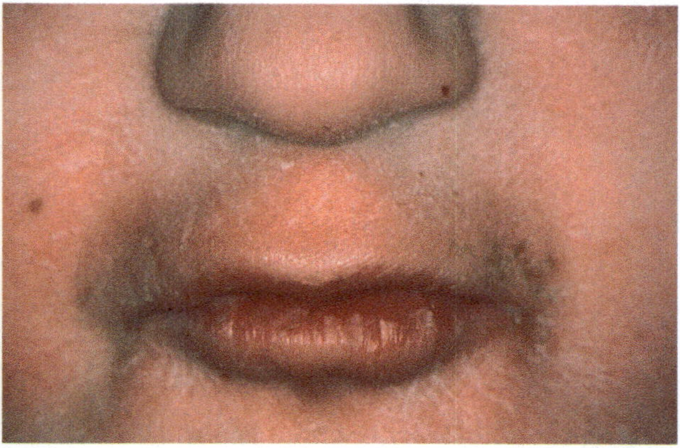

Fig. 9.4 Kawasaki's disease showing perioral redness, lip swelling and surrounding desquamation.

Reproduced courtesy of Jo Sowden, Consultant Dermatologist, UK

Box 9.1 Facial rashes and tumours by distribution

- *Acneiform*—predominately cheeks; chin and forehead (acne lesions—comedones, papulopustules, cysts; adenoma sebaceum).
- *Butterfly* (cheeks and across nose)—seen in SLE (Fig. 9.3) and rosacea.
- *Perioral*— ➲ see Chapter 10.
- *Perinasal*—see Box 9.2.
- *Periorbital swelling*—see Box 9.3.
- *Auricular* (ears)— ➲ see Ears, pp. 133–5.
- *Photosensitive*—spares eyelids; below nose and chin; hair margins; just behind the ears (➲ see Chapter 16, Fig. 16.1).
- *Eyebrows*—seborrhoeic eczema; dermoid cysts; ulerythema ophryogenes; Langerhans cell histiocytosis. Eyebrow hair loss in alopecia areata, Netherton's syndrome, leprosy (madarosis).
- *Cheeks alone*—slapped cheek syndrome (erythema infectiosum, ➲ see Fig. 22.4); erysipelas; SLE; von Frey's syndrome; KP; atrophoderma vermicularis.
- *Glabella area*—seborrhoeic eczema, rosacea. Tumours (nasal glioma, dermoid cyst).
- *Chin*—acne; dental sinus; angiofibromas (adenoma sebaceum), cutaneous TB.

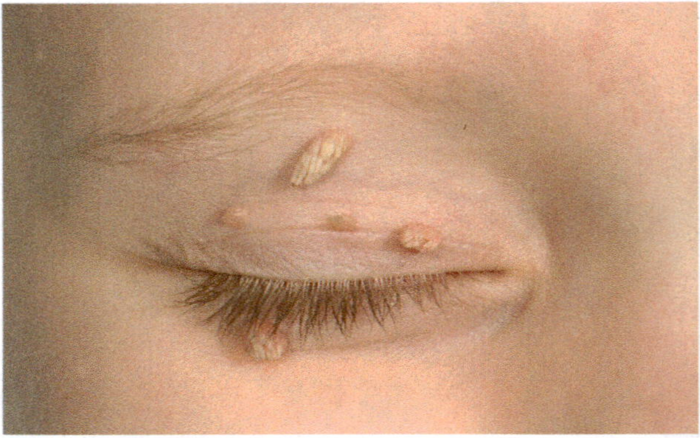

Fig. 9.5 Filiform warts around eye.

Reproduced courtesy of Susan Lewis-Jones, Hon Consultant Dermatologist, Ninewells Hospital and Medical School, Dundee, UK

Nose

Rashes and lesions particularly associated with the nose

- *Atopic crease*—horizontal crease accentuated by rubbing the nose in an upward direction as in hay fever (salute sign).
- *Comedones* and other acne lesions such as papules and pustules (➲ see Chapter 18).
- *Milia*—tiny white inclusion cysts of epidermal cells (Fig. 9.6 and ➲ Chapter 7).
- *Infantile haemangioma*—deep blue lesions on tip known as 'Cyrano nose' may cause disfigurement and cartilage loss. Those around nares can cause obstruction of breathing (➲ see Vascular tumours, pp. 94–9).
- *Lupus pernio*—seen in sarcoidosis (very rare).
- *Scarring*—especially from acne (➲ see Chapter 18) and photosensitive disorders, such as hydroa vacciniforme (➲ see Fig. 16.4).

Box 9.2 Rashes and lesions around alae nasae

- *Adenoma sebaceum* (angiofibromas)—seen in tuberous sclerosis complex; also around central chin.
- *Impetigo*—common around nostrils.
- *Herpes simplex infections*—common around nostrils often confused with impetigo.
- *Seborrhoeic eczema*.
- *Langerhans cell histiocytosis* (often confused with seborrhoeic eczema).
- *Warts* (Fig. 9.5) and molluscum contagiosum—from digital spread (Fig. 9.7).

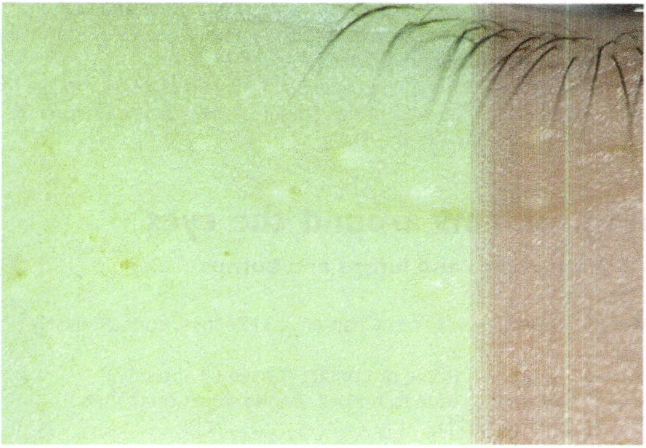

Fig. 9.6 Milia around eye.

Reproduced courtesy of NHS Tayside Clinical Photography, Dundee, UK

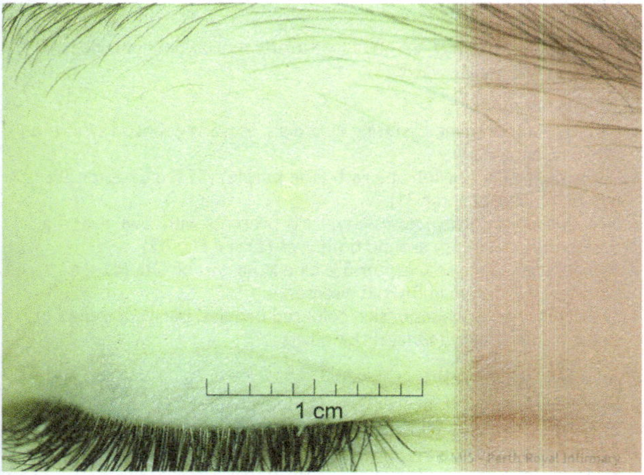

Fig. 9.7 Molluscum contagiosum around eyes.

Reproduced courtesy of NHS Tayside Clinical Photography, Dundee, UK

- *Photosensitive disorders* including sunburn (➲ see Chapter 16).
- *Impetigo*—often around the nares.
- *Recurrent*—herpes simplex: usually around the nares.
- *Rosacea* (rare in children).

- *Dilated pilosebaceous orifices (pores)*—common in acne and with seborrhoea (increased sebum excretion). Often a cause for complaint in dysmorphophobic patients (➲ see Chapter 24).
- *Snuffles*—perinasal rash seen in congenital syphilis (rare). Cartilage may be damaged causing sunken bridge (saddle nose) (➲ see Chapter 7, Congenital infections, pp. 88–9).

Skin problems around the eyes

Periorbital rashes and lumps and bumps

Common

- *Blistering conditions*—(➲ see Chapter 25) infective, contact allergy, or bites.
- *Eczema*—especially atopic or contact (➲ see Chapter 17).
- *Eczema herpeticum*—due to herpes simplex infection (➲ see Chapter 17, Fig. 17.11).
- *Insect bites*.
- *Impetigo*.
- *Psoriasis*—often occurs in children around eyes (Fig. 9.2) (rare in adults).
- *Pigmentation*—brown in moles or café-au-lait macules (➲ see Chapters 33 and 34).
- *Milia*—see Fig. 9.6.
- *Warts*—any types (Fig. 9.5) but particularly molluscum contagiosum (Fig. 9.7) and planar warts.

Uncommon to rare

- *Blisters*—autoimmune blistering disorders, Stevens–Johnson syndrome (➲ see Chapter 23).
- *Dermatomyositis*—heliotrope rash (lilac-purple) (➲ see Chapter 29, Fig. 29.11, and Chapter 31).
- *Neonatal lupus erythematosus*—typically presents with 'owl' eyes—a dusky red-brown rash around both eyes (➲ see Fig. 7.2).
- *Pigmentation*—(➲ see Chapter 33) blue in naevus of Ota (➲ see Chapter 35), brown in thyroid disease.
- *Syringoma*—small whiteish/skin coloured papules, benign tumours of sweat glands usually teenagers or adults.

Eyelashes and eyelids

- *Loss of eyelashes* in alopecia areata (➲ see Chapter 14), chronic infection or pulling (trichotillomania).
- *Inflammation and redness (blepharitis)*:
  - Usually due to chronic infection such *Staphylococcus aureus*.
  - Associated with allergy such as pollen or animal dander or contact dermatitis.
  - Rosacea (usually adults).
- *Stye (hordeolum)*—due to acute infection with *Staphylococcus aureus*.
- *Crab lice (Pediculosis palpebrarum)*— ➲ see Fig. 22.15 (uncommon).
- *White colour (poliosis)*—in vitiligo, albinism, and other rare genetic conditions (➲ see Chapter 31).

- *Long eyelashes*—occur with ciclosporin treatment, some topical agents for glaucoma, and a few rare genetic conditions.
- *Beaded papules on eyelids*—associated with hoarse voice in lipoid proteinosis. Very rare (➲ see Lipoid proteinosis, p. 448).

Pigmentation of the sclera or conjunctiva

- *Blue*—naevus of Ota, osteogenesis imperfecta.
- *Brown*—melanocytic naevi.
- *Yellow*—jaundice (raised bilirubin). Localized areas may be due to pinguecula, pterygium, or disseminated xanthoma.
- *Red*—bleeding into sclera occurs with raised pressure (e.g. whooping cough or may be spontaneous). Increased vasculature is seen in vascular anomalies and ataxia telangiectasia.

Box 9.3 Swelling of the eyelids

Eyelid swelling

- Infantile haemangiomas, vascular anomalies (➲ see Chapter 8), and tumours can all cause localized swelling of the eyelids although this is not oedema.

Periorbital oedema/diffuse swelling

- Angioedema (➲ see Chapter 21).
- Acute contact allergy (e.g. eye drops, make-up, hair dye).
- Dermatomyositis (➲ see Chapter 29).
- Heroin overdose.
- Infections such as cellulitis or erysipelas (redness).
- Infiltrative disorders (e.g. myxoedema, mucopolysaccharidoses).
- Insect bites.
- Trichinosis—intestinal nematode—associated fever, myalgia.
- Trauma—usually associated with bruising.
- Lymphoedema of any cause.
- Neonatal LE (➲ see Chapter 7).
- Nephritis.
- Rosacea—very rarely reported in children.
- Roseola infantum (exanthema subitum) 30% of cases (➲ see Chapter 22).

Ears

Rashes and other problems

Common

- *Allergic contact dermatitis*—usually caused by nickel allergy from earrings or antibiotic eardrops particularly neomycin.
- *Comedones (blackheads)*—common (➲ see Fig. 18.2) usually in association with acne.

- *Eczema*—itchy, redness, and scaling, may be atopic, seborrhoeic, or contact allergy and, if weeping from ear canal, look for otitis externa.
- *Fissuring*—common in atopic eczema, often with secondary impetigo behind ear and crease of lobe. Also occurs with psoriasis.
- *Insect bites*.
- *Juvenile springtime eruption*—blisters on ear rims after sun exposure (➲ see Chapter 16, JSE, p. 228).
- *Psoriasis*—red scaling behind, around and within ear canal (➲ see Fig. 22.2).
- *Red ears*—often seen in viral rashes, rarely relapsing perichondritis (see next section).
- *Seborrhoeic eczema*—red scaling, not usually itchy.
- *Traumatic tears*—especially from wearing earrings.

Uncommon to rare

- *Abnormal shape, size, and/or positioning*—think of genetic diseases.
- *Addison's disease*—dark pigmentation.
- *Chilblains*—(perniosis; ➲ see Fig. 31.9) follows cold exposure, rarely autoimmune.
- *Langerhans cell histiocytosis*—may present as aural discharge or rash.
- *Ochronosis*—black staining often from use of skin 'lightening' products containing hydroquinone or phenols (pseudo-ochronosis). Rare autosomal recessive endogenous form exists.
- *Purple ears*—seen in perniosis (chilblains, ➲ see Fig. 31.9), cryoglobulinaema, vasculitis (➲ see Fig. 38.3).
- *Relapsing perichondritis*—usually adults, ears initially swollen and red. Later floppy as cartilage is destroyed by autoimmune process.

Lumps and bumps of the ear

Common

- *Accessory auricles, sinuses/pits*—(➲ see Chapter 7).
- *Earring keloids*—following ear piercing, particularly if complicated by secondary infection or contact allergic dermatitis (Fig. 9.8)
- *Warts*.

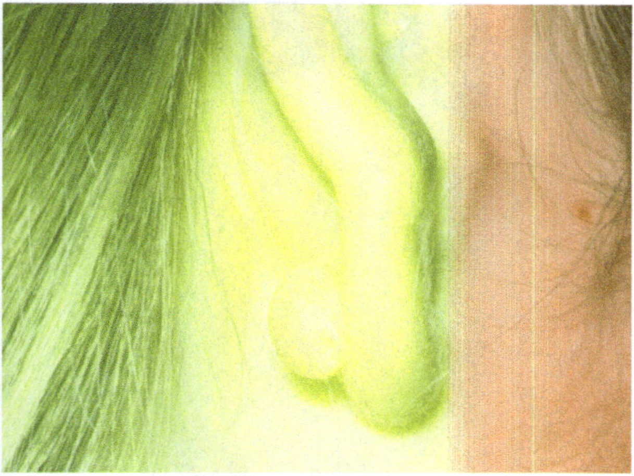

Fig. 9.8 Earring keloid.

Reproduced courtesy of Susan Lewis-Jones, Hon Consultant Dermatologist, Ninewells Hospital and Medical School, Dundee, UK

Uncommon to rare

- ***Cauliflower ear***—from constant trauma (e.g. rugby, boxing). Bruising causes swelling and fibrosis that becomes permanent.
- ***Chilblains***—tender, itchy purplish papules (➲ see Chapter 28 and Fig. 31.9)
- ***Darier's disease***—(➲ see Chapter 19) small warty papules.
- ***Epidermoid cysts***—look for a punctum (➲ see Chapter 28, Fig. 28.18).
- ***Granuloma annulare***—(Fig. 9.9) may present as hard irregular nodules on ears or scalp and is often confused with tumours. Skin biopsy will confirm the diagnosis if uncertain.

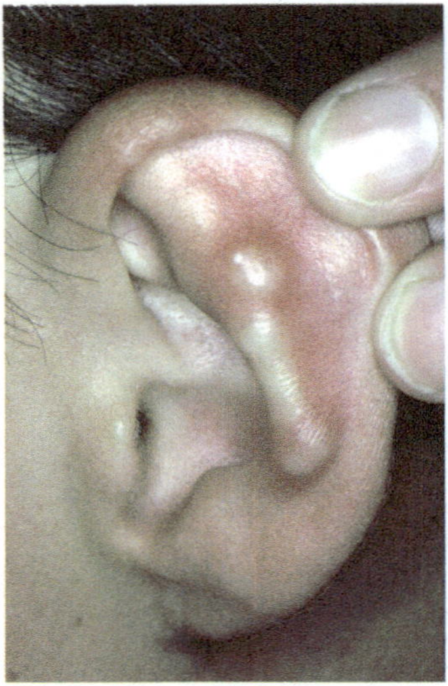

Fig. 9.9 Granuloma annulare of ear.

Reproduced courtesy of Susan Lewis-Jones, Hon Consultant Dermatologist, Ninewells Hospital and Medical School, Dundee, UK

References

1. NICE, Clinical Knowledge Summaries, *Cellulitis—Acute*, 2015, https://cks.nice.org.uk/cellulitis-acute

Chapter 10

Oral problems

Introduction

Sore and painful areas around or within the mouth are common in children. Many mouth lesions look similar making an exact diagnosis difficult to reach without a thorough medical history. Recurrent aphthous ulcers are common and may be associated with underlying inflammatory disorders such as coeliac disease or inflammatory bowel disease. Missing or abnormal teeth may be a clue to a genetic syndrome. Important diagnostic clues will be missed without carefully looking at the whole mouth and carrying out a general medical examination. Benign tumours such as warts or molluscum contagiosum can occur anywhere in the oral cavity and are relatively common, whereas malignant tumours are rare. Oral problems are grouped as follows by affected region.

Lips: cheilitis (inflammation of the lips)

Redness and swelling of the lips with or without fissuring and or crusts.

Common causes

Factitious

- *Lip licking*—a common presentation in children with atopic dermatitis and often worse in cold weather (Fig. 10.1). It can involve the whole lip and surrounding skin, usually with a well-demarcated cut-off beyond reach of the tongue. It is due to the irritant effect of saliva and has a habitual component.
  Treatment: use Vaseline or similar emollient and avoid licking/smacking.
  Note: coloured/flavoured lip salves may cause contact irritation or sometimes true contact allergy worsening the licking.

Infective

- *Bacterial*—common, often caused by staphylococcal (golden crusts and fissures) or streptococcal infection (painful fissures).
  Treatment: oral antibiotics (e.g. flucloxacillin or erythromycin), 10 days.
- *Viral*—herpetic gingivostomatitis is very painful and may be well-localized to the lip or involve the oral cavity with multiple, tiny painful blisters (up to 100) which leave ulcers. Child is often febrile and pain makes swallowing difficult. Consider hospital admission for parenteral fluids and analgesia. Healing occurs in 7–10 days without scarring.
  Cause: herpes simplex virus (HSV) usually type 1. Varicella-zoster and Coxsackie viruses cause similar presentations.
  Specific treatment: systemic aciclovir for 5 days.

Allergic

- *Angioedema (type 1)*—rapid onset of lip swelling sometimes involving the tongue and usually subsides in less than 24h (➲ see Fig. 21.2). May be associated with urticaria.
  Causes: acquired type I allergy (e.g. to latex or foods). *Note*: inherited C1 esterase inhibitor deficiency (➲ see Types of angioedema, pp. 309–10 and its management, Box 21.3) causes a firm, longer lasting oedema—ask

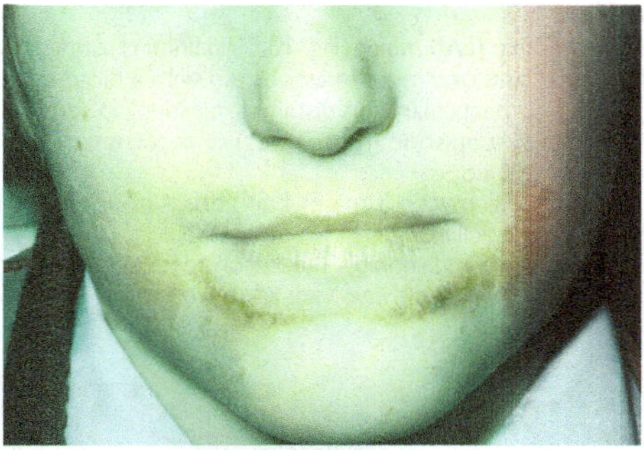

Fig. 10.1 Lick eczema.

Reproduced courtesy of Susan Lewis-Jones, Hon Consultant Dermatologist, Ninewells Hospital and Medical School, Dundee, UK

about family history and abdominal pain. It is unlikely in the context of urticaria.

- *Contact dermatitis (Type 4, delayed)*—e.g. to lipstick or toothpastes, presents with persistent lip dermatitis, often not itchy, and frequent recurrent bacterial infection may mask the underlying contact allergy. Consider referral to dermatology for patch testing.
- *Orofacial granulomatosis* (➲ see Rare lip problems, pp. 140–2) may present with angular cheilitis and indurated erythema of the adjacent skin.

Angular cheilitis

Dermatitis affecting the angles of the mouth only. Associated with iron deficiency and may be complicated by secondary bacterial or candida infection (may present as warty growths in mucocutaneous candidiasis, ➲ see Infection, pp. 144–5). If unilateral and recurrent, consider HSV. Angular thickening rarely occurs in bullous ichthyosiform erythroderma (➲ see Rare genetic ichthyoses, p. 408), and it can occur with orofacial granulomatosis.

Other presentations of lip problems

- *Vascular tumours*—e.g. infantile haemangiomas usually occur in the first weeks of life and may increase rapidly in size and/or ulcerate. Facial plaque-like haemangiomas may indicate PHACES syndrome or in beard area, may be associated with subglottic haemangioma(s) (➲ see PHACES syndrome, p. 99, and Fig. 8.8).
- *Fox–Fordyce spots*—small (1–3mm), uniform, white to yellowish coloured papules (sebaceous glands) or plaques on inner lips and buccal mucosa (Fig. 10.2). Often misdiagnosed as warts. They are commoner in adolescents. May also be present in the axilla and the glans penis or labia minora. Reassurance is required.

Rarer lip problems

- *Erythema multiforme (EM) major* (Fig. 10.3): painful crusting and ulceration of lips and oral mucosa associated with a blotchy red rash and target lesions, particularly on distal extremities (➲ see Fig. 4.12). It may be an acute first episode (most cases) or recurrent.
- *EM minor*: skin rash alone.
  Causes: infection, e.g. mycoplasma or HSV; drugs (much rarer in children than adults), e.g. penicillin.
  Treatment: supportive and monitor fluids, consider topical steroid mouth wash and IV fluids. If eyes are involved, ask for ophthalmic review; genital

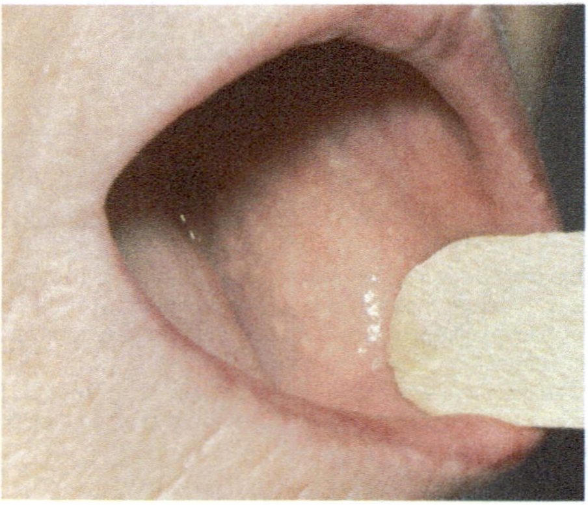

Fig. 10.2 Fox–Fordyce spots.

Reproduced courtesy of Susan Lewis-Jones, Hon Consultant Dermatologist, Ninewells Hospital and Medical School, Dundee, UK

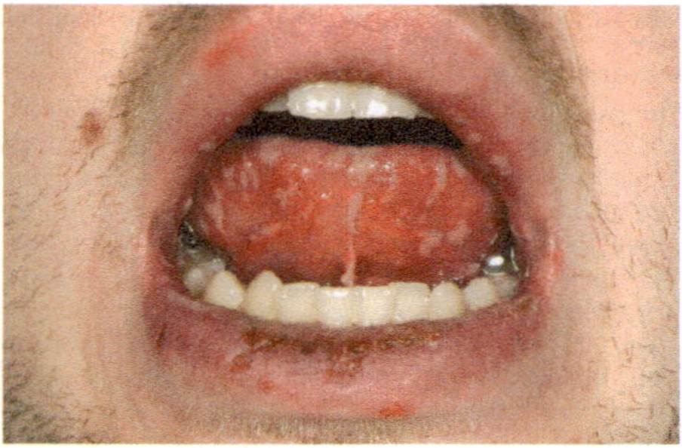

Fig. 10.3 Erythema multiforme with crusts on lips and erosions of tongue.

Reproduced courtesy of Ruth Murphy, Consultant Dermatologist, Royal Hallamshire Hospital, Sheffield, UK

skin involvement can rarely result in adhesions and phimosis. Recurrent episodes may be less severe and often associated with HSV. Look for trigger factors; suppress HSV with long-term oral aciclovir (e.g. 6 months).

- ***Stevens–Johnson syndrome (SJS) and toxic epidermal necrolysis** (TEN)* (see Chapter 23). These conditions represent two ends of a spectrum. The lips and oral cavity show extensive ulceration. The eyes and genitalia are often involved and affected individuals are constitutionally unwell.
  Causes: drugs (e.g. anticonvulsants) and less commonly infection.
  Treatment: withdraw any identified trigger. Give supportive care with parenteral fluids. Needs high dependency unit (HDU) or burns unit access (see Chapter 23, Fig. 23.4).
- ***Zinc deficiency***: severe perioral rash often with diarrhoea (see Figs. 7.4 and 13.4).
  Cause: primary (genetic) or secondary (see Zinc deficiency, pp. 179–82).
  Treatment: oral zinc replacement.
- ***Kawasaki disease***: (see Chapter 22) sometimes confused with SJS or EM since the lips are red and swollen but crusting is absent (see Fig. 9.4).
- ***Chronic granulomatous cheilitis***: chronic lip swelling and fissuring (Fig. 10.4)
  Causes: *Crohn's disease* (cobblestoned appearance of oral mucosa).
  Treatment: intralesional steroids and referral for gastrointestinal (GI) screening. If inflammatory bowel disease is identified treatment improves cheilitis.
- *Orofacial granulomatosis* (possibly a type 4 contact dermatitis to benzoates (E210–219), cinnamates, carvone, and cocoa).
  Treatment: refer to dietician for strict exclusion diet with emphasis on eating fresh food without preservatives.
- ***Melkersson–Rosenthal syndrome***: triad of recurrent/persistent facial swelling, facial nerve paralysis, and lingua plicata (tongue fissuring).
- ***Autoimmune blistering disorders***: pemphigus vulgaris, pemphigoid and chronic bullous disease of childhood are extremely rare (see Chapter 25) but may present with oral lesions. Pemphigus vulgaris will

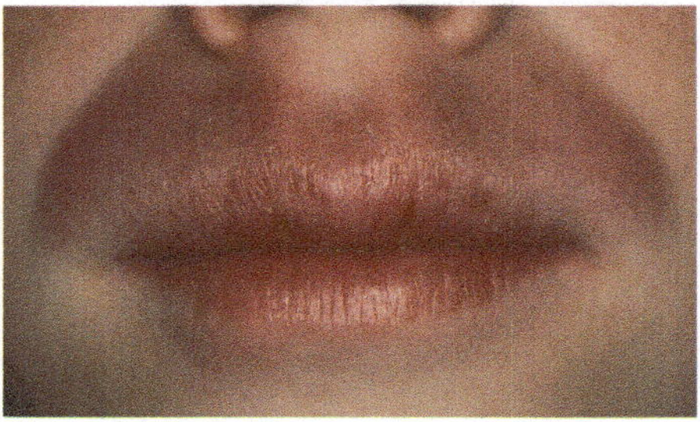

Fig. 10.4 Granulomatous cheilitis.

Reproduced courtesy of Susan Lewis-Jones, Hon Consultant Dermatologist, Ninewells Hospital and Medical School, Dundee, UK

sometimes present in a very localized form with non-healing erosions on the lips.

- *Artefactual cheilitis*: (Fig. 10.5) may appear as dermatitis, crusting, or blistering induced by deliberate trauma from biting or the application of irritants or known contact allergens, e.g. glues or caustic substances (➲ see Dermatitis artefacta, p. 371).

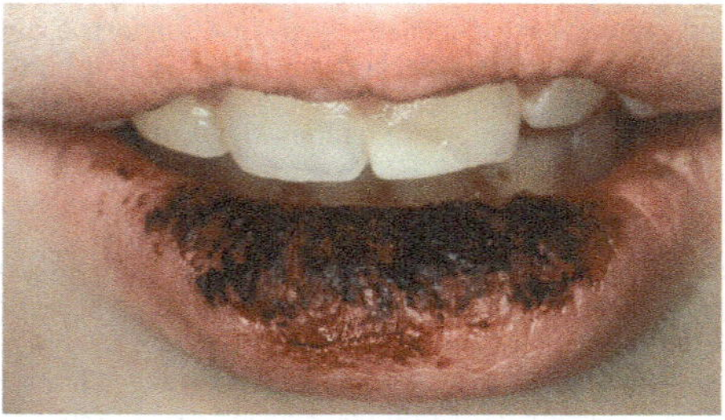

Fig. 10.5 Artefactual cheilitis (as a manifestation of dermatitis artefacta) caused by biting and rubbing (➲ see Chapter 24).

Reproduced courtesy of Susan Lewis-Jones, Hon Consultant Dermatologist, Ninewells Hospital and Medical School, Dundee, UK

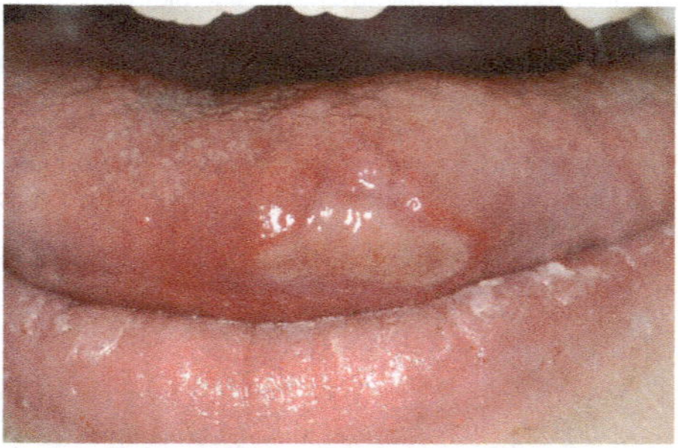

Fig. 10.6 Minor aphthous ulcer.

Reproduced courtesy of Ruth Murphy, Consultant Dermatologist, Royal Hallamshire Hospital, Sheffield, UK

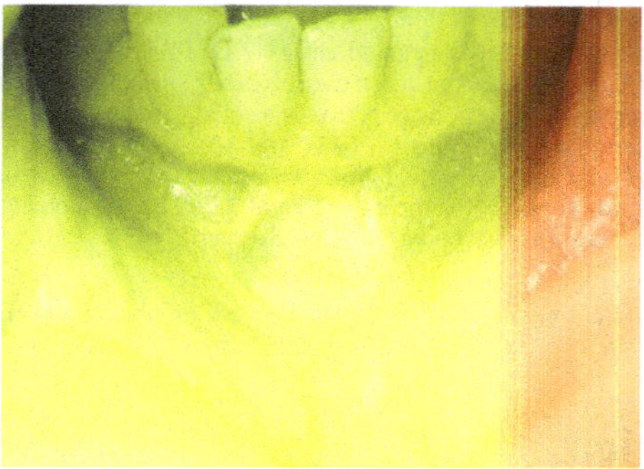

Fig. 10.7 Major aphthous ulcer with scarring.

Reproduced courtesy of Ruth Murphy, Consultant Dermatologist, Royal Hallamshire Hospital, Sheffield, UK

Buccal and labial mucosa and tongue: mouth ulcers

Commonly seen in:

- Aphthous ulceration (idiopathic or associated with underlying inflammatory bowel disease).
- Viral infection (HSV).
- Erythema multiforme.
- Systemic lupus erythematosus (➔ see Chapter 38).
- Neutropenia.
- Behçet's syndrome (rare).

Recurrent aphthous stomatitis (RAS) (oral ulceration)

- *Minor aphthae*—affect 20% of children, often with a family history of recurrent mouth ulcers. They occur anteriorly in the mouth and are mostly <10mm. Painful but do not usually result in malnutrition or dehydration. A low serum iron may cause exacerbation, so consider this if frequency or severity increases, particularly around menarche. Ask about abdominal pain and diarrhoea (association with coeliac or inflammatory bowel disease). Minor aphthae heal without scars in 7–10 days (Fig. 10.6).
  Treatment: identify and treat underlying causes (e.g. low serum ferritin). Prescribe analgesia (e.g. Difflam®) prior to eating and where indicated topical corticosteroids such as steroid inhalers directed to the ulcer.
- *Major aphthae*—are larger than minor apthae, often >10mm in diameter and heal with scarring (Fig. 10.7). Some children with RAS will go on to develop Behçet's disease (increased risk if HLA B51/52 positive).
  Treatment: may need local topical corticosteroid treatment. If difficult to control, thalidomide may be indicated.

Behçet's disease

A multisystem disorder diagnosed clinically by RAS occurring more than three times per year plus at least two of other site involvement including genital ulceration, eye lesions (e.g. uveitis, retinal vasculitis), and skin lesions (erythema nodosum, pseudofolliculitis, and acneiform pustules). Blindness may occur with ocular involvement and any history of visual disturbance warrants an urgent ophthalmology referral. HLA B51/52 positive individuals are at increased risk of systemic involvement.

Note: needs multidisciplinary input.

- ***Specific local treatment***: topical corticosteroid or steroid mouthwash. Colchicine, immunosuppression, and thalidomide may be indicated.

Infection

Viral

Common diseases include: HSV, chickenpox; (➲ see Disorders affecting the palate, p. 146) and viral warts (➲ see Tumours (lumps and bumps), p. 145).

Oral candidiasis (thrush)

Common in the newborn and after antibiotics. Appears as redness with white 'curd-like' deposits and soreness, usually on the palate and tongue but also affects the napkin area (➲ see Fig. 13.3). In older children consider immunosuppression or mucocutaneous candidiasis (Fig. 10.8).

Treatment: nystatin oral suspension. Immunosuppressed children may require systemic itraconazole or fluconazole.

Chronic mucocutaneous candidiasis

A group of very rare conditions of varying severity with tongue and lip involvement showing white coating and tongue fissuring (scrotal tongue, Fig. 10.8) causing severe soreness and difficulty eating. It also affects skin, nails, hair, and sometimes the lungs. It is associated with immunodeficiency

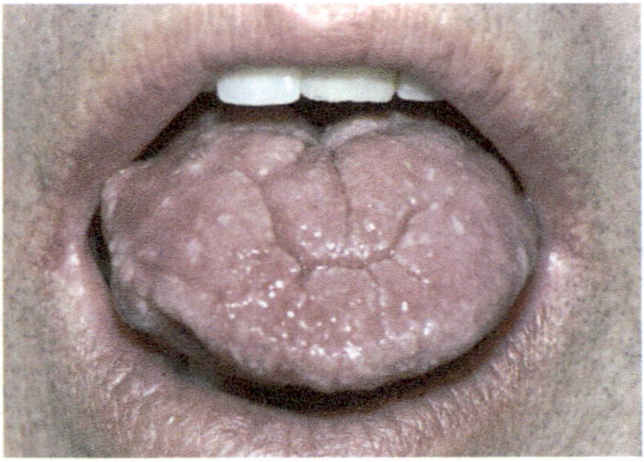

Fig. 10.8 Chronic mucocutaneous candidiasis involving the tongue.
Reproduced courtesy of Richard Williams, Betsi Cadwaladr University Health Board, Wales, UK

or immunosuppression and may be familial. Candida is found within the tissues rather than superficially and may only be evident on biopsy.

Treatment: systemic antifungal agents are usually required. Refer for dermatological opinion.

Tumours (lumps and bumps)

These may occur anywhere in the mouth although some have specific sites of predilection, e.g. epulis arises on the gum (➲ see Gum enlargement, p. 148) and lymphangiomas tend to arise on the tongue as clusters of fluid-filled lesions, some blood-filled (➲ see Chapter 28).

Commonly occurring:

- *Mucocoele*—slightly soft and translucent.
- *Viral warts* (Fig. 10.9) including molluscum contagiosum, often appearing white due to hydration of the keratin.
- *Vascular anomalies and haemangiomas* (➲ see Chapter 8).

Rarely

Tumours/infiltrates may be associated with systemic disease. Infiltrates may form plaques or lumps in the oral cavity. Consider:

- Oral fibromas (usually solitary) can occur on sides of tongue and cheek from chronic biting—usually adults or older teenagers.
- Leukaemia (vascular/bluish lesions).
- Langerhans cell histiocytosis (jaw swelling, gingivitis, loosening of teeth).
- Lichenoid lesions—graft-versus-host disease (➲ see Other oral changes, pp. 148–50, and Chapter 39).
- Mucosal neuromas in multiple endocrinopathy syndromes (thyroid carcinoma and phaeochromocytoma) (➲ see MEN syndromes, p. 66).

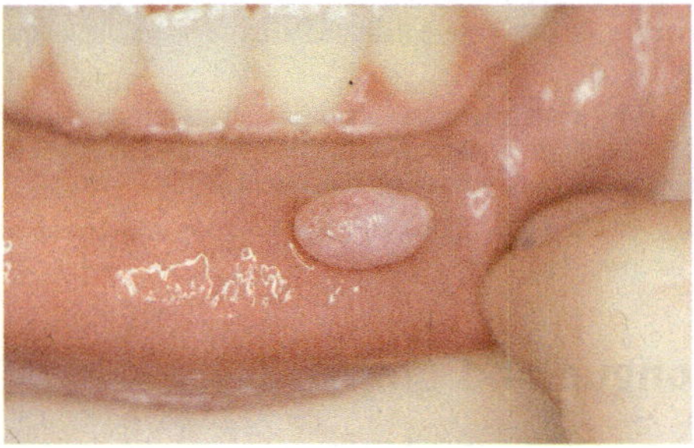

Fig. 10.9 Viral wart on mucosal surface of lip.

Reproduced courtesy of Susan Lewis-Jones, Hon Consultant Dermatologist, Ninewells Hospital and Medical School, Dundee, UK

Disorders affecting the palate

- *Petechial and or vesicular*—viral infections (hand, foot, and mouth disease; infectious mononucleosis, herpangina, varicella-zoster).
- *Ulceration*—neutropenia (cyclical, autoimmune, haematological).
- *Erythematous*—fungal (immunocompromised, HIV/AIDS, and multiple endocrine neoplasia syndromes, ➲ see MEN syndromes, p. 66).

Infective petechial or vesicular lesions

Hand, foot, and mouth disease

Mainly seen as small, red palatal blisters. Look for similar grey lesions with surrounding red flare on hands and feet. There is no gingival involvement and few symptoms (➲ see Figs. 4.1 and 12.2).

Cause: usually Coxsackie A16 virus, but many have been implicated. Differentiate from Koplik's spots; white spots on mucosa seen in measles and other viral infections.

Herpangina

Very painful, multiple, tiny vesicles quickly ulcerating to form aphthae with surrounding redness, on fauces, tonsils, and soft palate. Associated with high fever, vomiting, anorexia, and general malaise. Twenty per cent (20%) have abdominal pain.

Cause: Coxsackie A or echoviruses.

Infectious mononucleosis (glandular fever)

Commonly occurs in teenagers, occasionally prepubertal children.

Presentation: sore throat, petechial haemorrhage on the palate and an exudate on the fauces. Regional lymphadenopathy is usual, sometimes with systemic malaise, lymphocytosis, and hepatic abnormalities.

Cause: Epstein–Barr virus.

Chickenpox and varicella-zoster (VZV)

Chickenpox: very common (➲ see Varicella-zoster virus, p. 380) and presents with crops of oral and cutaneous vesicles (➲ see Fig. 9.1). Oral lesions occur anywhere including the palate and are usually multiple and cross the midline.

VZV: rare in children, appearing as unilateral palatal lesions that do *not* cross the midline. Usually preceded by oral discomfort and may be mistaken for toothache. Consider underlying immunosuppression.

Cause: reactivation of VZV following prior infection with chickenpox (which may have been *in utero*).

The tongue and gums

Tongue

The dorsum is the commonest affected site in children. Conditions affecting the lateral border such as erosive lichen planus and bullous pemphigoid are very rare.

Geographic tongue

Transient red patches with whitish surrounding tissue, which move around. Common, usually asymptomatic but may be associated soreness/burning. If worsening or severe, check iron levels, B_{12}, and folate.

Tongue fissuring (lingua plicata)

An autosomal dominant condition that does not affect function and is often associated with geographic tongue. Rarely found in association with Melkersson–Rosenthal syndrome: triad of recurrent/persistent facial swelling, facial nerve paralysis, and lingua plicata.

Black hairy tongue

Usually follows antibiotic therapy.
Treatment: brush tongue with toothpaste 2–3 times daily.

Macroglossia (large tongue)

Primary: due to muscular hypertrophy.
Secondary: many associations including infections, inflammatory disorders, chromosomal abnormalities (especially Down's syndrome, trisomy 21), tumours, vascular malformations, metabolic storage diseases, and congenital hypothyroidism.

Glossodynia (painful tongue)

Rare in children, consider infection, vitamin deficiencies, rough dental surfaces, contact allergic dermatitis to mouthwash, toothpastes, or chewing gum.

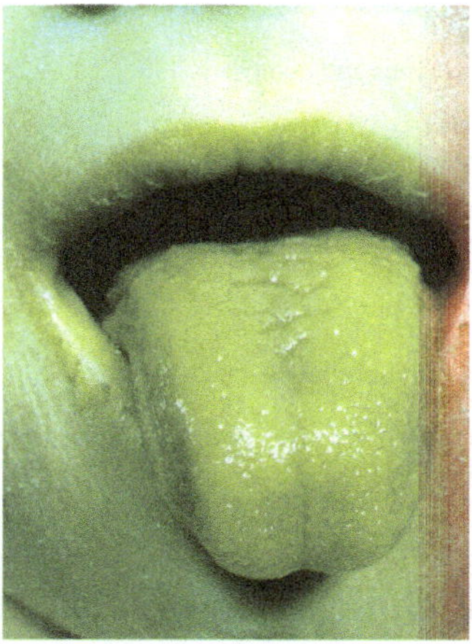

Fig. 10.10 Strawberry tongue.

Reproduced courtesy of Susan Lewis-Jones, Hon Consultant Dermatologist, Ninewells Hospital and Medical School, Dundee, UK

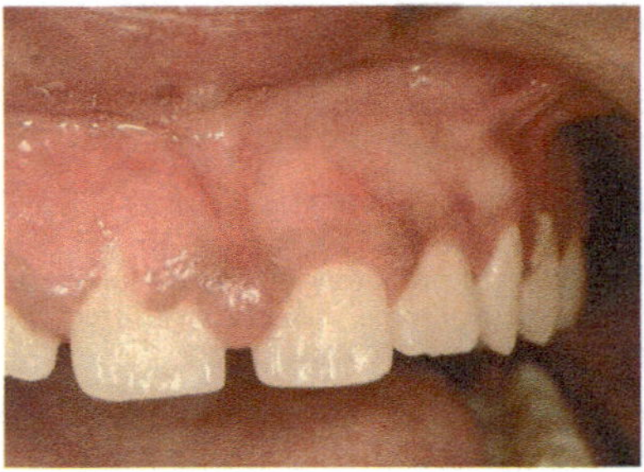

Fig. 10.11 Granulomatosis with polyangiitis presenting with gum infiltration.
Reproduced courtesy of Ruth Murphy, Consultant Dermatologist, Royal Hallamshire Hospital, Sheffield, UK

Infections
Candidiasis and mucocutaneous candidiasis (Fig. 10.8), HSV, chickenpox.

Strawberry tongue
Seen in Kawasaki's disease and streptococcal infections such as scarlatina (Fig. 10.10).

White tongue
Causes: Candida albicans infections, leukoplakia, lichen planus, white sponge naevus.

Tumours
- ➲ See Tumours (lumps and bumps), p. 145.

Gum enlargement
Due to hypertrophy or infiltration.

Always look for an underlying cause:
- Drugs (e.g. phenytoin, ciclosporin).
- Scurvy.
- Leukaemia.
- Sarcoidosis.
- Granulomatosis with polyangiitis (Fig. 10.11).
- Amyloidosis.
- Congenital epulis is a benign firm pink tumour arising from gum, which often regresses with time.
- Tuberous sclerosis complex (➲ see Chapter 32)—gingival fibromas.

Other oral changes

Dry mouth (xerostomia)
Rare in children and associated with impairment of salivary glands.
Congenital: hypoplastic salivary glands.

Acquired: dehydration, drugs, collagen vascular diseases especially Sjögren's syndrome, neurological, obstruction of salivary ducts, endocrine (hypothyroidism, diabetes mellitus), dietary (anaemia, vitamin deficiencies), post-irradiation, graft-versus-host disease.

Lichenoid reactions in the mouth

- *Allergy to dental products containing amalgam*—may cause lichenoid type reactions that mimic lichen planus. Seen adjacent to dental fillings on buccal mucosa and tongue. Refer to dermatology for patch testing to mercury salts.
- *Lichen planus*—rare in children and usually associated with underlying disease (e.g. hypothyroidism).
  Note: cheek biting is often mistaken for lichen planus. This occurs at the site of the occlusal ridge and is commonest on the buccal mucosa adjacent to the molars.
- *Systemic lupus erythematosus*—may present with lichenoid type reactions on the tongue, lips, and buccal mucosa with or without ulceration. Check antinuclear antibodies (ANA) and carry out multisystem enquiry (➲ see Chapter 38).
- *Graft-versus-host disease*—in chronic cases lichenoid oral lesions occur in conjunction with sclerodermatous skin changes. A history of blood and marrow transplantation identifies the diagnosis (➲ see also Chapter 39).

Pigmentary changes

- ➲ See also Chapters 31–37.

These changes are often diagnostic of underlying genetic or systemic disease. To aid diagnosis it is important to examine the whole skin especially the groin, axilla, and palms.

- *Brown/blue-black*.
  Generalized: Addison's disease, drugs.
  Focal: amalgam tattoo; lentigines (freckles)—particularly lips and perioral; Peutz–Jegher syndrome (➲ see Fig. 33.5); melanoma (very rare); naevus of Ota (➲ see Chapter 35); Carney complex (➲ see Chapter 33, Vitamin deficiencies, p. 494); leukaemic deposits.
  Drugs, e.g. minocycline, amiodarone. Lead and bismuth poisoning cause a blue line along gums.
  Metabolic, e.g. alkaptonuria with ochronosis (➲ see Chapters 9 and 35).
- *Red/blue or purple*—infantile haemangiomas (➲ see Chapter 8): vascular anomalies (e.g. port-wine stains, venous anomalies); hereditary haemorrhagic telangiectasia: purpura (➲ see Section 6); early viral lesions such as hand, foot, and mouth (➲ see Chapter 22); purple/blue lesions especially if palatal/uvular consider Kaposi's sarcoma in HIV caused by HSV-8; or blue rubber bleb naevus syndrome (➲ see Purple and non-blanching (purpuric) lesions, p. 424).
- *White*—vitiligo (➲ see Chapter 32); lip/cheek biting; lichen planus (rare), a lacey white appearance (➲ see Non-infective causes, pp. 285–8); Koplik's spots (➲ see Disorders affecting the palate, p. 146); leukoplakia (rare, usually teens) associated with many diseases including dyskeratosis congenita (usually X-linked); pachyonychia congenita (usually A/D) (➲ p. 389); candidiasis; tumours (e.g. white sponge naevus); skin diseases

(psoriasis, systemic lupus erythematosus, lichen sclerosus, Darier's disease); secondary syphilis.

Perioral skin disease

For causes of perioral skin disease, see Box 10.1 and ➲ Chapter 9.

Box 10.1 Perioral problems

Common

- Herpes simplex virus (primary and recurrent).
- Impetigo—golden crusts and fissuring.
- Eczema both atopic (lick eczema) and irritant/contact allergy.
- Factitious disease (dermatitis artefacta) (➲ see Chapter 24).
- Acne vulgaris (➲ see Chapter 18).
- Angioedema (➲ see Chapter 21).
- Angular cheilitis.
- Freckling (also rarely in some genetic disorders) (➲ see Chapter 33).
- Spider naevi, infantile haemangiomas, port-wine stains (➲ see Chapter 8).
- Moles (➲ see Chapter 34).
- Vitiligo (➲ see Chapter 32).
- Warts of all types including molluscum contagiosum.

Uncommon to rare

- Angiofibromas (*syn. adenoma sebaceum*) in tuberous sclerosis complex (➲ see Chapter 32).
- Child abuse.
- Dental sinus.
- Granulomatous cheilitis—swelling of lips and surrounding skin.
- Perioral dermatitis—red papules and pustules.
- Other vascular anomalies (e.g. venous or lymphatic or mixed).

Circumoral pallor

- Erythema infectiosum and other viral diseases.
- Scarlatina.
- Atopic eczema (➲ see Chapter 17).

Note: vitiligo (often perioral) is a true loss of pigmentation.

Chapter 11

Trunk and flexures

Introduction

Some truncal skin diseases are very distinctive, e.g. fir-tree pattern of rash in pityriasis rosea (➲ see Fig. 22.7), the whorls and swirls of the pigmentary phase of incontinentia pigmenti or the large brown, hairy patch, usually over the upper shoulder, of Becker's naevus (➲ see Fig. 33.2). This list is not all inclusive and omits many conditions which can occur anywhere on the body.

Red scaly truncal rashes

- ➲ See also Chapter 22.

Common

Eczema (➲ see Chapter 17)

- ***Seborrhoeic*** pattern on central chest and back plus flexures of trunk.
- *Atopic*—anywhere on trunk, usually also limb flexures and face.

Pityriasis rosea

A single red to salmon-coloured herald patch with fine scales, which predates oval pink lesions in 'fir-tree' pattern on back in the distribution of Langer's lines (➲ see Figs. 22.7 and 4.9) in a 'T-shirt and shorts' distribution, i.e. not on lower arms or legs and never on palms or soles (unlike syphilis). However, atypical, more widespread forms may occur in Africans and Asians. Some children feel unwell for a few days prior to developing the rash with headache, fever, and joint pain.

Cause: Viral aetiology but none yet identified.

Treatment: Rash is self-limiting, give reassurance and education in general. Erythromycin has been shown to reduce time to resolution.

Pityriasis versicolor

The colour of the rash varies with skin type from brown, pale pink to white patches (Fig. 11.1). It occurs on the upper trunk and upper arms in a 'T-shirt' pattern and does not usually extend below the waist. There

Fig. 11.1 Pityriasis versicolor.

Reproduced courtesy of Susan Lewis-Jones, Hon Consultant Dermatologist, Ninewells Hospital and Medical School, Dundee, UK

is very fine surface scaling. It is mainly seen in adults, occasionally adolescents. Wood's lamp examination shows a coppery orange fluorescence.

Cause: *Malassezia furfur* (a yeast). Skin scrapings treated with potassium hydroxide (KOH) and stained with diluted (10%) blue ink show the typical 'spaghetti and meatball' appearance of spores and hyphae on microscopy.

Treatment: topical imidazole cream (twice daily for 4 weeks) or undiluted selenium sulphide shampoo overnight (bright orange), repeated 1 week later. In extensive, resistant cases (e.g. due to immunosuppression), oral itraconazole or fluconazole may be used.

Note: the pale colour is due to 'bleaching' of the skin and will not disappear following treatment until further light-exposure occurs.

Psoriasis

- ➲ See Psoriasis, pp. 320–1.
- *Plaque type*: typically lumbar area, affecting elbows, knees, and scalp but can be very generalized in severe cases (➲ see Fig. 22.1).
- *Guttate (raindrop) type*: small red, scaly lesions on trunk, less on limbs (➲ see Fig. 22.3).

Scabies

Very itchy, often with generalized scaling, erythema, and sometimes hives (urticarial lesions). Burrows rarely occur on the trunk but usually hands, feet, and penis (➲ see Figs. 22.13 and 22.14). Nodules sometimes occur in axillae, groin, and genitals (➲ see Fig. 28.14). Typically spares the face and scalp except in babies.

Tinea corporis

Annular lesions with central clearing and red, scaly borders, sometimes with pustules, on trunk and limbs (➲ see Fig. 22.8).

Viral exanthems

Viral exanthems often start on the trunk (➲ see Red viral exanthemas, pp. 326–30).

Uncommon to rare

Mycosis fungoides

Cutaneous T-cell lymphoma. Pale to dusky red, oval, or digitate well-defined patches with slight surface scaling and a cigarette-paper wrinkling on lateral light (➲ see Mycosis fungoides, p. 340).

Pityriasis lichenoides

Small circular scaly purplish lesions healing to leave scars. Acute and chronic forms may coexist. Also affects buttocks and limbs, rarely face (➲ see Pityriasis lichenoides, p. 287).

Syphilis

Rash of secondary syphilis is very variable with macules, papules, pustules, sometimes plaques. The colour ranges from shades of pink to purplish or yellow/brown (➲ see Syphilis, p. 336).

Papular and pustular rashes

- ➲ See also Chapters 19 and 20.

Common

- *Acne vulgaris* (➲ see Chapter 18).
- *Folliculitis* (➲ see Chapter 20).
- *Insect bites* (➲ see Figs. 19.4 and 20.5).
- *Molluscum contagiosum* (➲ see Figs. 9.7 and 19.1).

Blisters

- ➲ See also Chapter 25.

Common

- *Varicella-zoster*
  - *Chickenpox:* mainly concentrated on trunk and face, less on limbs (➲ see Figs. 9.1 and 25.3).
  - *Shingles*: dermatomal distribution (➲ see Fig. 25.5).
- *Impetigo*: particularly in flexures (➲ see Fig. 25.1).
- *Insect bites* (➲ see Figs. 19.4 and 20.5).

Uncommon to rare

- ➲ See also Chapter 25.
- *Chronic bullous disease of childhood*—may concentrate around umbilicus.
- *Pemphigus vulgaris.*

Lumps, bumps, and other lesions

- ➲ See also Chapter 28.

Common

- *Accessory nipples*—in line below nipples. May be unilateral, bilateral, or multiple. More obvious after puberty and often mistaken for moles.
- *Haemangiomas and vascular malformations* (➲ see Chapter 8).
- *Moles*—several types of various colours (➲ see Chapter 34).
- *Neurofibromas* (➲ see Fig. 28.2) soft, fleshy lesions.
- *Warts*—particularly molluscum contagiosum (➲ see Figs. 9.8 and 19.1).

Uncommon to rare

- *Becker's naevus*—large, hairy brown patch commonest on posterior shoulder and mainly in young males (➲ see Fig. 33.2).
- *Connective tissue naevi*—firm lumpy skin-coloured areas (➲ see Fig. 29.14 and Colour, pp. 419–27).
- *Papular rashes*—e.g. lichen nitidus (➲ see Fig. 19.5).
- *Sternal pits*—sometimes associated with other syndromes, e.g. PHACES syndrome (➲ see Fig. 8.8)
- *Xanthomas*—various types, including eruptive (often on buttocks; ➲ see Figs. 5.3 and 37.2).

Colour changes

- See Section 6.
- *Red*—see Chapter 11. Whole trunk is red in erythroderma (see Fig. 22.17 and Chapter 22, Generalized redness, p. 341).
- *Blue*—Mongolian blue spots (always on dorsal trunk) (see Figs. 7.5 and 24.2); naevus of Ito (see p. 510) usually upper trunk (rare).
- *Black*—moles, malignant melanomas, and thrombosed lesions (see Chapters 34 and 35).
- *Brown*—moles, café-au-lait macules (see Fig. 33.3), pigmentary mosaicism (many causes—see Chapters 33 and 34).
- *White* (see Chapter 32) vitiligo, postinflammatory especially after eczema or psoriasis; scars; albinism; pityriasis versicolor (Fig. 11.1); leprosy; piebaldism (diamond shaped on anterior trunk) rare.
- *Yellow*—xanthomas and juvenile xanthogranulomas (see Figs. 28.11 and 37.3; see also Chapter 37).

Flexural skin problems

The flexures of the body include the neck, postauricular areas, axillae, groin, and natal cleft, antecubital and popliteal fossae, and anterior ankles and ventral wrists (Fig. 11.2). Some conditions such as atopic eczema (see Atopic eczema/dermatitis, pp. 245–52), flexural psoriasis (see Psoriasis—clinical variants, pp. 322–4, and Fig. 11.3), and hidradenitis suppurativa (see pp. 157–8) typically affect the flexures (Box 11.1). Most are dealt with elsewhere in this book. For diseases in the genital areas, see Chapter 13.

Intertrigo

Itchy/sore red rash in moist flexural areas often with secondary candidiasis. Commoner in diabetics or under appliances (e.g. tracheostomy tubes, colostomy bags).

Uncommon to rare flexural skin disorders

- *Acanthosis nigricans*—pigmentation of neck, groin, axillae (see Fig. 33.6).
- *Erythrasma*—rare in childhood (see Uncommon to rare causes, pp. 167–9).
- *Hidradenitis suppurativa* (see next section).
- *Hailey–Hailey disease*—rare genetic blistering disorder of flexures (see p. 389).
- *Langerhans cell histiocytosis*—may mimic seborrhoeic eczema (see pp. 182–3 and Fig. 13.5).
- *Rare acquired autoimmune blistering disorders* (see Chapters 12 and 25).
  - Chronic bullous disease of childhood: often around genital area.
  - Linear IgA disease.
  - Bullous pemphigoid: may present in genital area in children.
  - Pemphigus vulgaris: more typically trunk and mouth.

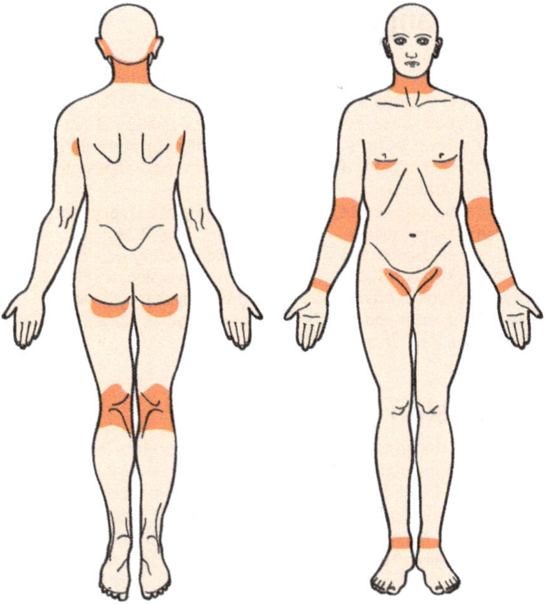

Fig. 11.2 Flexural distribution of skin disease.

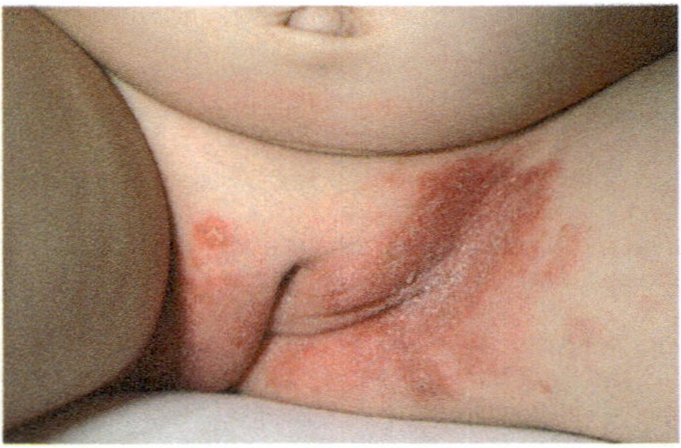

Fig. 11.3 Flexural psoriasis.

Reproduced courtesy of Susan Lewis-Jones, Hon Consultant Dermatologist, Ninewells Hospital and Medical School, Dundee, UK

Box 11.1 Common diseases affecting the flexures

- Atopic eczema (➲ see Chapter 17)—mainly limbs, neck, and retroauricular but not usually axillae and groin.
- Psoriasis—axillae, groin/genital area (➲ see Fig. 11.3), retroauricular.
- Seborrhoeic eczema—axillae and neck, sometimes groin (➲ see Infantile seborrheic eczema, p. 260).
- Hyperhidrosis (➲ see Disorders of sweating, pp. 11–13).
- Intertrigo (➲ see Intertrigo, p. 155).
- Impetigo (➲ see Infections causing blisters, pp. 378–82).
- Vitiligo (➲ see Chapter 32).
- Scabetic nodules (➲ see Chapter 19 and Fig. 28.14).

Hidradenitis suppurativa

Recurrent abscesses, boils, keloid scarring, and sometimes discharging sinus tract formation in anogenital, axillary, and submammary areas (may be localized to one area). Comedones are common and typically in adjacent interconnecting pairs (bridge comedones). It is mainly seen in postpubertal females, often overweight. There is significant morbidity and quality of life impairment associated with this chronic disease.

Cause: destruction of hair follicles, possibly due to comedonal occlusion with secondary bacterial infection. It is sometimes familial and may be associated with severe nuchal acne and conglobate acne and autoinflammatory syndromes SAPHO, PAPA, and PASH (➲ see Chapters 18 and 21).

Differential diagnosis: Crohn's disease; actinomycosis; lymphogranuloma venereum (*Chlamydia trachomatis*); granuloma inguinale syn. donovanosis (*Calymmatobacterium granulomatis*). All are very rare in children.

Management is very difficult:

First-line

- Take lesional and nasal bacteriological swabs to exclude *Staphylococcus aureus* carriage (although this may also be secondary event).
- It is vital to encourage weight loss and avoid smoking.
- Local hygiene measures and antiseptics for washing and in emollients and dressings.
- Topical clindamycin helps some mild cases. Try systemic antibiotics (e.g. erythromycin for at least 6 weeks).[1]
- Monitor improvement by using a patient diary of numbers and size of lesions. Assess quality of life (➲ see Chapter 2), as can cause severe loss of confidence and depression. May need psychosocial intervention. Refer to a dermatologist if no improvement.

Second-line (specialist only)

- Systemic retinoid therapy (isotretinoin) may help.
- Hormonal therapy, e.g. Dianette® (females only), especially if there is significant worsening perimenstrually.
- Dapsone 50–100mg daily with appropriate monitoring (side effects: haemolytic anaemia; methaemoglobinaemia; neuropathy).

- The biological anti-TNF agent, adalimumab, is licensed in the United Kingdom to treat patients from 12y with moderately severe unresponsive disease.[1]
- Surgery is a last resort, which should be avoided in children although local abscesses may require surgical lancing.

References

1. European Dermatology Forum, http://www.euroderm.org/edf/index.php/edf-guidelines/category/5-guidelines-miscellaneous

Chapter 12

Hands, feet, and limbs

Introduction

This chapter covers skin diseases that are typically found on the hands, feet, and limbs. For diseases of the nails, ➲ see Chapter 15.

Hands

Blisters

Common

- ***Bites***: particularly mosquito bites (➲ see Fig. 20.5).
- ***Burns, scalds, and non-accidental injuries*** (➲ see Chapter 24).
- ***Contact allergy*** (➲ see Chapter 17).
- ***Erythema multiforme***: target lesions in acral distribution sometimes blistered centrally (➲ see Fig. 4.12, Chapter 10, and Chapter 25, Varicella-zoster virus, p. 380).
- ***Herpes simplex infections***: painful and recur in same site (Fig. 12.1).
- ***Impetigo***: always check for underlying scabies (➲ see Infections causing blisters, pp. 378–82).
- ***Phytophotodermatitis***: from plants (➲ see Fig. 16.7).
- ***Pompholyx***: sides of fingers, very itchy (also on soles; ➲ see Fig. 17.14).
- ***Scabies***: itchy tiny vesicles in finger webs particularly and in infants typically on soles. It is often confused with pompholyx. Also look for burrows (➲ see Infestations, pp. 337–8 and Fig. 22.14).
- ***Stevens–Johnson syndrome*** (➲ see Chapters 10 and 23).
- ***Sunburn***: on dorsa with sparing between fingers, redness, and painful swelling which can blister if severe (➲ see Chapter 16).
- ***Viral exanthems***: e.g. hand, foot, and mouth (Fig. 12.2; ➲ see also Infections causing blisters, pp. 378–82).

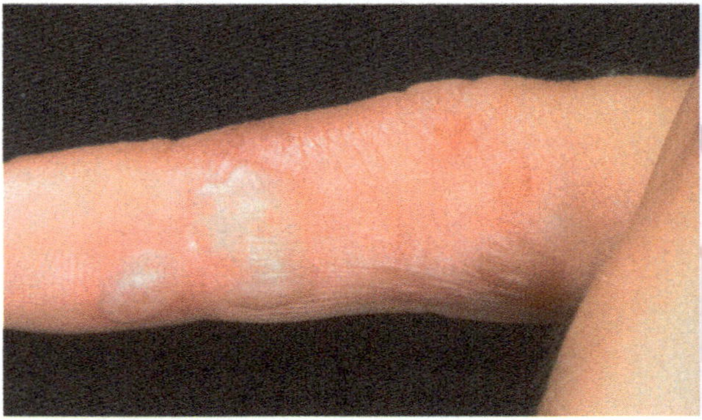

Fig. 12.1 Herpes simplex blisters on finger.
Reproduced courtesy of NHS Tayside Clinical Photography, Dundee, UK

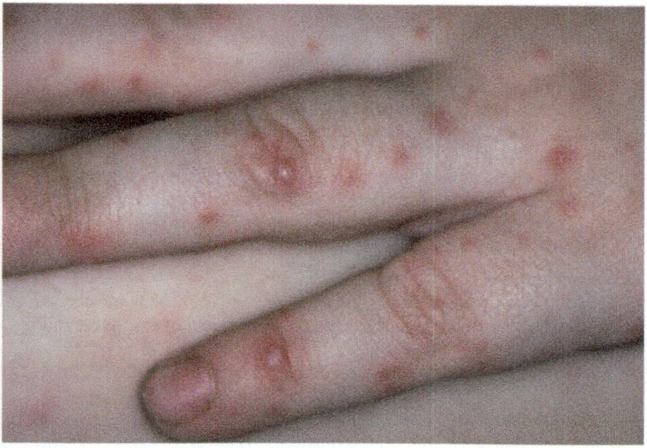

Fig. 12.2 Hand, foot, and mouth disease. Small, oval shaped pearly-grey blisters with surrounding erythema, all lesions are similar (monomorphic rash).

Reproduced courtesy of Susan Lewis-Jones, Hon Consultant Dermatologist, Ninewells Hospital and Medical School, Dundee, UK

Uncommon to rare

- *Epidermolysis bullosa dystrophica*: fusion of fingers (and toes) often occurs, giving a mitt appearance (➲ see Genetic causes of blisters, pp. 387–90).
- *Palmoplantar pustulosis*: yellowish blisters fading to brown as they heal, cause is usually psoriasis—very rare in children (➲ see Psoriasis, pp. 320–1).
- *DIRA and DITRA autoinflammatory disorders* (➲ see Chapter 38).
- *Porphyrias*: may present with blisters and erythema, usually on the dorsa of the hands (➲ see Chapter 16).
- *Poxvirus infections*: orf, Milker's nodules (cowpox is very rare) (➲ see Viral infections, pp. 398–401, and Fig. 26.4a and b).

Redness with or without scaling

- ➲ See also Chapter 22.

Common

- *Insect bites*: may be associated with swelling/urticaria and/or a punctum mark. Blisters and papules common (➲ see Figs. 19.4 and 20.5).
- *Drug rashes*: ➲ see Chapter 23.
- *Atopic eczema*: ➲ see Chapter 17. Atopic eczema is often associated with ichthyosis vulgaris (➲ see Fig. 27.2) and hyperlinear palms (➲ see Fig. 17.8).
- *Allergic contact dermatitis (eczema)* (➲ see Fig 2.4) and irritant contact dermatitis (eczema) (➲ see Chapter 17).

- *Peeling of fingertips and palms*:
  - *Poststreptococcal* (often peeling of hands and feet; Fig. 12.3) occurs 10–14 days after infection. Self-limiting. Treat with emollients.
  - *Kawasaki disease* (➲ see Fig. 22.16).
  - *Rare autosomal dominant trait* with recurrent fingertip peeling.
- *Psoriasis*: often affects hands including palms, which may be red and hyperkeratotic (➲ see Chapter 22). For nail changes, ➲ see Fig. 15.7.
- *Stings*: from insects or jellyfish. Associated redness, pain, and swelling. Jellyfish may cause bizarre linear lesions that could be mistaken for abuse (usually on legs while swimming).
- *Sunburn*: ➲ see Chapter 16.

Uncommon to rare

- *Candida*: white scaling, usually between finger-webs following chronic immersion in water; immunosuppression or mucocutaneous candidiasis (➲ see pp. 144–5).
- *Dermatomyositis*: ragged cuticles, redness over knuckles (➲ see Fig. 29.12).
- *Erythromelalgia*: episodic severe pain and burning feeling of hands, feet, and sometimes ears, triggered by heat and relieved by cold. Thought to be vasomotor in origin. Primary form due to *SCN9A* mutations. Secondary form has associations with underlying medical conditions including myeloproliferative disorders.
  Treatment: can include serotonin reuptake inhibitors, tricyclic antidepressants, anticonvulsants, or calcium channel inhibitors.
- *Tinea manuum*: hand ringworm (➲ see Chapter 22).
- *Syphilis*: secondary stage—circular erythematous scaly lesions on palms, soles, and body (➲ see Chapter 22).

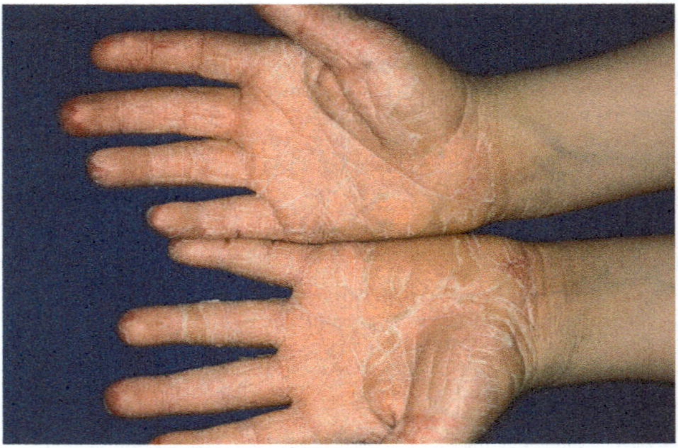

Fig. 12.3 Poststreptococcal peeling—extensive painless desquamation over palms, soles, and pressure areas of knees and anterior ankles.

Reproduced courtesy of Susan Lewis-Jones, Hon Consultant Dermatologist, Ninewells Hospital and Medical School, Dundee, UK

Box 12.1 Causes of palmar (and plantar) erythema (redness)

- Arteriovenous fistulae—associated thrill and warmth (➲ see Chapter 8).
- Atopic eczema (➲ see Chapter 17).
- Carotenaemia (usually more orange) (➲ see Chapter 37).
- Erythromelalgia (rare).
- Juvenile chronic arthritis (➲ see Chapter 38).
- Kawasaki disease (typically swollen sausage fingers, ➲ see Fig. 22.16).
- Liver and renal disease.
- Following streptococcal infections.
- Papular-purpuric 'gloves and socks' purpura (➲ see Chapter 31).
- Psoriasis (➲ see Chapter 22).
- Shoe dermatitis (➲ see Fig. 2.4).
- Autoinflammatory disorders (➲ see Chapters 18, 21, and 38).

Causes of palmar (and plantar) redness

See Box 12.1; for scaling and hyperkeratosis, see Box 12.2.

Other colour changes on hands

- ➲ See also Chapters 31–37.
- ***Whiteness***: vitiligo, lichen sclerosus, Raynaud's disease/syndrome, scars, and postinflammatory.
- ***Brown/black***: Addison's disease (flexural accentuation), café-au-lait macules, moles, freckles. Peutz–Jeghers syndrome (freckles on fingers and lips).
- ***Orange palms***: carotenaemia (common with frequent intake of puréed carrots and broccoli) (➲ see Fig. 37.1). Some hyperkeratotic conditions can appear slightly orange, especially pityriasis rubra pilaris (➲ see Chapter 22) and inherited palmoplantar keratodermas.
- ***Yellow lesions***: on palms—xanthomas (➲ see Metabolic, p. 520).
- ***Blue colour***: cyanosis, drug pigmentation, e.g. minocycline, Mongolian blue spots (rare on hands), blue naevi, vascular anomalies. Raynaud's disease/syndrome (recovery phase).
- ***Purple colour***: vasculitis, chilblains (more commonly feet, ➲ see Fig. 31.9), port-wine stains may appear purple rather than red, especially in the cold.

Box 12.2 Causes of palmoplantar scaling and thickening (keratoderma)

- Psoriasis.
- Some types of eczema (➲ see Chapter 17).
- Various forms of inherited ichthyoses (Fig. 12.4).
- Pityriasis rubra pilaris (rare) (➲ see p. 343).
- Tinea manuum or pedis—typically with *Trichophyton rubrum*.
- Norwegian/crusted scabies (Fig. 12.5; ➲ see also Infestations, pp. 337–8).
- Reactive arthritis (previously known as Reiter's syndrome) (very rare in children).

Palmoplantar keratoderma

Thickening of the skin with scaling and hyperkeratosis (see Box 12.2) may involve the palms, soles (Fig. 12.4), or both. It may be congenital, inherited (many types), or acquired. If severe, it is known as palmoplantar keratoderma (sometimes called tylosis) and this may be localized or include the whole palm or sole. Patterns of keratoderma include:

- Punctate.
- Linear.
- Honeycomb.
- Diffuse.

There may be associated erythema and sometimes the areas extend over the dorsa of hands and feet, and onto the wrists and ankles. This is known as transgrediens. In some inherited types thickened bands develop and constrict the digits, sometimes causing auto-amputation (ainhum). (For peeling of palms and soles, ➲ see Redness with or without scaling, pp. 161–2).

Lumps and bumps on hands

- ➲ See also Chapter 28.

Common

- ***Granuloma annulare***: skin-coloured or slightly purple nodules in annular pattern (➲ see Fig. 28.3).
- ***Knuckle pads***: from friction or biting (➲ see Fig. 24.7).
- ***Viral warts***: verrucae vulgaris (➲ see Fig. 9.5) or planar warts (➲ see Fig. 29.5).

Uncommon to rare

- ***Calcinosis***: occurs on fingers in systemic sclerosis and other connective tissues diseases and there may be associated Raynaud's disease (➲ see Chapter 38).

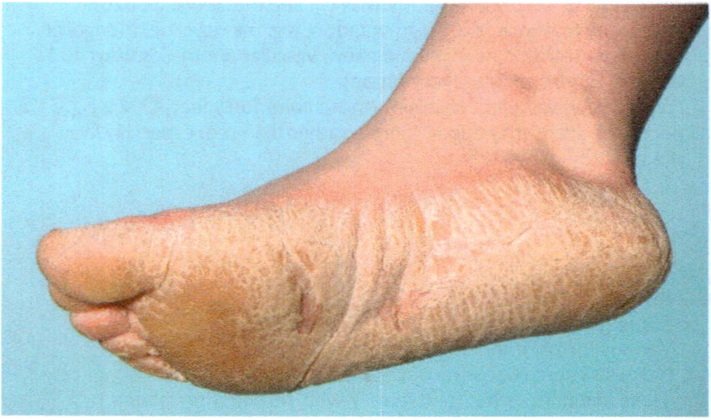

Fig. 12.4 Inherited plantar keratoderma.

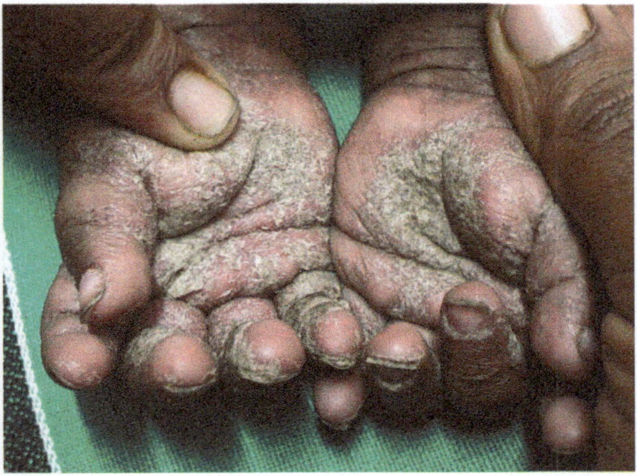

Fig. 12.5 Norwegian or crusted scabies.
Reproduced courtesy of Patrick Yesudian, Consultant Dermatologist, Chennai, India

- ***Fish tank granuloma***: red persistent nodule(s) (Fig. 12.6) which may weep or discharge pus. Rarely new lesions occur proximally along the arm (sporotrichoid spread), caused by *Mycobacterium marinum*. Ask about contact with tropical fish.
  Diagnosis: lesional skin biopsy including microbiological culture*.
  Treatment: long-term minocycline or co-trimoxazole (may require weeks or occasionally months).
- ***Subungual exostosis***: a hard lump usually on a digit or under a nail. There is often hyperkeratosis so may be mistaken for a wart. X-ray shows a bony exostosis (➲ see Fig. 15.10).
- ***Periungual fibroma***: firm nodules around proximal nail folds seen in tuberous sclerosis complex (➲ see TSC, pp. 483–4 and Fig. 15.11).
- ***Gottron's papules***: in dermatomyositis (➲ see Fig. 29.12).
- ***Arsenical keratoses***: seen in chronic exposure, e.g. contaminated water in Bangladesh (➲ see Chapter 33, p. 498).

Other changes

Palmar pits: seen in Darier disease and arsenic poisoning.

* Notify laboratory, as some species require growth at lower temperatures.

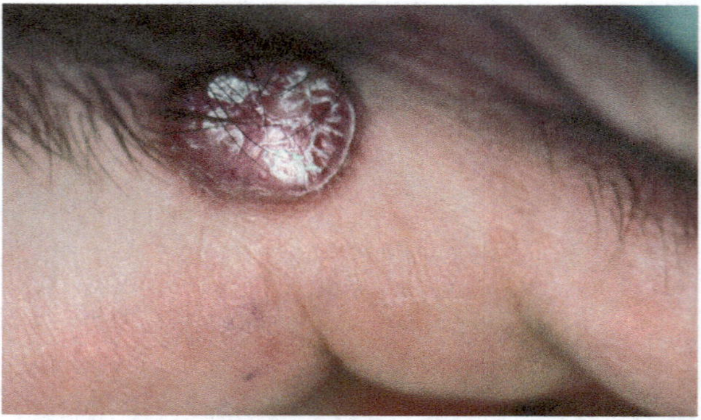

Fig. 12.6 Fish tank granuloma.
Reproduced courtesy of Susan Lewis-Jones, Hon Consultant Dermatologist, Ninewells Hospital and Medical School, Dundee, UK

Feet

Blisters

- See also Chapter 25.

Common

- *Insect bites*: particularly on dorsa and usually with associated redness (also presents as red papules).
- *Frictional*: e.g. shoes.
- *Hand, foot, and mouth disease*: see Fig. 12.2.
- *Impetigo*: often streptococcal, usually in toe-webs—look for underlying tinea pedis (athlete's foot) infection (see Rashes with or without scaling p. 169).
- *Pompholyx*: occurs *de novo* but sometimes associated with contact allergy or tinea pedis (see Fig. 17.14).
- *Scabies*: usually soles, sides of heels and ankles, particularly infants.

Uncommon to rare

- *Acute allergic contact dermatitis*: may blister if severe (see Fig. 2.4 and Chapter 17).
- *Epidermolysis bullosa* (see Chapter 25).
- *Infantile acral pustulosis* (see Chapter 20).
- *Palmoplantar pustulosis*: usually psoriasis (see Chapter 22)—rare in children.

Rashes with or without scaling

Common

- *Atopic eczema*, especially around ankles (see Chapter 17).
- *Chilblains*: mainly toes which look blue/purplish red and feel cold (see Fig. 31.9).

Box 12.3 Severe pain and redness when walking on beach with bare feet

Fish venom, e.g. Weaver fish (largely N. Wales coast in United Kingdom). Others mainly tropical, e.g. stone fish, lionfish, scorpion fish. *Pain is alleviated by hot water since venom is very heat labile.*

- ***Allergic contact dermatitis*** to footwear (➲ see Figs. 2.4 and 2.5).
- ***Foreign body***: usually soles from penetrating injury-painful red area (see also Box 12.3).
- ***Juvenile plantar dermatosis (forefoot eczema)***: affects soles, particularly balls of feet and heels with painful fissuring and scaling (Fig. 12.7) and sometimes shiny appearance. Toe-webs are spared, unlike tinea pedis. Thought to be due to use of modern occlusive footwear. It is commoner in atopics and some cases have associated allergic contact shoe dermatitis (➲ see Figs. 2.4 and 2.5).
  Management: leather shoes (avoid trainers), long cotton socks (to allow evaporation of sweat), emollients, cream impregnated bandages, topical corticosteroids if itchy.
  Investigations: patch testing (➲ see Patch testing, p. 25–6).
- ***Photosensitive rashes***: dorsa feet and toes, including sunburn (➲ see Chapter 16).
- ***Pitted keratolysis***: associated with sweaty feet (➲ see Fig. 1.5).
- ***Psoriasis*** (➲ see Chapter 22).
- ***Raynaud's phenomenon/disease***: usually transient colour changes (➲ see Chapter 29, see also Systemic sclerosis, p. 440).
- ***Sunburn***: mainly dorsa feet; toes may blister if severe.
- ***Tinea pedis***: ringworm of feet (Fig. 12.8; ➲ see Fungal infections of the skin, pp. 330–1) with toe-web scaling and maceration, usually teenagers and may include toenails (➲ see Figs. 15.5 and 15.6). More extensive disease may cause a moccasin pattern of redness and scaling. Differentiate from juvenile plantar dermatosis, which lacks toe-web scaling (➲ see pp. 166–7). Take scrapes for mycological examinations and culture (➲ see Other dermatological investigations, pp. 24–6).

Uncommon to rare causes

- ***Erythrasma***: orange/redness and scaling in toe-webs, (more commonly axillae, groins, and inframammary folds), usually teens and adults. Bright coral pink fluorescence under Wood's light (➲ see p. 19).
  Cause: *Corynebacterium minutissimum*.
  Treatment: topical antibiotics; oral erythromycin.
- ***Erythromelalgia***: episodic painful red/purple colour (➲ see Redness with or without scaling, pp. 161–2).
- ***Larva migrans***: occurs on feet, buttocks, back of legs, and trunk after walking, sitting, or lying unprotected on contaminated sand above the water line in endemic areas (usually Africa, W. Indies). May be caused by several types of hookworm larvae (usually cat or dog) that burrow through skin producing itchy, erythematous, serpiginous (snake-like) lesions, sometimes with blisters (➲ see Fig. 4.14).

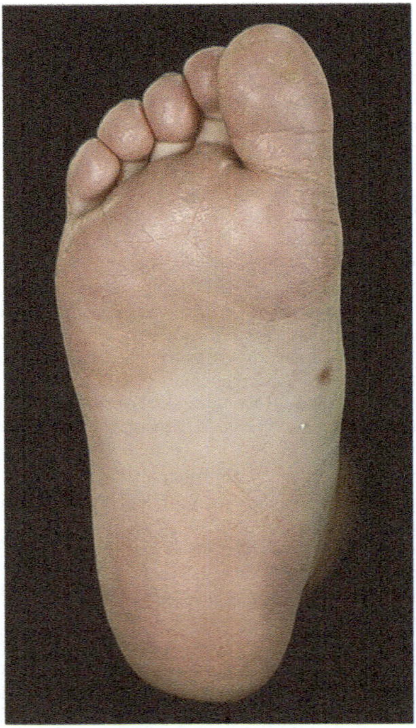

Fig. 12.7 Severe forefoot eczema.
Reproduced courtesy of NHS Tayside Clinical Photography, Dundee, UK

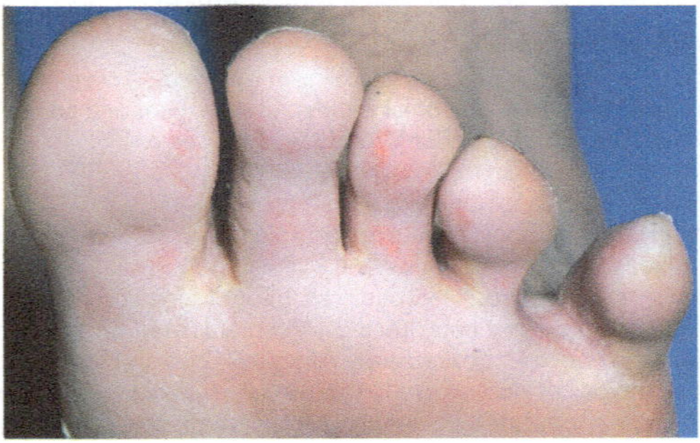

Fig. 12.8 Tinea pedis with involvement of toe-webs.
Reproduced courtesy of Susan Lewis-Jones, Hon Consultant Dermatologist, Ninewells Hospital and Medical School, Dundee, UK

Treatment: Single dose of ivermectin (12mg) is most effective or topical albendazole 10–15% twice daily for 10 days (when available); oral albendazole for 4 days.

- ***Keratoderma blenorrhagica***: often pustular lesions with a thick yellow crust found on the soles, a classical additional feature of reactive arthritis (previously Reiter's disease). Rare in children.
- ***Fish venom***: causes acute pain on venom injection from spines, see Box 12.3.

Redness of soles

- See Box 12.1.

Redness and hyperkeratosis affecting the soles

- See Box 12.2.

Other colour changes on feet

- ***Black heels***: (Talon noir) bleeding into skin due to constant trauma from footwear, particularly during sports (➲ see Chapter 35 and Fig. 35.3). Black spots in viral warts are due to thrombosed feeding capillaries (Fig. 12.9). Both may be mistaken for a mole or melanoma.
- ***Purple***: e.g. vasculitis and chilblains, ➲ see Chapter 31.
- ***White***: e.g. vitiligo; postinflammatory depigmentation, ➲ see Chapter 32.
- ***Brown***: e.g. moles; postinflammatory hyperpigmentation, ➲ see Chapter 33.
- ***Blue***: e.g. blue naevi (➲ Fig. 35.1); venous anomalies (➲ see Figs. 8.17 and 8.18; see also Chapters 8 and 35).
- ***Yellow/orange***: hyperkeratosis of soles; carotenaemia, ➲ see Chapter 37.

Swelling (oedema) of the feet

- ➲ See Lymphoedema, p. 191.

Lumps and bumps on feet

Common

- ***Corns***: painful slightly yellow hyperkeratosis distinguished from warts by paring, which shows no loss of skin ridge marks.
- ***Viral warts***: often painful on soles. They may be large and mosaic, sometimes having black dots on the surface (thrombosed vessels) that can cause confusion with moles and melanoma (Fig. 12.9).
- ***Granuloma annulare***: skin-coloured or red/purple nodules in annular distribution (➲ see Diabetes mellitus, pp. 60–2, see also Fig. 5.1 and Fig. 28.3).

Uncommon to rare

- ***Subungual exostosis***: hard bony lump, distorting the nail (➲ see Fig. 15.10).
- ***Digital fibromatosis***: firm, slow growing warty lesions usually on toes, which tend to recur after excision. Although considered benign, they can locally progress but surgery should be avoided (➲ see Chapter 29 and Fig. 29.15). Usually resolve spontaneously.
- ***Plantar fibromatosis (syn. Ledderhose's disease)***: very rare progressive fibromatosis similar to digital type but involving plantar fascia and causing

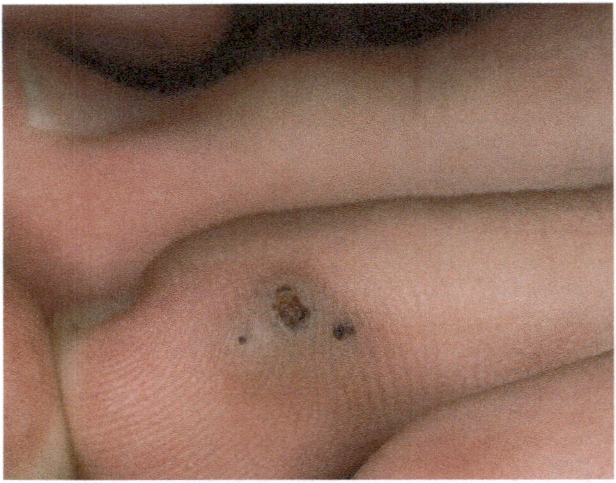

Fig. 12.9 Viral warts with thrombosed vessels.

Reproduced courtesy of Susan Lewis-Jones, Hon Consultant Dermatologist, Ninewells Hospital and Medical School, Dundee, UK

slowly progressive nodules on instep. Surgical intervention is difficult and lesions may recur.

- *Diffuse thickening or hyperkeratosis (keratoderma)*: several rare inherited types occur but it may also occur in certain skin diseases such as psoriasis (Box 12.2 and Fig. 12.4).
- *Jiggers (tungiasis)*: small intensely itchy pea-sized inflamed lesions on feet (97%) and other exposed sites after walking on infested sand (S. America, sub-Saharan Africa). Female sand flea burrows under skin, laying eggs over 2 weeks, then dies. Secondary infection common. Associated with poverty and much morbidity. Ask about foreign travel. *Treatment*: surgical removal often impractical. Use occlusion, e.g. 20% petroleum jelly. Benzyl benzoate. Treat secondary infection.

Arms and legs

Most skin rashes and lesions can present on the limbs. Those typically presenting on the wrists are shown in Box 12.4, and those on the arms in Box 12.5.

Colour changes on limbs

- ➲ See also Chapters 31–37.
- *White skin*: vitiligo, scars, and postinflammatory, ➲ see Chapter 32.

Box 12.4 Rashes typically found on wrists

- *Atopic eczema*—often affects whole wrists.
- *Scabies* (ventral)—look for burrows.
- *Lichen planus* (ventral)—rare in children.
- *Watch-strap dermatitis*—contact allergy to strap.
- *Self-inflicted scars*—white scars from attempted suicides or cutting in an obsessive-compulsive disorder, usually ventral forearms, wrists.

Box 12.5 Rashes typically found on arms

- *Keratosis pilaris*—small papules on upper outer arms.
- *Insect bites*.
- *Self-inflicted scars*—see Box 12.4.
- *Atopic eczema* is typically in the ante-cubital fossae and wrists but often in an extensor pattern in infants.
- *Freckles*—extensor aspects.
- *Photosensitive rashes*—extensor aspects arms.
- *Psoriasis*—classically extensor aspects, especially elbows
- *Dermatitis herpetiformis*—itchy blisters and redness on elbows.

- *Purple/blue*: perniosis, e.g. cold patches on lateral thighs—horse rider's chilblains (➲ see Chapter 31).
- *Redness*: vascular changes (➲ see Chapter 8).

Lumps and bumps

- ➲ See Chapter 28.

Diseases typically seen on lower legs

- *Ankles and lower legs*: see also Box 12.6 (shins) and Box 12.7 (calves)
- *Atopic eczema* (➲ see Chapter 17).
- *Capillaritis*: purple/brown pigmentation caused by capillary leakage (➲ see Fig. 31.6).
- *Drug rashes*: often start on trunk but migrate to legs as they clear.
- *Erythema nodosum*: usually shins but can occur elsewhere on body (Box 12.6 and Fig. 12.10; ➲ see also Chapter 28).
- *Folliculitis*: (➲ see pp. 293–4) commonly from shaving or waxing or wearing tight jeans. Also seen in association with atopic eczema, especially with occlusive bandages and the use of potent topical corticosteroids.
- *Infections*: such as cellulites, erysipelas, tinea, cutaneous tuberculosis, or necrotizing fasciitis (latter very rare).
- *Insect bites*: itchy papules or blisters, often clustered together (➲ see Figs. 19.4 and 20.5. See also Papular urticaria, p. 284).
- *Jellyfish stings*: uncommon in United Kingdom, usually seen in swimmers.
- *Lumps and bumps*: e.g. warts, dermatofibroma (➲ see Figs. 28.9 and 28.10).
- *Leg ulceration*: numerous causes (➲ see Chapter 30) mainly infective, neuropathic, traumatic, or vascular.

Box 12.6 Skin changes typically occurring on shins

- *Bruising* (➲ see Chapter 31).
- *Atopic eczema* (➲ see Chapter 17)
- *Contact dermatitis*, e.g. from shin guards—may be due to allergy or irritancy. Worse in atopics (➲ see Chapters 2 and 17).
- *Ehlers–Danlos syndrome*—may present with apparent bruises on shins and marked atrophic scars (➲ see Fig. 24.3).
- *Epidermolysis bullosa*—dominant dystrophic type-bruises and scarring as above (➲ see Chapter 25).
- *Erythema nodosum*—tender red nodules lasting about 10 days (Fig. 12.10).
- *Folliculitis*—with occlusive bandaging or after shaving.
- *Granuloma annulare*—unusual rare presentation with deep, hard often irregular, skin-coloured nodules; may be mistaken for tumours (➲ see Fig. 5.1 and Fig. 28.3).
- *Necrobiosis lipoidica diabeticorum*—annular lesions (➲ see Fig. 5.2).
- *Pretibial myxoedema*—redness and induration, exceptionally rare in children.

Box 12.7 Skin changes typically seen on calves

- *Erythema induratum*—rare in United Kingdom but common where tuberculosis (TB) is rife. Can be anywhere on lower legs (➲ see TB skin diseases, pp. 333–5).
- *Panniculitis*—several rare types (erythema nodosum is the only common childhood type but tends to be on shins).

- *Lichen aureus*: golden brown discoloured patch typically around ankles caused by localized capillaritis (➲ see Fig. 31.6).
- *Lymphoedema*:
  - *Primary*: several types, e.g. Milroy's disease (autosomal dominant)—swelling of leg usually from birth (➲ see also Chapter 8).
  - *Secondary*: rare in children. Caused by lymphatic damage or blockage, e.g. postsurgery or radiation, parasitic infections such as onchocerciasis (➲ see Infestations and parasites, pp. 283–5) or other filarial infections.
  - *Podoconiosis*: a non-infective type with genetic predisposition. Walking barefoot allows penetration of silica crystals damaging lymphatics, eventually irreversibly (highlands of tropical Africa, Central America, NW India, prevalence 5–10%). Causes much morbidity. *Management*: (➲ see also Chapter 8) using footwear is vital for prevention.
- *Non-accidental injury* (see Chapter 24).
- *Psoriasis*: typically knees but plaques often all over legs (➲ see Chapter 22).

- ***Purpura and vasculitis***: commonest sites are lower legs and feet (➲ see Cutaneous vasculitis, pp. 470–2).
- ***Vascular anomalies***: (➲ see Chapter 8) many types, e.g. Klippel–Trenaunay syndrome (capillary, venous, lymphatic malformation with port-wine stain and enlarged limb); arteriovenous anastomosis (look for warmth and thrill/bruit).

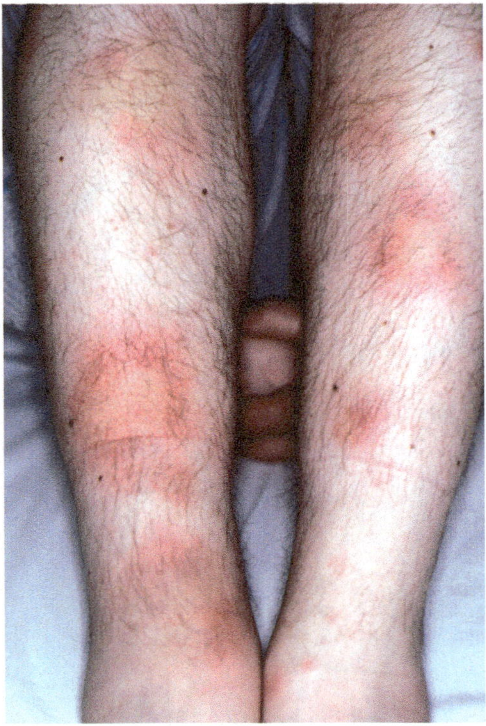

Fig. 12.10 Erythema nodosum of the shins showing typical red nodules.

Reproduced courtesy of Susan Lewis-Jones, Hon Consultant Dermatologist, Ninewells Hospital and Medical School, Dundee, UK

Chapter 13

Genital skin disorders

Introduction

Genital problems in childhood are less common than in adults and occur more frequently in females than males. The poorly oestrogenized skin of prepubertal females protects against chronic *Candida* infection but may predispose girls to conditions not seen in adulthood (e.g. labial adhesions).

Nappy rash (*syn.* napkin dermatitis)

A red rash in the genital area of infants and babies is common and can be due to many conditions (Table 13.1 and Box 13.1). Investigations are rarely warranted.

Napkin dermatitis

- ➲ See also Chapter 7.

Napkin dermatitis is a sore, itchy, sometimes eroded rash with relative sparing of the intertriginous folds (Fig. 13.1). Extremely common, although incidence is falling, due mainly to the introduction of disposable nappies.

Variants
- *'Tide-water' mark dermatitis*—mild, can be caused by friction from nappy borders along lower abdomen and inner thighs.
- *Jacquet's dermatitis* (Fig. 13.2) severe erosive form—rarely seen.
- *Gluteal granulomas*—seen in conjunction with potent topical corticosteroid use (➲ see Complications, p. 176).

Treatment: simple measures are best and avoid provoking factors:
- Change nappy frequently.
- Avoid tight fitting waterproof pants.
- Allow time without the nappy each day.
- Regular cleansing with water, avoiding soaps and antiseptic wipes.
- Regular use of barrier creams after cleansing (e.g. zinc cream/ointment).
- If very inflamed, use short-term mild topical corticosteroid (1% hydrocortisone cream) or corticosteroid/antiyeast preparation.

Complications
- Secondary infection with *Candida* (common).
- Contact allergic dermatitis to topical applications and/or nappies (uncommon)—requires patch testing (➲ see Chapter 2).
- Gluteal granulomata—purplish painless nodules regress spontaneously over weeks to months (rare). It is associated with the use of potent topical corticosteroids.

Box 13.1 Napkin dermatitis: main causative factors
- Prolonged contact with faeces, urine, and chemical irritants, particularly astringent wipes.
- Friction.
- Excessive hydration.
- Increased temperature.
- Infection.

Table 13.1 Differential diagnosis of nappy rashes

Condition affecting the nappy area	Distribution	Investigations	Pathogenesis	Treatment	Prognosis
Napkin dermatitis	Convex surfaces. Flexures spared	None	Irritant contact dermatitis	Barrier creams	Excellent
Candidiasis	Convex surfaces and flexures	Swab for yeasts. Microscopical examination of skin scraping in 20% KOH	Secondary candidal infection	Topical antiyeast creams, e.g. clotrimazole	Excellent
Seborrhoeic dermatitis	Flexures	None	*Pityrosporum ovale*	Emollients, mild topical corticosteroids, corticosteroid/antiyeast combination product	Excellent
Intertrigo	Flexures	None, bacterial and candidal swabs	Infection with yeasts	Careful hygiene, corticosteroid/antiyeast/antibacterial combination product	Excellent
Psoriasis	Any site, often confluent areas	None	Part of the spectrum of psoriasis	Emollients, topical corticosteroid/tacrolimus	Poor
Staphylococcal scalded skin syndrome	Inguinal areas initially	'Skin snip'	Proteases from *Staph. Aureus* or *Streptococcus pyogenes*	Systemic antibiotics	Excellent (if treated correctly)
Langerhans cell histiocytosis	Inguinal areas and flexures	Skin biopsy	Proliferation of Langerhans cells	Topical corticosteroids, for cutaneous disease	Varies depending on degree of organ involvement
Zinc or biotin deficiency	Flexures	Measure zinc and/or biotin levels		Replacement	Excellent

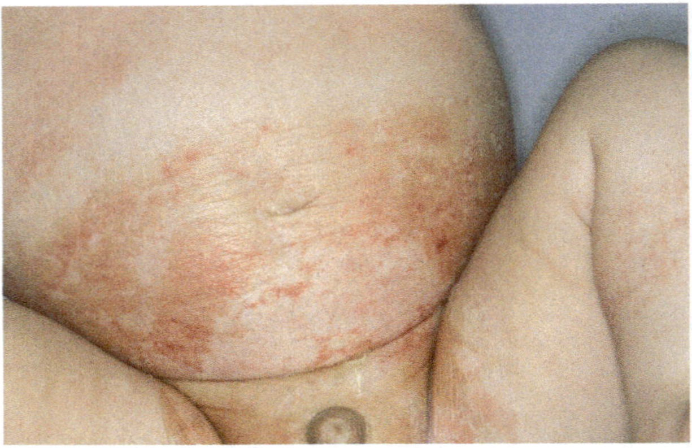

Fig. 13.1 Mild irritant napkin dermatitis with erythema and a slightly glazed appearance, with sharp borders of contact.

Reproduced courtesy of Susan Lewis-Jones, Hon Consultant Dermatologist, Ninewells Hospital and Medical School, Dundee, UK

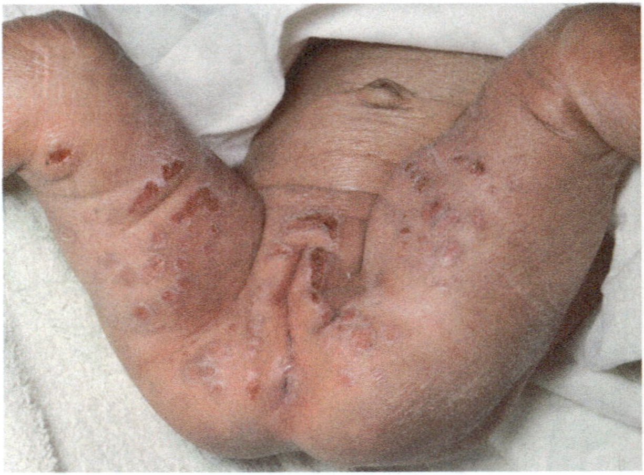

Fig. 13.2 Severe irritant napkin dermatitis with Jacquet's ulcers. Note shiny appearance and relative sparing of skin folds.

Reproduced courtesy of Susan Lewis-Jones, Hon Consultant Dermatologist, Ninewells Hospital and Medical School, Dundee, UK

Differential diagnosis

- See Box 13.2 and Table 13.1.

Candidiasis (*syn.* thrush)

Red, scaly napkin dermatitis which includes intertriginous areas (Fig. 13.3). Satellite pustules and scaly papules extend onto abdomen and inner thighs. Provoked by diarrhoea, or systemic antibiotics (see Tables 13.1 and 13.2). Caused by *Candida* species.

- Exclude oral thrush.
- Confirm by skin scraping and microscopy or culture.

Complications: widespread psoriasiform id eruption.

Treatment: topical antifungal agents (e.g. imidazole creams).

Seborrhoeic dermatitis

Starts with significant scalp scaling (cradle cap), then redness of flexures (genital area, axillae, neck, umbilicus). Usually not itchy and improves within a few months but may go onto develop atopic eczema (➲ see Infantile seborrheic eczema, p. 260).

Treatment: emollients, topical corticosteroids, or combination products (e.g. topical corticosteroid with antifungal preparation; ➲ see Table 3.3).

Staphylococcal scalded skin syndrome ⚑

An acute condition in the younger child (<5y). The groin is often the first place to be affected (➲ see Fig. 7.6 and Erythroderma, faltering growth, and recurrent infection, p. 346).

Psoriasis

Unusual in infancy but often targets the napkin area. Well-demarcated red, scaly plaques, symmetrically affecting any part of the genital area (➲ see Fig. 11.3). May be chronic and herald severe disease (➲ see Psoriasis, pp. 320–1). Look for psoriasis elsewhere or nail-pitting (rare in infancy; ➲ see Fig. 15.7).

Treatment: difficult. Use greasy emollients, intermittent short-term moderate potency topical corticosteroids (e.g. clobetasone butyrate 0.05%) or mild tar preparations.

Zinc deficiency (acrodermatitis enteropathica) ⚑

Rare. Consider in intractable, infantile seborrhoeic dermatitis. Severe, crusted, reddish-brown, well-demarcated plaques in the napkin area (Fig. 13.4) face (➲ see Fig. 7.4), fingers and toes. Child is often unwell, listless, with faltering growth, diarrhoea, and alopecia.

Box 13.2 Differential diagnosis of nappy rashes

- Candidal napkin rash—affects creases, satellite lesions (Fig. 13.3).
- Seborrhoeic dermatitis—flexural rash with cradle cap (➲ see Fig. 17.13).
- Bullous impetigo—large bullae, easily ruptured with yellow crusts (➲ see Fig. 25.1).
- Psoriasis—sharply demarcated red plaques (rare; ➲ see Fig. 11.3).
- Intertrigo—particularly in overweight infants, caused by sweating.

Atypical or recalcitrant nappy rash

Consider:

- Acrodermatitis enteropathica (zinc deficiency) (Fig. 13.4).
- Langerhans cell histiocytosis—(Fig. 13.5).

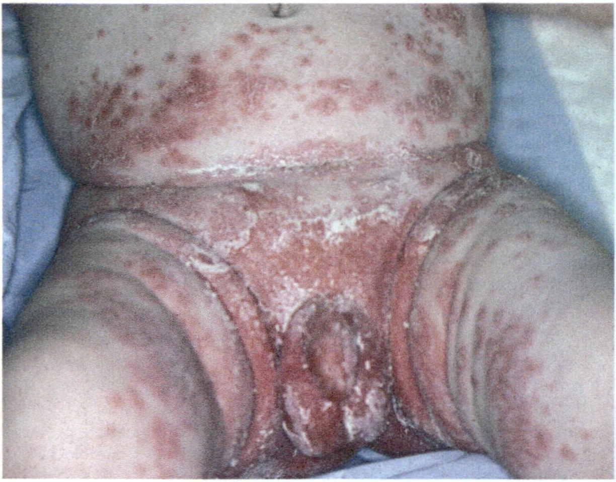

Fig. 13.3 Napkin candidiasis with erosions and white peeling areas over genitals. There are numerous pustular satellite lesions—it followed systemic broad-spectrum antibiotics.

Reproduced courtesy of Susan Lewis-Jones, Hon Consultant Dermatologist, Ninewells Hospital and Medical School, Dundee, UK

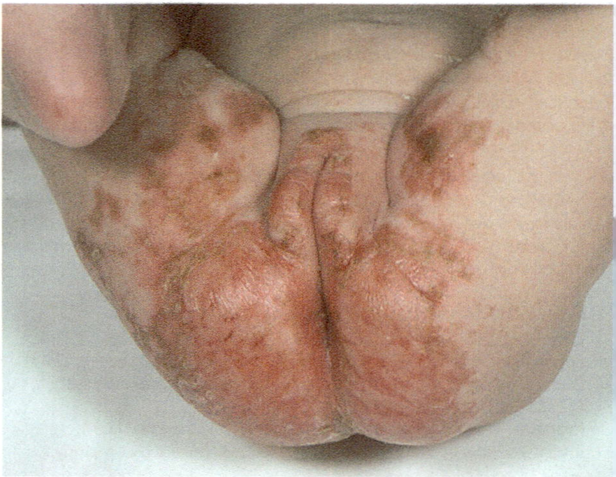

Fig. 13.4 Acrodermatitis enteropathica showing well-demarcated brownish red rash on buttocks.

Reproduced courtesy of Susan Lewis-Jones, Hon Consultant Dermatologist, Ninewells Hospital and Medical School, Dundee, UK

Primary: autosomal recessive (acrodermatitis enteropathica).

Acquired: nutritional; malabsorption; parenteral feeding; breastfeeding where milk is zinc deficient. Usually presents once the infant is weaned from breastfeeding.

Diagnosis: low serum zinc (<50 micrograms/ml; NR 70–110 micrograms/ml).

Management: skin lesions resolve rapidly with replacement therapy.

Differential diagnosis: for intractable periorificial eruption: biotin responsive multiple carboxylase deficiency, or cystic fibrosis.

Langerhans cell histiocytosis (LCH)

LCH is a rare disease of unclear aetiology. Consider as a differential diagnosis in any case of intractable seborrhoeic dermatitis in an infant.

- Due to a proliferation of Langerhans cells (LC) in the skin and other organs, notably the bones, bone marrow, liver, and lungs.
- Commoner in boys, incidence approximately 2–5 children per year in the United Kingdom.
- Skin lesions are common (40%). Typically it occurs in the intertriginous areas of the napkin area, the axillae and torso (Fig. 13.5). Look carefully for purpuric papules which are not usual in seborrhoeic dermatitis. Scalp lesions show yellowish scaly papules.

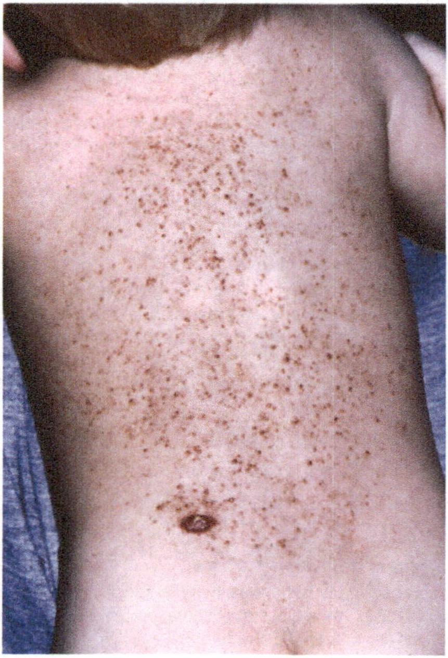

Fig. 13.5 Langerhans cell histiocytosis of back with widespread purpuric lesions.

Reproduced courtesy of Gina Kavanagh, Department of Dermatology, Lothian NHS Trust, Edinburgh, UK

Investigations: incisional skin biopsy shows proliferation of LC identified by immunohistochemistry (CD1a positive). Electron microscopy (Birbeck granules) are not always present. Further investigation for other organ involvement is necessary for staging.

Management: ideally with multidisciplinary team.

- Treatment depends on the extent of organ involvement.
- Systemic chemotherapy if three or more sites are involved.
- For isolated skin disease: topical emollients and mild topical steroids—rarely effective. Topical nitrogen mustard is used in symptomatic cases.

Red genital rash in the older child

Atopic eczema (AE, *syn.* atopic dermatitis)

Associated with itching, redness, and soreness, sometimes with dysuria and constipation. Usually involves the whole genital area including the flexures. Chronic cases show lichenification and scaling (➲ see Chapter 17). However, often spares napkin area with use of occlusive modern nappies.

Diagnosis: from clinical history and examine for signs of AE elsewhere.

Investigation: swab for microbiology.

Treatment: as for AE.

Psoriasis—flexural

Well-defined beefy-red plaques in the genital area affecting all surfaces, including flexures (➲ see Fig. 11.3). The typical silvery scale is only found at the periphery because it is a moist area. Look for psoriasis elsewhere, e.g. scalp, elbows, knees, sacral area, nails, and ears (➲ see Psoriasis, pp. 320–1). Often asymptomatic but can be itchy.

Treatment: often chronic and unresponsive. Emollients (Table 13.1) and moderately potent topical corticosteroid (intermittently) and/or tacrolimus.

Fungal infection (tinea cruris)

Erythematous, usually itchy, scaly lesions, which may extend onto inner thighs, often with pustules along the margins. Can involve the perianal area. Rare before puberty and usually seen in adolescent males (➲ see Fungal infections of the skin, pp. 330–1).

- Commonest organisms: *Trichophyton (T) rubrum, T. interdigitale, Epidermophyton (E) floccosum*.

Diagnosis: take skin scraping for fungal microscopy and culture.

Treatment: topical antifungal cream (e.g. imidazole, terbinafine).

Prognosis: excellent but concomitant nail involvement (➲ see Figs. 15.5 and 15.6) can cause recurrence.

Contact allergic dermatitis

A manifestation of Type IV hypersensitivity to specific allergens. Skin is itchy, sore, and red (➲ see Other types of eczema, pp. 259–62). Sometimes small blisters or crusts are present. Consider:

- When there is no personal or family history of atopic disease.
- With use of skin care products containing allergens such as perfumes, preservatives, and medicaments.

Investigation: patch tests (➲ see Patch testing, pp. 25–6).

Treatment: as for AE.

Infection

- *Group A streptococcus*: chronic perianal pain and itch with occasional bleeding and discharge. Well-localized perianal erythema and fissuring.
  Diagnosis: microbiological culture.
  Treatment: oral antibiotics.
- *Early infection* (preblisters, redness only): with either herpes simplex (extremely painful) or impetigo (*Staphylococcus aureus*).

Vulval itch

This is very common and sometimes no cause is found but the following should be excluded:

Threadworms

Extremely itchy: initially perianally, but may spread to whole perineum (rarely, severe perianal pain). Causes sleep disturbance. Skin changes are varied with excoriations, eczema, and nodular lesions.

Cause: Enterobius vermicularis.

Diagnosis: by the Sellotape test (applied to the perianal margin in the morning. Place on a glass slide for microscopy to view parasitic ova laid overnight).

Treatment: oral mebendazole or piperazine.

Eczema

- ➲ See Chapter 17 and Red genital rash in the older child, pp. 183–4.

Vulvovaginitis/vulvitis

Inflammation of the vulval and vaginal epithelia:

- If there is associated greenish discharge, then it is known as vulvovaginitis. This is generally due to a streptococcal infection.
- If no discharge, then it is vulvitis (see Table 13.2).

Scabies

Caused by *Sarcoptes scabiei* var. *hominis* (➲ see Infestations, pp. 337–8), a human host-specific arachnid transmitted by close physical contact (➲ see Fig. 12.5). Very common worldwide, particularly in infants/young children. Now a World Health Organization (WHO) Neglected Tropical Disease. Severe itch is the main symptom.

Clinical features: include widespread excoriations, often with eczematization (➲ see Fig. 22.13). Pathognomic burrows on the finger webs, wrists, sides of the feet and penis (➲ see Fig. 22.14). Nodules often occur on the penis and in the napkin area and/or axillae in infants (➲ see Fig. 28.14). Mites can be seen on dermoscopy (➲ see Fig. 2.1)

Treatment: antiscabetic applications—usually permethrin (total body excluding head, except in infants) to all household members and regular contacts (e.g. grandparents), on two occasions with a 1-week interval.

Table 13.2 Differential diagnosis of vulvitis and vulvovaginitis

	Cause	Symptoms	Differential diagnosis	Investigations	Treatment
Vulvovaginitis	Usually atopic dermatitis and secondary bacterial infection. If chronic consider foreign body	Irritation and vulval pain associated with discharge	Sexually transmitted infection	Examination, if necessary under general anaesthesia. Swab for microbiological culture	Extraction of foreign body. Treatment of secondary infection
Vulvitis	Irritants on the vulval skin, e.g. poor hygiene, sand pits, swimming, bubble bath, baby wipes	Irritation and inflammation of the vulval skin with redness and fissuring	All other causes of vulval itch and pain (➔ see Vulval itch, pp. 184–6)	Examination and swabs for microbiological culture	Wash with soap substitute, e.g. emulsifying ointment. Avoid irritants such as bubble bath. Emollients as barrier creams may help

Lichen sclerosus

A chronic genital dermatosis (Fig. 13.6) with white atrophic plaques, often with areas of purpura in a typical 'figure of eight' distribution around vulva and peri-anal area. Itching and soreness are common. Skin is fragile and the purpura may cause concern about sexual abuse* (➲ see Sexual abuse, pp. 366–7).

Complications

- Pain from fissures may cause dysuria and painful defaecation, often with secondary constipation/overflow incontinence.
- Scarring with loss of anatomical features and introital narrowing.

Cause: probably autoimmune, affecting prepubertal girls and older women.

Diagnosis: clinical—generally no need for biopsy in children. Differentiate from vitiligo (➲ see Changes in skin colour, pp. 186–7, and Chapter 30), which has no textural changes.

Treatment: very potent topical corticosteroids under specialist supervision.

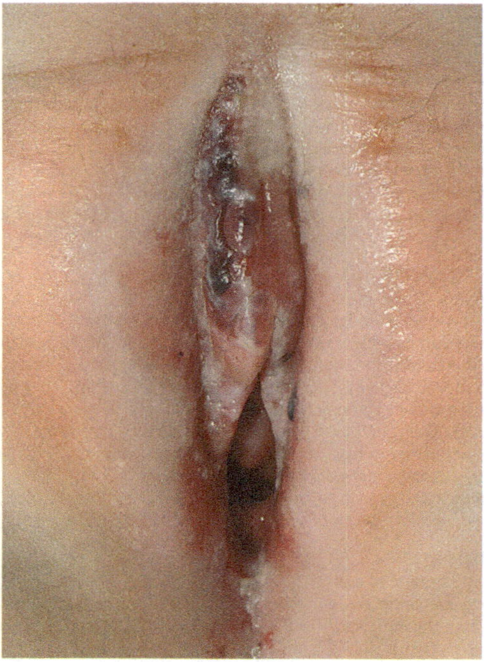

Fig. 13.6 Vulval lichen sclerosus with typical white areas and purpura affecting the labia.

Reproduced courtesy of NHS Tayside Clinical Photography, Dundee, UK

**Note:* both can rarely coexist and it may develop at sites of trauma. Extragenital involvement is rare in children (➲ see Fig. 32.5).

Long-term follow-up recommended: risk of local dysplasia and squamous cell carcinoma in later life in persistent cases.

Lichen sclerosus in boys is known as balanitis xerotica obliterans. It usually presents with phimosis in the uncircumcised and is often misdiagnosed. Potent topical corticosteroids can help but circumcision is usually curative. Dribbling and retention of urine under prepuce may be contributory.

Fusion of the labia

Relatively common in young girls and may be associated with an underlying vulvitis, causing itch. It should not be confused with an anatomical defect or lichen sclerosus.

Treatment: none if asymptomatic. Topical oestrogen cream may be applied once daily for 2–6 weeks.

Changes in skin colour

Hypopigmentation

- ➲ See also Chapter 32.
- Areas of whiteness.
- *Vitiligo*: asymptomatic, well-defined macular (flat), depigmented (white) areas, generally symmetrical. No textural changes. May be localized to the genital area but there are often patches elsewhere.
  Treatment: none in genital area.
- *Lichen sclerosus* (Fig. 13.6).
- *Postinflammatory*: usually follows a nappy rash. Paler areas with poorly demarcated margins, more obvious in dark skins (➲ see Fig. 32.2). Gradual spontaneous repigmentation.

Hyperpigmentation

- ➲ See also Chapters 33–35.
- *Melanocytic naevi*: congenital and acquired. Melanoma in childhood is very rare but has been reported in association with lichen sclerosus.
- *Postinflammatory*: follows fixed drug eruption and lichen planus (both uncommon). Also in association with vitamin deficiency, especially B_{12} or folate but is likely to be generalized.
- *Mongolian blue spot*: bluish discolouration most frequently on lower back/sacral area from birth, which fades over the first 2–4y of life. It may be misdiagnosed as child abuse (➲ see Figs. 7.5 and 24.2).
- *Lentigines*: rare, seen in association with genetic syndromes such as Carney complex (check heart), Peutz–Jegher (➲ see Chapter 33).

Bruising/purpura

- ➲ See Chapters 24 and 31.
- *Capillary malformation (port-wine stains)*: macular red/purplish marks, sometimes in association with other vascular malformations such as venous and lymphatic (➲ see Chapter 8).
- *Lichen sclerosus*: ➲ see Vulval itch, pp. 186–7.
- *Neonatal hemiscrotal bruising*: caused by high venous pressure during delivery.
- *Trauma*: accidental and non-accidental injury (NAI) should be considered.

Bruising in the genital area in non-mobile child should raise concerns of NAI.

- *Vasculitis*: usually causes purpura/petechia (see Purple colouration, pp. 463–77, and Chapter 38). It may be triggered by infection or drugs. Perform urinalysis to exclude renal involvement. Refer for specialist opinion.

Lumps and bumps

- See also Chapter 28.

Genital warts

- Flesh-coloured, benign epithelial papillomas—may be extensive. Can affect perianal area (Fig. 13.7), vulva, scrotum, penis, or urethral meatus. Usually asymptomatic but can cause itching, soreness, and bleeding with painful defaecation if perianal.
- Peak age: birth to 4y. Girls affected twice as often as boys. No accurate figures for childhood prevalence.

Transmission: individual assessment vital—several routes (Table 13.3). Look for associated findings suggesting sexual abuse, which is more likely in a child over 8y (see Sexual abuse, pp. 366–7). Include family history of

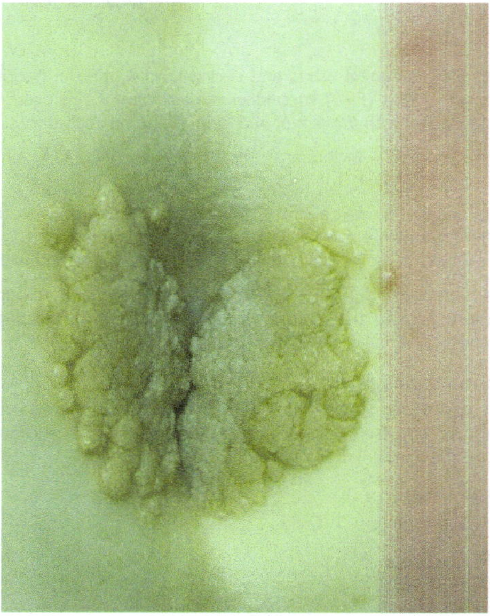

Fig. 13.7 Perianal warts.

Reproduced courtesy of Susan Lewis-Jones, Hon Consultant Dermatologist, Ninewells Hospital and Medical School, Dundee, UK

Table 13.3 Types of transmission of genital HPV infection in children

Types of transmission of genital HPV infection in children	Points to glean from the history	Associated clinical findings
Inoculation from cutaneous warts, e.g. hand warts	Personal or family history of hand warts or verrucae	Examine child for the presence of warts elsewhere
Vertical transmission prenatally and perinatally	Maternal history of cervical warts, or cervical intraepithelial neoplasia. Mother may be unaware of previous infection	Likeliest mode of spread in children with warts at birth and within 2y of life
Non-sexual transmission by innocent contact	For example, transmission via shared towels. Ask about family history of cutaneous/genital warts	Clinical history from parents and siblings required
Sexual transmission	Commonest mode of transmission between adults. Occurs in children but prevalence rates of anogenital warts in children confirmed as having been sexually abused is only 0.6–1.5%	Examine for other features of abuse. On the genitalia extension of the warts into the vagina or anal canal. Tears or bruising would support this suspicion. Assess urgently with child protection team

cutaneous and anogenital warts and cervical intraepithelial neoplasia. *Free human papilloma virus (HPV) vaccination is available for girls aged 12–18y in the United Kingdom with the aim of reducing risk of cervical cancer.*

Cause: variety of HPV including mucocutaneous HPV 6/11, HPV 16/18, and cutaneous HPV 1/4.

Treatment: usually none—await spontaneous resolution, or try 0.15% podophyllin cream (neurotoxic if taken orally so caution in toddlers) for 3 days per week. Refer to dermatologist for persistent genital warts.

Note: pearly penile papules are a normal variant with skin-coloured, often frondy lesions around the glans and coronal sulcus. They cause a lot of teenage 'angst' and may be mistaken for warts by the unwary.

Molluscum contagiosum

Common, benign self-limiting infection caused by molluscipox virus (➲ see Figs. 9.7 and 19.1). Often widespread and causes significant parental anxiety. Rare before the age of 1y.

Gluteal granuloma

- ➲ See Nappy rash, pp. 176–83.

Scabetic nodules

- ➲ See Fig. 28.14.

Median raphe cysts

Congenital, nodular, or elongated cystic lesions, along line of genitoperineal raphe, (from urethral meatus to anus, usually distal third of penis). Generally asymptomatic but can present with secondary infection.

Cause: developmental; incomplete urethral closure/or aberrant embryological epithelial buds.

Pyramidal perineal protrusion

Soft asymptomatic protrusion on the median raphe of baby girls. It resolves spontaneously.

Naevi (vascular/melanocytic/epidermal)

- *Vascular*: haemangiomas or vascular malformations (➲ see Chapter 8).
- *Melanocytic naevi* (➲ see Chapter 34).
- *Epidermal naevi*: usually follow Blaschko's lines so may be whorled or in a linear pattern (➲ see Figs. 4.5, 4.10, and 28.17), unlike genital viral warts.

Blisters

- ➲ See Infections causing blisters, pp. 378–82.

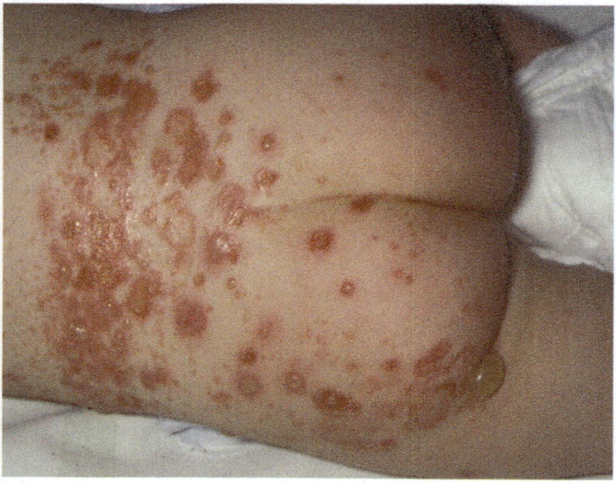

Fig. 13.8 Bullous impetigo of napkin area showing widespread erosions and a few large thin-walled bullae.

Reproduced courtesy of Susan Lewis-Jones, Hon Consultant Dermatologist, Ninewells Hospital and Medical School, Dundee, UK

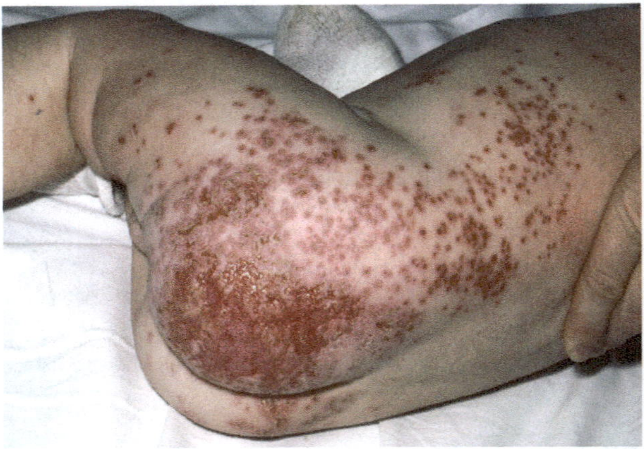

Fig. 13.9 Eczema herpeticum of napkin area in an atopic child. Mother had a herpetic whitlow on finger.

Reproduced courtesy of Susan Lewis-Jones, Hon Consultant Dermatologist, Ninewells Hospital and Medical School, Dundee, UK

Bacterial infections

- Bullous impetigo—usually *Staphylococcus aureus* (Fig. 13.8), occasionally *Streptococcus* spp. or both.

Viral infections

- *Herpes simplex* (HSV)—genital HSV is uncommon in children, a primary attack should be investigated for possible sexual abuse. Eczema herpeticum (➲ see Treatment of complications, pp. 256–7) can occur in this site (Fig. 13.9).
- *Varicella-zoster*—unilateral (but annular in perianal and buttocks area because it follows dermatomes).

Note: HSV is occasionally dermatomal.

Investigations: viral culture.

Treatment: oral aciclovir for 5 days.

Fixed drug eruption

- ➲ See Chapter 23, Fixed drug eruption, p. 356.

Mucosal and non-mucosal blisters, erosions, and erythematous annular lesions, which leave hyperpigmented areas. Genital lesions are often well-demarcated erosions recurring at the same site (e.g. glans penis).

Bullous erythema multiforme

Particular involvement of mucous membranes and sometimes confined to the genital area. It may leave scarring. Diagnose from history of recent bacterial/viral infection (e.g. HSV) or drug ingestion (less common cause in children). Onset is often abrupt with constitutional symptoms (➲ see Fig. 4.12).

Autoimmune blistering disorders

- ➲ See also Autoimmune blistering disorders, pp. 385–7.
  All are rare. Diagnosis is confirmed by biopsy and immunofluorescence.
- *Bullous pemphigoid*: may be localized to genital area as erosions rather than blisters. Ask for history of isolated 'blood' blisters or oral/ocular involvement. Rarer subtype: *mucous membrane pemphigoid* is associated with scarring and may mimic lichen sclerosus.
- *Chronic bullous disease of childhood*: predilection for genital area. Bullae characteristically cluster and form rosettes of blisters (➲ see Fig. 25.8). Usually remits spontaneously over a few years.
  Treatment: usually dapsone.
- *Dermatitis herpetiformis*: intensely itchy blisters deroofed by scratching to leave erosions. *Treatment* is usually dapsone.
- *Other immunobullous disorders*: e.g. epidermolysis bullosa acquisita, pemphigus vulgaris are extremely rare.

Swelling

Infection

- See Box 13.3.

Acute: secondary to streptococcal infection (redness, pain, and swelling).

Box 13.3 Causes of swelling of the genitalia in children

- Acute or chronic infections.
- Crohn's disease.
- Lymphoedema—idiopathic, secondary.
- Mastocytosis.
- Trauma—including testicular torsion.
- Tumours—such as sarcomas (rare).
- Urticaria, angioedema.
- Vascular anomalies or tumours (e.g. infantile haemangioma).
- Vasculitis—Henoch–Schönlein purpura, acute haemorrhagic oedema.

Box 13.4 Management of lymphoedema

- Treat underlying condition if possible—testicular torsion is an emergency.
- Avoidance of secondary infection—low-dose long-term antibiotics (e.g. erythromycin) have limited benefit.
- Compression/massage and support of the affected area—refer to lymphoedema nurse specialist.

Note: scrotal oedema can be permanent and have a significant morbidity; early intervention helps to reduce this.

Chronic: lymphogranuloma venereum, granuloma inguinale, filariasis, tuberculosis (found in certain endemic tropical areas).

Lymphoedema

Idiopathic: primary hypoplastic lymphatics. Local or general scrotal dysplasia which may present as lymphangiectasia or recurrent attacks of cellulitis.

Secondary: infective, Crohn's disease (often unilateral presentation initially).

Management: see Box 13.4.

Crohn's disease

Widespread, deep red, infiltrative granulomatous process of genital area and often lower abdominal wall. Secondary lymphatic obstruction leads to permanent genital lymphoedema. Early treatment is vital.

Transient scrotal oedema

Urticaria, angioedema, or mastocytosis (➲ see Chapter 21); Henoch–Schönlein purpura (purpura may be absent) or acute haemorrhagic oedema (➲ see HSP, pp. 471); trauma—including testicular torsion.

Ulceration/erosions

Secondary to blistering

- ➲ See Chapter 25.

Irritant dermatitis

Jacquet's ulceration (Fig. 13.2).

Ulcerated haemangioma

Often ulcerate in genital area because of rapid growth, napkin irritation, and secondary infection. Usually exquisitely painful requiring good pain management (➲ see Fig. 8.7).

Treatment: ➲ see Chapter 8, Treatment of haemangioma, p. 100.

Acute aphthous ulcers

Red areola with a yellow sloughy base. Uncommon in children but a more severe form in older prepubertal girls ('Lipschütz ulcer') is reported in association with Epstein–Barr virus and salmonella. There may be adjacent lesions 'kissing' ulcers.

Treatment: includes topical potent corticosteroids locally, or occasionally systemic corticosteroids.

Behçet's disease

Multisystem disease, rare in children. Diagnostic criteria include oral aphthae (➲ see Buccal and labial mucosa and tongue, pp. 143–4) with two of the following: genital aphthae, defined eye disease, skin disease, or pathergy (lesions arising in site of injection or injury).

Management: usually involves multidisciplinary input and includes potent topical corticosteroids, colchicine, thalidomide, and immunosuppressive drugs.

Crohn's disease

➲ See Swelling, pp. 191–2. Can also present with ulceration/erosions, especially perianally, and may precede the onset of gastrointestinal symptoms.

Chronic granulomatous disease

A group of inherited diseases characterized by severe recurrent infections, particularly skin, lungs, and perianal abscess, which may break down to form erosions.

Vaginal discharge

Common problem in young prepubertal girls and important to differentiate from exudates associated with vulvitis (see Table 13.2). Discharge may be non-purulent, purulent, or bloody. Vulval examination and taking of specimens should be done by a paediatrically trained practitioner and assessment by community paediatrician/genitourinary physician is recommended in persistent cases.

- In the majority discharge is non-purulent and is likely to be physiologic or bacterial vulvovaginitis (Table 13.2).
- Group A β-haemolytic *Streptococcus* and some Gram-negative bacilli are sometimes found as primary infection or secondary to foreign body.
- Isolation of *Trichomonas, Chlamydia*, and *Gonococcus* should initiate investigations for sexual abuse.
- Candidiasis is uncommon in prepubertal girls with thin, poorly oestrogenized tissue, but is more common in diabetics.
- Children with repeated infections or persistent purulent or bloody discharge should be referred for possible examination under anaesthetic to exclude a foreign body, most frequently toilet paper.
- Rare causes such as ectopic ureter should be considered if discharge is clear and mucoid.
- Rarely, vaginal involvement of pemphigus vulgaris or other rare cause of desquamative inflammatory vaginitis.
- Systemic infections: *Shigella* may cause gastrointestinal (GI) symptoms with bloody vaginal discharge.

Treatment: if symptomatic, give general advice about hygiene, avoidance of soaps, products containing fragrance or known irritants, and coloured toilet paper. Provide a barrier cream and emollient to wash with. Give appropriate oral antibiotics as indicated.

Chapter 14

Hair and scalp disorders

Introduction

Hair is found all over the body except for palms, soles, and mucosal surfaces. It is modified in different body sites to form scalp, eyebrow, eyelash, and nasal hairs all of which provide protection. At puberty, secondary sexual development causes a growth of body hair, particularly of pubic and axillary hair and in the male, increased coarse facial hair. The cycle of hair growth undergoes three phases, which are shown in Box 14.1.

In humans, hair mainly acts as a means of social and sexual communication and hair abnormalities of any degree may cause psychological effects. It is vital to recognize and manage this sympathetically. While young children may be unaffected by hair disorders, their parents may need support. Older children/teenagers may suffer a variety of problems including name-calling, social isolation, and bullying. Involvement of the school may be sufficient but in severe cases input from a paediatric clinical psychology service may be needed. Charities, such as Alopecia UK (https://www.alopecia.org.uk) and Changing Faces (https://www.changingfaces.org.uk) can also provide very helpful support.

Commonest hair and scalp problems in children include:

- Hair loss (➲ see Alopecia, pp. 197–8).
- Excessive hair (➲ see Hirsutism, p. 208 and Hypertrichosis. p. 209).
- Scalp scaling (cradle cap in eczema and psoriasis).
- Nits (head lice).
- 'Lumps and bumps' (moles and birthmarks).

Box 14.1 Hair cycle

- ***Anagen phase***: periods of active growth in which each individual hair reaches its maximum length. Scalp hair anagen may last for several years but elsewhere on the body it is very much shorter (weeks).
- ***Catagen phase***: a short phase of involution between anagen and telogen.
- ***Telogen phase***: follows catagen—a resting phase lasting a few weeks when hair growth stops.

Investigations

Hair sampling

- ***Hair plucking***: use if tinea (scalp ringworm) is suspected (➲ see Scalp infections, pp. 203–4).
- ***Cutting hair***: use if hair shaft abnormality suspected (➲ see Structural abnormalities of hair shaft, pp. 199–200) to prevent damage from pulling.
- ***Hair pull test***: pull gently but firmly on about 20 hairs. Test is positive if more than approximately six can be pulled out (seen in active phase of telogen effluvium, loose anagen syndrome, or alopecia areata).

Hair counts

A normal scalp will lose 50–100 hairs per day. Counting hairs, however, is not a very useful pursuit.

Direct microscopy

Useful to identify hair shaft abnormalities and absence of root sheaths in loose anagen syndrome (➲ see Structural abnormalities of hair shaft, pp. 199–200).

Dermoscopy

Useful for identifying nits and lice and exclamation hairs in alopecia areata (AA) (➲ see Examining the skin, pp. 18–9). Hair shaft abnormalities can often be identified and variation in thickness is seen in AA with yellow dots around follicular openings. Loss of follicular openings can be seen in scarring alopecias.

Hair loss (alopecia)

This may be localized or diffuse, scarring, or non-scarring. There are many causes of which the most common are:

Localized non-scarring

- *Alopecia areata*: (Fig. 14.1a) a chronic autoimmune inflammatory disease. Well-circumscribed areas of complete absence of hair. Exclamation mark hairs (Fig. 14.1b) indicate continued activity. They are very short hairs which are thicker at the top (like an exclamation mark!). More easily seen on dermoscopy which also shows hairs of different widths and short abnormal hairs. Spontaneous regrowth occurs in most over 6–12 months but alopecia may recur and progression to alopecia totalis (AT) or universalis (AU) occurs in some cases. Children with extensive patches at presentation have a worse prognosis and recovery is uncommon in patients with AT/AU. Some cases have generalized thinning without bald areas. Nail dystrophy, most commonly fine stippled pitting, occurs in a minority of cases, typically in association with more severe forms of hair loss. Atopic disease is a common association in childhood-onset AA. There is also an increased frequency of other autoimmune diseases such as thyroid disease and psoriasis.

(a) (b)

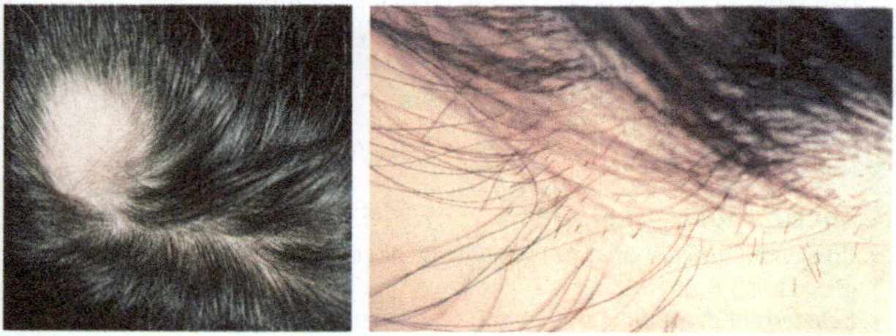

Fig. 14.1 (a) Alopecia areata. (b) Alopecia areata showing exclamation mark hairs.
Reproduced courtesy of Susan Lewis-Jones, Hon Consultant Dermatologist, Ninewells Hospital and Medical School, Dundee, UK

Treatment: there is no very effective local or systemic treatment. Potent topical steroids may help in milder forms of AA. Intralesional steroid injections are more effective but usually not appropriate in children. Some specialist centres use contact immunotherapy with diphencyprone but this is not widely used in children.

- *Hair-pulling disorder (previously Trichotillomania)*: (➲ see Self-inflicted artefactual disease, pp. 367–9 and Fig. 24.8) hair pulling/cutting produces hair loss often of varying lengths but rarely totally bald areas. Usually frontoparietal or parietal areas. Eyelashes are sometimes pulled out. Hair regrows on cessation of pulling but long-term pulling causes permanent alopecia. Often associated with stress, psychiatric disorders, particularly in older children/teenagers.

Hair twiddling in toddlers and young children is more likely a habit problem and considered normal behaviour.

- *Traction alopecia*: hair loss is caused by constant traction on hair. Relates to certain hairstyles such as tight ponytails or tight braids. Initially non-scarring but if persistent irreversible scarring may develop.
- *Infections*: tinea capitis (➲ see Scalp infection, pp. 203–4).

Localized scarring

- *Congenital scalp lesions*: ➲ see Scalp lesions, pp. 201–2.
- *Secondary to various extrinsic insults*: includes trauma, burns, infection, or intrinsic disorders, e.g. linear morphoea ('en coup de sabre' variant—➲ see Fig. 29.2 and Chapter 39).
- *Primary scarring alopecias*: e.g. lichen planopilaris; discoid lupus erythematosus (➲ see Chapter 38); folliculitis decalvans.

Diffuse non-scarring

- *Telogen effluvium*: short history of diffuse hair loss with increased hair shedding. Antecedent febrile illness, surgery, or major stress event causes hair to enter resting phase (telogen) of growth prematurely and is shed excessively 3 months later. No discrete bald patches. Regrowth occurs within a few months.
- *Pattern hair loss*: occurs in both sexes. Usually postpubertal but onset before puberty is well-recognized. In children, both boys and girls, the pattern is similar to female pattern hair loss in adults. An androgen-mediated aetiology is assumed but unproven.
- *Anagen effluvium*: hair shedding during chemotherapy.
- *Endocrine disorders*: e.g. hypothyroidism; hypopituitarism (➲ see Chapter 5).
- *Diffuse form of AA*.

Genetic causes of alopecia

- *Congenital atrichia* or *hypotrichia*: total absence or reduction in hair growth from birth.
- *Ectodermal dysplasia*: large group of disorders with associated defects such as clefting, nail and dental anomalies and poor sweating (➲ see Disorders of sweating, pp. 11–13).

Structural abnormalities of hair shaft

Hair shaft structural abnormalities may be caused by *environmental damage* including weathering from hair treatments such as bleach, heat, chemicals, and styling.

Others include *genetic hair shaft abnormalities* caused by alteration of the mechanical structure or chemical composition the hair shaft, leading to fragility and increased susceptibility to traumatic fracture. Some more common examples include:

- *Monilethrix*: autosomal dominant (Fig. 14.2). Sparse hair or even baldness. Associated prominent keratosis pilaris (➲ see Chapter 20) of nape is a helpful diagnostic clue. Hair shaft is regularly beaded—the constricted areas are weak points where breakages occur (Fig. 14.3). Diagnosis by dermoscopy or light microscopy of cut hair. No treatment but may improve with time.
- *Pili torti*: twisted hair with breaks through the irregular twists giving a spangled appearance (Fig. 14.4). Severity varies with some having widespread stubble/baldness while in others abnormal hairs are difficult to find. Presents in young children and may improve in teens. Associated with various syndromes but can also be acquired.

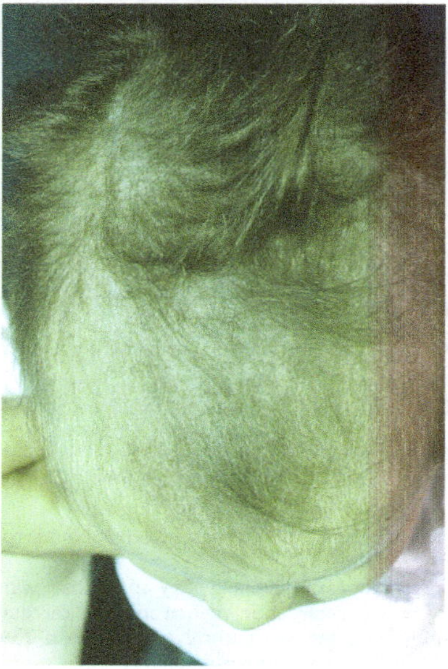

Fig. 14.2 Monilethrix.

Reproduced courtesy of Aileen Taylor, Department of Dermatology, Royal Victoria Infirmary, UK

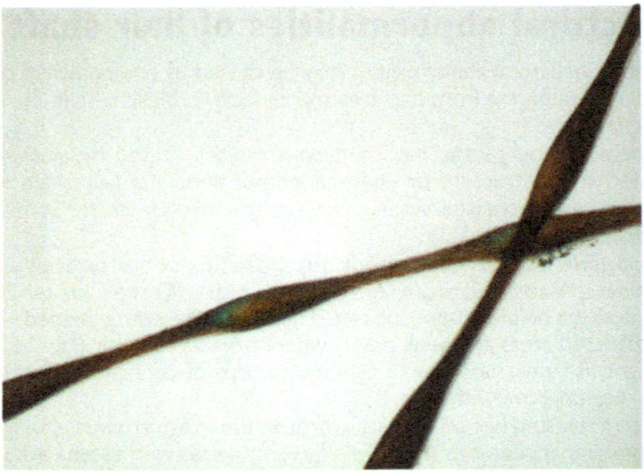

Fig. 14.3 Hair shaft showing monilethrix.
Reproduced courtesy of Aileen Taylor, Department of Dermatology, Royal Victoria Infirmary, UK

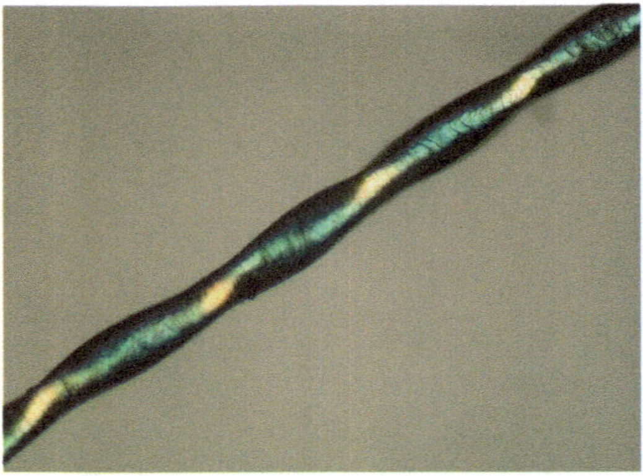

Fig. 14.4 Hair shaft showing pili torti.
Reproduced courtesy of Aileen Taylor, Department of Dermatology, Royal Victoria Infirmary, UK

- *Bamboo-hair* (trichorrhexis invaginata): seen in Netherton syndrome (➲ see Figs. 6.2 and 27.7).
- *Trichothiodystrophy*: rare, several types—sparse hair, with varying features of growth retardation, mental and physical retardation, photosensitivity (➲ see also Trichothiodystrophy, p. 236 and Syndromes with marked ichthyosis, pp. 411–12).

Others include woolly hair, uncombable hair, ringed hair—all with typical hair shaft abnormalities and some with associated anomalies.

Scalp lesions

- *Melanocytic naevi*: (moles, ➲ see Chapter 34): may be congenital or develop during childhood (acquired). If small, symmetrical with regular colour and outline, they are likely to be benign. For changes in size, shape, or colour, ➲ see Chapter 34.
- *Sebaceous naevi*: (*syn.* Naevus sebaceous of Jadassohn) well-demarcated yellowish plaques found on the head and neck of 0.3% of neonates. (Fig. 14.5). Usually on scalp and associated with localized alopecia. Become hyperplastic and raised with time. Possible local malignant change in adult life (e.g. basal cell carcinoma although histology of these tumours is contentious). If cosmetically possible, local excision can be carried out in teenagers.
- *Epidermal naevi*: benign lesions with a rough, warty, skin-coloured, or pigmented surface. Present at birth (not always obvious) becoming wartier with age. Represent genetic mosaicism appearing in linear

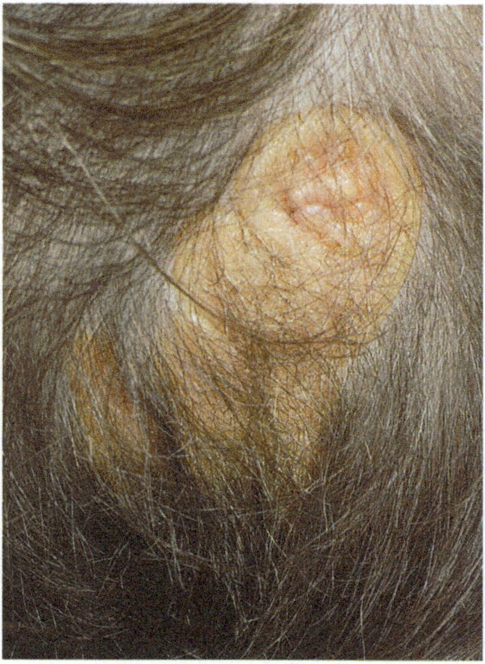

Fig. 14.5 Sebaceous naevus.

Reproduced courtesy of Susan Lewis-Jones, Hon Consultant Dermatologist, Ninewells Hospital and Medical School, Dundee, UK

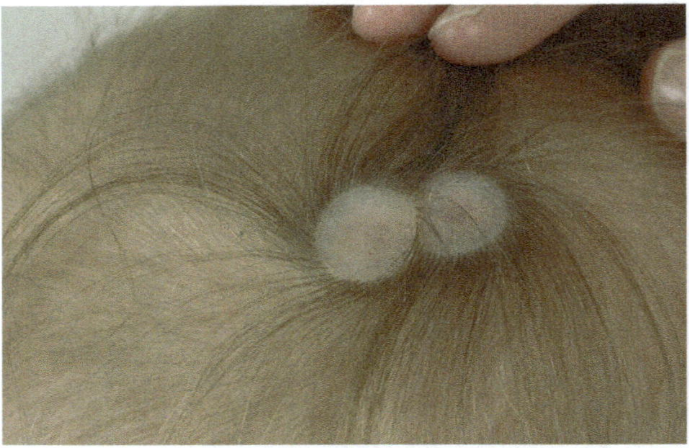

Fig. 14.6 Aplasia cutis with hair collar sign.
Reproduced courtesy of Susan Lewis-Jones, Hon Consultant Dermatologist, Ninewells Hospital and Medical School, Dundee, UK

streaks and whorls (Blaschko's developmental lines; ➲ see Fig. 4.5), ranging in size from small papules to much more extensive lesions (➲ see Fig. 28.17). Do not resolve but are benign. Very rarely associated with widespread epidermal naevi and the epidermal naevus syndrome with systemic manifestations.

- *Juvenile xanthogranuloma*: may develop in young children as solitary or multiple, firm yellow scalp nodules associated with nodules elsewhere on the body (➲ see Yellowish lesions, p. 426 and Translucent lesions, p. 427, and Figs. 28.11 and 37.3). Asymptomatic, resolve spontaneously (several years), and require no treatment.
- *Aplasia cutis*: (Fig. 14.6) total or partial absence of areas of skin at birth; most commonly on scalp but may occur at other sites and can be single (1–4cm) or multiple. Several different types have been delineated some with associated abnormalities. The defects are sharply demarcated bald areas, which may be ulcerated, bullous, or scarred at birth. May be mistaken for birth trauma. Sometimes hair collar sign is present (Fig. 14.6); ➲ see Localized hypertrichosis, p. 210.
  Cause: usually sporadic. Can be due to teratogenic effects of carbimazole taken during pregnancy.
  Prognosis: most heal without complication if trauma and infection are avoided but will remain permanently hairless. In 20% there will be other congenital defects, which include underlying bony defects, central nervous system associations, and limb/digit anomalies.
  Investigations: diagnostic imaging such as MRI to monitor defects.
  Treatment: usually none although small defects can be excised. Multidisciplinary care with neurology and an orthopaedic opinion may be required in those cases with associated abnormalities.

Scalp infections

Fungal (tinea capitis *syn.* ringworm)

Presents as bald, scaly patches with variable degrees of inflammation. May see pustules or black spots (Fig. 14.7). Three main types:

- ***Zoophilic***: animal source—usually cats/dogs. In the United Kingdom the commonest organism is *Microsporum (M) canis*. Usually scaling and hair loss or thinning with little inflammation. Occasional cause of *Kerion,* an inflamed boggy swelling with crusting and pustules more commonly caused by cattle ringworm (*Trichophyton (T) verrucosum*). Scarring can develop in untreated cases so needs prompt systemic therapy.
- ***Anthropophilic***: human-to-human infection. *T. tonsurans* is an increasing problem of inner cities, predominantly affecting children of African and, to a lesser extent, Asian ethnicity. Can manifest as grey scaling with patchy hair loss to a moderately severe inflammatory reaction producing hair loss and subsequent scarring. Contacts should be checked for subclinical infection (common). *T. violaceum* is another organism increasingly found.
- ***Geophilic***: from the soil—much less common (e.g. *M. gypseum*).

Investigations: Skin scrapings and hair plucking (➲ see Other dermatological investigations, pp. 24–6): should be undertaken for mycological identification of fungus.

Wood's light examination (➲ see Fig. 2.2): bright green fluorescence may be seen if the fungal infection is due to cat/dog ringworm (*M. canis*) or

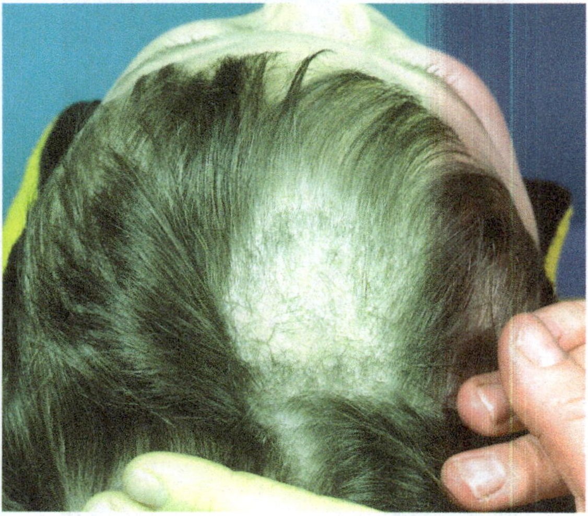

Fig. 14.7 Tinea capitis.

Reproduced courtesy of Aileen Taylor, Department of Dermatology, Royal Victoria Infirmary, UK

M. audouinii. Non-fluorescent species include *T. tonsurans* and *T. violaceum*, both now commonly seen in the United Kingdom.
Treatment: either systemic griseofulvin (10–20mg/kg) for 6 weeks or terbinafine, not yet licensed for children under 12y but frequently used because of effectiveness and shorter therapy time of 2 weeks. Itraconazole may also be used. *Topical agents are insufficient alone* but can reduce secondary infection and inflammation. Gently remove kerion crusts with saline soaks, and use antimicrobial therapy if secondarily infected (Fig. 14.8). See British Association of Dermatologists (BAD) guidelines.[1]

School exclusion: there is a risk of infection being transmitted by close classroom contacts. However, it is recommended that children should return to school once they have started systemic and topical medication. Ideally family members/close contacts should be screened.

Bacterial

Scalp impetigo: secondary infection with *Staphylococcus aureus* is common on eczematous or lice infested scalp (Fig. 14.9).
Treatment: treat underlying condition plus antiseptics (e.g. chlorhexidine containing lotions) and/or oral antibiotics (flucloxacillin or erythromycin).

Viral

Molluscum contagiosum: particularly around hairline and ***verrucae vulgaris*** *(common warts)* can occur anywhere on scalp.

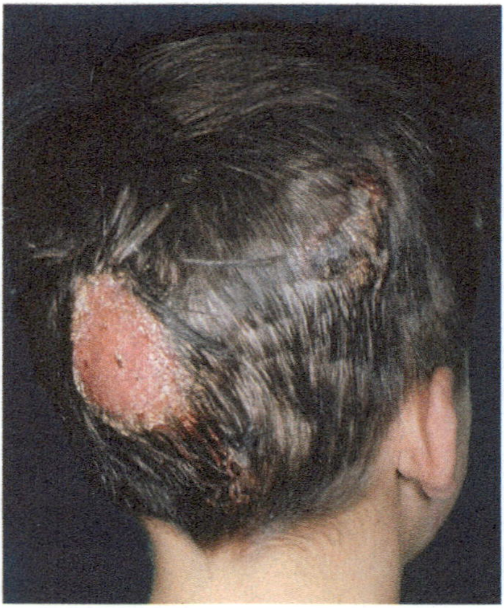

Fig. 14.8 Kerion with crust removed.
Reproduced courtesy of Aileen Taylor, Department of Dermatology, Royal Victoria Infirmary, UK

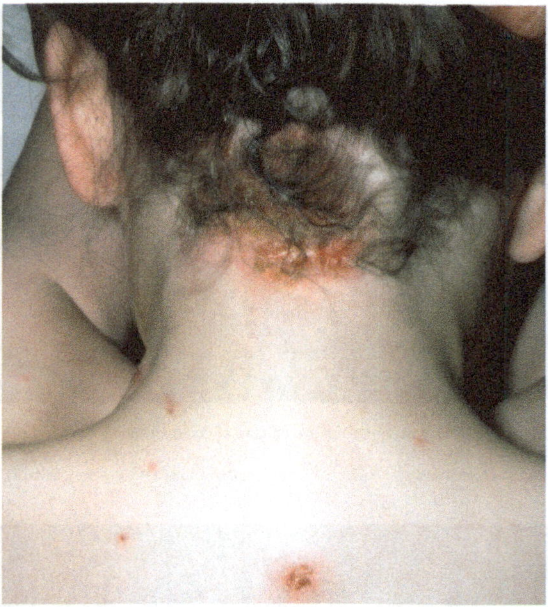

Fig. 14.9 Impetigo, secondary to head lice.

Reproduced courtesy of Susan Lewis-Jones, Hon Consultant Dermatologist, Ninewells Hospital and Medical School, Dundee, UK

Scalp infestations

Infestations

- *Pediculosis capitis (head lice)*: common in school children. Often asymptomatic, may cause itching, secondary eczematization and impetiginization (infection; Fig. 14.10). Adult lice are usually very few. Empty nit cases firmly adherent to hair shaft can be seen with naked eye whereas live nit cases tend to be hair-coloured (Fig. 14.10). Can be confused with hair casts, which are freely mobile collars of hyperkeratotic debris from hair follicle.

  Treatment: follow local guidelines (dimeticone, isopropyl myristate, malathion, wet combing). Treat severe eczema and infection with topical agents.

  Diagnostic tip: with scalp impetigo always consider head lice.
- *Ticks*: occasionally seen as large pinkish-grey sacs (Fig. 14.11). Take care when removing (twist through 180° with tick remover-available at pet shops/vets) not to leave mouthparts behind, which can cause persistent weeping and soreness. Try alcohol or heat topically or smother tick in Vaseline to prevent breathing.

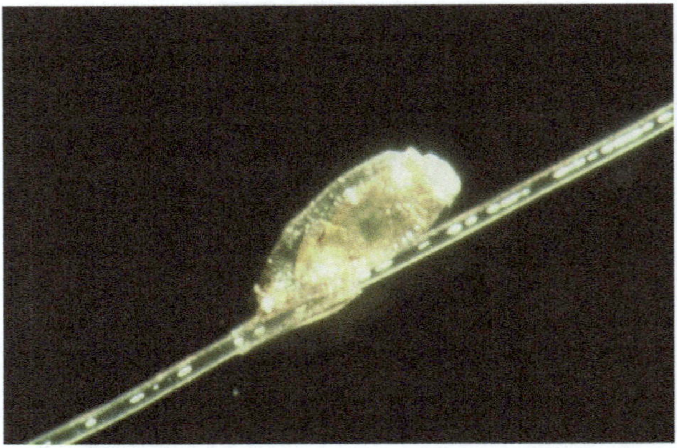

Fig. 14.10 Microscopical image of live nit case of *Pediculus capitis*, head louse—this is cemented to hair shaft.

Reproduced courtesy of Aileen Taylor, Department of Dermatology, Royal Victoria Infirmary, UK

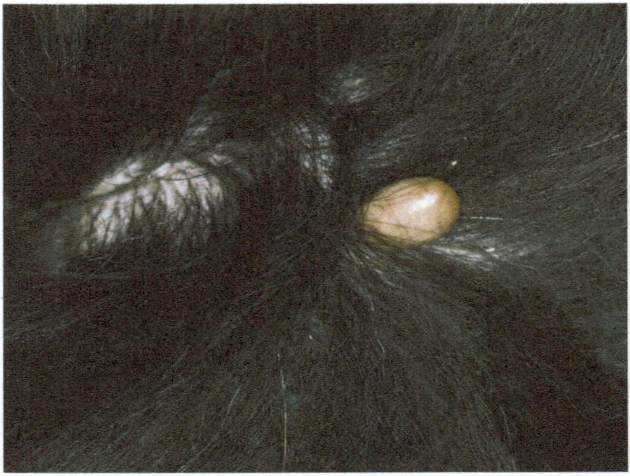

Fig. 14.11 Engorged tick on scalp.

Reproduced courtesy of Susan Lewis-Jones, Hon Consultant Dermatologist, Ninewells Hospital and Medical School, Dundee, UK

Inflammatory dermatoses of scalp

- *Atopic eczema*: common site as first manifestation in babies (cradle cap). May persist. Very itchy. In older children often becomes infected. *Treatment*: remove scales by soaking in oil for a few hours (e.g. olive or coconut oil). Avoid irritants/detergents. Use emollients and topical corticosteroids if itchy (start with hydrocortisone 1%).
- *Infantile seborrhoeic eczema*: presents as a yellow crusted cradle cap (➲ see Fig. 17.13 and Infantile seborrhoeic eczema, p. 260) and there may be flexural scaly erythema (commonly associated with atopic eczema). Treat scalp as for atopic eczema and topical imidazole cream to other lesions.
- *Psoriasis*: in children a solitary scaly plaque or more diffuse thick scale may be a presenting feature (Fig. 14.12; ➲ see also Psoriasis: clinical variants, pp. 322–4).
  Treatment: with tar-based preparations (e.g. Alphosyl®), and if thick scale present use keratolytic ointments first, e.g. salicylic acid in emulsifying ointment (see Table 14.2) (but avoid in young babies because of risk of salicylate toxicity, see ➲ Table 7.1, p. 80).
- *Rare causes*: lichen planus and systemic lupus erythematosus can both produce scarring alopecia.

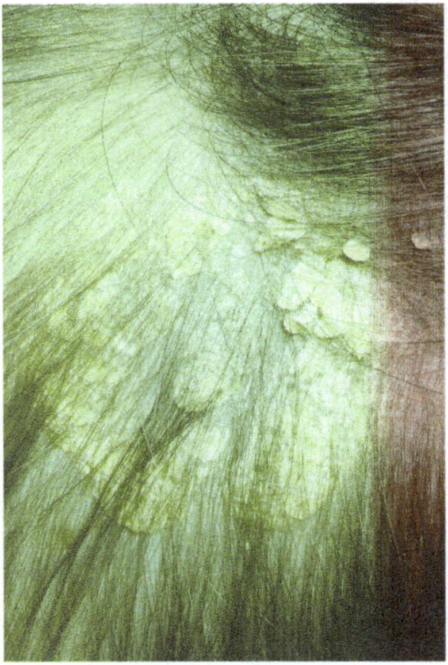

Fig. 14.12 Psoriasis of scalp.

Reproduced courtesy of Susan Lewis-Jones, Hon Consultant Dermatologist, Ninewells Hospital and Medical School, Dundee, UK

Box 14.2 Treatment of very scaly scalps

- Apply keratolytic (softening agent) first for 3h, e.g. 2–5% salicylic acid (avoid <2y) or proprietary one with tar, salicylic acid, and coconut.
- Wash out with tar-based shampoo and gently comb out loose scales.
- Apply antipsoriatic agent after drying hair, e.g. vitamin D analogue or topical corticosteroid (scalp preparation or cream.) Tar can be used overnight—messy to use but very effective.

Note: some scalp applications are alcohol-based and may cause stinging so best avoided when very sore (➲ see also Box 22.2).

Box 14.3 Differential diagnosis of thick scalp scaling (pityriasis amiantacea)

Sometimes called tinea amiantacea:

- Psoriasis.
- Tinea (ringworm) infections.
- Heavy infestation of nits (usually with secondary impetigo).
- Eczema: infants with eczema often have thick 'cradle cap'.

Changes in hair colour

- *White hair* occurs in vitiligo, albinism (➲ see OCA, p. 485 and Box 32.2) and other rare genodermatoses (e.g. white forelock in Waardenburg's syndrome and piebaldism). In AA, initial regrowth is often white.
- *Silver hair* is seen in rare genodermatoses such as Griscelli syndrome.
- *Red hair* may be inherited as a normal variant or appear in malnutrition (e.g. kwashiorkor, or in phenylketonuria).
- *Darker (or paler) areas of hair* may occur within melanocytic lesions (moles).

Hirsutism

Excess male-pattern hair in a female (i.e. excess facial hair or pubic hair escutcheon).

Causes

- Physiological—idiopathic, racial, hereditary.
- Biochemical/functional hyperandrogenism—drug induced, e.g. androgens or endocrine disorders, such as polycystic ovarian syndrome (PCOS), Cushing's syndrome, congenital adrenal hyperplasia, acromegaly.

Check for signs of virilization (male-pattern baldness, deep voice, clitoromegaly and shoulder hair) (➲ see Chapter 5).

Management

- ➲ See Hypertrichosis, pp. 209–11.

Polycystic ovary syndrome (PCOS)

Patients may present with hirsutes, acne, oligomenorrhoea, amenorrhoea and, in adults, infertility. Ultrasound of ovaries typically shows multiple peripheral ovarian cysts. Luteinizing hormone (LH) may be elevated and follicle-stimulating hormone (FSH) depressed with an increased LH/FSH ratio. For causes of PCOS, ➲ see Chapter 18.

Algorithm for excess hair

- See Fig. 14.13.

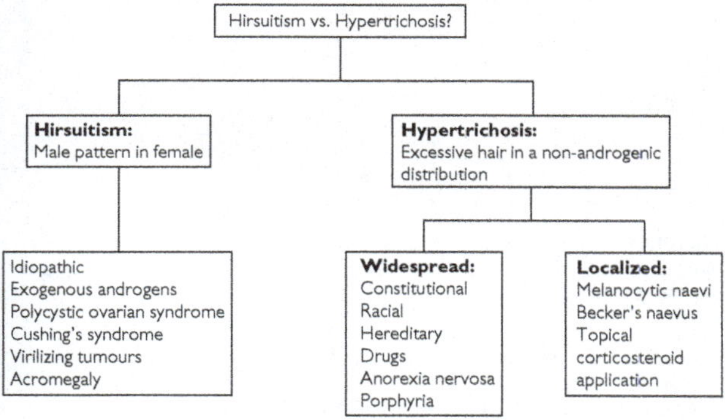

Fig. 14.13 Algorithm for excess hair.

Reproduced courtesy of Aileen Taylor, Department of Dermatology, Royal Victoria Infirmary, UK

Hypertrichosis

Excess hair growth in non-male pattern. It may be generalized or localized, congenital, or acquired.

Generalized

- *Constitutional or ethnic variation* (Fig. 14.14)—normal variation and usually not severe.
- *Congenital*: may be genetic; drug induced; or due to systemic disease.
- *Hereditary (genetic)*: hypertrichosis lanuginosae (can also be acquired); can be syndromal (e.g. Cornelia de Lange, Hurler's syndrome).
- *Drug induced*, particularly:
  - Cortisone.
  - Ciclosporin.
  - Phenytoin.
  - Diazoxide.
  - Minoxidil.
- *Porphyrias*: in some types. Usually there are other features, e.g. photosensitivity (➲ see Immediate photosensitive rashes, pp. 230–1 for cutaneous porphyrias).

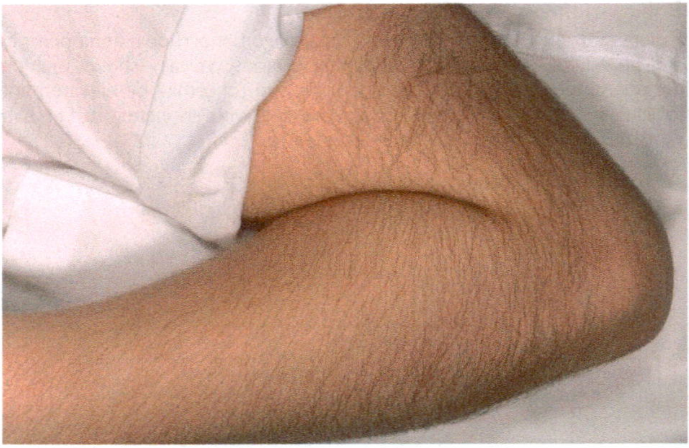

Fig. 14.14 Hypertrichosis—generalized (constitutional).
Reproduced courtesy of Susan Lewis-Jones, Hon Consultant Dermatologist, Ninewells Hospital and Medical School, Dundee, UK

- ***Endocrine disturbance***: e.g. thyroid dysfunction (➲ see Disorders of thyroid function, pp. 62–3).
- ***Acquired***: e.g. malnutrition; anorexia nervosa.

Localized

- ***Underlying naevus***: e.g.
  - *Melanocytic naevus* (mole): may be very pale and unapparent. Hair may contrast sharply in colour and texture with that of the normal scalp.
  - *Faun-tail naevus*: usually midline, overlying spine, may be a pointer to underlying neurological abnormalities (spinal dysraphism—spina bifida, cord tethering, and so on; Fig. 14.15).
  - *Becker's naevus*: pigmentation and hypertrichosis usually over upper back/shoulder area. Develops postpuberty, almost exclusively in boys (➲ see Fig. 33.2).
- ***Hair collar sign***: ring of increased, often darker hair around patch of alopecia such as aplasia cutis (Fig. 14.6) and can be marker for ectopic brain tissue or other neurological defect.
- ***Drug induced***: e.g. potent topical corticosteroids.
- ***Acquired***: e.g. chronic inflammation or friction such as scratching (which paradoxically can also cause alopecia—see under environmental causes of alopecia, ➲ see Structural abnormalities of the hair shaft, pp. 199–200).

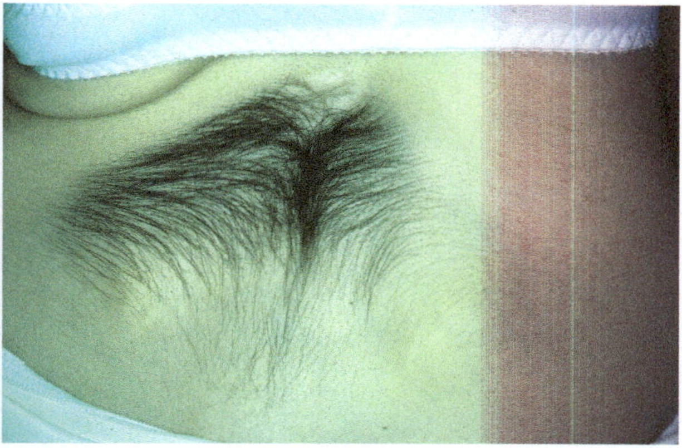

Fig. 14.15 Hypertrichosis—over lumbar spine (faun-tail)—localized (congenital) associated with spina bifida.

Reproduced courtesy of Susan Lewis-Jones, Hon Consultant Dermatologist, Ninewells Hospital and Medical School, Dundee, UK

Management of hirsutism/hypertrichosis

- *Physical methods* of shaving, bleaching, plucking, waxing, application of depilatory cream may be used but the hair will regrow. These methods may cause folliculitis (➲ see Chapter 20).
- *Electrolysis and laser treatments* may produce longer lasting results but are painful. Laser (e.g. long-pulsed ruby laser) is more effective with dark hairs and usually requires repeated treatments. Perifollicular postinflammatory hypo- and hyperpigmentation may occur (➲ see Other modalities of treatment, pp. 41–46).
- *Eflornithine cream*—reduces rate of hair growth but continued treatment needed to maintain the response.
- *Oral antiandrogen* (spironolactone, cyproterone acetate)—in children recommend management by paediatrician/endocrinologist.
- *Weight loss.*

References

1. Fuller, L.C., *et al.* (2014). British Association of Dermatologists' guidelines for the management of tinea capitis 2014. *Br J Dermatol* **171**:454–63.

Chapter 15

Nail changes

Introduction

Examination of the fingernails is part of the preliminary assessment of all patients. Nail changes can be indicative of systemic disease. Normal variants need to be recognized. Some signs are found on toenails.

Normal variants

- *Koilonychia*: spoon-shaped concavity of the nail most marked on the big toe. It has no clear association with iron deficiency in a healthy child (Fig. 15.1).
- *Lamellar splitting*: transverse lamellar fragmentation at free edge of the nail is a normal finding and often more marked in sucked digits.
- *Chevron nails*: chevron or herring-bone ridged surface markings on the nail seen on thumb and radial fingers.

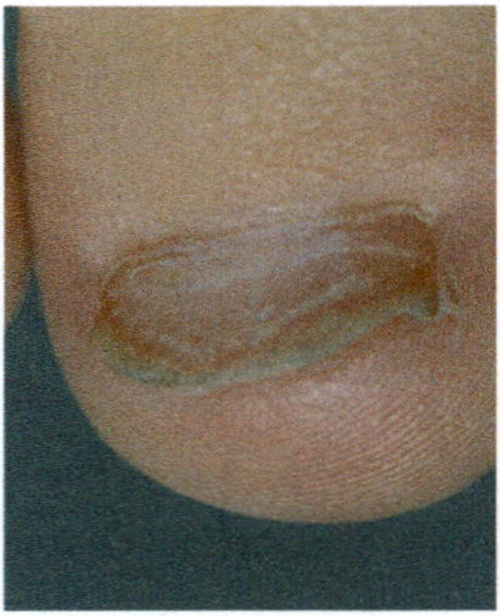

Fig. 15.1 Koilonychia.

Reproduced courtesy of David de Berker, Consultant Dermatologist, Department of Dermatology, Bristol Royal Infirmary, Bristol, UK

Thumb sucking

Causes paronychia with mild to moderate nail dystrophy, sometimes with secondary infection such as *Candida* (Fig. 15.2).

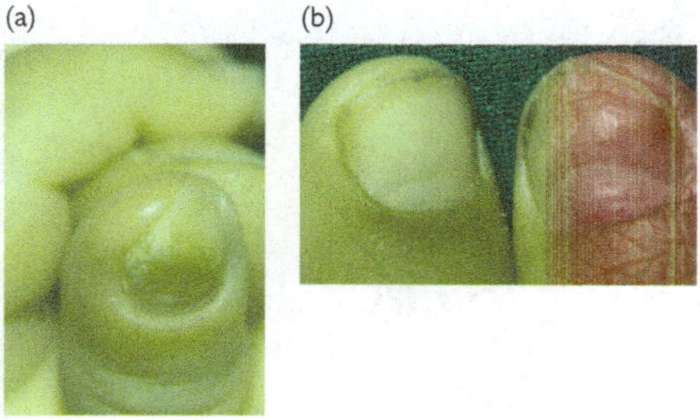

Fig. 15.2 (a) Chronic paronychia in an 8-month-old baby with secondary *Candida* infection. (b) Chronic paronychia through thumb sucking.

Reproduced courtesy of David de Berker, Consultant Dermatologist, Department of Dermatology, Bristol Royal Infirmary, Bristol, UK

Ingrowing nails

Infant

In the first year of life or with early mobility, distal ingrowing is the most common pattern, with the free edge of the toenail embedding in the soft tissues of the tip of the toe. Hypertrophy of the lateral nail fold can produce a similar lateral pattern.

Management: obtain bacteriology samples. Local treatment with potent topical steroid and local or systemic antibiotic for the acute episode. Leave the nail long enough for it to press flat the skin at tip of the toe.

Adolescent

- *Nail biting* (onychophagia) leads to ingrowing of fingernails at the distal and lateral margins.
  Management: occlusion with tape to stop biting may help, combined with same measures as for *infant ingrowing* nails.
- *Lateral ingrowing of the big toenail* is usually associated with sport (Fig. 15.3a), footwear, or faulty manner of cutting the nail.

  Management: as for *Infant* plus review of footwear and activities, keeping the nail longer, cut straight (Fig 15.3b) and antiseptic soaks, e.g. dilute (pale pink) potassium permanganate. Taping to draw the inflamed nail fold away from the advancing nail edge (Fig. 15.3c) Recurring episodes may require surgical treatment.
- *Rarer diagnoses*: congenital malalignment of the big toenails is seen with ingrowing at the lateral and distal margin as the nail becomes triangular, thickened, and yellow. Can resolve spontaneously or require surgical management.

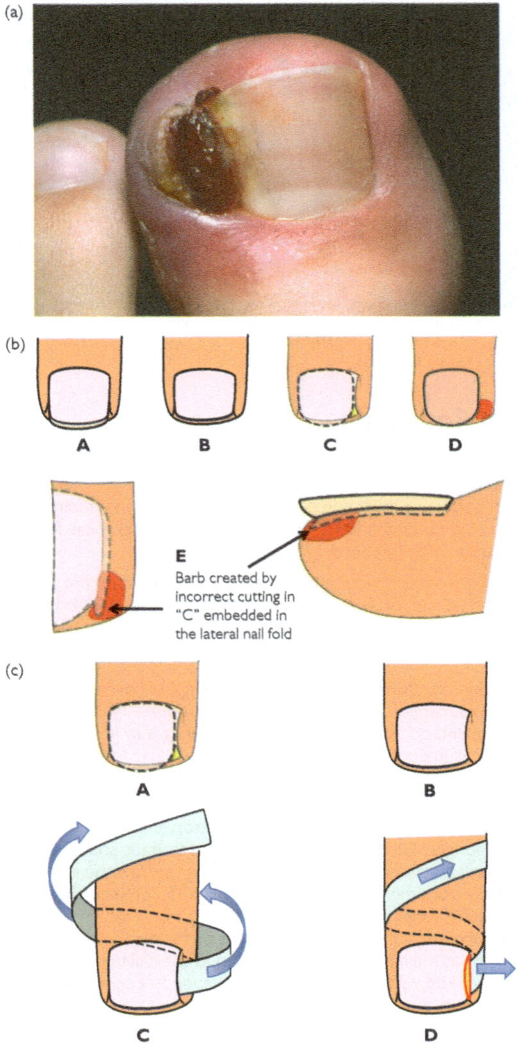

Fig. 15.3 (a) Ingrowing toenail with granulation tissue; (b) how to relieve it; and (c) how to relieve it with taping.

Reproduced courtesy of David de Berker, Consultant Dermatologist, Department of Dermatology, Bristol Royal Infirmary, Bristol, UK

Infection

Non-fungal infections

Often acute, painful, and primarily affect the soft tissues around the nail. Trauma is a predisposing factor. The nail may be shed or show signs of disturbed growth over months with transverse ridges and depressions.

Bacterial

- ***Acute paronychia***: infection of nail folds, usually staphylococcal or streptococcal, typically associated with sucking or nail biting (Fig. 15.4). ***Treatment***: take swabs for culture, drainage if possible, systemic flucloxacillin, daily washing, local dressing.
- ***Infected ingrowing nails***, ➲ see Ingrowing nails, p. 215.
- ***Blistering dactylitis*** with variable inflammation and no pus, on nail fold or digit pulp. Consider other causes of blisters, including herpes simplex. ***Treatment***: as for paronychia.

Viral

- ***Herpes simplex*** with vesicopustule with or without haemorrhage. Single digit. Clear vesicles coalesce with red margin and pain. May extend onto digit pulp and cause nail shedding.

  Treatment: self-limiting, but may warrant systemic antiviral therapy if diagnosed early.

Rarer diagnoses: epidermolysis bullosa (➲ see Genodermatoses and the nail, pp. 223–4).

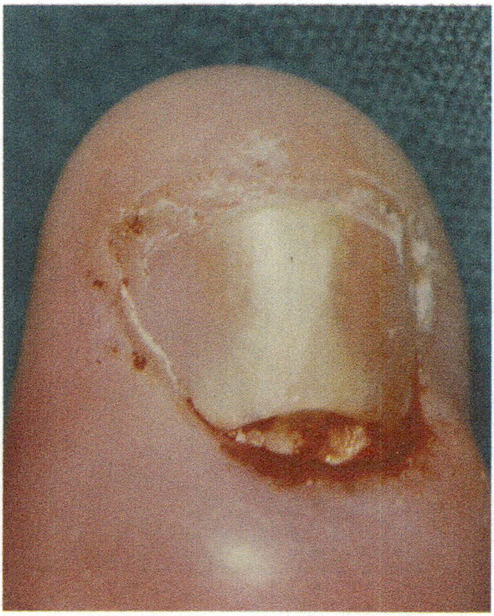

Fig. 15.4 Acute paronychia with drainage proximally and beneath the nail.

Reproduced courtesy of David de Berker, Consultant Dermatologist, Department of Dermatology, Bristol Royal Infirmary, Bristol, UK

Fungal infections

Fungal infections affect the nail bed and nail plate (tinea unguium). Pathogens are of two families—dermatophytes and non-dermatophytes. *Candida* (second category) is separate from the other non-dermatophytes ('moulds'). Dermatophytes are typical skin pathogens, whereas non-dermatophytes are rarely so and are more typically found in soil or as saprophytes.

Dermatophyte fungi

May be found with signs of fungal skin infection on soles of feet or between the toes (*qv. tinea pedis*). Rare, and seen in three patterns:

- ***Superficial white onychomycosis***—small white powdery areas on the nail surface (Fig. 15.5). Can be partially removed by scraping. Mycology typically *Trichophyton (T.) rubrum* or *T. mentagrophytes*. Do not confuse with other causes of leukonychia (whiteness of nails) (➲ see Genodermatoses and the nail, pp. 223–4).
  Treatment: can respond to topical therapy with amorolfine lacquer applied weekly coupled with surface debridement.
- ***Distal lateral subungual onychomycosis (DLSO)***—free edge and/or one side of the nail is discoloured, with nail plate thickening and scale

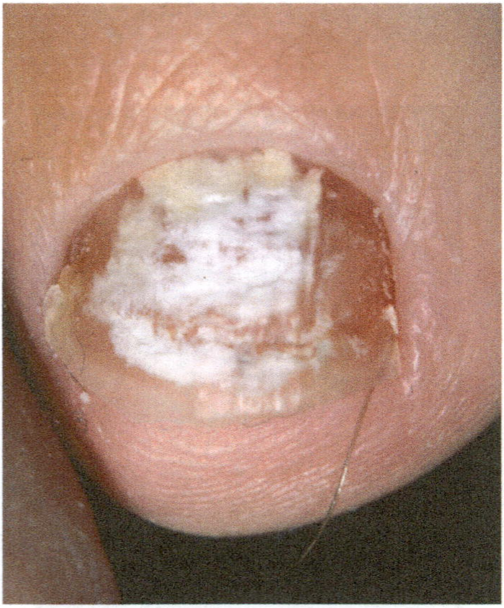

Fig. 15.5 Superficial white onychomycosis.

Reproduced courtesy of David de Berker, Consultant Dermatologist, Department of Dermatology, Bristol Royal Infirmary, Bristol, UK

accumulated beneath the nail. Involvement of nail in the lateral sulcus can compromise response to topical therapy.

- ***Total dystrophic subungual onychomycosis***—most or all of a nail is altered by the changes of DLSO (Fig. 15.6).
  Treatment: likely to need systemic therapy for cure. Chemical avulsion with 40% urea paste under occlusion can make area amenable to topical therapy. Chemical avulsion currently available through dedicated packaged kit with dressings and paste (Canespro™)

Non-dermatophyte fungi

- ***Candida* spp.**: often isolated from digits which are sucked and where there is onycholysis or inflammation. Rarely part of a true fungal infection and correction of contributory factors is usually effective. Where true fungal infection of the nail plate appears possible, cure may require systemic therapy.
- ***Moulds***: extremely rare in children from Western countries. *Fusarium* spp., *Scopulariopsis* spp., and *Aspergillus* spp. are the most common types. May have associated inflammation and tenderness of proximal nail fold. Seek local microbiology advice concerning suitable agents and prescribing guidance in children. Chemical avulsion coupled with topical therapy may be required due to lack of effective oral agents.

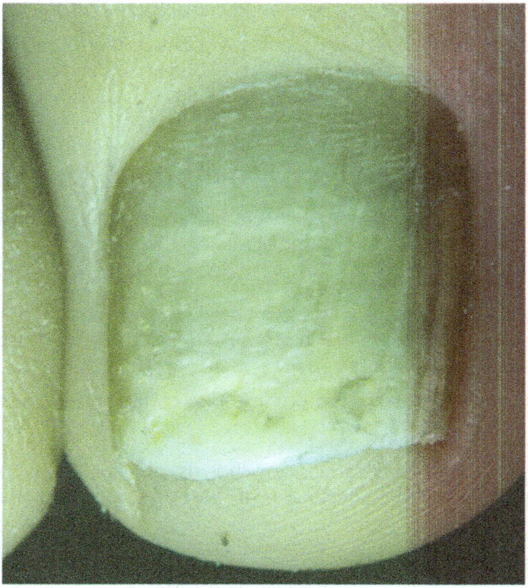

Fig. 15.6 Total dystrophic subungual onychomycosis.

Reproduced courtesy of David de Berker, Consultant Dermatologist, Department of Dermatology, Bristol Royal Infirmary, Bristol, UK

- *Rarer diagnoses* include:
  - Chronic mucocutaneous candidiasis, where there is a mix of bulky and crumbling nails on all or most digits associated with Candida at other sites, e.g. oral changes (➲ see Fig. 10.8).
  - Human immunodeficiency virus and other forms of immune deficiency can result in gross patterns of onychomycosis including the rare form of proximal subungual white onychomycosis.

Management

- *Mycology*: all onychomycosis treatments should be informed by taking samples for culture and microscopy. Take a large sample of dystrophic nail with associated crumbling material from affected area. If superficial white disease, scrape the surface for sampling.
- *Topical therapy* (e.g. amorolfine lacquer) can work in nails infected lightly on the superficial or distal aspect. Deep and more widespread infection responds poorly.
- *Systemic therapy*:
  - Griseofulvin is the only available treatment in most countries but it is slow and not very effective.
  - Oral terbinafine or itraconazole can be used with up to 80% efficacy, but are not licensed for this indication in children. Titrate doses by body weight.
- *Supplementary treatment* with amorolfine lacquer and topical therapy to relapses of tinea pedis may be needed in susceptible children.

Note: non-dermatophyte fungi are less responsive often requiring longer courses of systemic therapy, aggressive debridement, and supplementary topical therapy until the nail is cured.

Inflammatory dermatoses and the nail

The main dermatoses affecting skin and nail are eczema, psoriasis, and lichen planus (see Box 15.1 for rarer causes).

Atopic eczema (common)

Pits, ridges, surface irregularities associated with eczema of nail folds of same digit. Tends to affect nail in proportion to local skin disease and can present at all ages.

Local treatment: skin care and protection, topical corticosteroid, and emollient.

Psoriasis (common)

Pits, ridges, surface irregularities, onycholysis, and subungual hyperkeratosis (Fig. 15.7). Tends to affect nail in proportion to local skin disease. Can

Box 15.1 Rarer diagnoses of nail disorders

- Lichen striatus extending to nail (➲ see Chapter 17).
- Langerhans cell histiocytosis (➲ see Chapter 13).
- Ectodermal dysplasias (➲ see Chapter 14).
- Pityriasis rubra pilaris (➲ see Chapter 22).
- Graft-versus-host disease (➲ see Chapter 39).

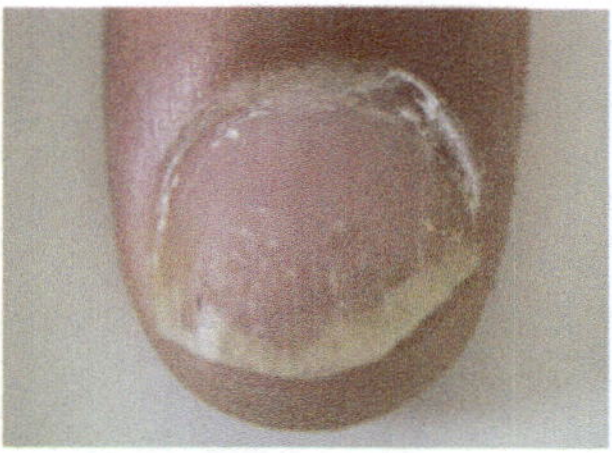

Fig. 15.7 Psoriasis showing typical thimble pits and onycholysis.

Reproduced courtesy of David de Berker, Consultant Dermatologist, Department of Dermatology, Bristol Royal Infirmary, Bristol, UK

present at all ages and also independently from other features of psoriasis in time and body site. Mild features are described from birth, but it usually gains prominence in early adulthood.

Treatment: as for eczema, but also with calcipotriol cream or ointment.

Lichen planus (uncommon)

Pits, ridges, surface irregularities may affect all nails, with ultimately fragmentation and loss of nail (Fig. 15.8). Other patterns include scarring, loss of nail with creation of prominent scar tissue forming between wings of nail creating a pterygium. Most typically presents as an isolated nail disease, but can be seen with involvement of skin and oral and genital mucosal surfaces.

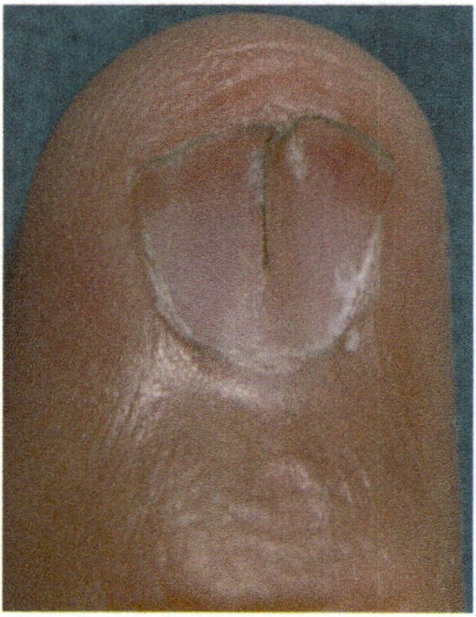

Fig. 15.8 Lichen planus with central splitting.

Reproduced courtesy of David de Berker, Consultant Dermatologist, Department of Dermatology, Bristol Royal Infirmary, Bristol, UK

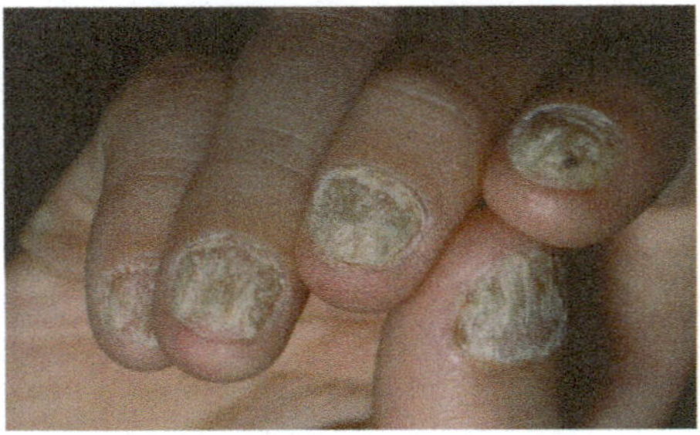

Fig. 15.9 Twenty-nail dystrophy.

Reproduced courtesy of David de Berker, Consultant Dermatologist, Department of Dermatology, Bristol Royal Infirmary, Bristol, UK

Treatment: may require systemic corticosteroid if progressive, where therapy would normally be guided by biopsy or corroborating clinical features elsewhere.

Twenty-nail dystrophy of childhood (uncommon)

Fine pits that may progress to fragment the nail plate. May affect up to 20 digits, hence the name (Fig. 15.9).

Treatment: usually self-limiting and reverses over 2–5y. Mild variants may respond to nail eczema therapy. Aggressive forms may need to be distinguished from lichen planus which can permanently destroy nails, and respond to systemic corticosteroid when deemed necessary.

Tumours and the nail

Viral warts

Usually self-limiting but can respond to treatments for warts at other sites. Made worse by nail and nail-fold biting, which may make topical therapies such as keratolytic agents difficult.

Treatment: wrapping in duct tape or surgical tape may make them more comfortable and help treatments. Salicylic acid products available in variety of formulations for topical use. Combination product of 0.5% 5-fluorouracil with salicylic acid in collodion is sometimes used off-license.

Subungual exostoses

Occasionally related to trauma, presenting as firm to hard nodules protruding from beneath the distal edge of the nail (Fig. 15.10). Typically affects the big toenail in those 10–20y of age. May cause painful ingrowing of nail into soft tissue due to displacement of nail.

Diagnosis: by combined plane and lateral X-ray.

Treatment: is surgical.

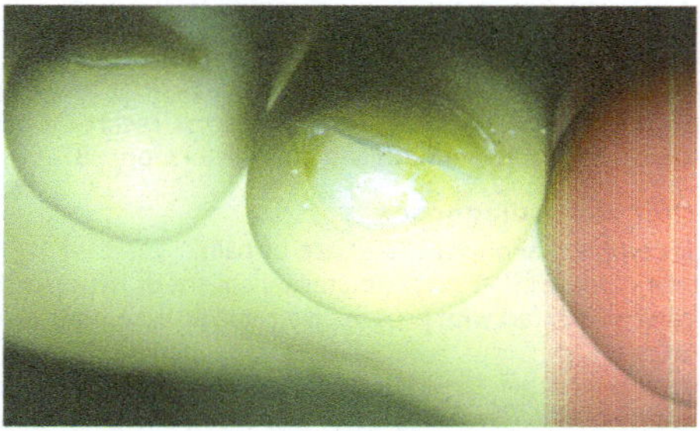

Fig. 15.10 Subungual exostosis.

Reproduced courtesy of David de Berker, Consultant Dermatologist, Department of Dermatology, Bristol Royal Infirmary, Bristol, UK

Genodermatoses and the nail

Nail features are rarely seen in infancy.

Periungual fibromata

Firm fibrous hamartomas of nail plate (Fig. 15.11) seen in tuberous sclerosis complex as well as an isolated finding in a single nail (see TSC, pp. 483–4). Cause longitudinal nail ridging.

Pachyonychia congenita

Rare. Prominent thickening of the nail bed, usually distinct from the nail plate. Appears as a wedge of nail-like material pushing up from the nail bed. Progressively affects all nails. Spectrum of phenotypes, broadly conforming to two types associated with cutaneous and mucosal features (see Pachyonychia congenita, p. 389).

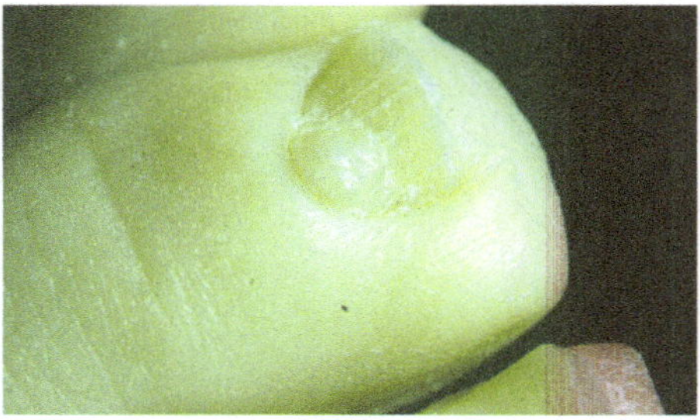

Fig. 15.11 Periungual fibroma in young child.

Reproduced courtesy of David de Berker, Consultant Dermatologist, Department of Dermatology, Bristol Royal Infirmary, Bristol, UK

Epidermolysis bullosa

Epidermolysis bullosa may cause blistering, nail shedding, and nail dystrophy—especially of big toes where trauma elicits the shedding and secondary scarring. Look for family history, chronic recurrent pattern, and blisters elsewhere (➲ see Genetic causes of blisters, pp. 387–90).

Some other rarer diagnoses

- Partial or complete anonychia (absence of nail).
- Nail patella syndrome—triangular lunulae, absent or hypoplastic nails, and patellae associated with progressive renal disease, glaucoma, and bony features.
- Ectodermal dysplasias—large group of disorders with various abnormalities of skin, sweating, hair, nails, teeth, and skeletal function.

Discolouration of nails

- *White nails* (leukonychia): often due to trauma but also seen after systemic illness or can be inherited. Superficial white onychomycosis (➲ see Fungal infection, pp. 218–20). Onycholysis may appear white or yellowish.
- *Blue nails*: seen in cyanosis, drug therapy especially high-dose minocycline which causes blue lunulae (rare), tumours such as glomus (➲ see Blue lesions, p. 423) or blue naevi, p. 511.
- *Yellow*: congenital malalignment of great toenails. Yellow nail syndrome—thickened nails curved longitudinally and horizontally associated with lung cysts and facial lymphoedema. A rare genetic disease usually seen in adults.
- *Redness*: splinter haemorrhages, usually traumatic but if numerous consider subacute bacterial endocarditis in those at risk.
- *Brown/black*: trauma is commonest cause. Melanocytic bands or streaks are not uncommon in black or Asian skin types but can rarely be malignant melanoma in Caucasians—rare in children. Congenital melanocytic naevi can involve the nail.
- *Green nails*: secondary *Pseudomonas pyocyaneus* under areas of onycholysis. Usually adults. Treat with gentamycin eye drops or clip back nail and use vinegar soaks 5min each night and dry with a hair dryer.

Chapter 16

Photosensitivity

Introduction

Ultraviolet (UV) light can affect the skin in several ways. An abnormal reaction to UV light (photosensitivity) may be caused by allergy, plants, drugs, or genetic disease and usually shows a typical distribution on exposed body sites (Fig. 16.1).

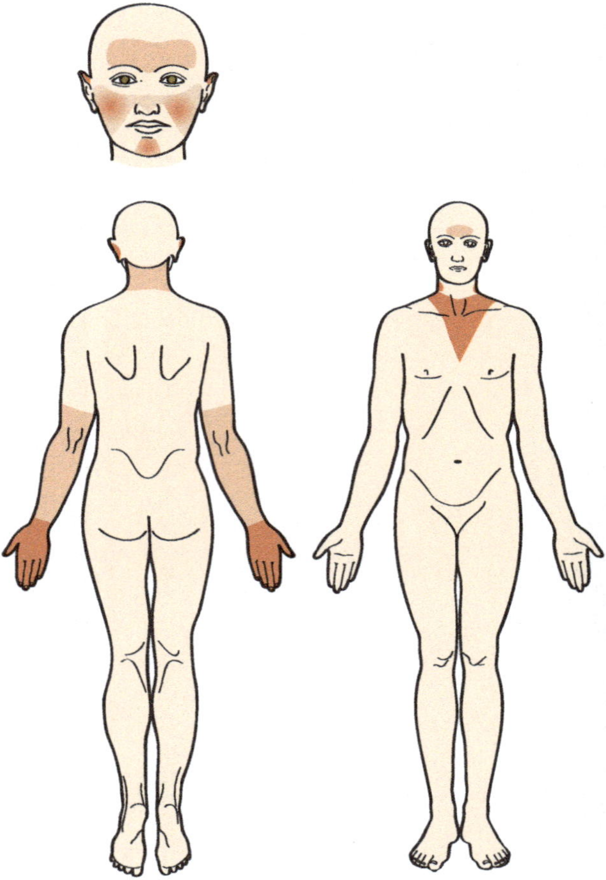

Fig. 16.1 Typical photosensitive distribution.

Ultraviolet light

Electromagnetic radiation from the sun reaching the earth's surface includes wavelengths greater than 290nm in the UV and visible ranges. The majority of UV and visible radiation is absorbed by skin with different wavelengths penetrating the skin to a greater or lesser extent depending on their absorption by cellular structures:

- UVB (280–320nm) and UVA2 (320–340nm) wavelengths are absorbed in the epidermis.
- UVA1 (340–400nm) wavelengths penetrate deeper, producing effects on the cellular structures of the dermis.

Chromophores and photoproducts

Different components of the skin (e.g. DNA and cell membranes) absorb specific wavelengths of light, and these are called chromophores. Upon absorption of light energy chromophores can become excited and convert to a photoproduct. Photoproducts then elicit immediate or delayed hypersensitivity reactions believed to be involved in the pathogenesis of many photosensitive rashes (photodermatoses) including solar urticaria (➲ see p. 230) and polymorphic light eruption (PLE) (➲ see p. 228).

Phototoxic and photoallergic reactions

Chemicals present in the skin after cutaneous absorption (such as in sunscreens/fragrances) or oral ingestion (commonly drugs, Box 16.1) can act as an exogenous chromophore absorbing radiation of wavelengths specific to that chemical (predominantly UVA) to become excited and produce a photoproduct. This can elicit a *phototoxic or photoallergic reaction*.

Box 16.1 Drugs commonly causing photosensitivity

Phototoxic rashes

- Thiazide diuretics.
- Fluoroquinolone antibiotics.
- Non-steroidal anti-inflammatory drugs (NSAIDs).
- Retinoids.
- Amiodarone.

Photoallergic rashes (rarer)

- Topical fragrance.
- Sunscreens.

Photosensitive rashes

The most common photosensitive rashes are less common in children than in adults. However, children in general receive 50% more sun exposure than adults, so it is not uncommon for these to present in childhood. In addition, certain photosensitive rashes have their onset in childhood and photogenodermatoses are present from birth. A rash which is related to sun exposure is usually delayed but may be immediate.

Delayed photosensitive rashes

Polymorphic light eruption (PLE)

- Appears as very itchy papules, plaques, or even blisters on exposed sites and fades in days without scarring (Fig. 16.2). Face and hands may be spared because of 'hardening' (see next bullet point).
- Worse in spring and summer; often improving as summer proceeds because pigmentation (tanning) and thickening of the skin in response to sun exposure provide protection known as 'hardening'. This protection is lost in winter.
- Affects 10–20% of individuals in temperate climates and generally has its onset during the first three decades.

Management: photoprotective measures (➲ see p. 238) with gradual sun exposure to produce hardening. In severe cases hardening can be induced (desensitization) by early season ultraviolet (usually narrow-band UVB) phototherapy. Topical corticosteroids may be helpful during the acute phase.

Juvenile springtime eruption (JSE)

- Occurs recurrently in summer as papules and vesicles on the rims of boys' ears in the 5–12y age group.
- May represent a form of PLE as a family history of both is common.

Management: it is usually self-limiting and prevented by a longer haircut with or without other photoprotective measures.

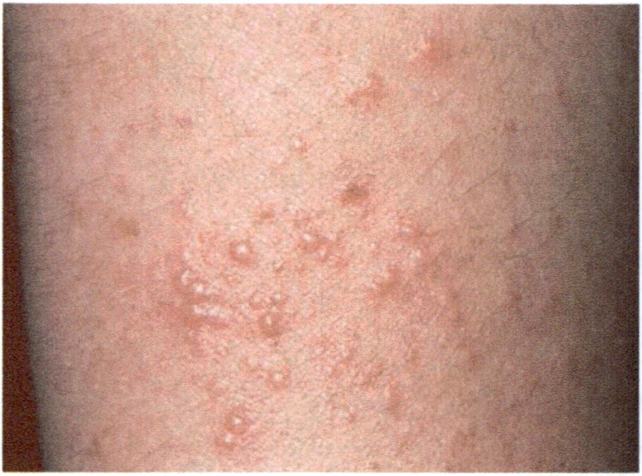

Fig. 16.2 Polymorphic light eruption.

Reproduced courtesy of James Ferguson, Emeritus Professor, University of Dundee, Dundee, UK

Actinic prurigo

- Chronic excoriated papules, plaques and scarring on exposed sites (Fig. 16.3), often affecting the lips and distal third of nose. Can affect covered sites. Conjunctivitis may also be present.
- Occurs throughout the year with a spring/summer exacerbation but hardening is uncommon.
- Rare in the United Kingdom, commoner in central and south America. Often familial. Affects four females for every male and 75–80% of cases present in the first decade.[1]
- HLA association (HLA-DR4 and DRB1*0407 subtype) but this is not essential for disease development.

Management: the same as for PLE but systemic therapy may be required.

Hydroa vacciniforme

- Characterized by itch, erythema, swelling, papules, haemorrhagic vesicles, and crusts that heal to leave varioliform scars (Fig. 16.4). There is often eye (conjunctival) and ear involvement.
- It affects only photoexposed sites.
- Rare, usually sporadic, and usually presents in the first decade.
- It resolves spontaneously after a mean duration of 9y.[2]

Management: systemic therapy may be required if photoprotection and desensitization therapy fail to provide adequate control.

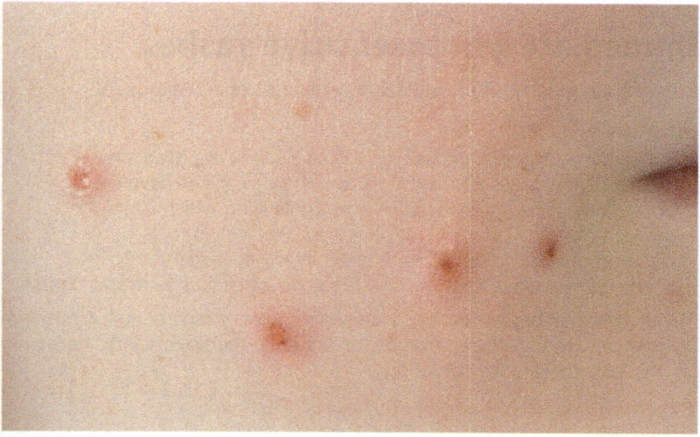

Fig. 16.3 Actinic prurigo.

Reproduced courtesy of Paula Beattie, Consultant Dermatologist, Department of Dermatology, Royal Hospital for Children, Glasgow, UK

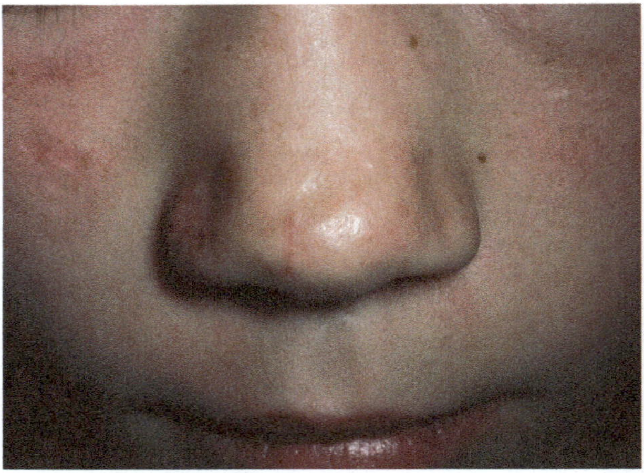

Fig. 16.4 Hydroa vacciniforme. A close-up of varioliform scars on nose and cheeks.
Reproduced courtesy of Susan Lewis-Jones, Hon Consultant Dermatologist, Ninewells Hospital and Medical School, Dundee, UK

Immediate photosensitive rashes

These occur quickly, often within a few minutes of sun exposure.

Solar urticaria

- Characterized by immediate itch and swelling of exposed areas.
- Most individuals are affected throughout the year and have their urticarial rash provoked by UVA and visible light, which filters through glass.
- Uncommon (3.1/100,000) with onset in any decade.[3]
- It may spontaneously resolve but in the majority runs a chronic course.

Management: photoprotection is important. Two-thirds benefit from antihistamines, but UV desensitization or systemic therapy may be necessary for this very debilitating condition.

Erythropoietic protoporphyria (EPP)

- Average age of onset is 2y.
- Presents as immediate burning and pain in sunlight with swelling and erythema, which often resolve with no sequelae but can cause purpura and scarring (Fig. 16.5).
- May be associated with gallstones and liver failure in later years.

Cause: inherited defect in the ferrochelatase enzyme in combination with a low expression allele. Provocation is by visible wavelengths.

Management: a specially formulated sunscreen is required for photoprotection. UV desensitization may be of benefit.

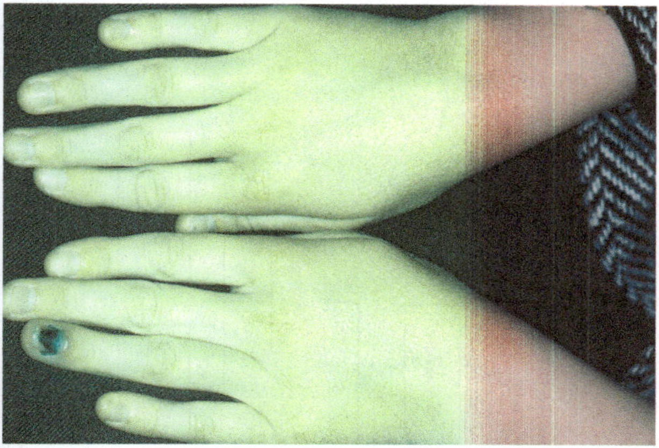

Fig. 16.5 Erythropoietic protoporphyria showing erythema and swelling of hands following a few minutes' exposure.

Reproduced courtesy of James Ferguson, Emeritus Professor University of Dundee, Scotland, UK

Note: EPP is one of a group of inherited disorders of porphyrin metabolism. Most others rarely present before puberty apart from the very rare Günther's disease (congenital erythropoietic porphyria) with extreme photosensitivity causing mutilation and scarring particularly of face and hands. For information and support, refer to https://www.porphyria.org.uk

Drug-related photosensitive rashes

These can be immediate or delayed, occur in response to a variety of drugs, and include phototoxic or photoallergic reactions (Box 16.1 and Fig. 16.6). There is a range of possible clinical presentations:

- Immediate prickling or burning sensation during exposure ± delayed erythema and pigmentation (amiodarone, chlorpromazine).
- Exaggerated sunburn (fluoroquinolone antibiotics, thiazide diuretics, and tetracyclines).
- Pseudoporphyria: increased skin fragility and blistering with trauma (nalidixic acid, naproxen, fluoroquinolone antibiotics, amiodarone, non-steroidal anti-inflammatories, and tetracyclines).
- Exposed site telangiectasia (calcium channel antagonists).
- ➲ See also Chapter 23.

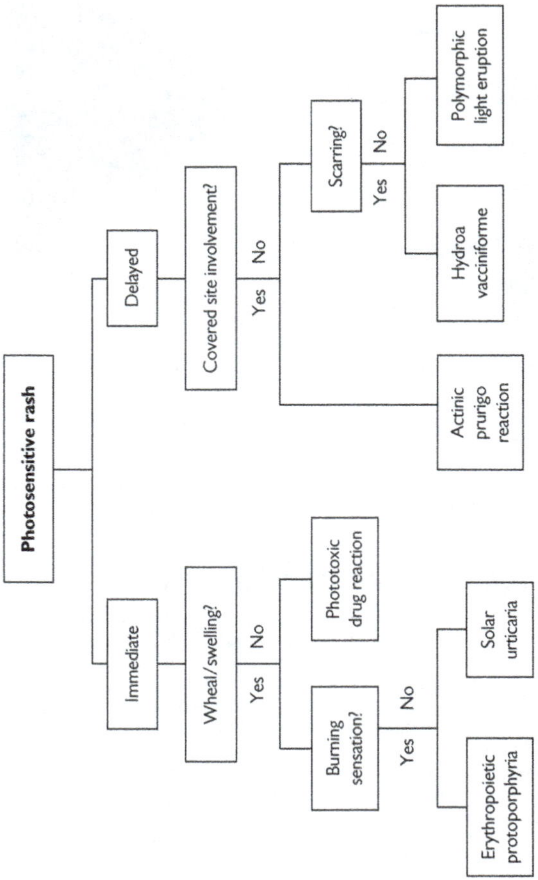

Fig. 16.6 Photosensitivity in childhood.
Reproduced courtesy of Paula Beattie, Consultant Dermatologist, Department of Dermatology, Royal Hospital for Children, Glasgow, UK

Phytophotodermatitis

A phototoxic reaction caused by exposure to plant products and UVA irradiation in sunlight. Presents as:

- Erythema, which may blister with subsequent hyperpigmentation (long-standing and may be a presenting feature).
- Linear, bizarrely shaped distribution in site of plant sap (Fig. 16.7).

Causative plants: contain psoralen, a phototoxic chemical defence against invading organisms. In the United Kingdom, giant hogweed (Fig. 16.8), an umbelliferous plant growing along riverbanks and waste land, causes the most severe reactions. Children often play with the hollow stems and commonly present to emergency departments in the summer months. May be mistaken for non-accidental injury.

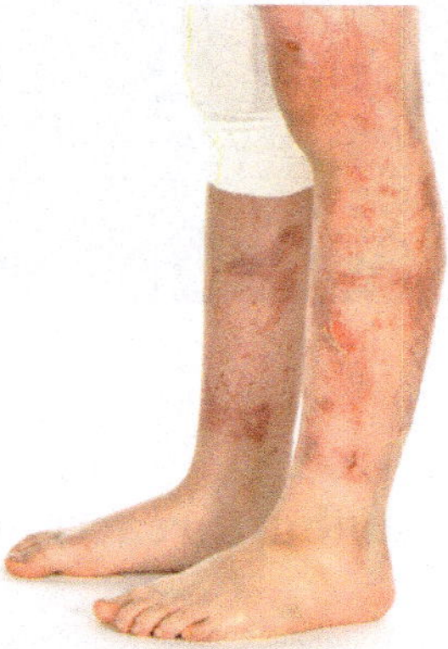

Fig. 16.7 Linear blistering on leg from contact with giant hogweed (phytophotodermatitis). This can be mistaken for non-accidental injury.

Reproduced courtesy of Paula Beattie, Consultant Dermatologist, Department of Dermatology, Royal Hospital for Children, Glasgow UK

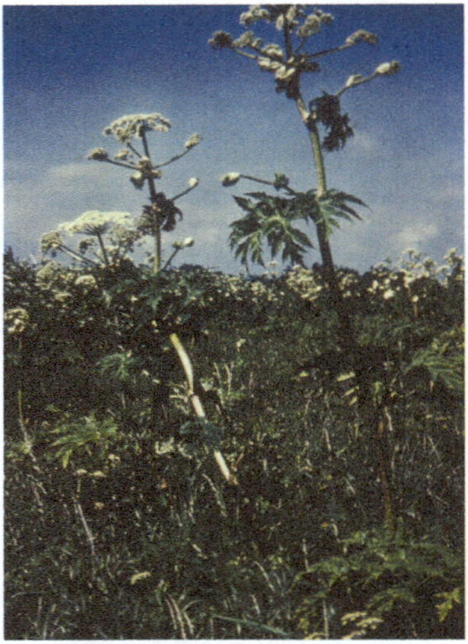

Fig. 16.8 Giant hogweed.

Reproduced courtesy of Susan Lewis-Jones, Hon Consultant Dermatologist, Ninewells Hospital and Medical School, Dundee, UK

Exaggerated sunburn reaction

Sunburn

Erythema, swelling, and occasionally blistering develop after excessive sun exposure as a result of UV-induced damage to nuclear DNA in keratinocytes. This fades as the damage is repaired in a variety of ways. Long-term sun exposure and severe or frequent sunburn predisposes to skin cancers in adult life, particularly in skin types I and II.

Any child exposed to the sun for an excessive period of time without adequate sun protection will develop sunburn. The severity depends on length of exposure, latitude, altitude, and Fitzpatrick skin type[1] (an arbitrary grading system giving a rough indicator of an individual's tendency to burn). This system grades skin as follows:

Skin type I—pale white skin that always burns and never tans.

Skin type II—fair skin that burns easily and tans poorly.

Skin type III—darker white skin that burns then usually tans well.

Skin type IV—light brown skin that burns minimally and tans easily.

Skin type V—brown skin that rarely burns and tans darkly.

Skin type VI—dark brown or black skin that never burns and always tans darkly.[1]

Exaggerated sunburn

Very rarely, the reaction may be exaggerated in severity and may be delayed, developing later and lasting longer than would normally be expected following exposure to sunlight. ***Long-term effects of sunburn include freckling, xerosis, and telangiectasia,*** which may also be exaggerated.

The commonest cause of an exaggerated sunburn reaction is drug ingestion (see Drug-related photosensitive rashes, p. 231) but other causes include the following rare genetic diseases:

Xeroderma pigmentosum (XP)

There are two main forms of this condition: classical and variant XP.

Skin manifestations result from deficient DNA repair after UV exposure.

Classical XP

A number of subtypes are associated with much clinical heterogeneity in terms of skin and neurological disease.[3] Types A, B, and D present in the first 3y of life with exaggerated sunburn (Fig. 16.9), followed by excessive freckling, xeroderma (dry skin), and premature skin ageing (Fig. 16.10; see also Fig. 32.6). Types C, E, and V (variant) present later because they do not develop an exaggerated sunburn but have a higher (increased up to 1000-fold) risk of developing skin cancers (basal cell cancers, keratoacanthoma, squamous cell cancer, and melanoma) than other types and these appear at a younger age, often before 10y. The eyes are also affected.

Management of XP

- Children should be managed by a specialist multidisciplinary team, including a paediatric dermatologist.
- Strict photoprotection with suitable hat, wrap-around sunglasses, long-sleeved clothes, and sun avoidance including photoprotective film on windows (including car and school) is essential. For information and support, refer to https://www.xpsupportgroup.org.uk.

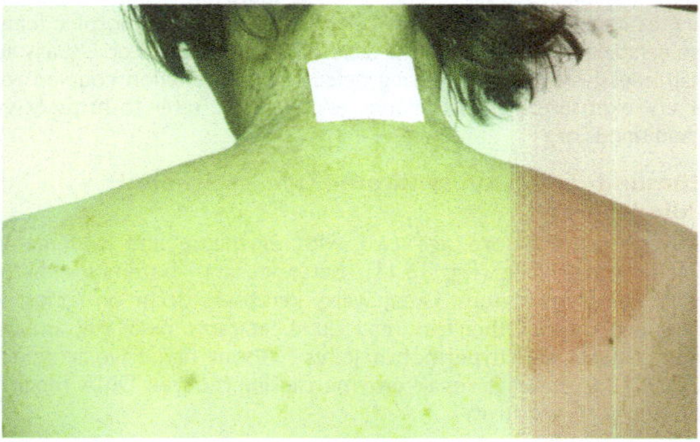

Fig. 16.9 Exaggerated sunburn response in xeroderma pigmentosum burning through white part of dress.

Reproduced courtesy of James Ferguson, Emeritus Professor University of Dundee, Scotland, UK

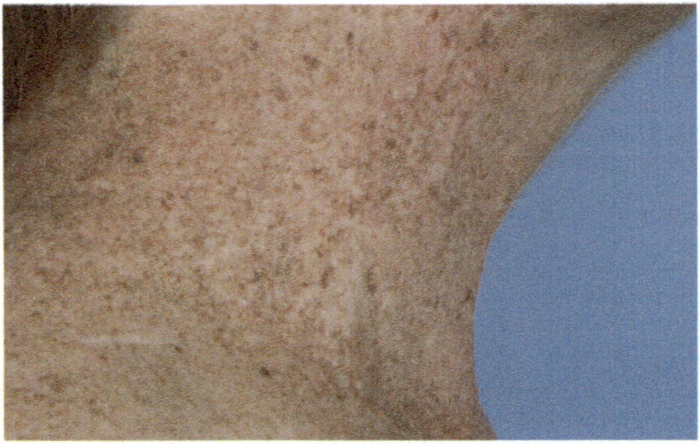

Fig. 16.10 Typical premature ageing with extensive freckling seen in xeroderma pigmentosum.

Reproduced courtesy of Paula Beattie, Consultant Dermatologist, Department of Dermatology, Royal Hospital for Children, Glasgow, UK

Trichothiodystrophy

Autosomal recessive condition also resulting from mutations in XPD/ERCC2 or XPB/ERCC3 causing deficient DNA repair. Some have photosensitivity. Other features include sulphur-deficient brittle/sparse hair (➲ see Chapter 14), ichthyosis, neurological disease, decreased fertility, short stature, a receding chin, protruding ears, and microcephaly.

Cockayne's syndrome

Classical type A presents in infancy with exaggerated and delayed sunburn then mottled pigmentation and atrophy. Other features include short stature, salt and pepper retinal degeneration, intellectual impairment, cataracts, central nervous system complications, and dysmorphic features (large ears and hands and bird-like facies). Milder types occur. Usually autosomal recessive condition causing defects in transcription coupled repair after UV exposure. For information and support, refer to https://www.amyandfriends.org

Rothmund–Thomson syndrome (*syn.* congenital poikiloderma)

Usually presents before age two with erythema and oedema then poikiloderma of face (Fig. 16.11), buttocks, and extremities, faltering growth, and short stature. Later, warty keratoses occur on hands, feet, elbows, and knees. Other features include cataracts, radial ray, and other skeletal defects and hypermobile joints.[4] About half have a defect in RECQL4 DNA helicase repair enzyme causing reduced DNA repair and associated UVA sensitivity.

Management: regular screening for osteosarcoma (seen in 30%) and other tumours including squamous cell carcinoma.

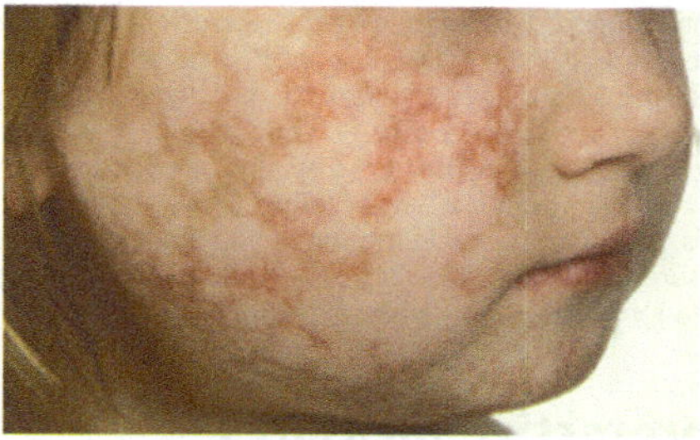

Fig. 16.11 Rothmund–Thomson syndrome showing facial poikiloderma.
Reproduced courtesy of James Ferguson, Emeritus Professor University of Dundee, Scotland, UK

Bloom's syndrome

Autosomal recessive condition associated with a DNA helicase mutation. Characterized by erythema and telangiectasia of exposed sites, severe growth retardation (intra- and postgestational) resulting in dwarfism and immunodeficiency (IgA). Other features include an elongated face and reduced fertility. Individuals are usually of normal intelligence but with a susceptibility to leukaemia, lymphomas, and carcinomas which may lead to premature death.

Photoaggravated dermatoses

Some inflammatory skin and connective tissue disease rashes can be exaggerated by sunlight exposure (Fig. 16.12).

- *Juvenile systemic lupus erythematosus*: most common childhood photoaggravated dermatosis, presents as a macular rash provoked

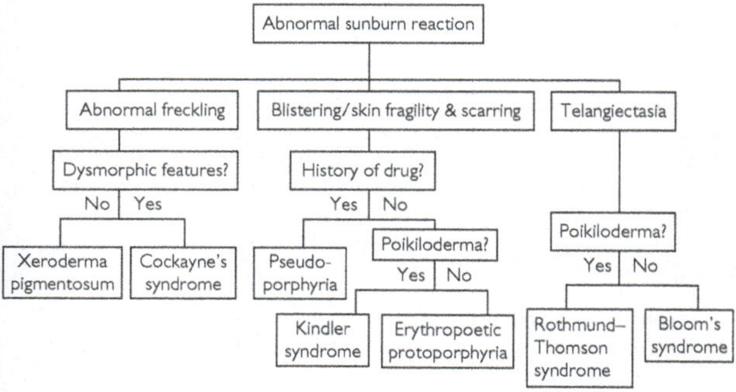

Fig. 16.12 Algorithm.
Reproduced courtesy of Paula Beattie, Consultant Dermatologist, Department of Dermatology, Royal Hospital for Children, Glasgow, UK

by sunlight and most prominent on exposed sites of face (➲ see Fig. 9.3), chest, and limbs. Mainly in girls. May be accompanied by arthritis, serositis, renal, neurological, haematological, or immunological involvement (➲ see Chapter 38).
- *Atopic eczema*: (➲ see Chapter 17) may also be photoaggravated, usually in teenagers with life-long eczema.
- *Psoriasis*: is usually improved in the sun but a few cases worsen on sun exposure (➲ see Psoriasis, pp. 320–1). Sunburn may cause koebnerization of psoriasis (➲ see Fig. 4.8).

Photoprotective measures

Preventative measures are the most vital part of the management plan of any photosensitive disorder (see Box 16.2).

Sunscreens

- ➲ See p. 40.

Rashes associated with sunscreen use

These are usually associated with either the sunscreen chemical or the added fragrance or preservatives. They may be:
- *Irritant contact dermatitis* (most common)—occurs without any sun exposure. Rash occurs soon after application. More likely if child reacts to multiple types of sunscreen.
- *Allergic contact dermatitis* (uncommon)—occurs without any sun exposure. Rash is delayed.
- *Photoallergic contact dermatitis* (rare)—only occurs with use of sunscreen followed by sun exposure (i.e. not where sunscreen has been applied to covered sites).

Investigation of photoallergy: includes patch testing (➲ see pp. 25–6) and photopatch testing. The latter involves applying duplicate panels of sunscreen chemicals to the back and irradiating one panel with UVA. Photocontact allergy is confirmed if an allergic reaction is seen on the irradiated panel only.

Box 16.2 Preventing sun damage to the skin

- *Avoid mid-day sun* (most UV is received between 11am and 3pm).
- *Seek shade*—but important to note that approximately a third of direct UV exposure occurs in shade (depending on object giving shade).
- *Wear protective clothing*—long sleeves, long trousers, or skirts in a tightly woven fabric.
- *Wide-brimmed hat.*
- *UV-protective sunglasses.*
- *Sunscreen* with a high sun protection factor (SPF), e.g. SPF50. Reapply hourly during sun exposure and after swimming or bathing.

References

1. Fitzpatrick, T.B. (1986). Ultraviolet-induced pigmentary changes: benefits and hazards, in Hönigsmann, H. and Stingl, G. (eds.), Therapeutic Photomedicine: Clinically Oriented Symposium, Organized by the European Society for Dermatological Research, Baden/Vienna, February 1985. *Curr Probl Dermatol* **15**:25–38.
2. Xeroderma Pigmentosum Support Group, https://www.xpsupportgroup.org.uk
3. British Association of Dermatologists (BAD), Patient Information Leaflets (PILs) are available for phototherapy; actinic prurigo; hydroa vacciniforme; solar urticaria; xeroderma pigmentosum (XP); erythropoietic protoporphyria and X-linked dominant protoporphyria; congenital erythropoietic protoporphyria (Günther's disease), http://www.bad.org.uk/for-the-public/patient-information-leaflets.
4. Rothmund–Thomson Syndrome Foundation, https://www.rtsplace.org

Section 4

Rashes

Chapter 17

Atopic eczema and related itchy rashes

Introduction

The eczemas are a group of itchy inflammatory skin diseases sharing some common clinical features. Dry skin is an important feature, particularly in atopic eczema (➲ see Atopic eczema (*syn.* atopic dermatitis), p. 245) and is a sign of poor barrier function, which often manifests itself from birth. The terms 'eczema' and 'dermatitis' are interchangeable.

Signs of acute eczema

- Redness (erythema) and warmth—due to vasodilatation, mediated by a cascade of inflammatory cytokines (Fig. 17.1).
- Swelling (oedema)—due to extravasation of serum from dilated vessels, sometimes with vesicle or bulla formation (blisters).
- Scratch marks (excoriations)—due to itching.
- Crusts—formed from dried serous exudate. Serous exudate encourages secondary bacterial infection, particularly with *Staphylococcus aureus*.

Signs of chronic eczema

- Lichenification—thickening of the epidermis producing an exaggeration of the normal skin creases. It is caused by chronic scratching and rubbing.
- Pigmentary changes—both hyper- and hypopigmentation may occur as a result of postinflammatory changes, in particular in ethnically pigmented skin.
- Follicular prominence—this is more common in those who are Asian or have black skin.

Box 17.1 lists the different types of eczema but there can be a degree of overlap between different types and some may coexist (e.g. irritant contact dermatitis is a common secondary event in those with atopic eczema).

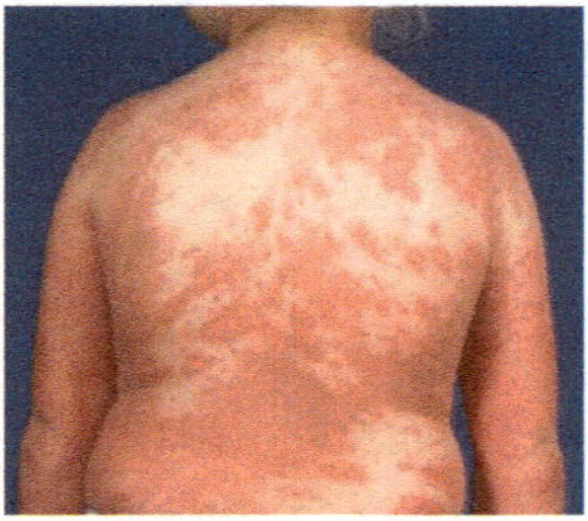

Fig. 17.1 Acute generalized atopic eczema.

Reproduced courtesy of Sivakumar Natarajan, Consultant Dermatologist, The James Cook University Hospital, Middleborough, UK

Box 17.1 Classification of eczema

Endogenous
- Atopic
- Seborrhoeic
- Discoid
- Pompholyx
- Varicose

Exogenous
- Allergic contact
- Irritant contact
- Photosensitive/photo-aggravated

Atopic eczema (*syn.* atopic dermatitis)

The commonest type of eczema in children affecting one in five in the United Kingdom. It usually starts in infancy and the majority have mild disease. There is an increased risk of subsequent food allergies, asthma, and later perennial rhinitis (hay fever)—the so-called atopic march, which is greater in those with severe eczema.

Diagnosis

The 2007 National Institute for Health and Care Excellence (NICE) clinical guideline for management of childhood atopic eczema[1] recommends using the refined Hanifin and Rajka diagnostic criteria from Williams *et al.*, 1994 (Box 17.2).[2]

Clinical features of atopic eczema

- Dry skin in the majority, reflecting impaired skin barrier function.
- Waxing and waning pattern with periodic flares and remissions, except in severe cases where it may be chronic.
- Flares are heralded by increased itching and development of poorly defined, dry red patches with subsequent scratching and further skin barrier damage.
- Sleep disturbance caused by itching is common and there can be marked impairment of quality of life for the child and family members.

Box 17.2 Diagnostic criteria

Itching, plus three or more of the following:
- Visible flexural dermatitis involving the skin creases*.
- Personal history of flexural dermatitis*.
- Personal history of dry skin in the last 12 months.
- Personal history of asthma or allergic rhinitis (or history of atopic disease in a first degree relative of children under 4y).
- Onset of signs and symptoms under the age of 2y (do not use this criterion in children under 2y).

**or visible dermatitis on the cheeks and/or extensor areas in children aged 18 months or under.*

Adapted with permission from Williams H.C. *et al.* (1994). The U.K. working party's diagnostic criteria for atopic dermatitis. Derivation of a minimum set of discriminators for atopic dermatitis. *Br J Dermatol.* 131(3):406–16. https://doi.org/10.1111/j.1365-2133.1994.tb08532.x.

- Pattern:
  - *Infants*—typically starts on face and neck (Fig. 17.2), often with cradle cap and usually clears after a few months but may spread more generally to trunk and extensor surface of the limbs (Fig. 17.3). The napkin area is usually spared due to the protective effect of modern nappy materials. Note, flexural involvement is often also seen in infants.
  - *Older children*—a flexural pattern predominates, particularly of the antecubital and popliteal fossae, wrists, hands, and ankles (Figs. 17.4–17.6) often with marked lichenification. In severe cases it may be generalized with marked excoriation and pigmentary changes (Fig. 17.7). Facial eczema often recurs, particularly around the eyes, ears, and neck, reflecting an airborne pattern of allergy or yeast colonization (Fig. 17.9).
- Secondary infection by *Staph. aureus* with golden crusting (impetiginization) is common.

Pathogenesis of atopic eczema

Atopic eczema is caused by a combination of complex genetic, immunological, and environmental factors, mostly linked to a 'Western' lifestyle.

Gene-environment interaction

- Polymorphisms occur in several genes regulating skin barrier function, located on chromosome 1q21 (the epidermal differentiation complex). Those causing deficiency of filaggrin (FLG), the cause of ichthyosis vulgaris appear to be particularly important (Box 17.3).
- Overproduction of serum total immunoglobulin E (IgE)—higher levels are linked to more severe disease and association with allergic sensitization (raised specific IgE levels to environmental allergens).
- Important environmental factors that contribute to the development of eczema in early life, especially in those who are genetically predisposed, are water hardness and exposure to antibiotics.

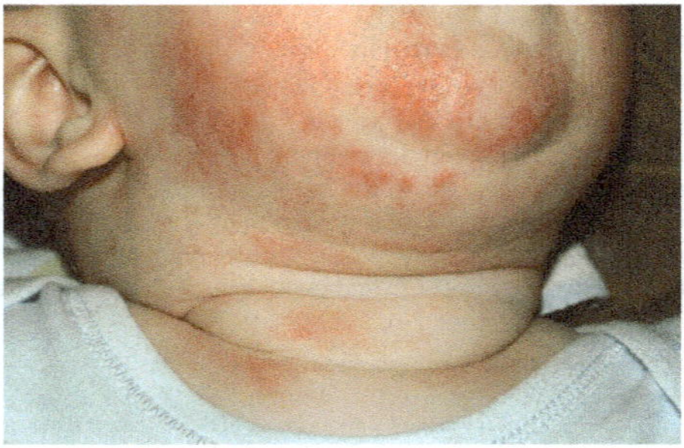

Fig. 17.2 Infantile eczema lower face.

Reproduced courtesy of Susan Lewis-Jones, Hon Consultant Dermatologist, Ninewells Hospital and Medical School, Dundee, UK

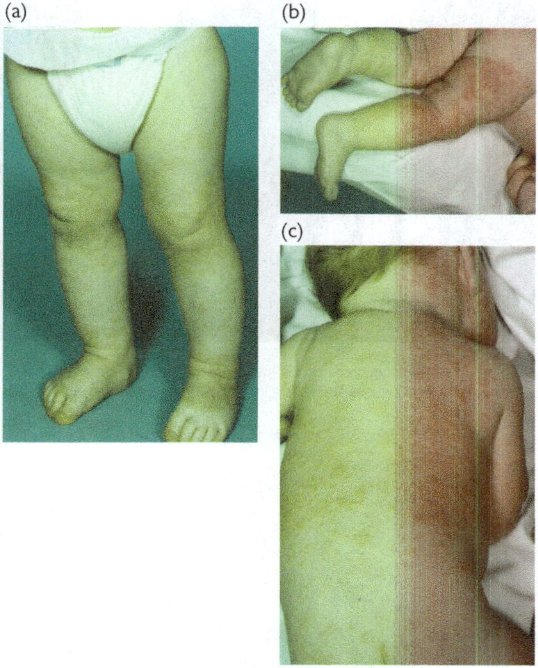

Fig. 17.3 Infantile pattern of rash on (a) extensor limbs. Sparing of (b) flexures and (c) napkin area.

Reproduced courtesy of Susan Lewis-Jones, Hon Consultant Dermatologist, Ninewells Hospital and Medical School, Dundee, UK

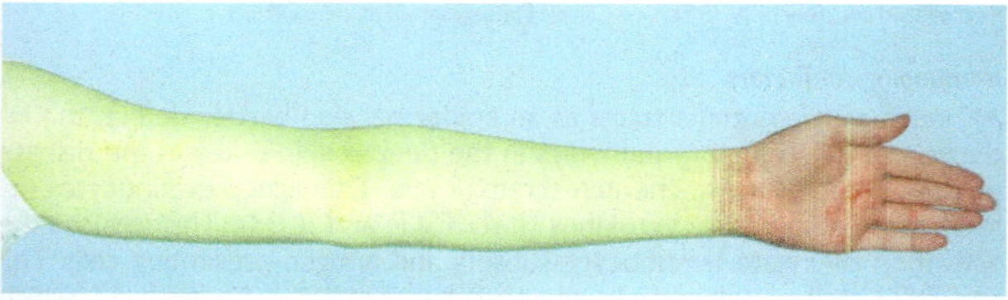

Fig. 17.4 Flexural atopic eczema in the older child involving antecubital fossa, wrists, and hands.

Reproduced courtesy of NHS Tayside Clinical Photography, Dundee, UK

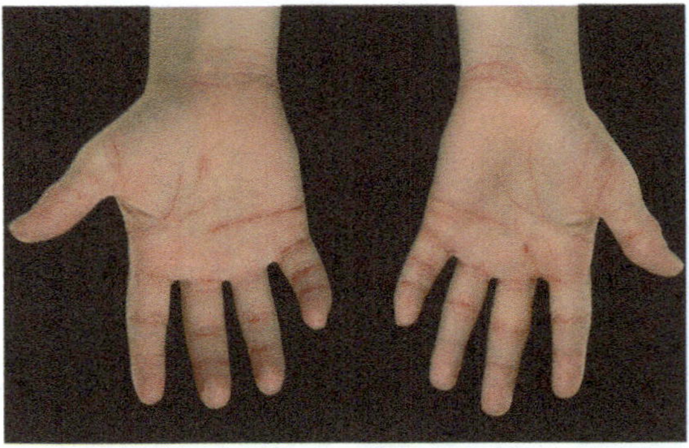

Fig. 17.5 Chronic atopic eczema of the hands with fissuring of creases, involvement of the wrists and hyperlinearity suggesting inheritance of mutation in the skin barrier gene filaggrin (*FLG*).

Reproduced courtesy of NHS Tayside Clinical Photography, Dundee, UK

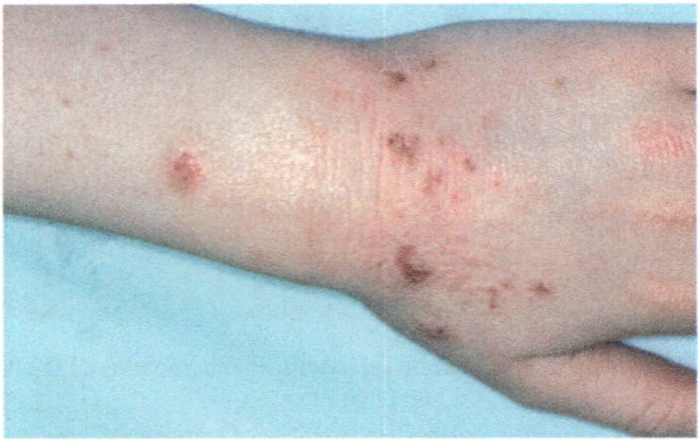

Fig. 17.6 Chronic lichenifed atopic eczema of dorsal wrists with crusted excoriations.

Reproduced courtesy of NHS Tayside Clinical Photography, Dundee, UK

Immunological factors

Although atopic eczema starts as an epidermal skin barrier defect, the induction of inflammatory pathways in the deeper skin is key in the disease process and closure of the itch-scratch cycle. Damaged keratinocytes release pro-inflammatory cytokines (IL-1, TSLP, and IL-33). This induces the activation of innate lymphocyte subsets and antigen-presenting cells Th2 and Th22 pathways, leading to an upregulation in Il-4, IL-5, and IL-13, which drives eosinophil and mast cell recruitment. Crosstalk between inflammatory cytokines and cutaneous nerves mediates itch, and the resulting scratching causes further damage to the skin barrier. There is now also evidence that the disrupted skin barrier in atopic eczema facilitates allergic sensitization to food and aeroallergens. Novel biologic therapies currently under investigation target the immunological pathways in eczematous skin, in particular Th2 cells and their cytokines (Box 17.4).

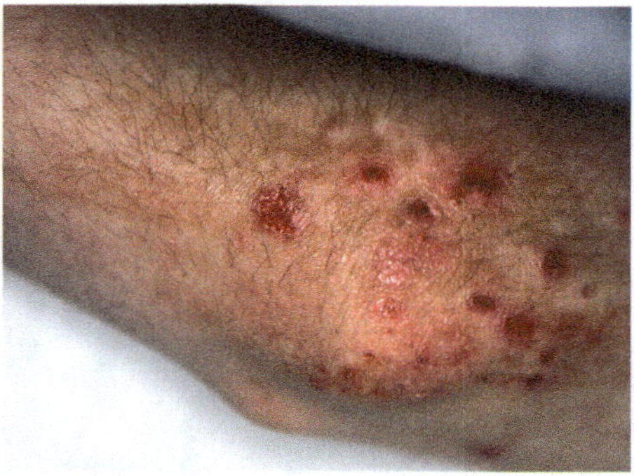

Fig. 17.7 Severely excoriated atopic eczema over elbow with postinflammatory hyperpigmentation.

Reproduced courtesy of Susan Lewis-Jones, Hon Consultant Dermatologist, Ninewells Hospital and Medical School, Dundee, UK

Box 17.3 Filaggrin deficiency and ichthyosis vulgaris

Filaggrin (FLG), formed in the keratohyalin granules (epidermal granular layer) is necessary for maturation of the corneal layer and production of natural moisturizing factor. Lack of FLG causes poor epidermal barrier function and a generally dry skin known as ichthyosis vulgaris.

- Heterozygosity for FLG null-mutations occurs in about 10% of the United Kingdom population. The skin may be normal or dry and there is a greatly increased risk of developing atopic eczema (odds ratio ~4).
- Homozygosity for FLG null-mutations occurs in about one in 90 and is strongly associated with early onset, more severe atopic eczema with a higher chance of persisting into adult life and often with concomitant allergic disease.

Clinical clues: extremely dry skin, especially on the shins with palmar hyperlinearity particularly over thenar eminence (Fig. 17.8). Keratosis pilaris is frequently associated.

History and examination

Thorough history taking is essential (➲ see Taking a dermatological history, p. 16). Key areas include whether there was erythroderma at birth (think of syndromes associated with eczematous rashes, such as Netherton) (➲ see Chapters 14 and 27), personal and family history of atopy, triggering, and relieving factors, diet and infant feeding, sleep disturbance, impact on quality of life and schooling, any severe medical illnesses or developmental problems, any severe infections (especially deep abscesses and pneumonia), current and past treatments and their effects, including use of alternative/over-the-counter therapies.

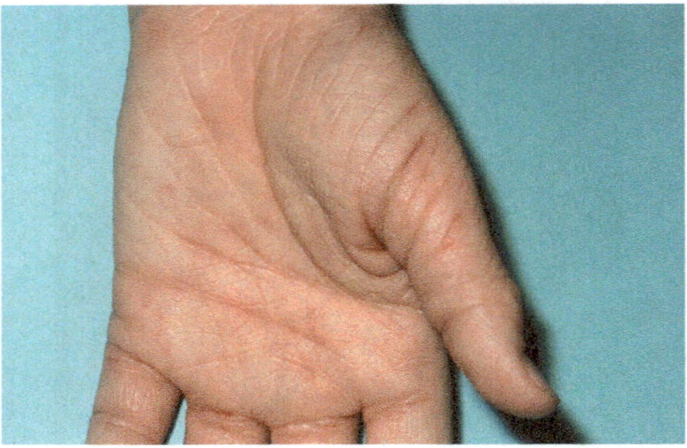

Fig. 17.8 Palmar hyperlinearity seen in those with a *FLG* loss-of-function mutation.
Reproduced courtesy of NHS Tayside Clinical Photography, Dundee, UK

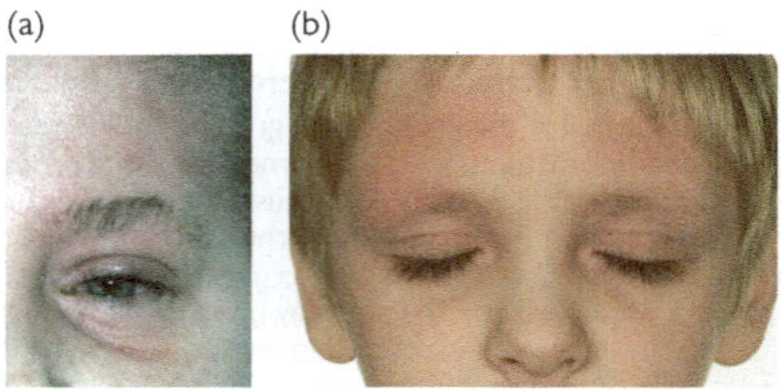

Fig. 17.9 Airborne allergy and atopic eczema around eyes. Note that this can also indicate a contact allergic dermatitis and be a feature in infected atopic eczema.
Reproduced courtesy of (a) Susan Lewis- Jones, Hon Consultant Dermatologist, Ninewells Hospital and Medical School, Dundee, UK and (b) Carsten Flohr, Professor and Head of Unit for Population-Based Dermatology Research, St John's Institute of Dermatology, St Thomas' Hospital, London, UK

Box 17.4 Chromosomal loci implicated in atopic eczema

- 1q21: epidermal differentiation complex, *FLG* locus.
- 5q31: shared loci with asthma and total IgE (RAD50/IL-13).
- 11q13: shared locus with food allergy and allergic rhinitis (C11orf30).

Examination

This should focus on the distribution and extent of involved skin and grading severity to mild, moderate, or severe (which may vary in different body sites[1]). Many scales exist for severity assessment but few are easy for clinical use and a global physician's assessment is probably sufficient. Look for evidence of secondary infection. Record growth parameters on standard charts to check for faltering growth.

Box 17.5 Assessing severity of eczema in clinic

Clear: normal skin. No evidence of active atopic eczema.

Mild: areas of dry skin, infrequent itching (with or without small areas of redness).

Moderate: areas of dry skin, frequent itching, redness (with or without excoriation and localized skin thickening).

Severe: widespread areas of dry skin, incessant itching, redness (with or without excoriation, extensive skin thickening, bleeding, oozing, cracking, and alteration of pigmentation).

Trigger factors

These should be actively sought (Box 17.6). Typical examples are:

- *Heat*: excessive heat from central heating or overwrapping causes sweating with irritation and increased itching.
- *Climate*: very dry skin tends to be worse in winter when humidity is low. Summer heat can increase itching but sunlight has an immunosuppressive effect and is usually beneficial, with appropriate sun protection measures.
- *Impaired barrier function*: is exhibited by dry skin—cells lose water (increased transepidermal water loss), the protective lipid bilayer is lost and irritants and allergens can penetrate through the epidermis. Soaps and detergents in particular worsen barrier impairment.
- *Infection*: secondary infection (impetiginization) with bacteria, particularly *Staph. aureus*, worsens atopic eczema, partly through production of super-antigens and endotoxins. Eczema herpeticum (caused by herpes simplex) is an uncommon but serious complication (➲ see Treatment of complications, p. 256 and Fig. 17.11). ⚑ Viral warts, chicken pox, and molluscum contagiosum tend to be more severe in children with atopic eczema.

Box 17.6 Trigger factors for flares

- Heat and climatic changes.
- Impaired barrier function—dry skin.
- Infection—especially *Staph. aureus* and yeast colonization.
- Stress.
- Allergens:
  - Food—mainly in infants with moderate/severe atopic eczema.
  - Airborne—more important from 5 to 7y.
  - Contact allergy.

High prevalence in:

- Urban settings and high-income countries. Also 'Western' lifestyle environments.

- *Specific allergens*:
  - *Dietary*: food allergens (in particular cow's milk, egg, and peanut) are mainly implicated in infants and young children up to about 5y (➲ see p. 252). They are a less common cause of atopic eczema in older children or adults.
  - *Airborne* allergens become increasingly important from early school age (i.e. house-dust mite, pet dander, tree and grass pollens, and some moulds).
- *Contact allergic eczema*: suspect in those reacting to multiple topical agents and in chronic facial or hand eczema (➲ see p. 259).
- *Stress*: may be an important contributory factor for flares.
- *Breastfeeding*: there is evidence that exclusive breastfeeding for 3 months (but not for longer) has a protective effect on atopic eczema.

Note: Parents should be informed that the causes of atopic eczema are multifactorial and that there are often many contributory factors.

Investigations in a child with atopic eczema

- Usually none are required.
- Take skin swab for bacteriology/virology if infection is suspected.
- Allergy testing (see rest of this section).

Note: parents should be informed that the majority of children with mild eczema do not need allergy testing and high street allergy tests are a waste of money.[1]

Food allergy as a trigger for atopic eczema

Research suggests that up to 30% of children with moderate to severe atopic eczema may have food allergy, but it is uncommon in the >80% with mild atopic eczema. Suspect food allergy in:

- ***Immediate (IgE-mediated) reactions***: such as hives, lip/facial swelling (angioedema) (➲ see Fig. 21.2), facial redness and itching, vomiting/diarrhoea, or anaphylaxis (difficulty breathing, limpness, cardiovascular collapse) within 2h after ingestion (➲ see Chapter 21). Most immediate reactions are caused by cow's milk, egg, peanut, cod fish, soya, and wheat. 🚩
- ***Delayed (non-IgE-mediated) reactions***: worsening of eczema within 24–48h in response to a particular food, especially if it occurs each time the food is ingested. Most are caused by cow's milk, egg, wheat, and soya.
- ***Gastrointestinal problems***: e.g. reflux, colic, and diarrhoea.
- ***Cases of faltering growth***: faltering growth and food allergy also occur in association with immunodeficiency syndromes (hyper IgE syndrome) and Netherton syndrome (➲ see Chapter 6).
- ***Severe atopic eczema***: in young children, especially if unresponsive to therapy of adequate potency.
- ***Severe generalized itching***: even when the skin seems clinically improved.

Investigation of food allergy in atopic eczema

It is important to realize that evidence for sensitization to an allergen does not necessarily imply actual clinical allergy and expert advice is usually required to interpret test results. The following tests may be helpful:

- Bloods for specific IgE antibodies.
- Skin prick testing to specific allergens*.
- Single-blind or open food challenges*.
- Double-blind placebo-controlled food challenges*—the 'gold standard' is available in only a few centres (open challenges more commonly used).
- Atopic patch testing: used in parts of Europe (and by some allergists in the UK). Reliability, sensitivity, and repeatability are not fully established.

Management of suspected food allergy in childhood atopic eczema

- In severe atopic eczema unresponsive to topical therapy a 6-week trial of hydroxylated amino acids can be tried while awaiting specialist opinion† (e.g. Nutramigen® or Neocate®). This is particularly the case in children under 6 months.
- Do not recommend diets based on unmodified proteins of other species' milk (e.g. goat or sheep milk†).
- All children placed on a restricted diet should be referred to a paediatric dietician.

  Note: childhood malnutrition associated with rickets and various skin disorders has been reported in association with unsupervised dietary restrictions.
- Refer children with moderate to severe atopic eczema suspected to be due to multiple food allergy for advice by a specialist.

Airborne allergens

Airborne allergens such as pollens, house-dust mite, pet dander, and some moulds appear to cause sensitization and exacerbation of atopic eczema in some children. This usually occurs from about 2y onwards. The pattern is typically of exposed sites such as face, neck, and periorbitally (Fig. 17.9) and there may be associated perennial rhinitis. The time of first allergen exposure may be important (e.g. contact with a household dog from birth seems to have a protective effect) but later initial exposure can lead to the development of allergic symptoms. House-dust mite reduction regimens have been disappointing in atopic eczema, although they sometimes benefit younger children and are worth trying, especially where children are shown to be house-dust mite allergic on formal specific IgE or skin prick testing.

General advice about airborne allergens

- In children with evidence of house-dust mite sensitization, reduce house-dust mite levels as far as is reasonably possible. Damp dust and vacuum mattress weekly.
- Avoid playing in long grass or with grass cuttings.
- Wash skin immediately after contact with pollens or other airborne allergens.

* Should be done by trained personnel with nearby resuscitation facilities.

† These recommendations are based on NICE guidance CGO57

- Avoid introducing a furry pet if children have established atopic eczema, especially if they react to pets outside the home.
- Keep pets out of bedrooms and also living areas (if possible). Avoid dusty environments (e.g. attics, cellars, and house renovations).

Management: general principles

- Establish diagnosis, severity, and extent of disease.
- Check growth parameters.
- Determine any possible trigger factors and investigate accordingly.
- Spend time with parents to explain what atopic eczema is and its management, advising that management is aimed at controlling disease and that symptoms in many children improve over time with optimized skin care.
- Good education is vital: give verbal and written advice and demonstration of treatment methods, with a clear written treatment plan. Nurse-led education, where available, is very helpful.
- For general measures see Box 17.7.
- Give advice on where to access further advice, e.g. a local nurse helpline (where available), National Eczema Society (UK), NICE guidelines CG057[1] (eczema); CG116 (food allergy).[3]
- Other support may be required especially for those with more severe disease (e.g. social, psychological, schooling, and so on.).
- Reduce allergen exposure as far as possible.

Improving barrier function

- *Treat dryness*: use emollients regularly (Box 17.6; ➲ see Emollients, p. 38 and Specific treatments for eczema, p. 255).
- *Avoid irritants*: e.g. soaps, detergents, and shampoo in the bath (wash hair separately), woollen clothing (except over cotton) or nylon.

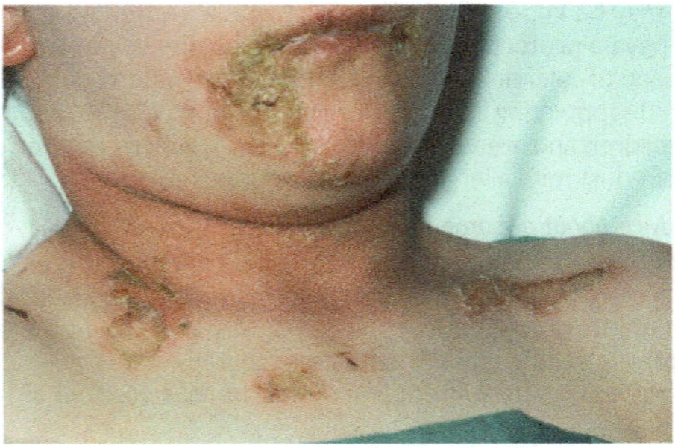

Fig. 17.10 Impetiginized atopic eczema.

Reproduced courtesy of Susan Lewis-Jones, Hon Consultant Dermatologist, Ninewells Hospital and Medical School, Dundee, UK

Box 17.7 General measures for treating atopic eczema

- Keep cool—use a fan in bedroom at night when necessary.
- Avoid soaps and detergents—wash with emollients. Reduce allergen exposure as far as possible (within reason; ➲ see Airborne allergens, p. 253).
- Use emollients regularly all over the body at least twice daily—even when the atopic eczema is clear. Children with significant atopic eczema will need 250–500 g per week.
- Keep nails cut short and filed to reduce scratching damage.
- Use cotton clothes and bed sheets (avoid nylon and wool).
- Use synthetic duvets and pillows (i.e. avoid feathers).
- Consider protective gloves or bandages or sleepsuit.
- Keep animals out of the bedroom and reduce dust levels.
- Use non-biological washing powder and avoid fabric conditioners.
- Avoid dusty environments like attics or house renovation.
- Avoid playing in long grass or walking among trees during pollen season.

Specific treatments for atopic eczema

It is vital to have a clear, written plan for maintenance therapy, flares, and episodes of infection. This should follow the stepped-care pathway (NICE Clinical Guideline CG057[1]) where treatment is tailored to severity.

First-line treatment

- *Emollients*: use liberally and frequently (at least twice daily and even when the atopic eczema is clear) (➲ see also Emollients, p. 38). Greasy emollients are best for dry skin and at night. Water-based creams are cooling for inflamed acute atopic eczema and more cosmetically acceptable. Consider emollients with antiseptics if recurrent infection is a problem.

NICE Quality statement 4: Provision of emollients states that: '*Children with atopic eczema are prescribed sufficient quantities (250–500g weekly) from a choice of unperfumed emollients for their daily use*'[1]

- ***Topical corticosteroids (TCS)***: (➲ see Anti-inflammatory treatments, p. 30) use once daily (*Note*: there is little evidence that twice daily is better) to red inflamed atopic eczema and for a few days after the skin has cleared to reduce flares and the itch-scratch cycle has been broken. Steroid phobia is a major cause of non-use of TCS, so explain that the benefits outweigh the risks when used correctly, and that side effects such as skin thinning will not be seen as long as the appropriate potency TCS is used[1] (Box 17.8). For quantities to use see finger-tip units (➲ see Fig. 3.1).
    - Use mild TCS for mild areas and the face and flexures.[1]
    - Use moderate TCS for moderate atopic eczema (~3–5 days on face and neck).[1]
    - Use potent TCS for severe atopic eczema (excluding face) for as long as needed initially and then in short bursts early on in flares (~1 week). Take care in vulnerable sites such as groin and axillae, and

avoid below 12 months of age except under specialist guidance. Refer if *'the atopic eczema is severe and has not responded to optimum topical therapy after 1 week'*.[1]
- Do not use very potent TCS preparations in children without specialist dermatological advice.[1]

- *Oral antihistamines*: non-sedating antihistamines can be helpful where airborne allergens are involved (especially head and neck predilection) and those with severe itching or associated urticaria. Continue if helpful but review 3-monthly. In those with marked sleep disturbance sedating antihistamines can be additionally helpful.

Treatment of complications

Infection: remember that moisturized skin is less prone to infection.
- *Bacterial* (common)—usually *Staph. aureus* or occasionally *Streptococcus pyogenes*. These cause golden crusts (impetiginization) and sometimes pustules (Fig. 17.10).

  Treatment: for very localized areas use topical antimicrobial agents for a maximum of 14 days together with a TCS. If severe or more generalized, use oral agents such as flucloxacillin or clarithromycin for 5–14 days as well as topical therapies.
- *Viral*—e.g. chickenpox can be widespread and severe (➲ Varicella-zoster virus, p. 380). Wart viruses including molluscum contagiosum can be spread widely by scratching. ***Eczema herpeticum*** is a serious complication of herpes simplex virus presenting with monomorphic (all lesions similar) small, circular blisters which quickly rupture to form erosions or crusts and often coalesce over large areas (➲ see Figs. 13.9 and 17.11). It may occur without active atopic eczema being present. ⚑

Management of eczema herpeticum

Commence systemic aciclovir if eczema herpeticum is suspected. Ask for urgent same day dermatological opinion (potentially lethal, e.g. from encephalitis).[1] ⚑ Valaciclovir may also be used.

Corneal scarring may result, so ask for ophthalmological advice if around eyes (Fig. 17.11).

- *Fungal*—tinea incognito is a fungal infection partially suppressed by TCS and may be missed (➲ see Fungal infections of the skin, p. 331). Look for red, sharply defined annular or arcuate margins (unusual in atopic eczema), sometimes with pustules.

Box 17.8 Note on topical corticosteroid usage

- When used correctly and monitored appropriately, corticosteroids are safe to use and usually very effective. Topical corticosteroids should always be used *as well as* emollients and *not instead of* emollients.
- Consider twice weekly ('weekend') treatment for flare prevention, once adequate control has been achieved. For 'weekend' therapy, TCS are applied even if the atopic eczema is well controlled. In the long-term this reduces the number of flares and amount of TCS used. This approach is particularly suitable where the atopic eczema tends to recur in the same places (➲ see also Anti-inflammatory treatments, p. 30).

Treatment: topical terbinafine and corticosteroid.

- *Erythrodermic atopic eczema*—a generalized inflammatory eczema covering >90% body surface area causing temperature dysregulation, fluid loss, protein loss, and rarely high-output cardiac failure. It is rare in children and requires immediate hospital admission (➲ see Generalized redness, p. 341).

Second-line treatment‡

- *Topical calcineurin inhibitors*: use only for moderate to severe atopic eczema and by physicians with a special interest and experience of dermatology. Can be used on the face for mild atopic eczema in those requiring long-term use of TCS (➲ see also Other topical immunosuppressants, p. 36).
- *Bandages or stockinette garments*: can be helpful for localized areas as protection from scratching or as short-term whole-body dressings, including wet-wrap therapy (➲ see also Other modalities of treatment, p. 41). Do not use over areas of obviously infected atopic eczema. Use with extreme caution on top of TCS because of increased systemic absorption. They should only be initiated by healthcare professionals trained in their use.

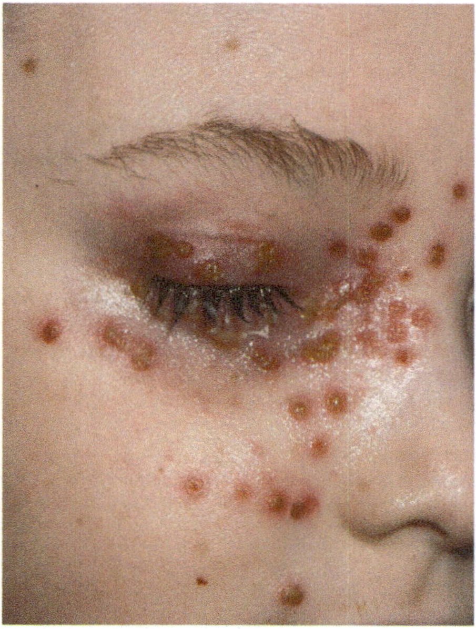

Fig. 17.11 Eczema herpeticum.

Reproduced courtesy of NHS Tayside Clinical Photography, Dundee, UK

‡Requires specialist expertise in dermatology.

Third-line treatment‡

- *Phototherapy*—ultraviolet (UV) light is only available in specialist units, but can be a useful third-line treatment, especially in children with racially pigmented skin.
- *Systemic therapies* such as ciclosporin, azathioprine, methotrexate, or mycophenolate mofetil are used for recalcitrant atopic eczema and only under specialist dermatological advice. Historically, ciclosporin and azathioprine have been used most but methotrexate has become the first-line systemic therapy in many centres based on a favourable side effect profile and randomized controlled trial (RCT) data suggesting comparable effectiveness. In addition to conventional systemic immunosuppressive therapy, dupilumab is the first biologic licensed for the treatment of moderate to severe atopic eczema in adolescents and adults. Further biologics and small molecules will enter clinical practice over years to come.

When to refer for specialist help

- See Box 17.9.

Box 17.9 Indications for referral (for specialist advice)

Immediate
- Suspected eczema herpeticum.

Urgent
- Severe atopic eczema unresponsive to 1-week topical therapy.
- Infected atopic eczema unresponsive to treatment.

Other
- Diagnosis uncertain.
- Child or parent/carer feels the atopic eczema remains uncontrolled (see Box 17.10).
- Suspected contact allergy.
- Significant associated social or psychological problems.
- Severe recurrent infections (e.g. pneumonia, deep abscesses).
- For specialist advice on treatment application (e.g. bandaging).
- Atopic eczema associated with faltering growth.
- Moderate to severe atopic eczema suspected to be due to food allergy.

Psychological assessment
- If severe impairment of quality of life and psychosocial well-being.

‡ Requires specialist expertise in dermatology.

Box 17.10 Useful guidance for parents/children with atopic eczema

- Eczema Outreach Scotland: http://www.eos.org.uk/
- National Eczema Society: http://www.eczema.org
- NICE Clinical Guideline [CG134]—*Anaphylaxis: Assessment and Referral After Emergency Treatment*: https://www.nice.org.uk/guidance/cg134
- NICE Clinical Guideline CG057—*Management of Childhood Eczema*: https://www.nice.org.uk/guidance/CG57
- NICE: *Testing for Food Allergy in Children and Young People*, https://www.nice.org.uk/
- NICE Quality Standards for Eczema Care: https://www.nice.org.uk/standards-and-indicators
- NICE (2011). Clinical Guideline [CG116]—*Food Allergy in Under 19s: Assessment and Diagnosis*: https://www.nice.org.uk/guidance/cg116
- Nottingham Support Group: http://www.nottinghameczema.org.uk

Prognosis

Most children with mild atopic eczema will clear during childhood with overall clearance of approximately 50% by the age of 5y and 60% by the age of 10y. However, in severe atopic eczema clearance is much less and there is a high risk of development of food allergies, asthma, and perennial rhinitis. In those with homozygous filaggrin deficiency (➔ see Ichthyosis vulgaris, p. 406) the atopic eczema is highly likely to persist into adulthood (Box 17.3). See Box 17.10 for further guidance.

Other types of eczema

Discoid eczema

The childhood pattern is different from adult discoid eczema and usually presents in infancy as extremely itchy round/oval areas often on the trunk and proximal limbs (Fig. 17.12). Serous exudate encourages secondary impetigo from *Staph. aureus* with golden crusts. Many cases have concomitant atopic eczema or go on to develop it. It usually resolves over several months but in older children, usually those with atopic eczema, there may be more chronic discoid lesions, particularly on the legs.

Treatment: often responds poorly to mild TCS and requires moderate/potent or in older children even intermittent ultrapotent TCS (*specialist advice required if using ultra-potent TCS in children for longer than a few days*). Topical antiseptics or short-term antibiotics may be useful for recurrent secondary infection.

Contact eczema

There are two types: contact allergic and contact irritant eczema. Both may coexist and contact irritancy (e.g. from soaps and detergents) is a common exacerbating factor in hand dermatitis in those with atopic eczema.

- ***Contact allergy***: suspect contact allergy if eczema is present in an atypical distribution, or has recurred later in childhood, especially on the face and hands or in those with no previous history of eczema. It may

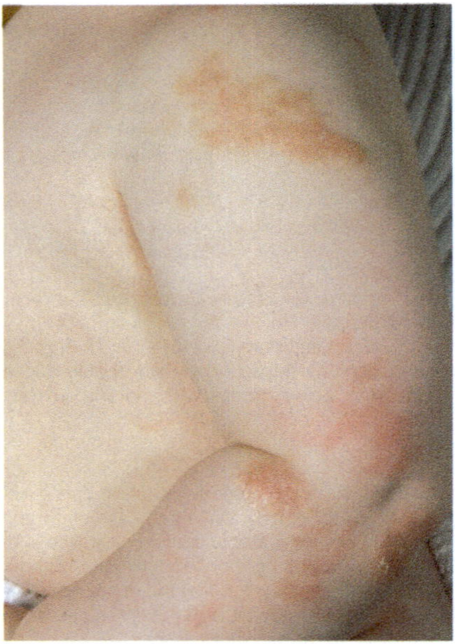

Fig. 17.12 Infantile discoid pattern of eczema.

Reproduced courtesy of Susan Lewis-Jones, Hon Consultant Dermatologist, Ninewells Hospital and Medical School, Dundee, UK

be well-demarcated in the site of contact (e.g. shoe dermatitis). The commonest allergens are nickel (cheap metal earrings, buckles, jean studs); fragrances; preservatives in cosmetics and medicaments; latex; rubber accelerators; and colophony (in fabric sticking plaster, violin rosin, pine trees).

Investigation: Patch testing; ➲ see Chapter 2 and Figs. 2.4 and 2.5.

Infantile seborrhoeic eczema

Yellowish-red flexural eruption with greasy scales, classically presenting with cradle cap and involving eyebrows, neck, axillae, and napkin area, with a strong association with yeast colonization (Fig. 17.13). Antifungal topical corticosteroid combination treatment can be very effective.

Seborrhoeic eczema can be confused with Langerhans cell histiocytosis (➲ see LCH, p. 180). In severe cases also consider HIV infection. Many go on to develop atopic eczema and some probably represent a form of infantile psoriasis.

(a) (b)

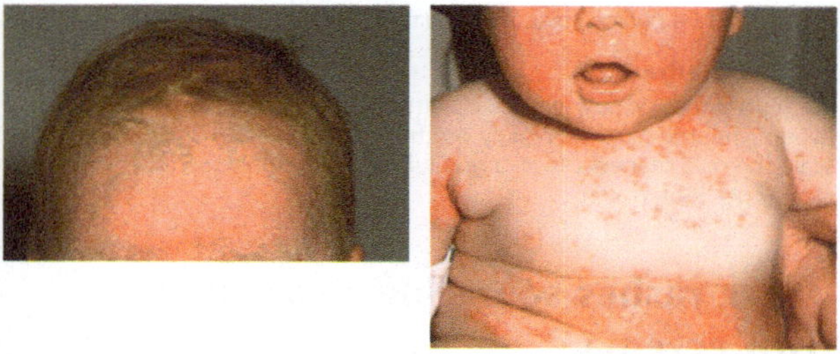

Fig. **17.13** Infantile seborrhoeic eczema with very psoriasiform rash.

Reproduced courtesy of Susan Lewis-Jones, Hon Consultant Dermatologist, Ninewells Hospital and Medical School, Dundee, UK

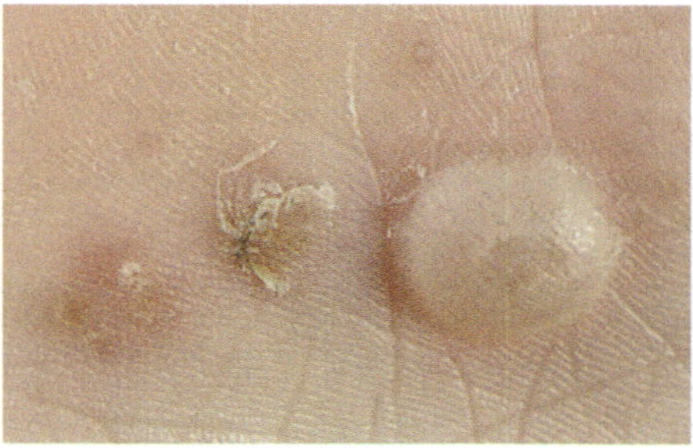

Fig. 17.14 Pompholytic eczema of sole.

Reproduced courtesy of Susan Lewis-Jones, Hon Consultant Dermatologist, Ninewells Hospital and Medical School, Dundee, UK

Pompholytic eczema (pompholyx)

Extremely itchy small blisters (vesicles) and occasionally larger bullae which tend to locate on hands and feet, particularly sides of fingers, palms, and soles (Fig. 17.14). It is commoner in spring and autumn and often recurrent. Often no cause is found but it is occasionally seen in association with acute tinea pedis (mainly in adults). Patch testing is important to exclude contact allergic eczema.

Treatment: moderate to potent TCS as necessary.

Varicose eczema

- Eczema of legs associated with venous insufficiency and varicose veins. Very rare in children.

Hyperimmunoglobulin-E syndrome

- Severe eczema, recurrent infections, skeletal and dental abnormalities, and very high IgE (➲ see Chapter 22). Very rare.

Forefoot eczema (*syn.* juvenile plantar dermatosis)

- Dry, fissured skin on soles, mainly balls of feet and heels (➲ see Fig. 12.7).

Pityriasis alba

An inflammatory low-grade eczematous process presenting as pale hypopigmented patches, mainly on the face (➲ see Fig. 32.3). Fine surface scale and mild redness can also occur. More commonly seen in children with racially pigmented skin.

Other rashes sometimes confused with eczema

- *Drug rashes* (➲ see Chapter 23).
- *Pityriasis rosea and other viral exanthems* (➲ see Chapter 22).
- *Pityriasis lichenoides* (➲ see Chapters 19 and 22).
- *Scabies* (➲ see Chapter 22). Eczema may also mask scabies.
- *Tinea infections (ringworm)*: may also complicate atopic eczema (➲ see Chapter 22).
- *Immunodeficiency syndromes*: consider in atypical eczema responding poorly to therapy, especially if associated with multiple allergies and severe or unusual infections (➲ see Table 6.2).
- *Mycosis fungoides*: a T-cell lymphoma which can look eczematous, usually not itchy but can be so (➲ see Mycosis fungoides, p. 340). Very rare in children (➲ see Chapters 11, 22, and 32).
- *Nodular prurigo*: very pruritic nodules, often on a background of atopic eczema, particularly located on the distal limbs and associated with chronic scratching. More common in children with racially pigmented skin.

  Treatment: difficult but potent or even ultra-potent TCS with or without occlusive bandaging can be tried. Other systemic therapies such as thalidomide have been used in adults.
- *Lichen striatus*: uncommon linear papular rash, following Blaschko's lines (➲ see Fig. 4.6) usually on limbs or trunk (Fig. 17.15). Red or skin coloured initially it is generally self-limiting over 1–2y leaving hypopigmentation that fades slowly without scarring. The histopathological process is of chronic eczematous change and TCS are helpful.

Itching

Itching is a common distressing symptom of many skin diseases, especially inflammatory skin diseases. Itching without evidence of skin disease is known as pruritus. Itching is perceived by itch receptors in the skin producing a release of cytokines (in particular IL-31) and the resultant desire to scratch so that scratch marks (excoriations) are seen in many itchy skin diseases. Scratching damages the epidermis causing release of inflammatory cytokines which exacerbate itching, the so-called itch-scratch cycle, seen particularly in atopic eczema and which often becomes habitual. Scratch

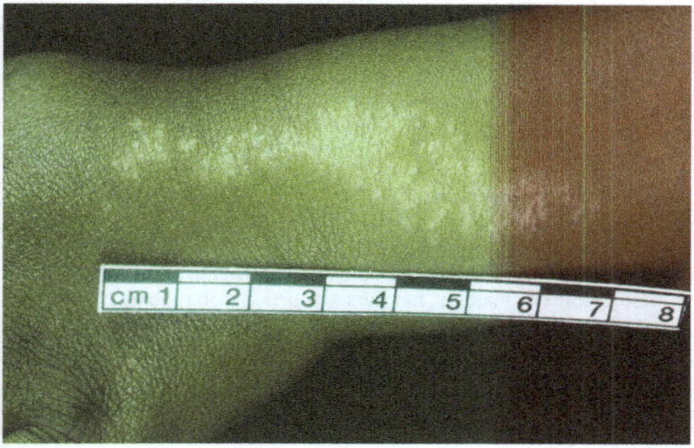

Fig. 17.15 Lichen striatus.

Reproduced courtesy of Cameron Kennedy, Consultant Dermatologist, Departments of Dermatology, Bristol Royal Infirmary, and Paediatric Dermatology, Bristol Royal Hospital for Children, Bristol, UK

marks present as small circular or linear lesions with crusting, superficial erosions, or ulcers. Scarring occurs if lesions involve the dermis. Scratching impairs barrier function and allows a portal of entry for infections such as viral warts, molluscum contagiosum, or impetigo. Scratching may cause koebnerization (➲ see Chapter 4) whereby diseases such as lichen planus or psoriasis occur within the damaged area.

Itching may occur in the following circumstances:

- Pruritus—itching without a skin rash.
- Itchy dermatoses—including drug reactions.
- In association with dry skin.
- Some skin lesions, e.g. insect bites, some 'lumps and bumps' (➲ see Chapters 19, 20, and 28).
- Neurotic excoriations (➲ see Chapter 24).

Itching without a rash (pruritus)

The most likely possibilities are:

- Hepatitis or renal disease that may be subclinical.
- Iron deficiency—although there is no good evidence to support this.
- Metabolic and endocrine disorders, e.g. thyroid disease or diabetes.
- Sign of underlying disease, e.g. lymphoma (very rare).
- Neuropraxis—partial nerve damage or crush injuries may produce an itchy sensation, e.g. peripheral neuropathy, spina bifida.
- Drugs, e.g. those causing subclinical hepatitis or renal disease.
- A delayed type food allergy (see earlier under food allergies).

Sometimes no cause is found but all cases need careful general examination.

Investigations: biochemical studies, including urea and electrolytes, liver function and thyroid function tests, full blood count, and iron studies. Food allergy testing. Chest X-ray may be necessary but should not be routine in children.

Management: appropriate to cause. Antihistamines and emollients can help. Topical and systemic corticosteroids have been used short-term and UV light phototherapy (➲ see Chapter 3) helps recalcitrant cases.

Itchy rashes (dermatoses)

A large number of skin rashes can be itchy the most common of which in children are listed in Box 17.11.

Other itchy skin lesions

Itching may be an occasional feature of any 'lump or bump' such as moles, but some are almost always itchy, e.g.:

- Keloid and hypertrophic scars—often intensely itchy initially.
- Mastocytomas—mast cell tumours that urticate on rubbing (➲ see Fig. 28.6).
- Insect bites.
- Scabetic nodules.
- Nodular prurigo (➲ see also Chapter 28).

Box 17.11 Examples of some itchy rashes

Common:

- Atopic eczema.
- Scabies.
- Urticaria.
- Viral exanthems.
- Drug reactions.
- Insect bites.
- Lichen simplex (uncommon in children).
- Psoriasis (sometimes itchy).

Rare:

- Lichen planus.
- Cutaneous T-cell lymphomas—may be very itchy.
- Epidermolysis bullosa—some types.

References

1. NICE (2007). *Clinical Guideline [CG57]. Atopic Eczema in Under 12s: Diagnosis and Management*, https://www.nice.org.uk/CG057.
2. Williams H.C., *et al.* (1994). The U.K. working party's diagnostic criteria for atopic dermatitis. Derivation of a minimum set of discriminators for atopic dermatitis. *Br J Dermatol* **131**(3):406–16.
3. NICE (2011). *Clinical Guideline [CG116]. Food Allergy in Under 19s: Assessment and Diagnosis*, https://www.nice.org.uk/guidance/cg116

Further reading

NICE (2013). *Support for Commissioning for Atopic Eczema in Children*, https://www.nice.org.uk/guidance/qs44/resources/support-for-commissioning-for-atopic-eczema-in-children-pdf-253673821

Chapter 18

Acne and acneiform rashes

Introduction

Almost all teenagers will develop some acne lesions. Approximately 5% develop clinical acne which requires medical intervention. Related acneiform rashes are also discussed.

Clinical features of acne vulgaris

Presentation varies but includes:

- Comedones, open (blackheads) and closed (whiteheads) (➲ see Examination findings, p. 267).
- Papules and pustules (➲ see Investigations, p. 268).
- Deep nodulocystic lesions (less common) (➲ see Investigations, p. 268).
- Secondary scarring (➲ see Examination findings, p. 267 and Investigations, p. 268).

Sites:

- See Box 18.1.

Causes

- There appears to be a strong genetic link especially in more severe cases.
- Acne lesions occur as a result of:
  - Sebaceous gland hypersensitivity to androgens (hormone levels are usually normal*).
  - Increased sebum excretion (seborrhoea), and ductal hypercornification, leading to blockage of the duct opening.
  - Increased bacterial colonization with skin commensal flora. *Propionibacterium acnes,* Gram-positive bacilli, which prefer anaerobic conditions.
  - Inflammation.

Prognosis

- In 80% of cases, acne clears by the twenties.

Exacerbating/modifying factors

- *Hormonal*: around 70% of females notice worsening of acne just before and during menstruation. PCOS and other endocrinological disorders (see next).
- *Stress*: may increase sebum excretion rate and alters lipid profile. Some patients tend to pick at/excoriate lesions.
- *Drugs*: e.g. antiepileptics, topical and oral corticosteroids (particularly in transplant patients), anabolic steroids, ciclosporin, rifampicin, isoniazid, iodides—all may induce or exacerbate acne.

Box 18.1 Sites of involvement of acne

- *Face*—usually the first site to be affected.
- *Back and chest*—often in a shield or V-shape, predominately upper trunk but may extend to the waist on the back (Fig. 18.1).

*A few do have abnormal hormone levels—enquire about onset and frequency of menstruation, hirsutism, alopecia, and weight gain in females indicating possible polycystic ovary syndrome (PCOS) and hyperandrogenism (➲ see Hirsutism, p. 208 and Examination findings, p. 267).

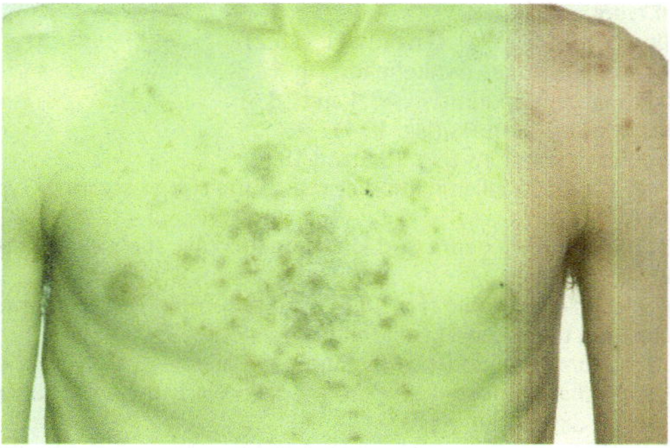

Fig. 18.1 V-shaped distribution of acne on the anterior chest showing inflammatory pustules, old purple lesions, and depressed scarring.

Reproduced courtesy of Sheila Clark, Consultant Dermatologist, The Leeds Teaching Hospital and Mid Yorkshire Hospitals NHS Trust, UK

- *Oil pomades*: commonly used by some ethnic groups and causes acne around the scalp margin (oil or pomade acne).
- *Other topical preparations*: cosmetics, moisturizers, sunscreens.
- *Diet*: evidence is limited but studies report improvement with a low-glycaemic index diet (slowly absorbed carbohydrates, e.g. most fruit, and vegetables, whole grain cereals, pulses).
- *Sun*: ultraviolet light can improve acne.

Association with other disorders

- Polycystic ovarian syndrome (PCOS)—association between polycystic ovaries, obesity, hirsuitism, and oligo- or amenorrhoea. Mild forms are relatively common. Up to 70% of patients with PCOS have acne. There are abnormalities in the metabolism of androgens and oestrogens and in the control of androgen production. It is associated with peripheral insulin resistance and hyperinsulinaemia (➲ see Hirsutism, p. 208).
- Congenital adrenal hyperplasia (CAH).
- Androgen secreting tumours.
- Cushing's syndrome.
- Hyperprolactinaemia.
- Acromegaly.
- Apert's syndrome (rare hereditary craniofacial dysostosis).
- Autoinflammatory syndromes:
  - SAPHO—synovitis, acne, pustulosis, hyperostosis, and osteitis.
  - PAPA—pyogenic arthritis, pyoderma gangrenosum, and acne.
  - PASH—pyoderma gangrenosum, acne, suppurative hidradenitis.
  - PAPASH—pyogenic arthritis, pyoderma gangrenosum, acne, suppurative hidradenitis.

Examination findings

- *Seborrhoea*: the degree of seborrhoea often relates to acne severity.

- *Lesion types*:
  - Open comedones (blackheads; Fig. 18.2)
  - Closed comedones (whiteheads; Fig. 18.3)
  - Inflammatory papules (Fig. 18.4 and 18.6)
  - Inflammatory pustules (Fig. 18.4)
  - Nodulocystic lesions (Fig. 18.5 and 18.6)
- *Scarring*: increasing inflammation increases the risk of scarring. Types include:
  - *Ice-pick* (Fig. 18.7) depressed, punctate atrophic scars with reduced or damaged collagen.
  - *Hypertrophic and keloid* (Fig. 18.8)—most common on the upper trunk, due to increased collagen production.
  - *Perifollicular elastolysis* (fragmentation of elastin)—usually on the trunk.
- *Pigmentary change* (postinflammatory), particularly hyperpigmentation, is common in darker skin types.
- *Features of hyperandrogenicity* (rare): androgenetic alopecia (frontal recession thinning of vertex) and hirsutism (➲ see Hirsutism, p. 208), cliteromegaly.

Investigations

None required in most cases.

- Swab the skin if bacterial folliculitis is considered.
- Hormone screen—only if clinically indicated.
  - Free testosterone, DHEAS, LH:FSH (if suspicion of PCOS).
  - 17-hydroxyprogesterone (CAH).
- Relevant investigation of underlying disease if suspected.

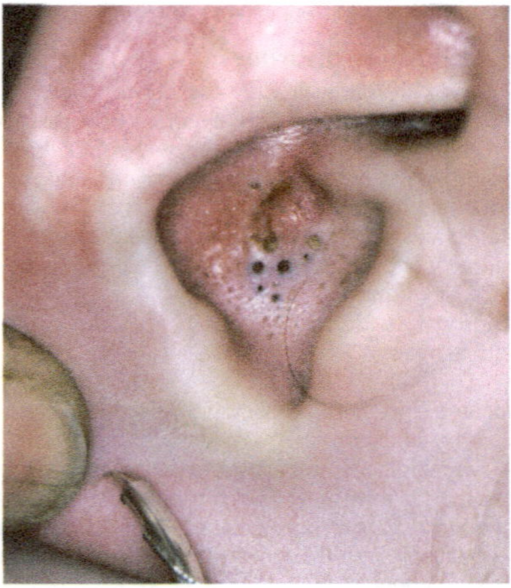

Fig. 18.2 Close-up of open comedones (blackheads) in ear.

Reproduced courtesy of Susan Lewis-Jones, Hon Consultant Dermatologist, Ninewells Hospital and Medical School, Dundee, UK

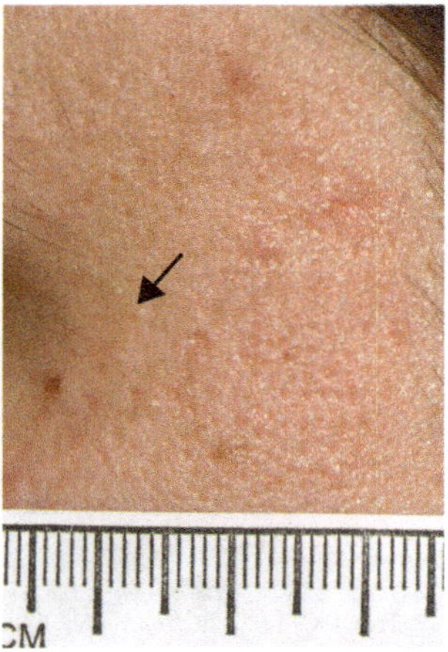

Fig. 18.3 Closed comedones (whiteheads).

Reproduced courtesy of Susan Lewis-Jones, Hon Consultant Dermatologist, Ninewells Hospital and Medical School, Dundee, UK

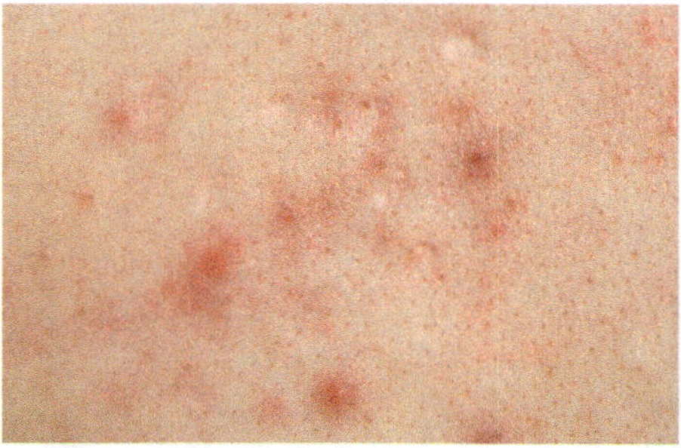

Fig. 18.4 Close-up of papules and pustules with some old scars.

Reproduced courtesy of Susan Lewis-Jones, Hon Consultant Dermatologist, Ninewells Hospital and Medical School, Dundee, UK

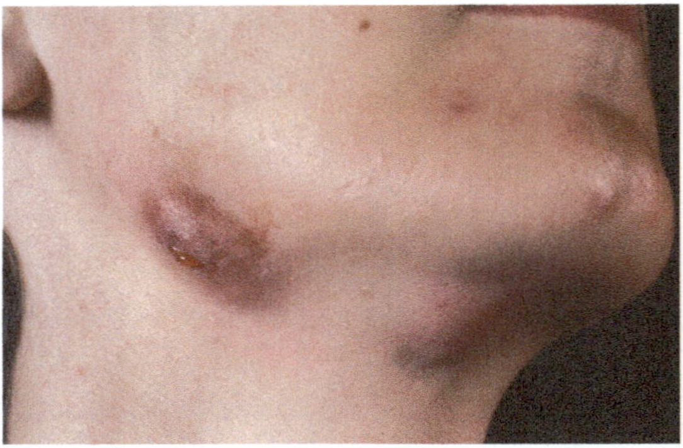

Fig. 18.5 Acne cyst jawline.

Reproduced courtesy of Sheila Clark, Consultant Dermatologist, The Leeds Teaching Hospital and Mid Yorkshire Hospitals NHS Trust, UK

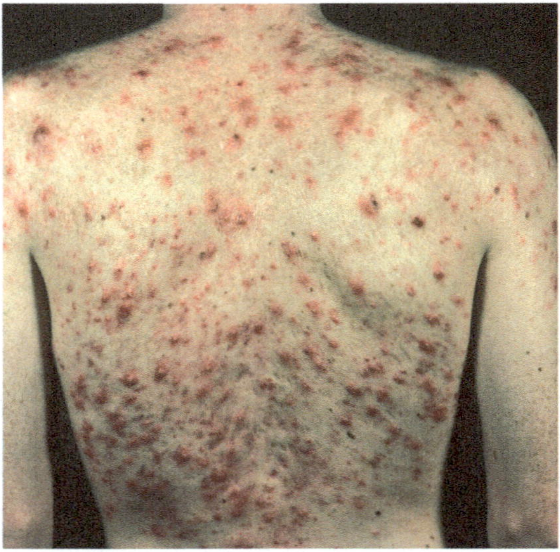

Fig. 18.6 Severe nodulocystic acne over the whole back.

Reproduced courtesy of Sheila Clark, Consultant Dermatologist, The Leeds Teaching Hospital and Mid Yorkshire Hospitals NHS Trust, UK

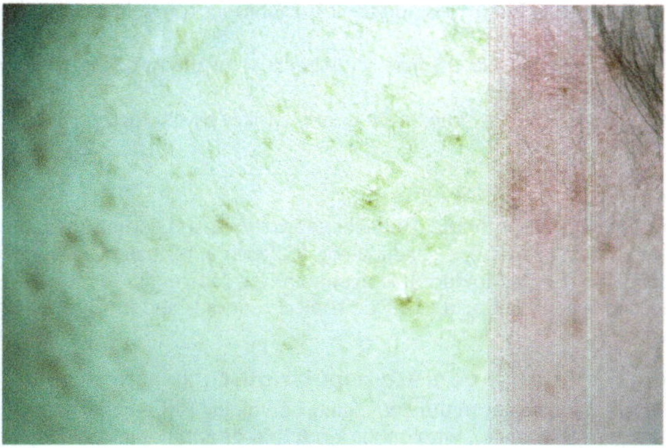

Fig. 18.7 Ice-pick scarring with some inflammatory papules.

Reproduced courtesy of Susan Lewis-Jones, Hon Consultant Dermatologist, Ninewells Hospital and Medical School, Dundee, UK

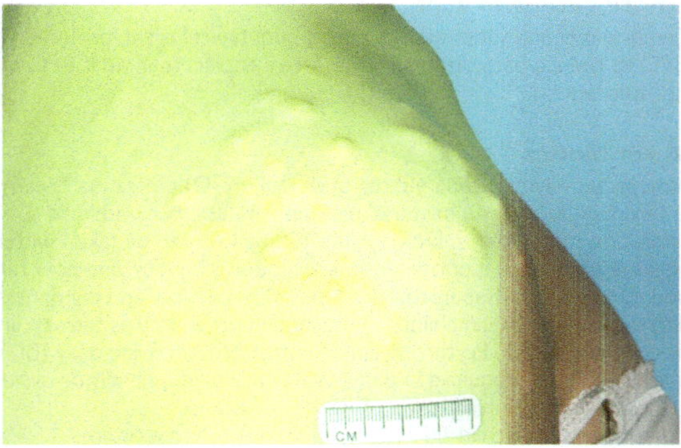

Fig. 18.8 Acne keloids.

Reproduced courtesy of NHS Tayside Clinical Photography, Dundee, UK

Management

General

- Provide appropriate patient information leaflet.
- Acne grading can be helpful to document severity and treatment response (e.g. Leeds and Comprehensive Acne Severity Scales).
- Inform that response to treatment is usually slow and treatment should be used for 3 months if tolerated.
- Several different agents may have to be tried alone or in combination.

- Avoid using dissimilar oral and topical antibiotics to minimize risk of bacterial resistance.
- Avoid tetracyclines in children <12y because of the risk of permanent staining of the teeth.
- Acne can significantly impact on quality of life/psychological stress.

Step 1: Comedonal acne

- *First line*: topical retinoid. Reduces seborrhoea and comedones (avoid in pregnancy), e.g. adapalene (Differin®), adapalene + benzoyl peroxide (BPO) (Epiduo®), isotretinoin (e.g. Isotrex®).
- *Second line*: azelaic acid or BPO. Topical retinoids and BPO cause dry skin and often irritation.

Step 2: Mild to moderate papular/pustular acne

- *Topical combination treatment*, ideally containing BPO (reduces bacterial resistance), with either a retinoid or antibiotic, e.g. adapalene + BPO (Epiduo®), clindamycin + BPO (Duac®), clindamycin + tretinoin (Treclin®), or BPO erythromycin combinations—Aknemycin®, Isotrexin®.

Step 3: Non-responsive to the previous recommendations or more extensive acne

- *Combine oral antibiotics with an appropriate topical agent*, preferably BPO to reduce bacterial resistance. Use a topical retinoid if BPO is not tolerated.

Oral antibiotics

- *Tetracyclines*—lymecycline 408mg once daily (OD) (Tetralysal®) can be taken with food and bacterial resistance is less than with first generation tetracyclines. Doxycycline 100mg OD can be taken with food (occasionally causes a photosensitive eruption). Minocycline now rarely used due to risk of hepatotoxicity, lupus-like reaction, and pigmentation.
- *Macrolides*—first line in children <12y and in pregnancy as tetracyclines are contraindicated. Erythromycin or clarithromycin twice daily (BD)—smaller doses are required in patients <12y. *Should generally be avoided >12y of age* due to high levels of *P.acnes* resistance.
- *Trimethoprim*—for children <12y who do not tolerate or are unresponsive to macrolides, or in older patients where tetracyclines have been inadequately effective, lost benefit, or are contraindicated or not tolerated.
- Continue oral antibiotic treatment for 3 months then switch to alternative oral antibiotic if response is inadequate. Longer-term treatment may increase *P.acnes* resistance.
- If there is inadequate response to two different antibiotics, consider options for severe acne.

Step 4: Women with moderate to severe acne

- If no contraindications, consider adding Dianette® contraceptive to the aforementioned treatments.

Step 5: Severe acne

- See also Acne conglobata and Acne fulminans in this chapter.

Options include:

- *High-dose oral antibiotics* (lymecycline 408mg BD or trimethoprim 300mg BD).
- *Oral isotretinoin* (retinoid). Doses usually 0.5–1mg/kg/day.
- *Oral steroid*—short course for severe inflammatory acne (in combination with other treatments).
- *Other*—phototherapies. Not currently routinely available. There is moderate evidence of the benefit of methyl aminolaevulinate photodynamic therapy (PDT) (red light) and low evidence on the use of aminolaevulinic acid PDT (blue light) as therapies for moderate to severe acne.

Acne in pigmented skin

- Postinflammatory hyperpigmentation is often significant and may persist long term, so consider early more aggressive treatment. Also irritant topical therapies (e.g. retinoids/BPO) may worsen it, so use less frequently and wash off at night.
- Secondary acne—from cultural practices, e.g. hair oil/pomades (➲ see Acne cosmetica, p. 275) and skin lightening products containing topical corticosteroids.

Management of scarring

- Around 50% of scars improve naturally over 12 months.
- Treating established scars is difficult.
  - Laser resurfacing: response variable and availability limited.
  - Excision of small 'ice-pick' scars.
  - Silicone gels may reduce lumpy erythematous scars.
  - Erythematous keloid/hypertrophic scars; steroid (topically and injected), cryotherapy, and pulsed dye laser have all been tried with variable success.

Differential diagnosis

- *Papular rashes*: especially keratosis pilaris (➲ see Facial problems, p. 124); angiofibromas seen in tuberous sclerosis complex (➲ see TSC, p. 483) concomitant acne is worsened by antiepileptic therapies.
- *Pustular rashes*: see Box 18.2.
- *Boils and abscesses* from any cause, including hidradenitis suppurativa which may coexist with acne (➲ see Hidradenitis suppurativa, p. 157).

Rarer presentations of acne

Neonatal acne (benign cephalic pustulosis)

- ➲ See Transient benign neonatal dermatoses, p. 81.

Infantile acne

Often presents between 18 months and 4y and is more common in boys. Lesions are usually localized to the cheeks, rarely elsewhere on the face (Figs. 18.8 and 18.9). Comedones, inflammatory lesions scarring, and rarely cysts may all occur. Hormone screens are usually normal but check for precocious puberty.

Box 18.2 Pustular rashes

- ➲ See also Chapter 20.

Pustular rashes of the head and neck

Common

- Perioral dermatitis.
- Gram-negative folliculitis.

Rarer

- Acne keloidalis nuchae (usually adults).
- Folliculitis barbae (usually adults).
- Rosacea (usually adults).
- Eosinophilic pustular folliculitis— note infantile variant.

Pustular rashes of the trunk and limbs

Common

- Gram-positive and Gram-negative folliculitis.
- Scabies.

Rare

- Pustular psoriasis (➲ see Fig. 22.18).
- Subcorneal pustular dermatosis (Sneddon–Wilkinson disease).
- Eosinophilic pustular folliculitis.
- Hot tub (pseudomonal) folliculitis.

Acral pustulosis

- ➲ See also Chapters 4 and 12.

Common

- Scabies.

Rare

- Acral pustulosis of infancy.
- Palmoplantar pustular psoriasis (pustular bacteroid of Andrew).
- Eosinophilic pustular folliculitis.

Differential diagnosis: aseptic facial granuloma (➲ see Red lesions, p. 420).

Treatment: topical erythromycin or benzoyl peroxide. Severe cases will require oral erythromycin or occasionally trimethoprim for a few months. Rarely oral isotretinoin has been used (under specialist supervision).

Acne excoriée

Usually affects young females with significant picking and scratching of lesions, often without significant acne (➲ see Fig. 24.9).

Comedonal acne

Due to topical follicular occlusion, both closed and open comedones are seen. Comedonal acne may occur with use of oily products such as sunscreens, greasy moisturizers, and make-up and pomades.

Naevus comedonicus

A rare, well-circumscribed, persistent naevus with grouped hair follicles filled with horny plugs. It is often linear and may present at birth or up to the

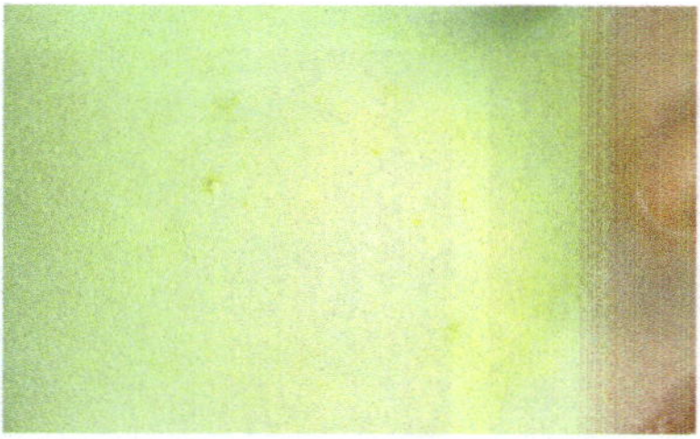

Fig. 18.9 Infantile acne with mild inflammatory papules and comedones (commonest presentation).

Reproduced courtesy of Susan Lewis-Jones, Hon Consultant Dermatologist, Ninewells Hospital and Medical School, Dundee, UK

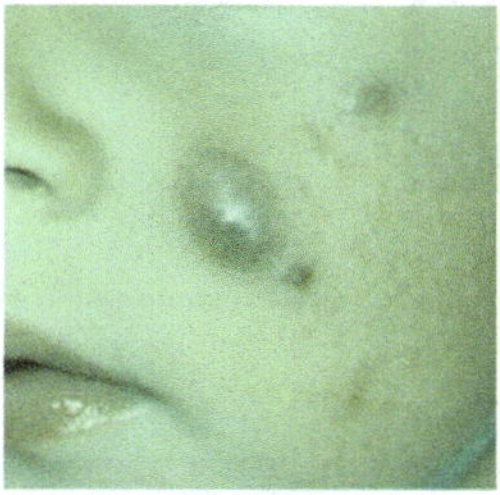

Fig. 18.10 Infantile acne with a large cyst and smaller inflammatory lesions.

Reproduced courtesy of Susan Lewis-Jones, Hon Consultant Dermatologist, Ninewells Hospital and Medical School, Dundee, UK

mid-teens, usually on the face, neck upper trunk, or upper arms. It is a localized mosaic form of Apert's syndrome (hereditary craniofacial dysostosis).

Pomade acne

Seen around scalp margins with oily hair pomades as multiple papules and sometimes pustules (Fig. 18.11).

Acne cosmetica

Similar to those already mentioned—women with a history of acne appear most susceptible.

Acne conglobata

A chronic suppurative form with bridge (paired) comedones, abscesses, and sinus tracts, usually in teenage boys and young men, and often associated with pilonidal sinus and/or hidradenitis suppurativa, ➲ see Hidradenitis suppurativa, p. 157.

Management: oral isotretinoin (see Step 5, severe acne, earlier in this chapter). Relapse is common and retreatment is frequently required.

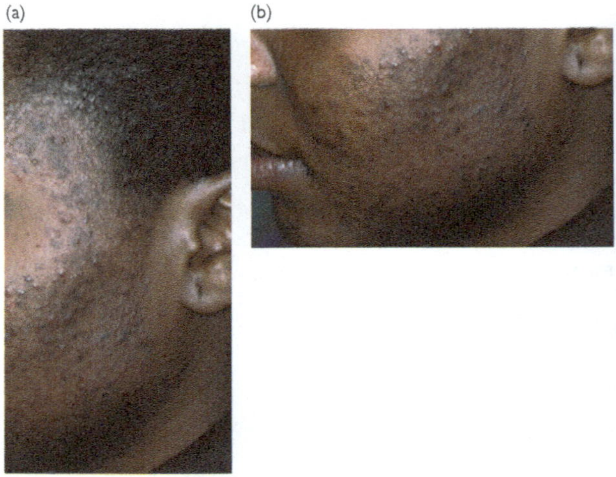

Fig. 18.11 Severe pomade acne.

Reproduced courtesy of Sheila Clark, Consultant Dermatologist, The Leeds Teaching Hospital and Mid Yorkshire Hospitals NHS Trust, UK

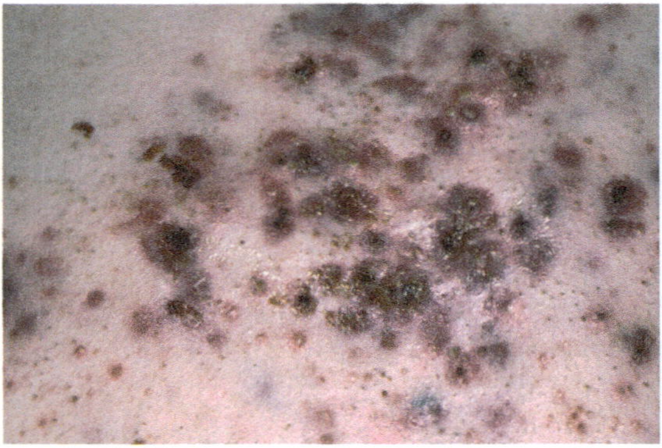

Fig. 18.12 Acne fulminans.

Reproduced courtesy of Sheila Clark, Consultant Dermatologist, The Leeds Teaching Hospital and Mid Yorkshire Hospitals NHS Trust, UK

Acne fulminans

A rare, severe ulcerative form of acne most common in adolescent boys (Fig. 18.12). Onset is acute with systemic symptoms including fever, weight loss, arthralgia, myalgia, erythema nodosum, hepatosplenomegaly, and osteolytic bone lesions.

Management: requires urgent dermatological review and occasionally hospitalization:

- Exclude any systemic complications.
- Oral prednisolone, commencing at 0.5–1mg/kg/day—often required for 2–3 months.
- Oral isotretinoin, with or without oral antibiotics are usually added once the inflammation has settled, starting at 0.5mg/kg/day, with close observation—rarely isotretinoin itself can precipitate the condition.

Pyoderma faciale

Rosacea variant. Usually affects females in their twenties. Pregnancy may trigger. Sudden onset, fulminating facial form with abscesses, sinus tracts, and background cyanotic colour. Scarring may be prominent. Seek early dermatological opinion.

Nuchal acne

Acne keloidalis nuchae is a chronic condition characterized by inflamed papules, pustules, nodules, and scars on the back of the neck around the occipital hair line (Fig. 18.13). Extensive keloid scarring and alopecia may occur. It is most common in young men of Afro-Caribbean skin type, less

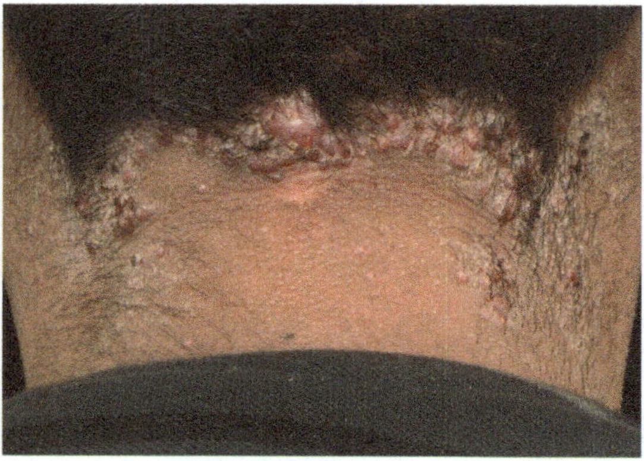

Fig. 18.13 Acne keloidalis nuchae

Reproduced courtesy of Sheila Clark, Consultant Dermatologist, The Leeds Teaching Hospital and Mid Yorkshire Hospitals NHS Trust, UK

commonly Asian or Latino descent. It is very uncommon in females and rarely seen prior to puberty.

Management: similar to acne vulgaris. Topical, intralesional, or oral steroids may be required to reduce significant inflammation. If extensive, liquid nitrogen cryotherapy or surgical excision of the affected area may be used.

Further reading

British Association of Dermatologists (BAD), patient information leaflets (PILS) acne, https://www.bad.uk

Cochrane reviews: Topical antibiotics for acne 2018; light as therapy in acne 2016; Complementary therapies in acne 2015; Treatment for acne scars 2016; Effect of birth control pills on acne in women 2012; Oral isotretinoin for acne 2011, https://www.cochrane.org

Nast, A., *et al.* (2016). European evidence-based (S3) guideline for the treatment of acne — update 2016—short version. *J Eur Acad Dermatol Venereol* **30**(8):1261–8.

O'Brien, S.C., Lewis, J.B., and Cunliffe, W.J. (1998). The Leeds revised acne grading system. *J Dermatolog Treat* 9:215–20.

Chapter 19

Papular rashes

Introduction

Papular rashes may occur due to infections, non-infective causes such as infestations or primary skin diseases. Common presentations are listed in Box 19.1. They may be found in association with other lesions such as pustules. Localized papular rashes on the face of a neonate may be due to sebaceous gland hyperplasia, milia or neonatal acne (➲ see Transient benign neonatal dermatoses, p. 81; see also Chapter 28). The texture may be helpful in making a diagnosis (Box 19.2).

Infective causes

- Molluscum contagiosum.
- Viral warts (➲ see Figs. 9.5, 12.9, 29.4, and 29.5).
- Viral exanthems (➲ see Chapter 22).
- Gianotti–Crosti disease.
- Congenital candidiasis (➲ see Chapter 22).

Infestations and parasites

- Scabies (➲ see Figs. 2.1, 22.13, 22.14).
- Insect bites (➲ see Fig. 20.5).
- Papular urticaria.
- Cercarial dermatitis (swimmers itch) (rare in the UK).
- Leishmaniasis (rare in the UK) (➲ see Figs. 26.4a and b).
- Onchocerciasis (rare in the UK).

Non-infective causes

- Acne papules and closed comedones (➲ see Examination finding, p. 267).
- Eczema (➲ see Introduction, p. 244).
- Keratosis pilaris (➲ see Facial problems, p. 124).
- Lichen planus.
- Lichen nitidus.

Box 19.1 Common presentations in children

Acute presentations

- Insect bites—usually exposed sites.
- Gianotti–Crosti—pink/red papules on acral sites of elbows, knees, buttocks, and sometimes cheeks.
- Other viral exanthems.

Longstanding papular rashes

- Molluscum contagiosum—skin-coloured with dimpled centre, may be inflamed, sometimes eczematized (red, itchy patches).
- Viral warts—skin-coloured/brownish; irregular surface.
- Keratosis pilaris—non-itchy papules on upper outer arms.
- Papular urticaria—purple lesions, mainly lower legs, very itchy.
- Acne—face, chest, and back, usually with pustules and comedones (➲ see Chapter 18).

Scabetic nodules

- Usually axillae, groin, and genital areas.

Box 19.2 Types of papular rashes by texture

- ➲ See also Chapter 28.

Smooth

- *Skin-coloured*—lichen nitidus, molluscum contagiosum (dimpled or plugged centre), elastosis perforans serpiginosa (rare).
- *Pink/red*—acne, insect bites, papular urticaria, swimmers itch, Gianotti–Crosti syndrome, scabetic nodules, Gottron's papules (dermatomyositis, ➲ see Chapter 29).
- *Blue/purple*—some acne lesions, lichen planus (white Wickham's striae on surface), papular atopic eczema.
- *Yellow/reddish-brown*—mastocytomas/urticaria pigmentosa, histiocytic diseases, eruptive xanthomas.

Rough or warty

- Viral warts, keratosis pilaris, Darier's disease, epidermal naevi (➲ see Figs. 4.5 and 4.10).

Scaly

- Pityriasis lichenoides, some viral exanthemata.

Crusted

- Any excoriated papule may develop a serous crust.

- Pityriasis lichenoides.
- Urticaria pigmentosa (➲ see Non-infective causes, p. 285 and Differential diagnosis of urticarial rashes, p. 313).
- Histiocytic disorders (➲ see LCH, p. 180 and The histiocytoses, p. 287).
- Darier's disease.
- Eruptive xanthomata (➲ see Fig. 5.3 and Eruptive xanthomas, p. 288).

Infection

Molluscum(a) contagiosum(a)

- Common, benign self-limiting infection caused by molluscipox virus (Fig. 19.1; ➲ see also Fig. 9.7). Often widespread and causes significant parental anxiety. Rare before the age of 1y. May be large and numerous in HIV infection.
- Incubation—2 weeks to 6 months, transmission by close contact.
- Dome-shaped, flesh-coloured pearly papules with umbilicated centre. Usually numerous. Size between a few mm to about one cm. Atypical lesions resemble fibroepithelial polyps (skin tags).
- Usually last 6–9 months but can last for 2y or more.
- Often become inflamed prior to involution—usually leave no mark but can leave depressed atrophic scars or anetoderma.

Treatment: Parental reassurance and allow natural resolution. For persistent lesions, 1–5% hydrogen peroxide cream or weak (12.5%) salicylic acid mixture applied daily. **Do not extrude contents** (packed with poxvirus). Cryotherapy—avoid in young children (painful). Curettage of individual lesions can be considered in older children.

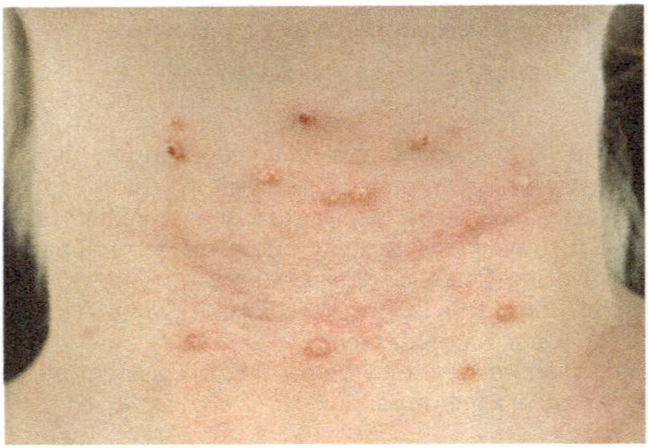

Fig. 19.1 Molluscum contagiosum—papules have indented (umbilicated) centres. Some are excoriated and surrounding erythema suggests secondary eczematous changes.

Reproduced courtesy of NHS Tayside Clinical Photography, Dundee, UK

Viral warts

These may be skin-coloured or brownish papules and have a rough surface (➲ see Figs. 9.5, 12.9, and 29.4). May be very extensive in immunosuppressed children such as those with transplants or HIV infections.

Gianotti–Crosti disease *(papular acrodermatitis of childhood)*

Occurs in infants and young children presenting with monomorphic, small, flat, firm erythematous papules or papulovesicles mainly on the face, limbs, and buttocks (Figs. 19.2 and 19.3). Lesions may be oedematous and rarely purpuric and may form erythematous plaques on the cheeks. There may be a low-grade fever and malaise.

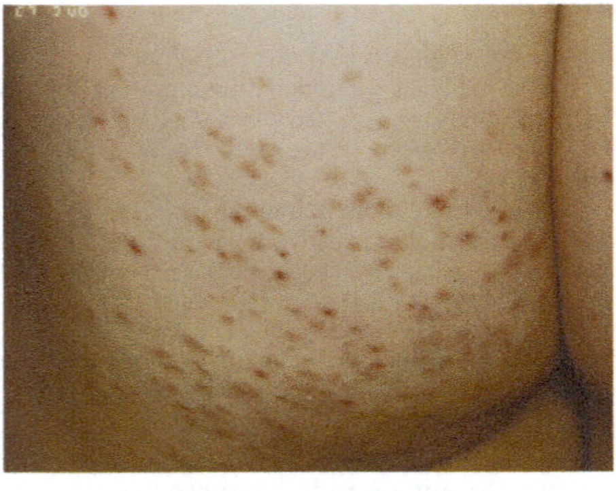

Fig. 19.2 Gianotti–Crosti showing papular lesions on buttock.

Reproduced courtesy of Susan Lewis-Jones, Hon Consultant Dermatologist, Ninewells Hospital and Medical School, Dundee, UK

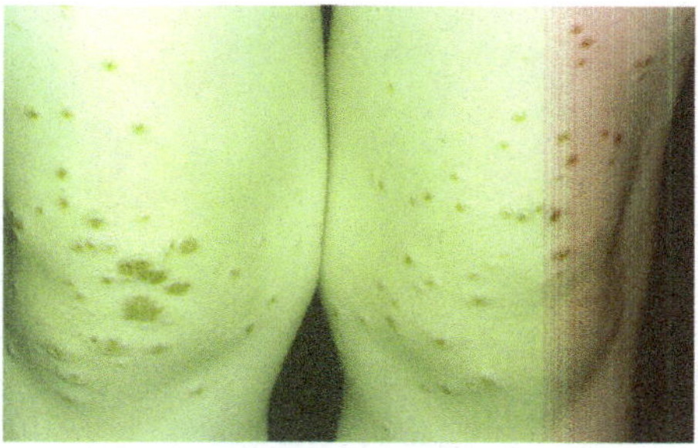

Fig. 19.3 Gianotti–Crosti: close-up of papules over knees and anterior thighs.
Reproduced courtesy of Susan Lewis-Jones, Hon Consultant Dermatologist, Ninewells Hospital and Medical School, Dundee, UK

Cause: most commonly *hepatitis B* or *Epstein–Barr* virus but others have been implicated. Jaundice is rare and prognosis is usually good.
Treatment: supportive.

Viral exanthems

Many viruses cause rashes (exanthems) with scattered erythematous papules and associated malaise, with or without fever. It is not usually possible to differentiate these clinically and unless the child is severely ill there is no necessity for diagnostic blood tests. These rashes can occasionally last for a week or more (➲ see Chapter 22 for some common viral rashes).

Infestations and parasites

Scabies

Papules and nodules occur particularly in axillae, groin, and penis (➲ see Fig. 28.14; see also Pustular rashes of the trunk and limbs, p. 296; and Infestations, p. 337).

Insect bites

Itchy red papules with surrounding urticarial flare of varying sizes, sometimes showing a puncture mark or occasionally blisters, which can be large (Fig. 19.4; ➲ see also Fig. 20.5). Usually occur in crops on exposed skin, although some bite through (mosquitoes) or under clothing (fleas), and some burrow under the skin (myiasis, e.g. bot flies) see also tungiasis (Jiggers) (➲ see Lumps and bumps on feet, p. 169). Some insects are vectors of serious infections such as malaria so protect children, especially when abroad, and always ask about holidays and animal contact. Occasionally persistent insect bite reactions occur: usually from retained mouthparts, e.g. ticks; or infection, e.g. leishmaniasis, ➲ see p. 285 (➲ see Figs. 26.4a and b). Bites are less likely in winter months in the United Kingdom.

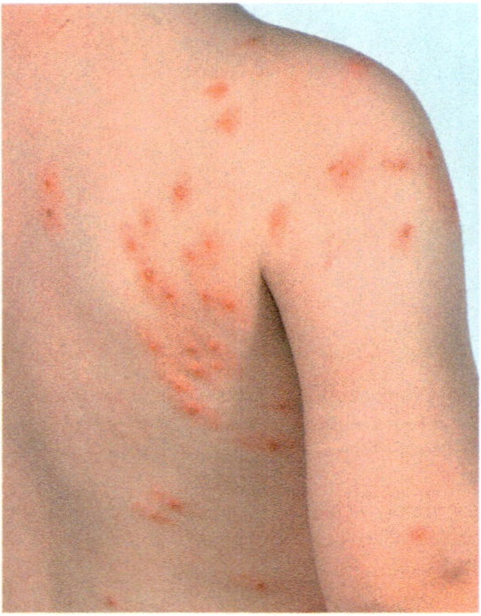

Fig. 19.4 Insect bites.
Reproduced courtesy of NHS Tayside Clinical Photography, Dundee, UK

Common causes

- Flying gnats, midges (order—Diptera, includes mosquitoes and sandflies)—these often cause blisters.
- Cat and dog fleas (*Ctenocephalides*).
- Human fleas (*Pulex irritans*): uncommon in the United Kingdom except for vagrants.
- Harvest mites (*Trombicula autumnalis*).
- Bed bugs (*Cimex lectularius*): large painful lesions usually on face.
- Tick bites: ticks may remain attached, their bodies bloated with blood before they drop off (➲ see Fig. 14.11). Ticks can transmit a number of diseases including Lyme disease (➲ see Spirochaete infections, p. 336).

Treatment of papular bites: oral antihistamines and topical corticosteroids may be helpful. Topical antihistamines are effective but not recommended because of possible contact allergy, so limit use to short periods only.

Papular urticaria

Intensely itchy and usually excoriated, dome-shaped red papules in crops mainly on lower legs. Sometimes with surrounding flare. Typically leave small circular purple scars taking up to 12 months to fade.

Cause: thought to be a sensitization reaction to bites and stings.

Usually in young children in the summer, older children becoming desensitized. Typically only one member of the family may be affected. Treat as for insect bites.

Swimmer's itch (cercarial dermatitis)

Itchy red papules occurring after swimming in waters infested with cercarial stages of several non-human schistosomes. Often starts as tingling in contact with the water. Treatment is symptomatic. Rare in the United Kingdom.

Leishmaniasis

Protozoal infections transmitted by sand flies. Several species from old world (N. Africa and Mediterranean but not United Kingdom) and new world (S. America) causing systemic and cutaneous manifestations. Presentation varies from: self-healing papules; large nodules; eschars (➲ see Figs. 26.4a and b); indolent scarring areas with multiple small papules at edges resembling lupus vulgaris (recidivans type); or non-healing indolent ulcers (➲ see Chapter 30). Typically, *Leishmania (L.) major* causes small, red, abscess-like lesions occurring on exposed parts about 2 months after bites, becoming crusted and sometimes ulcerated, before healing slowly to leave a scar. *L.donovani infantum* is commonest in Europe and N. Africa, causing visceral disease in infants but self-healing lesions in older children.

Treatment: depends on type—consult an infectious disease specialist, see the Centers for Disease Control and Prevention (CDC) website: https://www.cdc.gov/dpdx/leishmaniasis/index.html

Onchocerciasis

Common in endemic areas, mainly Africa. It presents as a papular rash in children >5y on lower trunk and legs. Late stages (adults) show nodules, depigmentation on shins and lax, dry skin (lizard skin). Blindness is common.

Cause: hypersensitivity reactions to microfilaria of *Onchocerca volvulus* a nematode transmitted by river black fly (*Simulium*).

Treatment: ivermectin with prior doxycycline. Consult an infectious disease specialist. See CDC website: https://www.cdc.gov/dpdx/onchocerciasis/index.html

Non-infective causes

Atopic dermatitis

May be papular, especially in chronic cases and particularly in black skin and those of Asian descent (➲ see Chapter 17). Always extremely itchy.

Keratosis pilaris

Commonly associated with atopic eczema and ichthyosis vulgaris. Usually just feels like rough skin on upper, outer arms (sometimes cheeks and legs) but often as small skin-coloured/pinkish papules, ➲ see Facial problems, p. 124).

Lichen nitidus

Regarded as a childhood variant of lichen planus and more common. Small skin-coloured, non-irritant flat-topped papules occur in groups on the skin. The trunk is the commonest site. Resolves spontaneously. See Fig. 19.5.

Treatment: none required.

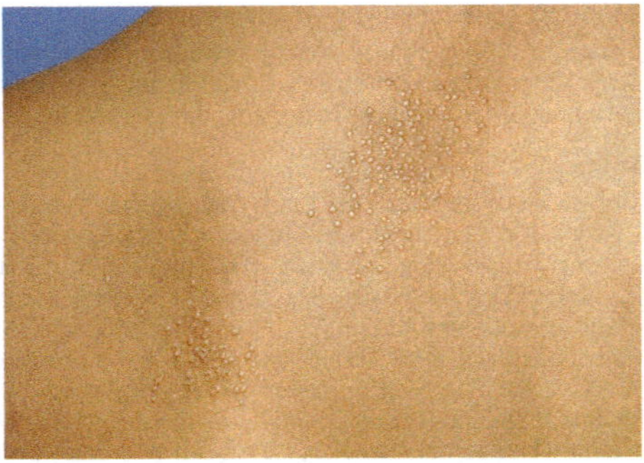

Fig. 19.5 Lichen nitidus.

Reproduced courtesy of NHS Tayside Clinical Photography, Dundee, UK

Lichen planus

Very uncommon in children, usually occurring in those of Asian descent. Itchy, flat-topped, polygonal, violaceous papules with a fine linear white scale on the surface (Wickham's striae; Fig. 19.6). They can occur anywhere but have a predilection for the ventral wrists and legs. A rare bullous form exists. A white lace-like pattern may be seen on the buccal mucosa. Nail dystrophy (➲ see Fig. 15.8) and localized scarring alopecia are uncommon.

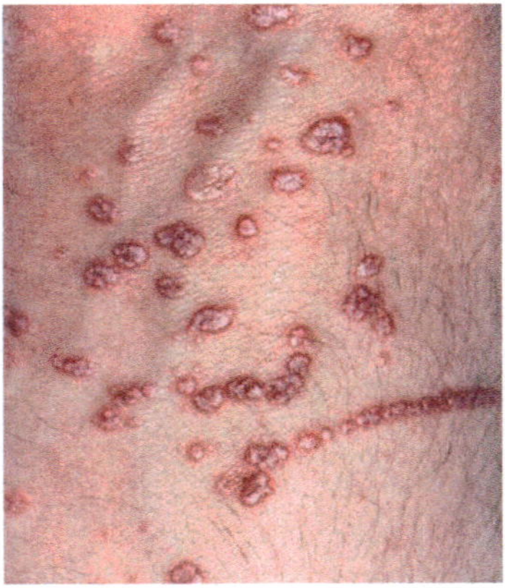

Fig. 19.6 Close-up of lichen planus; note koebnerization with linear arrangement of papules.

Reproduced courtesy of Susan Lewis-Jones, Hon Consultant Dermatologist, Ninewells Hospital and Medical School, Dundee, UK

Treatment: moderately potent/potent topical corticosteroids. Generalized disease may require a short course of systemic therapy with oral corticosteroids.

Pityriasis lichenoides

Affects children of all ages. Reddish-brown papules develop in crops over the trunk and limbs. There are acute and chronic variants which may coexist:

- ***Acute form***: lesions become haemorrhagic with occasional necrosis, ulceration, and small eschars. Systemic symptoms may occur. May be confused with chickenpox.
- ***Chronic form***: more common (Fig. 19.7). The papules have an adherent silvery (mica) scale. New lesions may appear every few weeks over long periods of time.

Aetiology: unknown, although sensitization to a virus is postulated.

Treatment: systemic erythromycin may be helpful in the acute variant. Sunlight helps and ultraviolet phototherapy (➲ see Chapter 3) can be helpful.

The histiocytoses

Reddish-brown papules are present in several of the cutaneous histiocytoses. These are a complicated group of disorders recently reclassified into five groups (L, C, M, R, and H).

Group L includes Langerhans cell histiocytosis (➲ see Fig. 13.5).

Group C: The cutaneous and mucocutaneous forms of histiocytosis include:

- ***Juvenile xanthogranuloma*** (➲ see Figs. 28.11 and 37.3).
- ***Benign cephalic histiocytosis***: small yellow-brown papules on head and neck of infants which gradually resolve to form pigmented, atrophic macules.
- ***Generalized eruptive histiocytomas***: usually seen in adults.

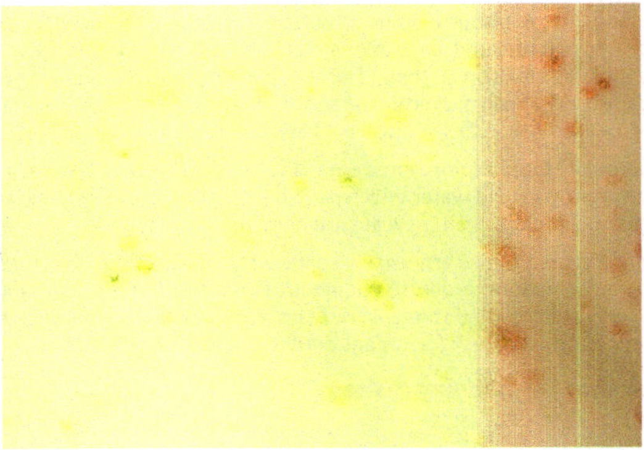

Fig. 19.7 Pityriasis lichenoides chronica.

Reproduced courtesy of Susan Lewis-Jones, Hon Consultant Dermatologist, Ninewells Hospital and Medical School, Dundee, UK

- *Papular xanthomas*: small yellowish papules (skin and mucous membranes). Differentiated from true xanthomas by normal lipid profile.
- *Xanthoma disseminatum*: widespread yellow or red-brown lesions—may be associated with diabetes insipidus. Can be difficult to distinguish from true xanthomas.

Eruptive xanthomas

Crops of yellowish papules often with narrow red halo, usually buttocks or extremities/pressure areas (➲ see Fig. 5.3).

Cause: most commonly associated with diabetes mellitus but check for hereditary forms of hyperlipoproteinaemias and nephrotic syndrome.

Elastosis perforans serpiginosa

Rare papular rash occurring in arcuate or serpiginous pattern often on the neck associated with connective tissue disorders, drugs (e.g. D-penicillamine), Down's syndrome, and Wilson's disease (copper storage disorder).

Darier's disease

Warty, reddish-brown greasy papules, particularly backs of hands (acrokeratosis verruciformis), face, neck, trunk, and flexures. May be hypopigmented in those with racially pigmented skin. Usually mild in children. Nail changes are common (longitudinal ridging, splitting, or notching) and palmar pits. Worsened by heat, sweating, and the sun. There may be associated neuropsychiatric disease such as epilepsy and mental impairment.

Differential diagnosis: seborrhoeic eczema.
Cause: autosomal dominant gene mutation—chromosome 12q23–q24.

Urticaria pigmentosa

A type of cutaneous mastocytosis usually starting in the first year of life. Numerous red-brown or yellowish macules, papules, and occasionally scattered nodules or plaques occur anywhere in varying numbers (Fig. 19.8). Darier's sign (unrelated to Darier's disease) is the elicitation of a wheal (which may blister) on rubbing. Flushing and abdominal pain can occur. It generally runs a benign clinical course with lesions and symptoms gradually resolving over years (➲ see also Fixed annual urticated rash, p. 315).

Management: avoid aspirin, ibuprofen, and other histamine-releasing drugs and immersion in cold water which can precipitate attacks. Systemic antihistamines and sodium cromoglycate are helpful.

Variants: mastocytomas are usually solitary (➲ see Fig. 28.6) but there can be up to five lesions; a diffuse cutaneous form is extremely rare and presents with cutaneous thickening/nodules with erythema and blistering in the neonatal period (ask for urgent dermatological opinion). ⚑

Algorithm for papular rashes

- See Fig. 19.9.

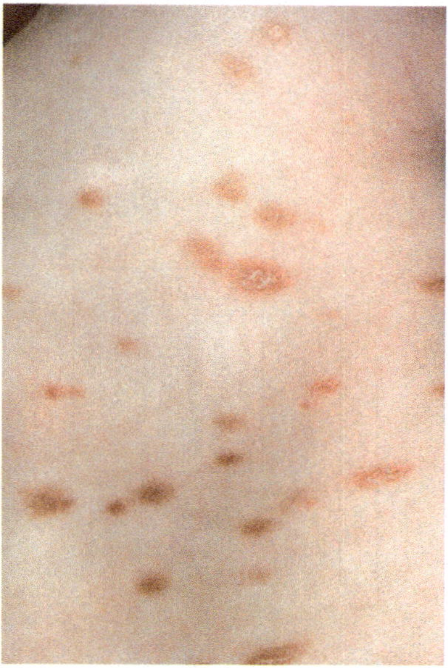

Fig. 19.8 Urticaria pigmentosa.

Reproduced courtesy of Susan Lewis-Jones, Hon Consultant Dermatologist, Ninewells Hospital and Medical School, Dundee, UK

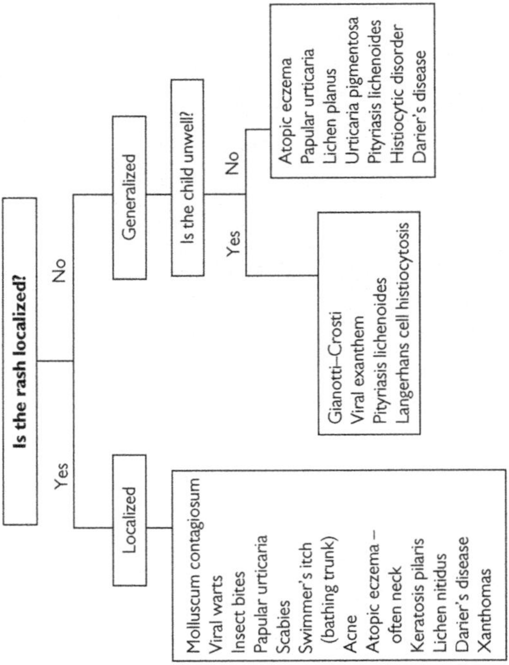

Fig. 19.9 Algorithm for papular rashes.

Reproduced courtesy of Malobi Ogboli, Consultant Dermatologist, Sandwell and West Birmingham Hospitals NHS Trust, UK

Chapter 20

Pustular rashes

Introduction

Pustules (Fig. 20.1) are elevations of the skin filled with neutrophils or occasionally other white cells such as eosinophils and they may arise from blisters. They can occur within the epidermis or below the dermoepidermal junction or in the adnexal structures such as hair follicles (folliculitis). They are most often due to bacterial, viral, yeast, and fungal infections. They also occur secondary to mechanical trauma (e.g. scratching or shaving) and are common in eczema. Sterile pustules can also occur and are seen in association with skin diseases such as acne, psoriasis, or rarely with drug reactions and systemic diseases such as Beçhet's and Crohn's (➲ see Chapter 38).

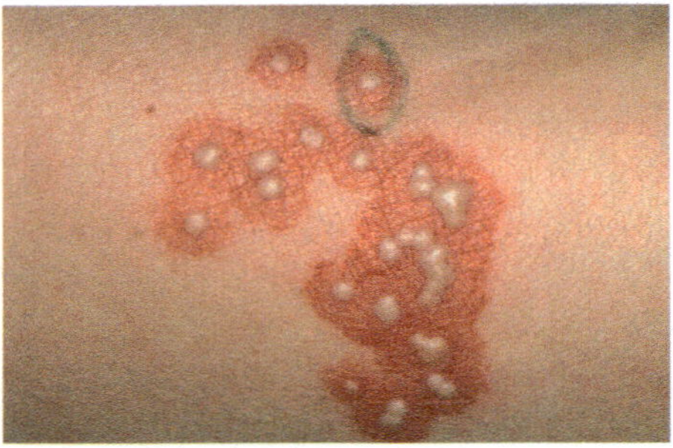

Fig. 20.1 Superficial pustules.

Reproduced courtesy of Susan Lewis-Jones, Hon Consultant Dermatologist, Ninewells Hospital and Medical School, Dundee, UK

Skin problems presenting with pustules

Infective causes

- Bacteria—*Staphylococcus, Streptococcus, Pseudomonas.*
- Fungi—dermatophytes (ringworm) especially animal types (➲ see Chapter 22).
- Parasites—scabies (➲ see Pustular rashes on trunk and limbs, p. 296 and Infestations, p. 337).
- Viruses—herpes simplex, varicella-zoster, molluscum contagiosum.
- Yeasts—mainly *Candida* species.

Non-infective causes

- Acne (➲ see Chapter 18).
- Acne keloidalis nuchae, *syn.* nuchal acne (➲ see Fig. 18.13).
- Drug reactions—acute generalized exanthematous pustulosis (➲ see Chapter 23).
- Incontinentia pigmenti (➲ see Genetic causes of blisters, p. 387).
- Infantile acral pustulosis (➲ see Acral pustular rashes, p. 297).

- Insect bites (➲ see Infestations and parasites, p. 283).
- Miliaria pustulosa (➲ see Pustular rashes in neonates and infants, p. 298).
- Perioral dermatitis (➲ see Pustular rashes of head and neck, p. 293).
- Pseudofolliculitis barbae (➲ see Pustular rashes of head and neck, p. 293).
- Pustular psoriasis—localized or generalized (➲ see Chapter 22).
- Pustular rashes in the newborn, including erythema toxicum neonatorum (➲ see Transient benign neonatal dermatoses, p. 81).
- Rosacea (➲ see Pustular rashes of head and neck, p. 293).

Investigations: take swabs for microscopy and culture or skin scrapes for fungal infections if an infective cause is suspected. Direct fluorescent antigen testing and real-time polymerase chain reaction (PCR) for viral infections where available. A skin biopsy may be required.

Pustular rashes of the head and neck

- See Box 20.1.

Acne vulgaris

Mixture of pustules, inflamed papules, sometimes with deeper lesions and/or cysts and comedones. Affects face, neck, anterior upper chest, and back (➲ see Chapter 18).

Perioral dermatitis

Symmetrical inflammatory papules and pustules with sparing of the vermilion border. May be triggered by topical corticosteroids or contact irritancy. Commoner in young females.

Treatment: stop topical corticosteroids; 6-week course of oral tetracyclines (erythromycin if under 12y).

Folliculitis

- *Gram-negative*—can occur with long-term antibiotics. Lesions on the alae nasi, face, and trunk.
  Treatment: may require oral trimethoprim or isotretinoin (topical or systemic).

Box 20.1 Common pustular rashes of the face and neck

- Infections—herpes simplex.
- Acne vulgaris (➲ see Chapter 18).
- Candidiasis—only common in the immunosuppressed, especially with oral candidiasis (➲ see Chapter 10).
- Dermatophyte infections (ringworm).
- Folliculitis.
- Insect bites (➲ see Fig. 19.4).
- Perioral dermatitis (teenage girls).

Note: impetigo, although common, only rarely causes pustules. More usually presenting as eroded areas with peeling edges and golden crusts and occasionally a few flaccid, thin-walled blisters.

- *Gram-positive*—usually staphylococcal. More common with atopy and dry skin. Lesions that may be tender on the trunk or limbs. Often small 1–2mm pustules (Fig. 20.2), sometimes with golden crusting and occasionally larger boils.
- *Pseudofolliculitis barbae*—occurs in males who shave, usually from penetration of shaved hairs into the skin often with secondary *Staph. aureus* infection. There is a genetic tendency.
  Management: avoidance or care with shaving or use of other hair removal methods; emollients and topical antibiotic or topical isotretinoin therapy. Oral antibiotics may be required.

Furuncle

A painful deep infection of the follicle, common in hair-bearing areas of the neck and groin (Fig. 20.3).

Cause: *Staphylococcus aureus*. A carbuncle is much larger and involves a group of follicles.

Molluscum (*pl.* -a) contagiosum (*pl.* -a)

These are papules rather than true pustules, but they often become inflamed and discharge pus as they resolve (➲ see Infection, p. 281).

Dermatophyte infections (*syn.* ringworm)

Pustules are frequently present at lesional edges, especially in animal ringworm, e.g. in tinea faciei (Fig. 20.4), also beard area (postpubertal males) and kerion that occur in scalp (➲ see Fig. 14.8, Scalp infections, p. 203 and Fungal infections of the skin, p. 331).

Miliaria pustulosa

More inflammatory form of miliaria (➲ see Chapter 7, Transient benign neonatal dermatoses, p. 81). Usually seen in the tropics in neonates.

Rosacea

Primarily an adult disease but seen rarely in teenagers who present with facial redness, especially cheeks, nose, and central forehead, with

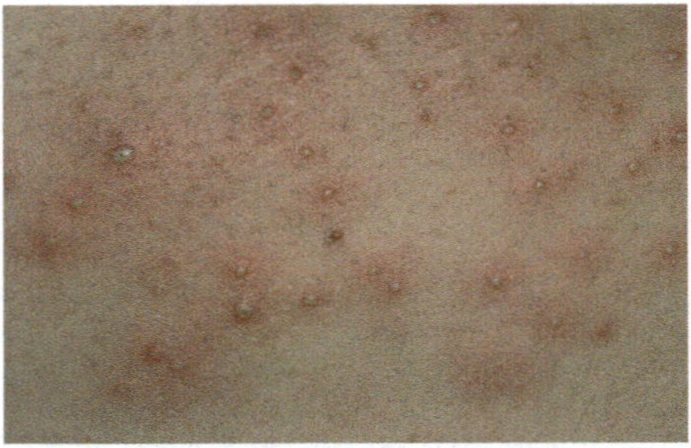

Fig. 20.2 *Staph. aureus* folliculitis showing follicular pustules and inflammation.
Reproduced courtesy of Susan Lewis-Jones, Hon Consultant Dermatologist, Ninewells Hospital and Medical School, Dundee, UK

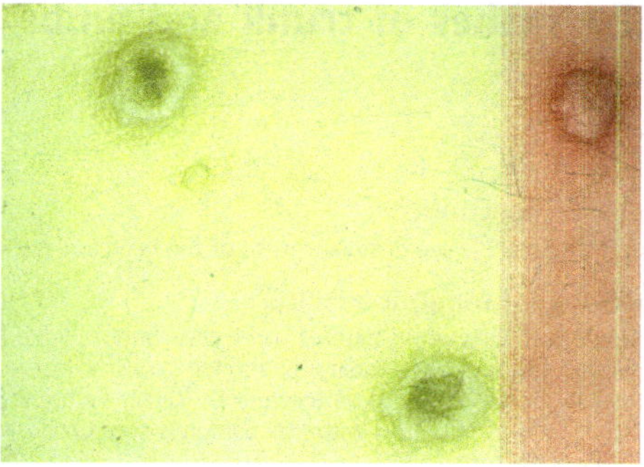

Fig. 20.3 Severe streptococcal folliculitis (furuncle) in HIV-positive patient.
Reproduced courtesy of Susan Lewis-Jones, Hon Consultant Dermatologist, Ninewells Hospital and Medical School, Dundee, UK

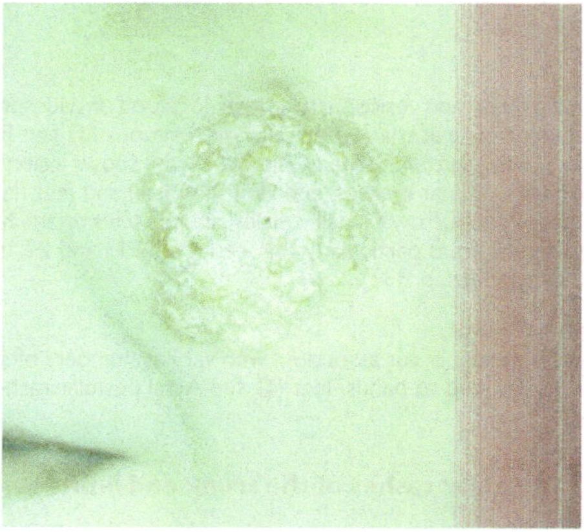

Fig. 20.4 Tinea faciei caused by cattle ringworm showing pustular reaction.
Reproduced courtesy of Susan Lewis-Jones, Hon Consultant Dermatologist, Ninewells Hospital and Medical School, Dundee, UK

inflammatory papules and pustules on a background of easy blushing, erythema, and telangiectasia.

Acne keloidalis nuchae

Firm papules and nodules on nape of neck, often with folliculitis (➲ see Rare presentation of acne, p. 285 and Fig. 18.13). Lesions coalesce to form large unsightly keloid-like plaques. Mainly adolescent males with black skin.

Pustular rashes of trunk and limbs

- See Box 20.2.

Acne vulgaris

- ➲ See Chapter 18.

Gram-positive folliculitis

Usually staphylococcal (➲ see Pustular rashes of the head and neck, p. 293).

Hot tub (pseudomonal) folliculitis

Pruritic, papulopustular rash in bathing trunk distribution, linked to use of hot tubs, whirlpools, and occasionally swimming pools or home baths and showers (usually occurs within days to weeks). Rarely systemic symptoms are associated. Due to infection with *Pseudomonas* spp. Occlusion by tight swimwear is contributory.

Treatment: usually self-limiting but can occasionally persist.

Insect bites

Only rarely present as pustules from secondary infection (Fig. 20.5). More usually as red papules or clear blisters (➲ see Fig. 19.4). Tend to occur in crops.

Scabies

Eczematized papular and vesicopustular rash, localized or widespread, often with an element of urticaria (type 1 allergic reaction) (➲ see Fig. 22.13). Caused by the mite *Sarcoptes scabiei*. Almost always shows lesions on hands (between fingers, palmar creases, and ventral wrists) and feet (lateral sides and soles). Look for burrows, small vesicles, and pustules on the hands, feet, axillae, and genital areas particularly (➲ see Figs. 22.13 and 22.14; Scabies, p. 184 and Infestations, p. 337).

Pustular psoriasis

Erythematous plaques occur associated with varying numbers of sterile pustules. May be localized to hands/feet (➲ see Acral pustular rashes, p. 297)

Box 20.2 Pustular rashes of the trunk and limbs

Common

- Acne vulgaris.
- Gram-positive folliculitis.
- Insect bites.
- Scabies.

Uncommon to rare

- Hot tub (pseudomonal) folliculitis.
- Pustular psoriasis.
- Eosinophilic pustular folliculitis.
- Pustular drug rashes.
- Subcorneal pustular dermatosis.
- Eosinophilic pustular folliculitis (of infancy).

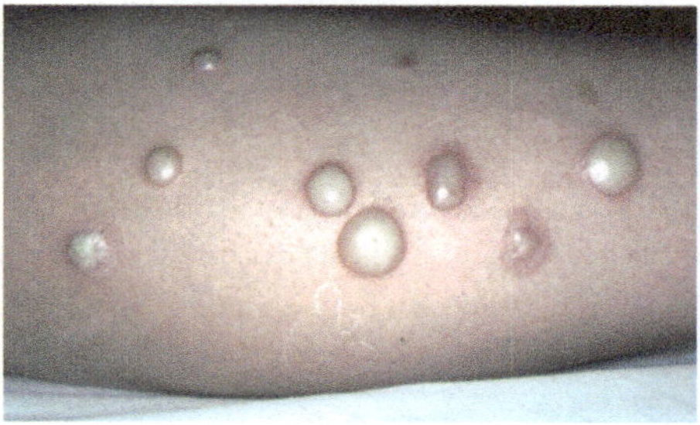

Fig. 20.5 Insect bites on a leg infected with *Staph. aureus* showing large pustules in a typically cropped distribution.

Reproduced courtesy of Susan Lewis-Jones, Hon Consultant Dermatologist, Ninewells Hospital and Medical School, Dundee, UK

but sometimes associated with systemic malaise and erythroderma (➲ see Fig. 22.18 and Features of specific causes of erythroderma, p. 343). May be precipitated by drugs, e.g. topical or oral corticosteroids, β-blockers, infection, pregnancy. Very rare but serious—seek dermatological advice.

Pustular drug reactions

Rare in children (➲ see Chapter 18).

Subcorneal pustular dermatosis (*syn.* Sneddon–Wilkinson disease)

Extremely rare, chronic vesicopustular disorder with annular and/or serpiginous arrangement of very superficial, flaccid pustules on trunk, axillae, and groins. Lesions may be itchy and resolve after 5–7 days. There may be fever and leucocytosis with remission and exacerbation in some.

Cause: unknown—some cases are associated with drugs and infection.

Treatment: topical or systemic corticosteroids; oral dapsone.

Eosinophilic pustular folliculitis (of infancy)

Follicular papules and pustules of unknown cause. Sites include face, trunk, and extremities. May be associated blood eosinophilia or leucocytosis. Often spontaneous remission and exacerbation. Rare.

Treatment: responds to topical corticosteroids.

Note: thought to differ from adult form (Ofuji's syndrome) which often has an annular/serpiginous pattern and is associated particularly with HIV infection.

Acral pustular rashes

Acral rashes are seen on hands, feet, and sometimes ears and nose (Box 20.3; ➲ see also Box 4.1 and Chapter 12).

Box 20.3 Causes of acral pustulosis

- Scabies.
- Acral pustulosis of infancy.
- Palmoplantar pustular psoriasis.
- Eosinophilic pustular folliculitis.
- Infections (e.g. congenital herpes simplex and syphilis).

Note: blisters in hand, foot, and mouth disease are greyish and may resemble pustules.

Scabies

Almost always shows lesions on hands (between fingers, palms, and wrists) and feet (soles) (➲ see Pustular rashes of trunks and limbs, p. 193 and Chapters 12, 13, and 22).

Acral pustulosis of infancy

Onset birth to 2y. Crops of very itchy vesicopapules and pustules (containing neutrophils and or eosinophils) that appear for 7–10 days then remit and relapse. More common in boys and black skin types. It has been linked to scabies in many cases. Uncommon (➲ see Chapter 7).

Treatment: usually unresponsive to topical corticosteroids. Severe cases may respond to oral erythromycin or dapsone.

Palmoplantar pustular psoriasis

Yellowish-green pustules that resolve to a brown scale. Look for evidence of psoriasis elsewhere (➲ see Psoriasis—clinical variants, p. 322). Rare in children.

Eosinophilic pustular folliculitis of infancy

- ➲ See Pustular rashes of trunks and limbs, p. 193.

Pustular rashes in neonates and infants

- For list of causes, see Box 20.4; ➲ see also Transient benign neonatal dermatoses, p. 81.

Scabies

- ➲ See Pustular rashes of trunks and limbs, p. 193.

Bacterial folliculitis

- ➲ See Pustular rashes of the head and neck, p. 193.

Erythema toxicum neonatorum

Inflamed pustules, mainly trunk—so-called flea-bitten appearance (➲ see Fig. 7.1). Contain eosinophils, easily seen by microscopy of a smear from pustule—allows fast diagnosis in florid cases.

Miliaria pustulosa

More inflammatory form of miliaria (➲ see Transient benign neonatal dermatoses, p. 81), usually in tropics.

Box 20.4 Pustular rashes in neonates and infants

Common

- Scabies.
- Bacterial folliculitis.
- Erythema toxicum neonatorum.
- Miliaria pustulosa.
- Benign neonatal cephalic pustulosis (neonatal acne).

Uncommon to rare

- Congenital or neonatal candidiasis.
- Neonatal herpes.
- Transient neonatal pustular melanosis.
- Incontinentia pigmenti (see Genetic causes of blisters, p. 387).

Neonatal herpes infections

Vesicopustules may be present. Take viral swabs. Tzanck smear gives quick answer but requires special training. Real-time PCR tests and direct fluorescent antigen tests may be used if available (see Chapter 7, Congenital infection, p. 88).

Congenital or neonatal candidiasis

May be systemic or non-systemic. Moist, 'beefy red' rash with satellite vesicopustules often in the napkin area (see Fig. 13.3; see also Chapter 11).

Benign neonatal cephalic pustulosis (neonatal acne)

Neonatal non-follicular pustulosis. Common sites are the face, neck, and scalp.

Cause: possibly due to *Malassezia* species. Self-limiting but responds to topical ketoconazole (see Transient benign neonatal dermatoses, p. 81).

Transient neonatal pustular melanosis

Rare, benign, self-limiting disorder of unknown aetiology. Sterile neutrophilic vesicopustules (chin, neck, back) that rupture easily and evolve into hyperpigmented macules. Often present at birth.

Chapter 21

Urticarial rashes

Introduction

Urticaria or hives is a common itchy, blotchy, red skin rash without scaling (Fig. 21.1). Lesions are usually annular but may also be arcuate. Individual lesions last less than 24h and fade without leaving bruising. Bruising following urticarial lesions suggests urticarial vasculitis. A number of rashes have an urticarial appearance sometimes described as urticated (➲ see Differential diagnosis of urticarial rashes, pp. 313–16).

Around 20% of the population will develop urticaria during their lifetime. Incidence is increased in those with an atopic diathesis. In children most cases resolve in <6 weeks.

(a) (b)

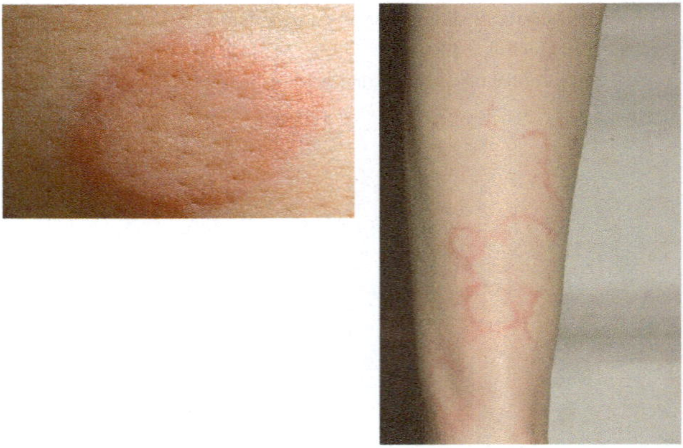

Fig. 21.1 (a) Urticarial wheal. (b) Urticaria showing annular and arcuate lesions.
Reproduced courtesy of Dr Sheila Clark, Consultant Dermatologist, The Leeds Teaching Hospital and Mid Yorkshire Hospitals NHS Trust, UK

Definitions

Urticaria (wheals)

Superficial, raised, itchy, red skin lesions due to vasodilation, increased blood flow, and vascular permeability with transient plasma leakage from small blood vessels. Wheals vary in size from mm to several cm and may be single or numerous (Fig. 21.1).

Angioedema

- Deeper swellings of the subcutaneous tissues, which may involve the skin, particularly lips and eyelids, respiratory and gastrointestinal tracts. Swellings may be painful rather than itchy and last longer than wheals (days). There are several different types of angioedema (➲ see Types of angioedema, pp. 309–10) (Fig. 21.2).

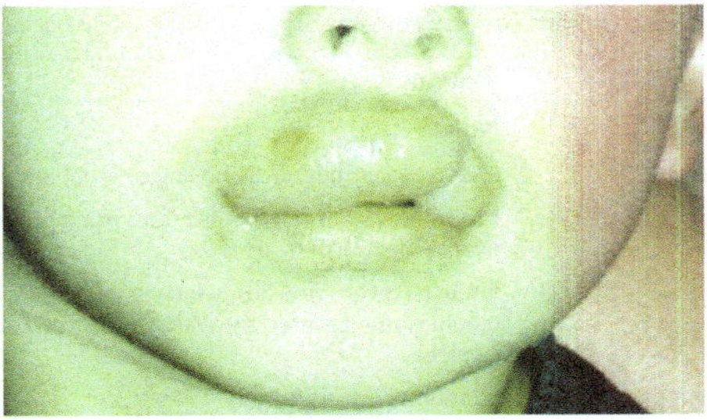

Fig. 21.2 Angioedema of the lips due to acute allergy to fish protein.

Reproduced courtesy of Susan Lewis-Jones, Hon Consultant Dermatologist, Ninewells Hospital and Medical School, Dundee, UK

- Urticaria alone occurs in 50% and angioedema alone in 10% of cases. Wheals and angioedema occur together in 40% of cases (Fig. 21.2).
- Urticaria and angioedema have been divided into:
  - Acute—symptoms lasting <6 weeks.
  - Chronic—daily or almost daily symptoms >6 weeks.
  - Episodic—acute intermittent symptoms lasting hours or days and recurring over months or years.

Dermographism

Dermographism is an exaggerated whealing tendency when the skin is stroked firmly causing a type 1 histamine response. It has been noted in around 5% of the population. It can occur alone and with urticaria and may also persist after urticaria clears (Fig. 21.3).

The Urticaria Activity Score (UAS) and UAS7 can be used to assess severity and response to treatment (Table 21.1).

Fig. 21.3 Dermographism.

Reproduced courtesy of Susan Lewis-Jones, Hon Consultant Dermatologist, Ninewells Hospital and Medical School, Dundee, UK

Table 21.1 The Urticaria Activity Score [UAS7] for assessing disease activity in CSU*

Score	Wheals	Pruritus
0	None	None
1	Mild (<20/24h)	Mild (present but not annoying or troublesome)
2	Moderate (20–50/ 24h)	Moderate (troublesome but does not interfere with normal daily activity or sleep)
3	Intense (>50/24h)	Intense (severe pruritus, which is sufficiently troublesome to interfere with normal daily activity or sleep)
Score: 0–6 for each day = maximum 42 over 7 days		
* CSU = chronic spontaneous urticaria		

Reproduced with permission from Zuberbier T. et *al*. (2018). The EAACI/GA²LEN/EDF/WAO guideline for the definition, classification, diagnosis and management of urticaria. *Allergy* 73(7):1393–414.

Pathogenesis

These reactions are due to allergic or non-allergic mast cell stimulation resulting in release of histamine and inflammatory cytokines such as IL4, IL5, and IFNγ, which in turn results in vasodilatation, vasopermeability, itching, and a wheal and flare response. Systemic symptoms may occur (Box 21.1) including anaphylaxis (➲ see Anaphylaxis, pp. 311–13).

Box 21.1 Systemic symptoms which may occur with urticaria or angioedema include:

- Flushing.
- Headache.
- Wheeze.
- Breathlessness.
- Palpitations.
- Vomiting.
- Diarrhoea.

If severe then anaphylaxis may occur.

Anaphylaxis

- Hypotension.
- Syncope.
- Complete airway obstruction.

Note: it is extremely rare for anaphylaxis to occur in association with common (ordinary) urticaria (➲ see Causes of urticaria, p. 305).

Causes of urticaria

In many cases no obvious cause/trigger is identified. There are a number of different possible trigger factors (Box 21.2).

In children common causes include:

- *Acute urticaria (AU)*—infections, IgE-mediated allergic reactions to foods, airborne allergens, drugs, bites/stings.
- *Chronic urticaria (CU)*—categorized in to two main types
  - Chronic spontaneous urticaria (CSU).
  - Physical or inducible urticaria: 25% of CU cases (➲ see Physical urticarias, pp. 305–7).

CU is not a manifestation of IgE-mediated food allergy; however, food allergy may occur independently from CSU.

Spontaneous (idiopathic) urticaria

In most patients with urticaria, no underlying trigger factor or associated disease is found and the condition is self-limiting. Spontaneous remission with relapses is common. Symptoms may persist for up to 1y in 70% and up to 5y in >10% of cases.

Circulating autoimmune antibodies have been found in some and familial autoimmune thyroid disease is associated in around 10%. CU may be exacerbated by infections, aspirin, and related drugs including ibuprofen.

Physical or inducible urticarias

Aquagenic urticaria and aquagenic pruritus

Aquagenic urticaria: water contact with the skin at any temperature may result in itching alone, or urticaria with small wheals similar to cholinergic urticaria.

Aquagenic pruritus (in the absence of urticaria) may be idiopathic, or occur in association with polycythaemia rubra vera, myelodysplastic disorders, Hodgkin's disease, and the hypereosinophilic syndrome.

Box 21.2 Urticaria—trigger factors

- *Idiopathic*.
- *Infections*: multiple (viral, bacterial, parasitic).
- *Drugs*: aspirin, NSAIDS, codeine, antibiotics, anaesthetics, radiocontrast media.
- *Contact*: food, pollens, plants, bites, stings.
- *Allergic*: food, drugs, pets, pollens, bites, stings, and venoms.
- *Physical*: heat, cold, sunlight, pressure, vibration, water, exercise (cholinergic) (➲ see Physical urticarias, pp. 305–7).
- *Systemic disease*: autoimmune—particularly thyroid disease, SLE (➲ see Management of urticarias, pp. 309–10).

Source: data from Zuberbier, T. et *al*. (2018). The EAACI/GA²LEN/EDF/WAO guideline for the definition, classification, diagnosis and management of urticaria. *Allergy*. 73(7):1393–1414.

Cholinergic (or heat-induced urticaria)

Develops after an increase in core temperature (e.g. after bathing, exercise, fever, etc.). Small, itchy, 1–2mm wheals surrounded by erythema. Occasionally angioedema and/or systemic symptoms occur. Increased incidence in those with an atopic diathesis and rarely familial. Some cases may result from an autoantibody to an antigen in sweat.

Cold

May be inherited dominantly or acquired (idiopathic or secondary to cold agglutinins or cryoglobulins). Often occurs within minutes of cold exposure (cold water, wind, air, direct contact, etc.) but may appear only after rewarming. May be associated with angioedema and systemic symptoms,

Ice-cube test (5–20min)

(a)

(b)

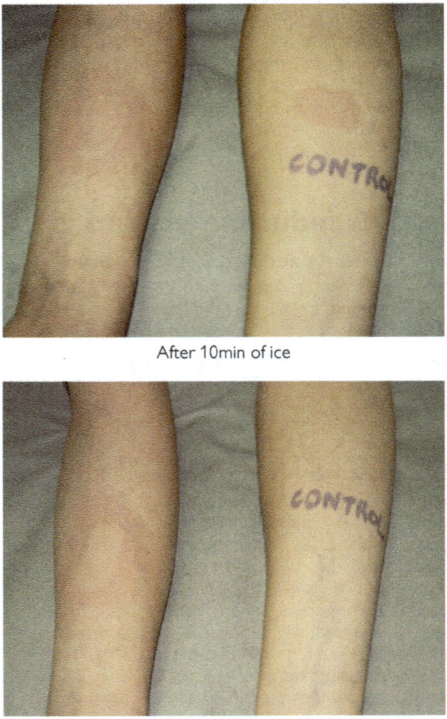

After 10min of ice

5min later – control normal

Fig. 21.4 Positive ice-cube test in cold urticaria.

Reproduced courtesy of Susan Lewis-Jones, Hon Consultant Dermatologist, Ninewells Hospital and Medical School, Dundee, UK

sometimes life-threatening if the whole body is cooled. Specific investigation: ice-cube skin challenge test eliciting wheal and flare (Fig. 21.4).

Exercise induced

Distinct from cholinergic urticaria. Pruritus, urticaria, angioedema, and syncope may occur. Increased incidence in those with an atopic diathesis. Around 30% of cases are food dependent (food-dependent exercise-induced anaphylaxis), e.g. wheat, shellfish. The reaction is triggered in combination and not with either exercise or food (or other) alone.

Pressure

Dermographism—the most common form of urticaria. A wheal and flare response is elicited at the site where the skin is stroked firmly (Fig. 21.3).

Delayed pressure—occurs 4–8h after local skin pressure and may persist for longer than 24h. Rare in childhood.

Solar

Pruritus, erythema, wheals, and occasionally angioedema. Develops within minutes after exposure to sun or artificial light. Very disabling and occasionally systemic features occur. Rare in children. Usually idiopathic, rarely associated with polymorphic light eruption (➲ see Chapter 16), systemic lupus erythematosus, or erythropoietic protoporphyria (➲ see Chapter 16).

Vibration

May be idiopathic, occur secondary to repeated vibration exposure, or may rarely be familial.

Management of urticaria and angioedema

- See Box 21.3.

Box 21.3 Guidelines

- Powell et al. (2015). BSACI guideline for the management of chronic urticaria and angioedema. *Clin Exp Allergy* **45**(3):547–65. doi: 10.1111/cea.12494. https://www.bsaci.org/guidelines/chronic-urticaria-and-angioedema
- Zuberbier et al. (2018). The EAACI/GA^{2}LEN/EDF/WAO guideline for the definition, classification, diagnosis and management of urticaria. *Allergy* **73**(7):1393–414. doi: 10.1111/all.13397.

General

- Explain that the cause is unlikely to be found.
- Written advice sheets (e.g. British Association of Dermatologists).[1]
- Exclude precipitating factors.
- Minimize non-specific aggravating factors (stress, overheating).
- Avoid exacerbating drugs (e.g. non-steroidal anti-inflammatory drugs (NSAIDs)).
- Cooling antipruritics (e.g. 1–2% menthol in emollient cream).
- Medi-alert bracelet—if relevant.

First-line treatments

- ***Second-generation non-sedating oral antihistamine*** in the daytime.
- Start at licensed doses. There is relatively little to choose between different antihistamines but individuals may vary in their response to different agents. *Up to four times* the recommended dose may be required to adequately control symptoms. Use continuous medication if attacks occur regularly. Use fast-acting antihistamines as required for sporadic attacks. If there is no response to one agent after 6 weeks, try a second and then a third.
- ***Sedative antihistamine*** at night in addition to the above only if need for sedation.
- ***Prednisolone*** 0.5–1mg/kg/day as a stat dose or for 1–2 weeks for severe symptoms. Avoid long-term use.
- ***Adrenaline*** for anaphylaxis or severe angioedema (Tables 21.2 and 21.3.)

Second-line treatments

Second-line treatments should be limited for use in difficult cases in children with CSU and only considered in specialist centres.

- ***Leukotriene receptor antagonists*** (montelukast). Patients not responding to antihistamines alone should be offered a 1–4-week trial (continue longer in chronic cases if beneficial). These are most effective in combination with antihistamines especially if there is a clear trigger (food, NSAID, physical, autoimmune).
- ***Anti-IgE.*** Omalizumab (Xolair®) is a monoclonal antibody directed against IgE. Very effective in treating CSU refractory to high dose antihistamines. Omalizumab has an excellent safety profile and is well tolerated in adults with increasing evidence for use in paediatric patients. Xolair® is licensed for children >6y, however current NICE guidelines recommend its use in children >12y.
- ***Ciclosporin*** should be used only in difficult cases because of risk of nephrotoxicity, hypertension, and frequent blood tests.

Table 21.2 IM adrenaline dosage according to child's age

Age	Dose of 1:1000 adrenaline
>12y	500mcg (0.5ml)
6–12y	300mcg (0.3ml)
<6y	150mcg (0.15ml)

Table 21.3 IM or slow IV chlorpheniramine and hydrocortisone dosage according to child's age

Age	Chlorpheniramine	Hydrocortisone
>12y	10mg	200mg
6–12y	5mg	100mg
6 months–6y	2.5mg	50mg
<6 months	250mcg/kg	25mg

Table 21.4 Management of angioedema

Ordinary	Attention to airway patency, otherwise as for urticaria ± adrenaline.
*Hereditary**	*Acute:* • Intubation and surgical airway should be considered early in progressive angioedema. • Plasma-derived human C1-INH concentrate Berinert® is approved in the United Kingdom in children <12y, dose 20 IU/kg IV. Cinryze® is licensed in adolescents and adults, dose 1,000 units IV (can repeated after 1h). • Plasma-derived kallikrein inhibitor, ecallantide (Kalbitor® in the United States) can be used in patients >16y, dose 30mg (3ml). The bradykinin-2 receptor antagonist icatibant (Firazyr®) is unlicensed in children in the United Kingdom. • Fresh frozen plasma (FFP) should only be used if the other therapies are not available. FFP has occasional paradoxical effect of making angioedema acutely worse and clinician must be prepared to intubate the patient if required. • Recombinant C1-INH, conestat alpha (Ruconest®) is unlicensed in children. • Antihistamines, steroids, and adrenaline are often unsuccessful. *Prophylaxis:* • Preprocedural—recommended for medical, surgical, and dental procedures: plasma derived C1 inhibitor; short course of attenuated androgens if C1 inhibitor is not available. *Long-term prophylaxis:* • Plasma-derived human C1 inhibitor Cinryze® 1,000 units twice weekly. • If not available, tranexamic acid and long-term androgens, e.g. Danazol, Oxandrolone (not recommended prior to Tanner stage V)#.
ACEI-induced	*Adrenaline and avoid all angiotensin converting enzyme inhibitors (ACEI).*

*NES, airway nebulizers; # Tanner stage; V Adult body

- **Other treatments:** Little evidence for use in children (e.g. mycophenolate mofetil, methotrexate).
- For management of angioedema, see Table 21.4.

Types of angioedema

Ordinary

Often associated with urticaria (for trigger factors, see Box 21.2). In children acute attacks of type 1 allergy are usually provoked by food (Fig. 21.2) or drug allergy. Often no cause is found for chronic angioedema with ordinary urticaria.

Hereditary angioedema (HA)

- Most commonly affects limbs, face, intestinal tract, and airway.
- Swelling common without known trigger (e.g. stress, infection, trauma, alcohol, menstruation, or pregnancy).
- Firm, indurated swelling, often extensive (e.g. whole limb).

- Intestinal involvement causes abdominal pain (may be severe), nausea, and vomiting. Restricted breathing from airway involvement can be life-threatening (mortality 20%). Urinary symptoms may occur.
- There is no urticaria, but around a third develop a non-itchy rash during an attack.
- Symptoms begin in childhood and worsen at puberty. Frequency of attacks varies but can be every 1–2 weeks and episodes often last several days.

Linked to genetic mutations affecting either C1 esterase inhibitor (C1-INH) or coagulation factor XII. C1-INH binds to and blocks activity of plasma kallikrein and activated factor XII (factor XIIa) which are both involved in bradykinin production. Bradykinin promotes inflammation by increasing blood vessel wall permeability.

Three reported types of HA

- *Type I*—85%. Deficiency or reduced level of normally functioning C1 esterase inhibitor (C1-INH). Autosomal dominant. Mutations in *SERPING1* gene, chromosome 11q12.1. 25% of cases result from new mutations.
- *Type II*—15%. Normal or increased levels of dysfunctional C1-INH. Autosomal dominant. Mutations in *SERPING1* gene.
- *Type III*—very rare. Normal levels and functioning C1-INH. Inheritance unclear —may be X-linked dominant. Mutations in the *F12* gene leading to increased coagulation factor XII with increased bradykinin triggered inflammation. Oestrogen dependent, so usually seen in women (e.g. with oral contraceptives and pregnancy).

Acquired angioedema

- Acquired C1-INH deficiency. Rare.
- *Type I*—associated with lymphoproliferative disorders and autoimmune diseases.
- *Type II*—autoantibody against C1-INH.
- *Other*—ACE inhibitor induced angioedema.

Investigations of urticaria and angioedema

None are necessary for the majority of cases (see also British Society for Allergy and Clinical Immunology (BSACI) guidelines, Box 21.3)

- *Skin prick tests/specific IgE* (food/animals/insects)—testing is warranted if the clinical history suggests a candidate allergen. Food allergy is usually obvious and trigger factors are usually easily identified. *These tests are not useful as a screening test for potential allergens in CU.*
- *Testing for physical or contact factors*—contact and physical urticarias are general suggested by the history. Tests include ice-cube test for cold urticaria, phototesting for solar urticaria, pressure testing for delayed pressure urticaria.
- *Blood tests—if clinically indicated in CU*: FBC, ESR, CRP, LFT, TFTs, autoantibodies including thyroid and coeliac screen.

- **Complement studies**—C1-INH (level and function) and C4 level in patients with angioedema without wheals. C4/C3 levels should be measured in patients with suspected urticarial vasculitis.

Note: patch testing is not usually helpful for investigating urticaria.
Note: <1y of age, C1-INH levels may be lower than in adults, therefore confirm the diagnosis after this age.

Adrenaline injection: dose and administration

- Three prefilled disposable devices are licensed in the United Kingdom (1mg/ml):
  - EpiPen®
  - Emerade®*
  - Jext®
- Dosage varies dependent on weight:
  - >30kg 300 micrograms
  - <30kg 150 micrograms
- The dose can to be repeated after 5–15min if needed. Check expiry date regularly (24 months for Jext®, 18 months for EpiPen®, and Emerade®)[2]
- Please see the British National Formulary (BNF) for further guidance, https://bnfc.nice.org.uk/

Note: A dosage <150 micrograms cannot be administered with sufficient accuracy in children weighing <15kg and use is therefore not recommended unless during a life-threatening situation and under medical advice.

Anaphylaxis

An acute severe life-threatening generalized or systemic reaction induced by an IgE-mediated allergic reaction. For symptoms, see Box 21.4.

Box 21.4 Symptoms of anaphylaxis

Allergy
- Itching/rash.
- Angioedema.
- Vomiting.
- Abdominal pain.
- Diarrhoea.
- Pale and sweating.

Anaphylaxis

Any allergy symptom +
- Angioedema of airways.
- Cough, wheeze, breathlessness, stridor.
- Restlessness.
- Hypotension.
- Floppiness/collapse.
- Loss of consciousness.
- Cardiac arrest.

* Emerade® also have 500 microgram pens for adults and children 12–17y.

Management of anaphylaxis

Non-medical environment

1. Call for help (UK emergency services 999)
2. Check Airway, Breathing, Circulation, Disability, and Exposure
3. Remove the cause/allergen if possible.
4. Give adrenaline via pen if vial not available:
   - Take off cap.
   - Place tapered end onto anterolateral mid-third thigh.
   - Press hard until it 'clicks' and continue to press for slow count to 10.
   - Massage the area.
5. Give inhaler if available and patient able to use.
6. If not breathing give CPR.
7. If no response at 5–15min repeat adrenaline administration.

Note: Record the time of adrenaline administration(s).

Hospital environment

1. Establish airway—high-flow oxygen (O_2).
2. Adrenaline—IM. Repeat every 5min if necessary.
3. IV fluids—sodium chloride 0.9% (normal saline) 20ml/kg IV bolus.
4. Chlorpheniramine—IM or slow IV.
5. Hydrocortisone—IM or slow IV.
6. ± salbutamol 2mg nebulized for bronchospasm, nebulized adrenaline. 400 micrograms/kg, 0.4 ml/kg ml of 1: 1,000, for croup.
7. Consider blood for mast cell tryptase if cause is drug- or venom-related or idiopathic.
8. After emergency treatment offer referral to a specialist allergy service.

Note: Approximate guide to a child's weight in kg = (Age + 4) × 2 (assuming child's weight is in normal range).

Adrenaline injection: dose and administration

Three prefilled disposable devices are licensed in the United Kingdom (1mg/ml) (Table 21.5).

The dose can to be repeated after 5–15min if needed. Check expiry date regularly (24 months for Jext®, 18 months for EpiPen® (Fig. 21.5) and Emerade®).[2]

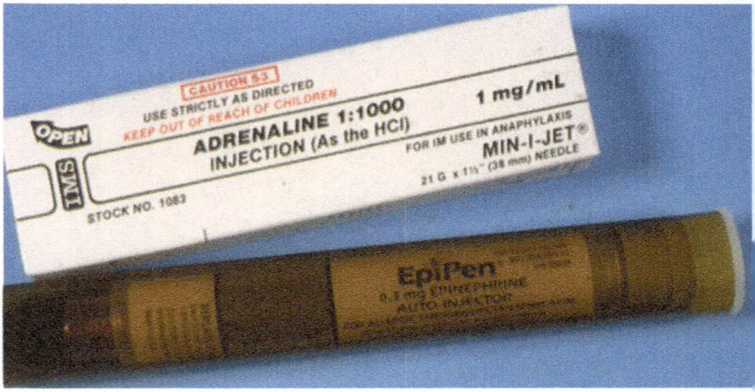

Fig. 21.5 EpiPen.

Reproduced courtesy of NHS Tayside Clinical Photography, Dundee, UK

Table 21.5 Selection of correct adrenaline dose in prefilled pens

Adrenaline pen brand	>30 kg	<30 kg
EpiPen® (Fig. 21.5)	300 micrograms	150 micrograms
Emerade®	300 micrograms (500 micrograms adults and children 12–17y)	150 micrograms
Jext®	300 micrograms	150 micrograms

Source: data from British National Formulary (BNF), https://bnf.nice.org.uk/

Actions of adrenaline

- Alpha-receptor agonist.
- Reverses vasodilatation.
- Reduces oedema.
- β-receptor agonist.
- Dilates airways.
- Increases myocardial contraction force.
- Suppresses further histamine and leukotriene release.

Differential diagnosis of urticarial rashes

Neonatal and infantile urticated rashes

Common

Erythema toxicum neonatorum (syn. urticaria neonatorum)

Common transient rash in healthy neonates, usually 1–2mm red macule ± central papule or pustule containing eosinophils (➲ see Fig. 7.1).

Scabies

Eczematized papular rash, which may be localized or widespread. There is often an associated urticated rash particularly on the trunk. Look for burrows on the hands, feet, axillae, and genital area (➲ see Chapter 20, Pustular rashes of the trunk and limbs, p. 296 and Infestations, pp. 337–8).

Rare

Neonatal lupus erythematosus

Photosensitive 'owl-eye' and urticated rash (➲ see Figs. 7.2 and 7.3).

Congenital infections

CMV, rubella, syphilis, toxoplasmosis (➲ see Congenital infection, pp. 88–9 and Red viral exanthems, pp. 326–30).

Acute haemorrhagic oedema of infancy

An immune-complex mediated vasculitis with oedema of face and often hands and feet (➲ see Chapter 32 and Fig. 31.5).

Annular erythema of infancy

A benign, self-limiting condition with onset in the first month. It may be a manifestation of maternal autoimmune disease. It presents as a slowly enlarging non-scaly, annular erythema which resolves to leave normal skin.

Metabolic disorders

Very rare, e.g. autoinflammatory syndromes such as familial Mediterranean fever syndrome, Muckle–Wells/familial cold urticaria, chronic infantile neurological cutaneous articular (CINCA) syndrome (*syn.* neonatal onset multisystem inflammatory disease (NOMID)).

'Moving' annular urticated rash

Common

Tinea (ringworm)

Active edge with scale ± pustules (➲ see Fig. 22.8).

Granuloma annulare

Asymptomatic dermal nodules (granulomatous reaction), without surface changes (➲ see Fig. 28.3). It very slowly expands over months and is often on acral sites of hands and feet.

Rare

Systemic lupus erythematosus (SLE)

Photo-exacerbated/induced rash, which may also occur on photo-protected sites (➲ see Fig. 9.3 and Systemic disease, pp. 340–1).

Other 'annular erythemas'

Several types are described, the best known of which is erythema annulare centrifugum, a slowly migrating annular erythema with an edge of fine scale. Thought to be a reaction to infection (fungal, viral, parasites) or rarely malignancy or autoimmune disorders.

Erythema marginatum

An annular migratory erythematous rash with a raised, demarcated, irregular edge and paler centre. Most commonly found on the trunk and often asymptomatic. Coalescent rings appear and disappear over hours and may persist for months. There is often an associated carditis. Skin-coloured painless nodules on the extensor surfaces may also be seen with rheumatic fever but are less common.

Cause: an autoimmune reaction to Group A *Streptococcus pyogenes* in the early stages of acute rheumatic fever, in children <16y. A similar eruption also reported preceding hereditary angioedema (➲ see Red viral exanthems, pp. 326–30).[3]

Erythema chronicum migrans

Lyme disease (*Borrelia burgdorferi*; ➲ see Fig. 22.12).

Familial annular erythema

A rare autosomal dominant condition with lesions that tend to persist into adulthood but lessen in frequency and severity over time. There are no significant associations.

Metabolic: ➲ see Differential diagnosis of urticaria, pp. 313–16.

'Fixed' annular urticated rash

Erythema multiforme

An acute, self-limiting condition with abrupt onset of symmetrical fixed urticated/target-like lesions in acral distribution. Central zone epidermal damage may cause bullae/crusts (➲ see Fig. 4.12). Can involve lips, buccal mucosa, and tongue (➲ see Fig. 10.3).

Triggers: infection (e.g. herpes simplex virus (HSV), atypical pneumonia), drugs (uncommon in children).

Cutaneous mastocytosis

Mastocytosis: a group of disorders characterized by mast cell proliferation and accumulation within various organs, most commonly the skin (➲ see also Chapter 19). Classification of cutaneous mastocytosis includes:

- Solitary mastocytoma (➲ see Fig. 28.6).
- Urticaria pigmentosa (most common type; ➲ see Fig. 19.8).
- Diffuse cutaneous mastocytosis.

Lesions often develop in early childhood and typically urticate on rubbing, rarely with blisters. *Darier's sign* is positive when a wheal and surrounding erythema develop in a lesion after rubbing. Diagnosis is usually clinical.

Systemic symptoms: result from histamine release and include flushing, abdominal pain, diarrhoea, wheeze, and rarely severe, anaphylactoid reactions.[4] These can result from significant skin disease without systemic involvement.

The condition persists for years but there is 75% spontaneous resolution of purely cutaneous disease.

Treatment: most do well with oral antihistamines and or mast cell stabilizing agents such as sodium cromoglicate; rarely phototherapy for older patients. Topical corticosteroids: use with caution for limited areas if very itchy and may speed involution of mastocytomas.

Cause: rarely familial. C-kit mutations are reported with systemic mastocytosis (see 'Other types').

Other types (all exceedingly rare in children):

- Indolent systemic mastocytosis.
- Systemic mastocytosis with an associated (clonal) haematologic non-mast cell lineage disease.
- Aggressive systemic mastocytosis.
- Mast cell leukaemia.
- Mast cell sarcoma.
- Extracutaneous mastocytoma.

Urticarial rash with angioedema (rare)

Acute haemorrhagic oedema of infancy

- ➲ See Cutaneous vasculitis, pp. 470–2.

Urticarial vasculitis

This may occur in conjunction with SLE and drugs. Lesions are painful, persist for days to weeks and heal with bruising. Can be associated with arthralgia, angioedema, uveitis, myositis, abdominal and renal involvement.[5]

Diagnosis: investigation of underlying cause. Skin biopsy with immunofluorescence may be helpful.

Treatment: systemic corticosteroids, antimalarials, and immunosuppressive therapy, depending on cause and severity.

Urticarial rash with systemic symptoms (rare)

Mastocytosis (cutaneous or systemic)

Histamine release may result in flushing, abdominal pain, diarrhoea, wheeze, hypotension and rarely anaphylactoid (➲ see Fixed annular urticated rash, pp. 314–15).

Juvenile idiopathic arthritis

- ➲ See Chapter 22, pp. 340–1.

Autoimmune disorders

- For example, rheumatoid arthritis, thyroid disease, SLE (➲ see Chapter 38, p. 530).

Urticarial vasculitis

- ➲ See Urticarial vasculitis, p. 315.

Dermatitis herpetiformis

Vesicles on a urticated base, quickly excoriated due to itching (➲ see Inflammatory skin diseases, p. 384–5).

Kawasaki disease

- ➲ See Infestations, pp. 337–8 and Figs. 9.4, 10.10, and 22.16.
- Recurrent febrile attacks, with elevated inflammatory markers, cardiac aneurism, arthralgia/arthritis, GI, and other symptoms (➲ see Chapter 22, pp. 339–40).

Malignancy and metabolic disorders

- Lymphoma, leukaemia.
- Erythropoietic protoporphyria (➲ see Chapter 16, pp. 230–1).
- Autoinflammatory disorders (periodic fevers)—see next.
- Other—autosensitization to oestrogen or progesterone—very rare.

Periodic fever syndromes

- See also Table 21.6.

Urticaria is the main cutaneous presentation

Cryopyrin-associated periodic syndromes. Family of rare autosomal dominant syndromes associated with mutations in cryopyrin, now termed NLRP3. Patients typically fall into one of three clinical syndromes:

- *Familial cold autoinflammatory syndromes (FCAS)*:
  - Type 1: recurrent episodes of fever and urticarial rashes along with arthralgias, conjunctivitis, thirst, headache, and nausea. Attacks usually occur following exposures to cold and last <24h.
  - Type 2: rare disease, *NLRP2* gene mutation. Recurrent episodes of fever, associated with urticaria, arthralgia, lymphadenopathy, abdominal pain, sensorineural hearing loss, and headaches following exposure to cold. Episodes last 2–7 days.
- *Muckle–Wells syndrome*: usually occurs during childhood and adolescence with urticarial rash, arthralgia, myalgia, and conjunctivitis. Symptoms last 12–36h. Sensorineural hearing loss begins in childhood and can lead to complete deafness in adolescence. Risk of amyloidosis as adult.
- *CINCA-NOMID syndrome* (chronic infantile neurologic cutaneous and articular syndrome, also called Neonatal onset multisystem inflammatory disease), characterized by urticaria, severe arthropathy, and central nervous system disorders. Risk of amyloidosis as adult.

Note: Schnitzler syndrome—an autoinflammatory syndrome of unknown aetiology, with onset in adulthood, characterized by urticaria, angioedema, monoclonal gammopathy, fever, arthralgia, bone pain, lymphadenopathy, and organomegaly.

Table 21.6 Features of autoinflammatory syndromes

Syndrome	Gene	Inheritance	Duration attacks	Rash	Other features	Amyloid risk	Therapy
FMF	*MEFV*	Recessive	<3 days	Yes	Serositis	+++	Colchicine
					Arthritis		IL-1 inhibition
HIDS	*MVK*	Recessive	3–5 days	Yes	Adenopathy	-	Prednisolone
					Abdo pain		Etanercept
					Arthritis		IL-1 inhibition
					Headache		IL-6 inhibition
TRAPS	*TNFRS1A*	Dominant	7–10 days	Yes	Myalgia	++	As for HIDS
					Serositis		
					Eye symptoms		
Cryopyrin-associated periodic syndromes (CAPS)							
FCAS	*NLRP3*	Dominant	<1 day	Urticaria	Arthralgia	_	Cold avoidance
							IL-1 inhibition
MWS	*NLRP3*	Dominant	5–7 days	Urticaria	Arthritis	++	IL-1 inhibition
					Headache		
					Hearing loss		
NOMID	*NLRP3*	Dominant	Constant	Urticaria	As for MWS	NOMID	NLRP3
					Papilloedema		

FMF, familial Mediterranean fever; HIDS, hyper-IgD syndrome; TRAPS, tumour necrosis factor receptor-associated periodic syndrome; FCAS, familial cold urticaria syndrome; MWS, Muckle–Wells syndrome; NOMID, neonatal onset multisystem inflammatory disease.

Source: data from British National Formulary (BNF), https://bnf.nice.org.uk/

References

1. British Association of Dermatologists (BAD), *Patient Information Leaflets (PILs)*, http://www.bad.org.uk/for-the-public/patient-information-leaflets/urticaria-and-angioedema
2. Medicines and Healthcare Products Regulatory Agency, http://www.mhra.gov.uk
3. [No authors listed] (1992). Guidelines for the diagnosis of rheumatic fever. Jones Criteria, 1992 update. Special Writing Group of the Committee on Rheumatic Fever, Endocarditis, and Kawasaki Disease of the Council on Cardiovascular Disease in the Young of the American Heart Association. *JAMA* **268**(15):2069–73.
4. National Institute for Health and Care Excellence (NICE), *Angio-oedema and Anaphylaxis* (revised November 2018), https://cks.nice.org.uk/angio-oedema-and-anaphylaxis
5. Powell, R.J., *et al.*; British Society for Allergy and Clinical Immunology (2015). BSACI guideline for the management of chronic urticaria and angioedema. *Clin Exp Allergy* **45**(3):547–65. https://www.bsaci.org/Guidelines/chronic-urticaria-and-angioedema

Chapter 22

Red rashes and erythroderma

Introduction

Red rashes are very common in children and may be due to a variety of processes, including:
- Primary skin diseases
- Infections
- Infestations
- Drugs
- Dietary insufficiency and metabolic disorders

A few may become generalized (erythroderma) (see Generalized redness, p. 341).

Red, scaly, or dry rashes in children

Common
- Eczema (see Chapter 17):
  - Atopic eczema
  - Discoid eczema
  - Seborrhoeic eczema
  - Contact eczema
- Psoriasis
- Viral exanthems: including measles, rubella, roseola, pityriasis rosea
- Tinea (fungal) infections
- Bacterial infections, especially *Staphylococcus aureus* and *Streptococcus pyogenes* spp.
- Yeast infections:
  - Pityriasis versicolor (teenagers only)
  - Candidiasis
- Infestations (e.g. scabies)

Uncommon to rare
- Lichen planus
- Pityriasis lichenoides (chronica and acuta)
- Pityriasis rubra pilaris
- Cutaneous T-cell lymphoma (mycosis fungoides)
- Dietary insufficiency*
- Spirochaetes: secondary syphilis, Lyme disease, yaws (tropical)*

Psoriasis

Epidemiology and pathogenesis

Psoriasis is an inherited, chronic, inflammatory condition of the skin that affects about 2% of the population. It is diagnosed prior to the age of 2y in 2% of cases and before 10y in 10% of cases. The inheritance is polygenic and not fully understood. Psoriasis may occur in association with psoriatic arthropathy, which may sometimes precede the skin lesions.

* *Common in some geographic areas.*

Clinical signs

The hallmark of psoriasis is a deep (beefy) red plaque, well-demarcated from normal skin, and often covered in adherent, silver-coloured scale (Figs. 22.1 and 22.2). In children the presentation may be less typical with narrower plaques and finer scale sometimes presenting on the face. The lesions may also present in hidden sites such as the scalp, natal cleft, groin, and umbilicus. Scratching off the scale may lead to surface bleeding. For particular sites, see Box 22.1. The clinical course is unpredictable, characterized by remissions and relapses.

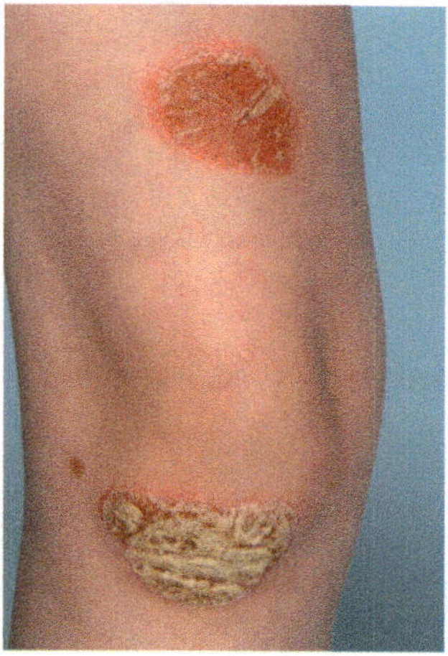

Fig. 22.1 Psoriasis, chronic plaque-type knee.

Reproduced courtesy of NHS Tayside Clinical Photography, Dundee, UK

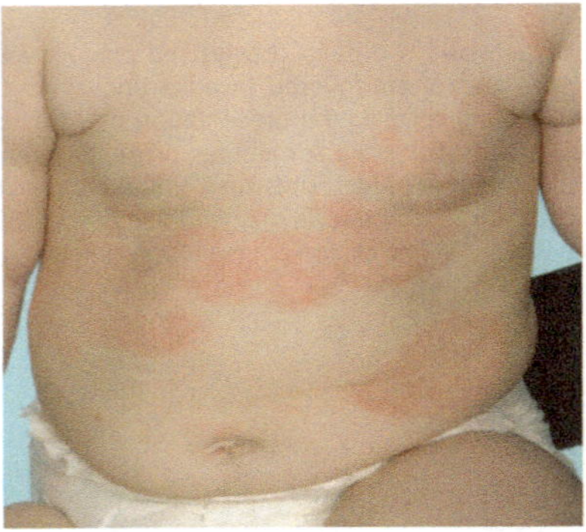

Fig. 22.2 Plaque psoriasis in an infant.

Reproduced courtesy of Susan Lewis-Jones, Hon Consultant Dermatologist, Ninewells Hospital and Medical School, Dundee, UK

Box 22.1 Sites of predilection for plaque psoriasis

- Elbows.
- Knees.
- Lumbar area.
- Scalp and scalp margins including ears.
- Nail changes often seen.

Note: in children psoriasis may present on the face, particularly around the eyes (➲ see Fig. 9.2)—this is uncommon in adults.

Psoriasis—clinical variants

Flexural psoriasis

Particularly common in infants. The napkin area is frequently the first site affected with well-defined erythema devoid of scale, although some scaling may be seen at the periphery (➲ see Fig. 11.3).

Plaque psoriasis

The most common variant in children (see Figs. 22.1 and 22.2). Typical lesions are 5–10cm in diameter, symmetrically located over extensor limb surfaces. Facial and scalp involvement are particularly common in children and either may be the only manifestation.

- Facial psoriasis can either be well-defined red scaly plaques, particularly around the eyes (➲ see Fig. 9.2), ears, or small circular thick, conical lesions (rupioid variant).
- Scalp psoriasis (➲ see Fig. 14.12) may be isolated plaques of thick scaling and redness or a more diffuse scaling. Very thick adherent scaling is one cause of pityriasis amiantacea (➲ see Box 14.3) and can cause traction alopecia.

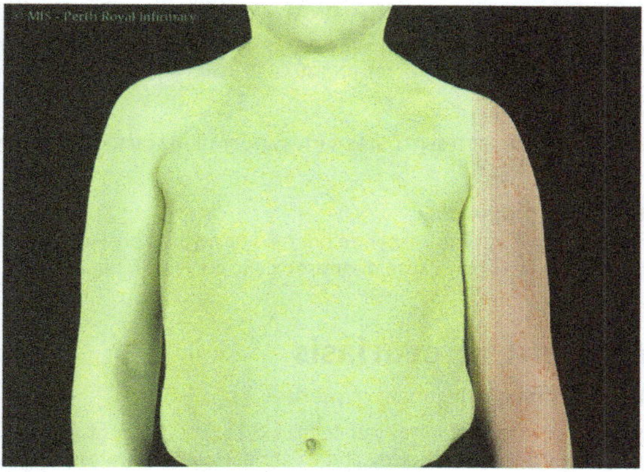

Fig. 22.3 Guttate psoriasis.

Reproduced courtesy of NHS Tayside Clinical Photography, Dundee, UK

Psoriasis of the nails

Superficial pits, onycholysis and subungual hyperkeratosis may occur (➲ see Fig. 15.7).

Guttate psoriasis

Usually develops suddenly, often in response to a streptococcal infection of the throat or skin. Characterized by the eruption of multiple papules 0.5–1cm in diameter over face, trunk, and limbs (Fig. 22.3). Take a throat swab culture and check serum antistreptolysin-O titre.

Generalized pustular psoriasis

Rare in childhood but potentially life-threatening. The pustules, which are superficial and sterile, may be generalized (erythrodermic) or localized (Fig. 22.19). General malaise, pyrexia, and anorexia are frequent accompaniments. ***Urgent same-day referral to a paediatric dermatologist is necessary as these patients may require systemic therapy.***

Table 22.1 Differential diagnosis of psoriasis

Type of psoriasis	Common differential diagnosis
Plaque psoriasis	Discoid eczema, tinea corporis
Scalp psoriasis	Seborrhoeic dermatitis or tinea capitis
Nail psoriasis	Fungal infection
Napkin psoriasis	Irritant contact dermatitis and seborrhoeic dermatitis
Guttate psoriasis	Pityriasis rosea and discoid eczema

Localized palmoplantar pustulosis

Very rare in children. Pustules on palms and soles are very resistant to therapy and often require potent topical corticosteroids.

Koebnerization

Psoriasis may occur at trauma sites such as operation scars, other injury, or sunburn (➲ see Fig. 4.8).

Differential diagnosis

Psoriasis is usually easy to recognize but mild or atypical presentations, particularly of the face, may cause diagnostic difficulty (see Table 22.1).

Treatment of psoriasis

- ➲ See also Topical treatment of psoriasis, pp. 37–8.

A realistic objective is control rather than cure. Education of children and parents about disease chronicity and treatment options are essential. Give information leaflets, e.g. British Association of Dermatologists (BAD) (see Further reading).

- *Emollients* reduce scaling and relieve itch and can reduce fissuring. They can also minimize koebnerization through reducing the likelihood of skin irritation. Use at least 1–2 times daily.
- *Topical vitamin D analogues* (e.g. calcipotriol) are clean and odour free so compliance is reasonable. Calcipotriol 50 micrograms (Dovonex®) is licensed for use in children at a maximum dose of 50g/week in those aged over 6y and 75g/week in those over 12y. However, the maximum safe dose has not been established and these are guidelines only.
- *Topical corticosteroids* are useful when itch is a major symptom. Mild corticosteroids can be used as monotherapy or combined with tacalcitol on the flexures, face, or scalp. On stable plaques on trunk and limbs, potent corticosteroids may be combined with topical vitamin D analogues for short periods (maximum 6 weeks). Risks of long-term sequelae include striae and telangiectasia and psoriasis may rebound following treatment cessation (➲ see Chapter 3).
- *Topical tars* are widely used in the treatment of psoriasis in adults but less so in children. Odour and tendency to stain limit acceptability.
- *Dithranol* (anthralin) is very effective, particularly for large, thick plaques but stains skin and clothing and is very irritant, especially on the flexures, face, genital areas, and healthy perilesional skin, where it should be

Box 22.2 Treatment of scalp psoriasis

- ➲ See also Chapter 3.
- Apply heavy oil-based preparation (e.g. olive oil, coconut oil or proprietary preparation) for 3h or overnight—daily until clear, then as necessary.
- Gently remove pieces of scale as they soften.
- Consider the use of a vitamin D analogue or a topical corticosteroid agent on dry scalp daily to help suppress recurrence.
- Avoid salicylic acid in children <2y.

avoided. It is available in many concentrations. Start with the weakest first and increase slowly to the maximum tolerated strength. Short contact (1h) treatment reduces the risk of burning and can be used for small plaques where it is not possible to avoid normal areas of skin. More suitable for inpatient use in children.

For treatment of scalp psoriasis, see Box 22.2.

Second-line therapies (specialist prescription only)

- *Topical calcineurin inhibitors*, e.g. Tacrolimus® 0.03% or 0.1% or Pimecrolimus® 1% cream are an effective alternative to topical corticosteroids on thin facial skin although this is an off-licence treatment. Topical calcineurin inhibitor is applied twice daily until satisfactory improvement and this is usually expected within the first month of treatment.
- *Phototherapy* (UVB or rarely PUVA) (➲ see Chapter 3, Other modalities of treatment, pp. 41–46) may be combined with topical treatment in older children with more extensive disease. Particular concerns about an increased risk of photocarcinogenesis limit use in children, as do the practical difficulties of administering the treatment in very young children and the frequent visits to attend the phototherapy department.
- *Systemic therapy*: none of the standard systemic therapies are licensed for the treatment of psoriasis in children. However, methotrexate, ciclosporin, and acitretin are all used under specialist direction and with caution (➲ see also Chapter 3).
- *Biologic therapies*: to date, etanercept (Enbrel®) and adalimumab (Humira®) both tumour necrosis factor (TNF) –alpha inhibitors, and ustekinumab (Stelara®) an inhibitor of interleukin-12 and 23, are

Box 22.3 Viral rashes

Localized viral rashes

- Papular acrodermatitis of childhood (also known as Gianotti–Crosti syndrome) (➲ see Chapter 19, Infection, pp. 282–3).
- Unilateral latero-thoracic exanthem (*syn.* asymmetric periflexural exanthem of childhood (APEC)).
- Hand, foot, and mouth disease (➲ see Infection causing blisters, p. 378 and Fig. 12.2).
- Gloves and socks purpura (➲ see Chapter 31, Sepsis, pp. 467–70).
- Herpes infections (➲ see Infection causing blisters, p. 378).

Generalized viral rashes

- Cytomegalovirus.
- Enterovirus infections.
- Epstein–Barr (infectious mononucleosis).
- Erythema infectiosum.
- German measles (rubella).
- Measles (rubeola).
- Morbilliform rashes.
- Pityriasis rosea.
- Roseola (exanthem subitum).

Note: This is not an exhaustive list and many other viral rashes are seen throughout the world but rarely present in the United Kingdom (e.g. Rocky Mountain spotted fever, typhus, typhoid).

licensed for the treatment of psoriasis in the paediatric population. In 2016 the Food and Drug Administration (FDA) approved the use of etanercept in children aged 4–17y (see Further reading for additional information).

Red viral exanthems

Many viral rashes cannot be ascribed to a particular virus without laboratory confirmation (unnecessary in most cases) and are simply described as viral exanthems. Although some have a characteristic clinical picture (Box 22.3), it is important to remember that some can present atypically. Also several different viruses may cause similar patterns of exanthem, e.g. a morbilliform rash (measles-like), and slapped cheeks which may occur with viruses other than *parvovirus*.

All viruses causing high fever may be associated with febrile convulsions. Viral exanthems may be localized or generalized and can take many forms:

- Redness—with or without scaling.
- Papules (➲ see Chapter 19).
- Blistering eruptions (➲ see Chapter 25).
- Purpuric/haemorrhagic rashes (➲ see Chapter 31).

The following are brief accounts of the typical presentation of common viruses. For congenital and neonatal presentations (➲ see Congenital infection, pp. 88–9).

Cytomegalovirus

Skin rashes are mainly seen in congenital infections not acquired, except in the immunocompromised where generalized exanthematous rashes or ulceration are commonest. Rarely, urticarial, or petechial rashes are seen.

Epstein–Barr virus (EBV); *syn.* infectious mononucleosis)

Ubiquitous member of the *herpes* family infecting over 90% of humans, usually asymptomatic in young children.

Presentation: fever, sore throat, and lymphadenopathy. Greyish-white pharyngeal exudate. Sometimes palatal purpura is seen. Flu-like symptoms with malaise, headache, myalgias, anorexia, and fatigue. Less commonly: gastrointestinal (GI) symptoms, hepatomegaly, and jaundice. Rarely splenic rupture.

Rash: morbilliform (measles-like) in 15–20%, sometimes urticarial, vesicular, or purpuric (Box 22.4).

Box 22.4 Causes of morbilliform rashes

- *Measles* (Rubeola)
- *Rubella* (German measles)
- *Enteroviruses:* coxsackie, enterovirus, echovirus
- *Respiratory viruses:* adenovirus, respiratory syncytial, rhinovirus
- *Epstein–Barr* (infectious mononucleosis)
- *Human herpes viruses*: HHV 6 and 7 (roseola subitum)
- *Parvovirus B19* (erythema infectiosum)
- *Drugs:* particularly antibiotics, anticonvulsants

Treatment: supportive; 33–80% of those treated with ampicillin will develop a morbilliform rash (original 1960s reports of 80–100% were not borne out in a recent *New England Journal of Medicine* study).

Erythema infectiosum ('Fifth' disease)

Common in winter and spring and often asymptomatic. Caused by human parvovirus B19.

Note: child is not infectious once rash appears.

Incubation: approximately 4–14 days.

Prodrome: low-grade fever and myalgia, headaches, malaise.

Rash: occasionally pruritic; three stages:

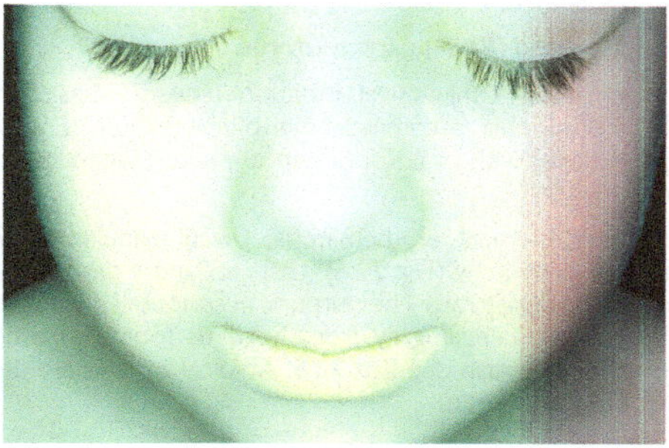

Fig. 22.4 Slapped cheeks in erythema infectiosum.

Reproduced courtesy of Susan Lewis-Jones, Hon Consultant Dermatologist, Ninewells Hospital and Medical School, Dundee, UK

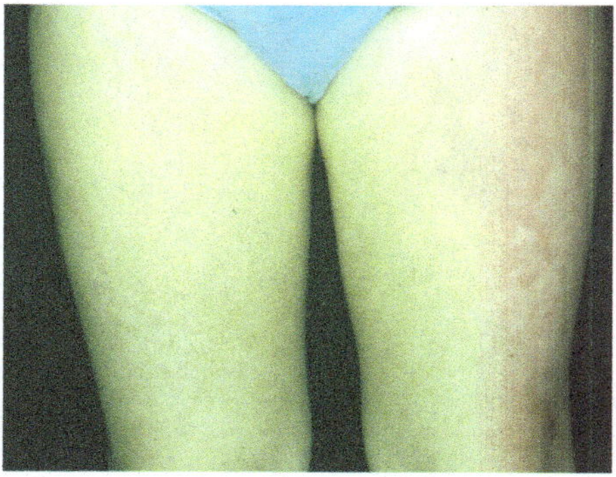

Fig. 22.5 Rash of erythema infectiosum—faint dull red, rash over proximal thighs.

Reproduced courtesy of Susan Lewis-Jones, Hon Consultant Dermatologist, Ninewells Hospital and Medical School, Dundee, UK

- 'Slapped cheeks'—bright red confluent on cheeks with circumoral pallor (Fig. 22.4).
- One to four days later—rash develops on proximal extremities (Fig. 22.5). It varies from morbilliform to a lacy, red pattern and spreads to trunk but spares palms and soles.
- Waxes and wanes over one or more weeks (usually biphasic).

Complications: arthralgia and arthritis uncommon in children. Non-immune pregnant mothers are at risk of fetal complications including hydrops fetalis, fetal loss (5%), and intrauterine death.

Measles (rubeola)

Becoming more common since parental anxiety (unproven) about measles, mumps, rubella (MMR) vaccine has reduced routine vaccination rates.

Incubation: approximately 14 days.

Cause: ribonucleic acid (RNA) paramyxovirus.

Prodrome: high fever, conjunctival injection (severe), nasal congestion, and cough. Photophobia is commoner in older children. *Enanthem* (mucosal manifestations) with oral Koplik's spots—small white spots on a red background.

Rash (*exanthem*): classical erythematous, maculopapular (morbilliform) rash—not particularly itchy (Fig. 22.6). Lasts around 4 days, darkening and often desquamating (may rarely be purpuric in serious cases). Starts around hairline and spreads centrifugally from head to foot. For other viruses causing a morbilliform rash, see Box 22.5. Atypical variants are described in those previously immunized.

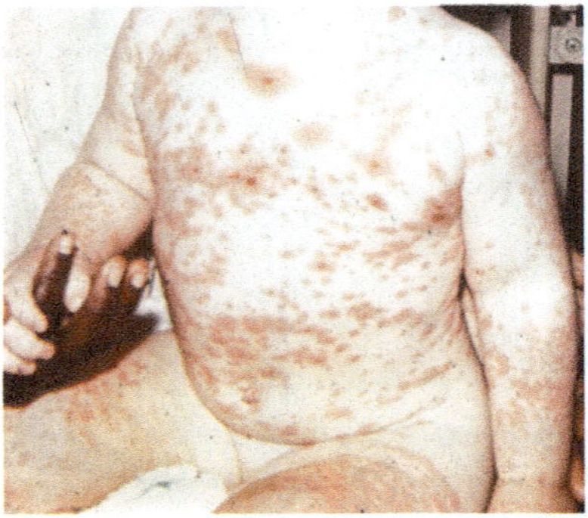

Fig. 22.6 Severe case of measles: child had photophobia and injected sclera and some lesions show early haemorrhagic centres.

Reproduced courtesy of Susan Lewis-Jones, Hon Consultant Dermatologist, Ninewells Hospital and Medical School, Dundee, UK

Complications: especially infants <1y and immunocompromised—pneumonia, encephalitis, cardiac, death. Rarely causes subacute sclerosing panencephalitis (1/100,000).

Treatment: supportive.

German measles (rubella)

Benign self-limiting disease; 50% subclinical especially in children. However, intrauterine infection causes severe congenital problems including deafness and central nervous system (CNS) effects (➲ see Congenital infection, pp. 88–9).

Incubation: 16–18 days.

Prodrome: 1–5 days before rash, mild fever, headache, conjunctivitis, upper respiratory tract infection. Tender posterior cervical lymphadenopathy is common.

Rash: red/pink macules with tiny papules which start on face and neck (particularly behind ears) moving caudally then fading in 2 days. Non-contagious 7 days after rash.

Treatment: supportive.

Vaccination: part of MMR UK vaccination schedule given at 12–15 months and again at school-age.

Roseola (*syn.* exanthem subitum)

Ubiquitous infection occurring in infants 6 months to 3y.

Cause: human herpes virus—HHV-6 or HHV-7.

Incubation: approximately 9–10 days.

Prodrome: high fever that subsides in a day, occasionally upper respiratory symptoms, abdominal pain, and malaise.

Rash: appears within 24–48h. Pale pink non-itchy macules and papules, fades over a few days. Eyelid oedema in 30%.

Complications: rarely encephalitis or encephalopathy.

Treatment: supportive. In immunosuppressed children ganciclovir and foscarnet are possible treatment options.

Unilateral laterothoracic exanthem

(*Syn.* asymmetric periflexural exanthem of childhood (APEC); superimposed lateral exanthem of childhood). Fairly common, seen in infants (range 1–5y). Commoner in girls.

Prodrome: fever from a few days to several weeks.

Rash: 95% have a solitary patch on the chest with variable morphology from pink papules to more eczematous areas. It spreads centrifugally and may become generalized, gradually fading over a 6-week period. There is sometimes an associated mild adenopathy and low-grade fever.

Cause: unconfirmed but has been associated with EBV, adenovirus, and parvovirus B19.

Treatment: resolves spontaneously. No treatment necessary. Emollients +/– mild topical corticosteroids if itchy.

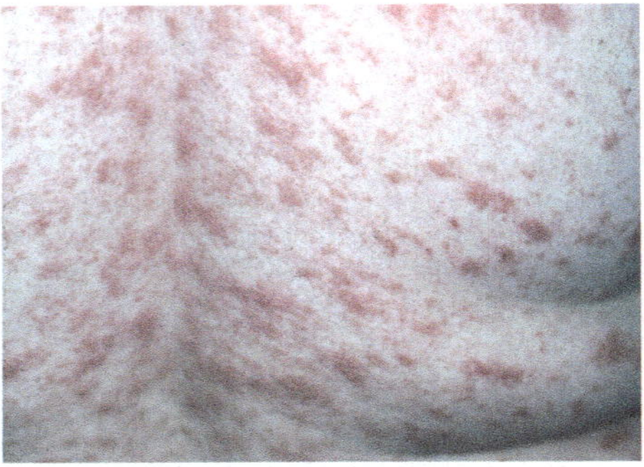

Fig. 22.7 Pityriasis rosea—erythematous macules with scaling in a 'fir tree' distribution.

Reproduced courtesy of Susan Lewis-Jones, Hon Consultant Dermatologist, Ninewells Hospital and Medical School, Dundee, UK

Pityriasis rosea

A self-limiting papulosquamous rash.

Prodrome: characterized by an initial red, scaly 'herald patch' commonly on the trunk (often missed).

Rash: follows a few days later by the development of smaller, oval, red, scaly patches in a 'fir tree' arrangement on the trunk, neck, and proximal limbs (Fig. 22.7). Lesions usually have a fine collarette of scale at the periphery, the free edge of which opens inwards. It resolves within 2–3 months. Occasionally itchy, it does not involve palms or soles (unlike syphilis), but tends to be on trunk and proximal limbs ('T-shirt and shorts' distribution). Atypical forms are very common in Africa and Asia and may be more severe and extensive.

Cause: exact cause unknown but believed that some strains of herpes virus (not *H. simplex*) may trigger it. Not thought to be contagious.

Complications: uncommon. Rarely severe itching. Postinflammatory pigmentation in darker skin types may be prolonged.

Treatment: supportive only.

Fungal infections of the skin

A large number of fungi, moulds, and yeasts can affect the skin, particularly in the immunocompromised. Most are uncommon to rare and only the dermatophyte infections (tinea *syn*: ringworm) are considered here. Immigrant or immunosuppressed children may present with unusual or extensive lesions.

Tinea infections

Caused by a dermatophyte fungus from human (anthropophilic), animal (zoophilic) or soil (geophilic) sources. Dermatophytes metabolize and rely upon keratin found in skin, hair, and nails.

Rash: Characterized by enlarging annular red scaly patches (Fig. 22.8) sometimes with pustules, particularly in animal ringworm where there is a more aggressive host response. It is named in Latin after the body part affected, e.g.

- ***Tinea corporis*** (trunk): ringed lesions with central clearing (Fig. 22.8) and an advancing edge with redness, scaling, and pustules. Partial clearance often results in arcuate shapes. Satellite lesions are common. Diagnosis depends upon a high index of suspicion.
- ***Tinea capitis*** (scalp): ➲ see Fig. 14.7. Zoophilic strains cause may cause a kerion (➲ see Fig. 14.8).
- ***Tinea manuum*** (hand): uncommon in children, always check the feet.
- ***Tinea pedis*** (feet): ➲ see Feet, pp. 166–70.
- ***Tinea cruris*** (groin): uncommon in children; differentiate from other flexural rashes such as psoriasis and seborrhoeic eczema (➲ see Box 11.1).
- ***Tinea faciei*** (face): ➲ see Fig. 20.4. even reported in young infants.
- ***Tinea unguium*** (nails): ➲ see Infection, pp. 217–20.
- ***Tinea incognito***: occurs in any site when topical corticosteroids have been used inappropriately to treat a rash. These partially suppress inflammation but allow widespread lesions with serpiginous (snake-like) edges, with little scaling or pustules.

Diagnosis is confirmed by skin scraping from the active edge of lesion for fungal microscopy and culture (➲ see Other dermatological interventions, pp. 24–6; for differential diagnosis of ringed (annular) lesions, see Box 4.2).

Treatment: topical antifungal agents (for localized disease without nail involvement); scalp lesions or extensive or refractory cutaneous infections or nail disease require oral antifungal agents (➲ see Chapters 14 and 15).

Note: nystatin is not effective treatment for dermatophyte infections.

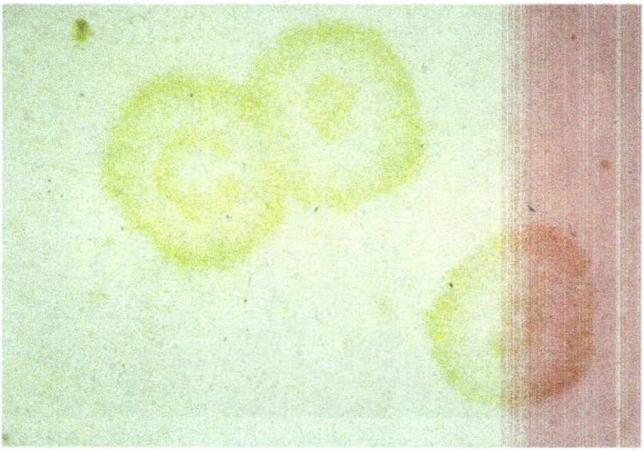

Fig. 22.8 Annular ringworm from *M. canis*.

Reproduced courtesy of Susan Lewis-Jones, Hon Consultant Dermatologist, Ninewells Hospital and Medical School, Dundee, UK

Bacterial infections

Many bacterial infections cause red rashes e.g.:

- Impetigo (➲ see Infections causing blisters, p. 378–82).
- Scarlatina (➲ see Erythroderma, faltering growth, and recurrent infection, p. 346).
- Staphylococcal scalded skin syndrome (➲ see Infection causing erythroderma, p. 345).

Hansen's disease (*syn.* leprosy)

Cause: mycobacterium leprae.

Chronic infection affecting mainly skin, peripheral nerves, upper respiratory tract mucosa, and eyes. Young children may be affected but more common in older children/teenagers. Mainly seen in those from high risk areas. Clinical pattern depends on host immune response. Two main patterns are seen:

- *Tuberculoid leprosy* (high-mediated cell immunity)—may present with infiltrated plaques or hypopigmented macules (Fig. 22.9). Plaques are hairless, dry and show reduced pain and temperature sensations (nearby nerves may be thickened).
- *Lepromatous leprosy* (low-mediated cell immunity)—lesions often widespread, symmetric, and polymorphic; macules, papules, diffuse infiltration, and nodules, often involving face and ears. Loss of eyebrows (madarosis) common.
- *Borderline disease* also occurs with features of both.

Diagnosis and investigations: based on clinical findings and split skin smear results (ideal). Negative smears from all areas = paucibacterial leprosy (PB). Positive smears at any site = multibacillary leprosy (MB).

In the field (WHO): if no split skin smears possible base diagnosis on number of lesions 1–5 = PB; 6 or more = MB.

Skin biopsy: often not done in endemic areas. Should be deep enough to contain a nerve fibre bundle.

Fig. 22.9 Leprosy with hypopigmented macule.

Reproduced courtesy of Susan Lewis-Jones, Hon Consultant Dermatologist, Ninewells Hospital and Medical School, Dundee, UK

Histopathology: typical epithelioid granulomas are seen in tuberculoid leprosy. Acid-fast bacilli are numerous in the lepromatous type but often difficult to find in the tuberculoid type.

Treatment: consult an expert in lepromatous disease. Drugs include dapsone (1mg/kg/day); rifampicin (10mg/kg/day), the most bactericidal drug available for treatment of leprosy; clofazimine (1mg/kg/day), major side effect is skin pigmentation. World Health Organization (WHO) guidelines suggest multidrug therapy (MDT) to reduce resistance; however, the duration of therapy is less than previously thought. For MDT include a single dose for a single lesion, or two drugs for lesions that contain more than one bacterium. A daily regimen for 1y of three drugs is necessary for more widespread multibacillary disease (Box 22.5).

Lepromatous leprosy is subject to reactions even after 1y of therapy and patients must be educated to return for diagnosis and appropriate therapy promptly as acute Lepra reactions can cause severe nerve damage and may require hospitalization.

Box 22.5 WHO recommended treatment for leprosy

Multibacillary leprosy in children (10–14y)

- *Once a month*: On day 1, two capsules of rifampicin (300mg + 150mg) plus three capsules of clofazimine (50mg × 3) plus one tablet of dapsone (50mg).
- *Once a day*: On days 2–28, one capsule of clofazimine every other day (50mg), plus one tablet of dapsone (50mg) daily.
- *Full course*: 12 blister packs over 12 months.
- For children younger than 10y, the dose must be adjusted according to body weight.

  Paucibacillary leprosy in children (10–14y)
- *Once a month*: on day 1, two capsules of rifampicin (300mg + 150mg) plus one tablet of dapsone (50mg).
- *Once a day*: On days 2–28, one tablet of dapsone (50mg).
- *Full course*: six blister packs over 6 months.

Tuberculosis (TB)—skin diseases

Clinical presentation depends on portal of entry (whether from systemic disease or cutaneous injury) and host response (whether previously infected or immunosuppressed). Causative organisms include *Mycobacterium (M.) tuberculosis*. Rare in United Kingdom and the West but common in Indian subcontinent and parts of Africa. Non-tuberculous environmental (atypical) mycobacterium such as *M. marinum* (fish tank granuloma; ➲ see Fig.12.6) are more common.

Types:

1. Those caused by inoculation:
   - ***Tuberculosis verrucosa cutis***: occurs by direct inoculation into the skin in those previously infected or vaccinated with Bacillus

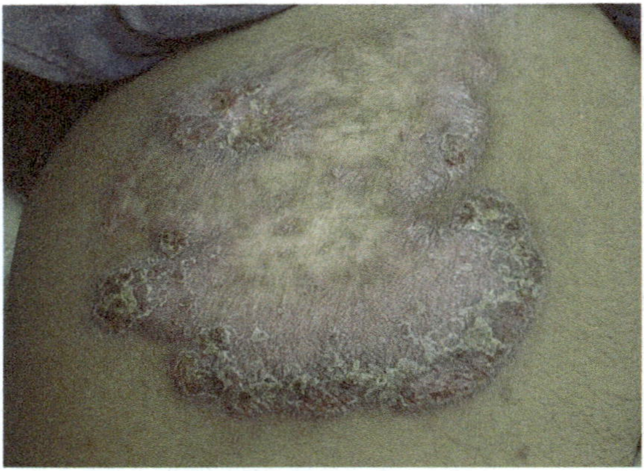

Fig. 22.10 Tuberculosis verrucosa cutis.
Reproduced courtesy of Patrick Yesudian, Consultant Dermatologist, Chennai, India

Calmette-Guérin (BCG). Localized purplish warty plaques or nodules develop, commonly on hands, feet, buttock, knees, or elbows and may take months to heal (Figs. 22.10 and 22.11).

- *Lupus vulgaris*: seen mainly on the face. A primary red-brown papule progresses to a well-defined reddish-brown plaque with typical apple-jelly nodules seen when pressed with a glass slide. There is often some central healing, but ulceration may also occur.

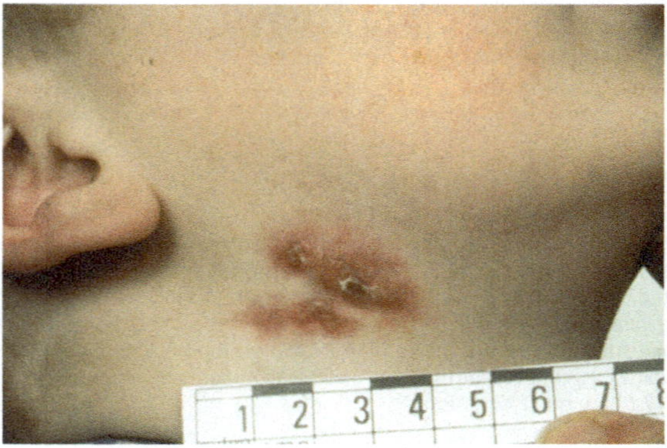

Fig. 22.11 Scrofuloderma of the neck due to tuberculous lymph gland.
Reproduced courtesy of Susan Lewis-Jones, Hon Consultant Dermatologist, Ninewells Hospital and Medical School, Dundee, UK

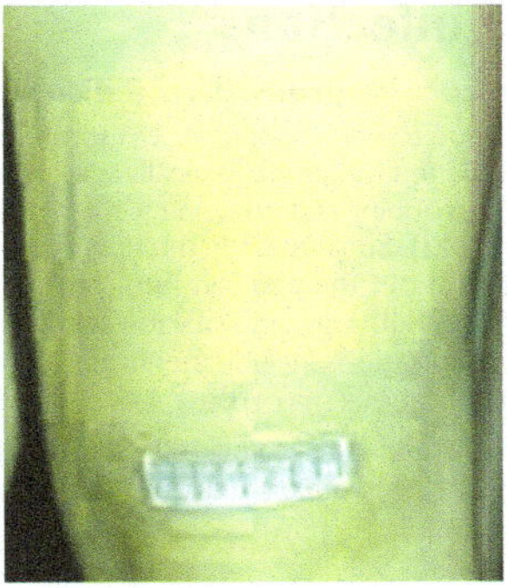

Fig. 22.12 Erythema chronicum migrans.

Reproduced courtesy of Susan Lewis-Jones, Hon Consultant Dermatologist, Ninewells Hospital and Medical School, Dundee, UK

- ***Scrofuloderma***: skin involvement secondary to underlying lymph node, joint, or bone involvement. It may be associated with pulmonary infection (Fig. 22.12).

2. Those caused by haematogenous spread:
   - ***Disseminated tuberculosis (miliary TB)***: occurs in the immunosuppressed due to blood-borne dissemination from underlying TB (usually pulmonary), to multiple organs including the skin. Presents as small papules developing into abscesses or ulcers.
3. Others:
   - ***Papulonecrotic tuberculids***: occurs as small, crusted papules on the extensors of the limbs and lower trunk.
   - ***Erythema induratum (syn. Bazin's disease)***: large nodules/ulcers are seen on calves usually in adolescents. These may postdate papulonecrotic tuberculids.
   - ***Erythema nodosum***: tender red nodules on legs (➲ see Fig. 12.10 and Colour, pp. 419–27). TB is just one cause of this disease.
   - ***Swimming pool and fish tank granulomas***: caused by atypical environmental mycobacterium mainly *M. marinum*. Usually an isolated nodule (➲ see Fig. 12.6) but sporotrichoid spread may occur (new, individual lesions occurring more proximally usually along a limb).
   - ***BCG vaccination***: local reactions are common, often with red nodules that may ulcerate before healing. Regional adenopathy can occur.

Diagnosis: skin TB is diagnosed by skin biopsy, Mantoux test, QuantiFeron-TB gold test, chest X-ray, sputum cultures.

Treatment: the commonly used antibiotics are isoniazid; rifampicin; pyrazinamide; streptomycin; and ethambutol, usually in triple combination. Consult an infectious disease expert.

Spirochaete infections

Erythema chronicum migrans (Lyme disease)

A tick-borne disease due to *Borrelia burgdorferi*† spread by the *Ixodes* species found on deer in the United Kingdom. Typically walkers may be affected and a red papule with an expanding red ring (up to 30cm) is seen around the site of the tick bite (Fig. 22.12). Subsequently multiple rings may develop. There may be central clearance but the papule often remains obvious. Untreated cases may develop fever, lethargy, and malaise with myalgia and arthralgia. Later neurological complications include meningitis and cranial nerve palsies and cardiological complications may arise.

Diagnosis: usually confirmed by serological tests but also skin biopsy. For differential diagnosis of ringed annular lesions (➲ see Box 4.2).

Treatment: doxycycline (avoid <12y), penicillin, azithromycin, or cefuroxime are effective.

Syphilis

Maternal transmission of *Treponema pallidum* can give rise to congenital syphilis which may present with variety of rashes (➲ see Congenital infection, pp. 88–9).

Primary stage: acquired syphilis manifests as a primary chancre between 1 week and 3 months, often with local lymphadenopathy. Usually heals spontaneously.

Secondary stage: generalized lymphadenopathy, influenza-like symptoms, mucocutaneous lesions (oral erosions and moist intertriginous lesions—condyloma lata) and a coppery papulosquamous rash that classically affects the palms and soles (unlike pityriasis rosea with which it may be confused). Also annular papulonecrotic lesions occur, especially in those with concomitant HIV infection. Scalp lesions and patchy alopecia occur.

Tertiary stage: cutaneous gummata occur in adults.

Treatment: single dose of benzyl penicillin intramuscularly (IM) or oral erythromycin for 3 weeks. In penicillin allergy, high-dose doxycycline or tetracycline may be used in older children and adults.

Yaws

Endemic in the tropics, *Treponema pallidum* subsp. *pertenue* gains entry through skin to skin transfer via abrasions causing destructive skin and soft tissue lesions. Predominately affects children.

- A crusted ulcerated primary papule occurs at the inoculation site healing to leave atrophic scar. Commonest sites are buttocks or extremities.
- Later small multiple secondary lesions resembling raspberries (framboesiform) develop and wide range of skin changes and bone involvement (e.g. osteoperiostitis) may occur. Periorificial and mucosal lesions are common.
- In the tertiary stages gummata may occur in skin, joints, and bone and hyperkeratotic lesions on the palms and soles. Typically no cardiac or neurological complications are seen.

† Various *Borrelia* species are common to different geographic locations worldwide and clinical features vary (e.g. in neurotoxicity and cardiotoxicity).

Diagnosis: *T. pallidum* particle agglutination assay or rapid plasma regain assay.

Treatment: 0.6 million units IM benzathine benzylpenicillin. Azithromycin is effective, less toxic, and easy to deliver in tropics but resistance may be a future problem.

Recognized as a neglected tropical disease by WHO; eradication strategies are in place.

Infestations

Scabies

Itchy contagious eruption caused by *Sarcoptes scabiei* var. *hominis* which often presents as a diffuse eczematous/urticated rash (Fig. 22.13).

Signs occur 4–6 weeks after infestation and include burrows which resemble fine, white cotton threads, especially on finger webs, wrists, ankles, soles, and penis (see Fig. 22.14); red papules or scabetic nodules seen in axillae and groin and penis (➲ see Fig. 28.14); excoriations; vesiculopustular or bullous lesions (especially hands and soles); urticaria; secondary eczema and impetigo. The extent is extremely variable and findings may be subtle. Rash spares the face and scalp (except in neonates). *Ask if any close contacts have an itchy rash.* ➲ See Dermoscopy, p. 19, which may be helpful for diagnosis.

Norwegian or crusted scabies: an uncommon, highly contagious hyperkeratotic variant, which may not be particularly itchy, found in immunocompromised or neurologically impaired individuals. Hands in particular show marked hyperkeratosis (➲ see Fig. 12.5).

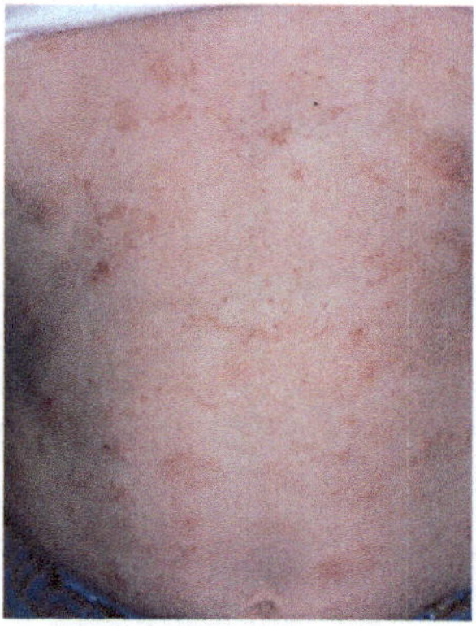

Fig. 22.13 Scabies: generalized eczematous excoriated rash on trunk—a very typical presentation in young children.

Reproduced courtesy of Susan Lewis-Jones, Hon Consultant Dermatologist, Ninewells Hospital and Medical School, Dundee, UK

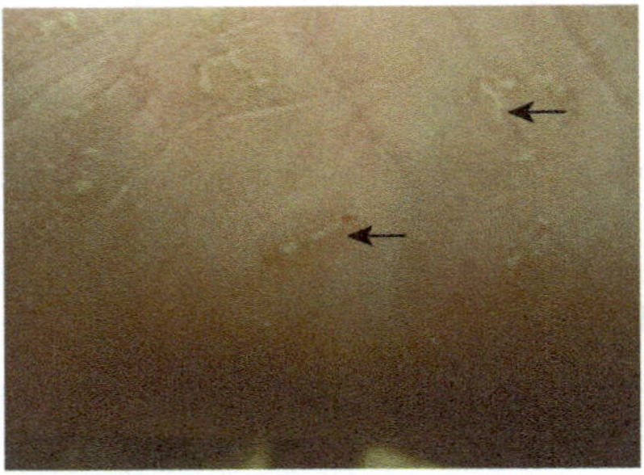

Fig. 22.14 Close-up of scabies burrows.

Reproduced courtesy of Susan Lewis-Jones, Hon Consultant Dermatologist, Ninewells Hospital and Medical School, Dundee, UK

Lice (pediculosis)

- ***Pediculosis capitis*** (head lice): ➲ see Fig. 2.3. Often associated with scalp impetigo (➲ see Fig. 14.10).
- ***Pediculosis corporis***: caused by *Pediculus humanus* (body lice) it is rare in the UK. The lice live in the seams of clothing. It may be seen in the context of neglect (e.g. homeless teenagers). Bites may or may not cause itching. Chronic cases show brownish red scaly rash, multiple excoriations, (vagabond's skin)—usually truncal and there may be regional adenopathy. Treat clothing (and bedding) at high temperatures (above 65°C [149°F]) for 15–30min and skin with topical 5% permethrin cream.
- ***Pediculosis pubis***: caused by *Pthirus pubis* (pubic or crab lice), which attach firmly and feed for long periods. Seen in context of close physical contact. Treat all hairy areas including scalp with permethrin cream. Unusual in young children but can affect eyelashes (*Pediculosis palpebrum*, Fig. 22.15) where safest treatment is with Vaseline 3–5 times daily for 8–10 days to kill hatching nymphs or oral trimethoprim for 10 days.

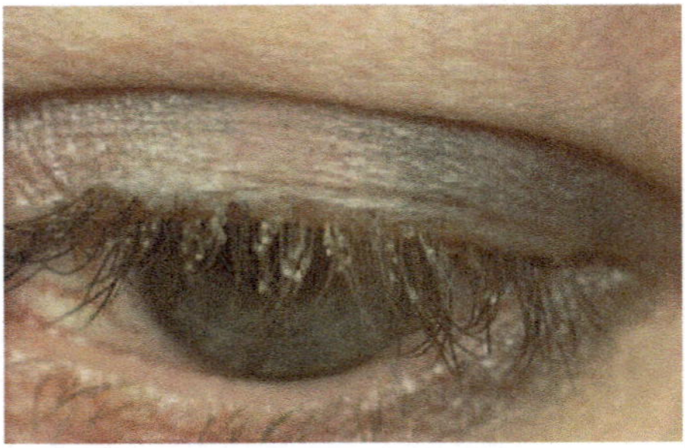

Fig. 22.15 Crab louse eggs on the eyelashes.

Reproduced with permission from Burns, T. *et al.* (Eds.) (2004). *Rook's Textbook of Dermatology*, Seventh Edition. Oxford, UK: Wiley Blackwell

Rare skin diseases causing red rashes

Erythema annulare centrifugum

Annular, red, expanding lesions with scaly edges. A descriptive term for a number of annular lesions of unknown cause (drugs and infections have been implicated) without systemic symptoms. It may be confused with ringworm or Lyme disease. If there is associated fever, then think of rare periodic fevers (➲ see Chapter 21).

Lichen planus

Characterized by very itchy polygonal, violaceous papules with fine white streaks, referred to as Wickham's striae (➲ see Fig. 19.6). Very rare in children (➲ see Chapter 19).

Pityriasis lichenoides

Acute and chronic forms (➲ see Chapter 19 and Fig. 19.7).

Kawasaki disease

Generalized erythema, with a predilection for palms and soles. Involvement of mucous membranes is usual with perioral erythema, swollen lips (➲ see Fig. 9.4) and strawberry tongue (➲ see Fig. 10.10). The child is ill with a spiking fever and (commonly) marked cervical adenopathy. Sometimes indurated oedema of the hands is seen with 'sausage fingers' (Fig. 22.16). Peeling of the palms is a *late* sign. Request urgent paediatric specialist help

Diagnosis: there is general acceptance of the following [1,2]:

Fever for 5 days or more.

Plus four of:

1. Bilateral conjunctival injection without exudate.
2. Cervical lymphadenopathy of at least 1.5cm.
3. Polymorphic rash.
4. Changes in lips and oral mucosa, strawberry tongue.
5. Changes in extremities:
   - Reddening of palms or soles.
   - Indurative oedema of hands or feet.

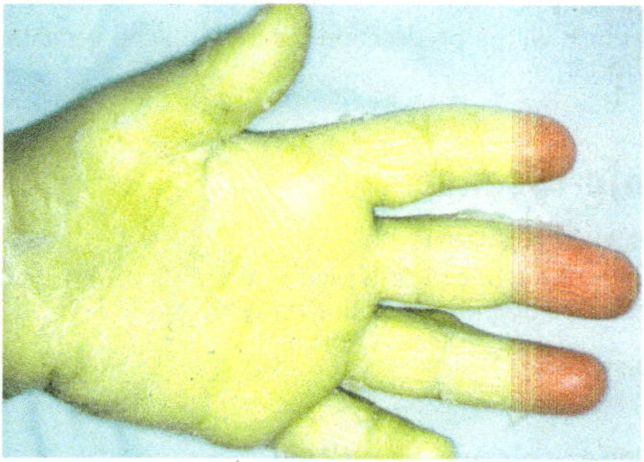

Fig. 22.16 Swollen hands in Kawasaki disease

Reproduced courtesy of Jo Sowden, Consultant Dermatologist, UK

Treatment: high-dose aspirin and intravenous immunoglobulin reduces risk of complications. Suspect in cases of unexplained fever with some signs and start treatment early.

Complications: coronary artery dissection and myocarditis are key complications caused by an acute inflammatory vasculitis.

Mycosis fungoides (cutaneous T-cell lymphoma)

Very rare in children. Often misdiagnosed as eczema but may not be itchy. Patches of dusky erythema, often oval with relatively poorly defined edges occur mainly on trunk and limbs. There may also be hyperkeratotic (thick scaling), particularly on hands and feet and sometimes a digitate pattern with finger-shaped macular lesions is seen on the trunk. Lesions look slightly atrophic and wrinkled (cigarette paper wrinkling). There may be associated systemic symptoms such as night-time sweating and lethargy.

Investigation and management: requires skin biopsy with special stains, PCR amplification, and interpretation by a specially trained histopathologist (it may take several biopsies over time before diagnosis is certain). Referral to paediatric dermatologist is essential and care should be multidisciplinary. Disease staging should be undertaken (see Further reading).

Prognosis: generally good in children although it depends on the stage.

Treatment: lesions (and systemic symptoms) often respond to potent topical corticosteroids and phototherapy, although they usually recur some time after stopping.

Dietary insufficiency

- ➲ see Vitamin deficiencies, p. 494.

Pellagra

Niacin (vitamin B_3 or nicotinic acid) deficiency. Pigmented brownish-coloured dermatitis, seen on photo-exposed sites (e.g. around neck). May be associated confusion and diarrhoea in severe cases.

Zinc deficiency

Psoriasiform rash with a predilection for perioral and genital area (➲ see Figs. 7.4 and 13.4).

Systemic disease

Erythema marginatum

A pale pink fleeting urticarial rash seen in association with rheumatic fever (➲ see Differential diagnosis of urticaria rashes, pp. 313–16).

Dermatomyositis

- ➲ See Dermal thickening, pp. 448–50.

Juvenile idiopathic arthritis (JIA)

JAC (arthritis that causes joint inflammation and stiffness for more than 6 weeks in a child of 16y of age or less) is sometimes associated with a transient erythematous rash and fever. Refer to paediatric rheumatologist. It is important to exclude other causes of juvenile arthropathy such as infection, other inflammatory connective tissue diseases and rarer causes such as haemoglobinopathies and chondrodysplasias (➲ see Chapter 38).

Systemic lupus erythematosus (SLE) ⚑

- ➲ See also Chapter 38.

Classically presents as a photosensitive rash with erythema in a butterfly distribution over cheeks and nose (➲ see Fig. 9.3). There may also be a reticulate rash in photo-exposed sites (➲ see Photoaggravated dermatoses, pp. 237–8). It is a multisystem disorder (mainly joints, renal, cardiovascular, pulmonary, and neurological) which may progress over a period of years. For diagnostic criteria (➲ see Table 38.1). For investigations, management, and monitoring, ➲ see pp. 526–7. For neonatal LE, ➲ see p. 82 and Figs. 7.2 and 7.3.

Generalized redness (erythroderma)

Children who are affected with an inflammatory rash covering more than 90% of their body surface area described as erythrodermic. It is relatively rare and potentially life-threatening and may be complicated by hypothermia (shivering), dehydration, and high output cardiac failure. There may be associated blistering or scaling with some types.

Always ask for an urgent dermatological opinion in cases of suspected erythroderma. ⚑

Causes of erythroderma

Generalized redness without blisters

The most likely are:

- Eczema.
- Drug rash (suspect any drug taken in the last 21 days) (➲ Chapter 23).
- Bacterial toxins (usually *Staphylococcus aureus* or *Streptococcus pyogenes*).
- Viral exanthem (usually patchy redness).

Rarer diagnoses include:

- Generalized psoriasis (Fig. 22.17).
- Kawasaki's disease.
- Pityriasis rubra pilaris.
- Cutaneous T-cell lymphoma (mycosis fungoides).
- Non-bullous ichthyosiform erythroderma (➲ see Chapter 27).
- Netherton syndrome (➲ see Figs. 6.2 and 6.3; see also Chapter 27).
- Graft-versus-host disease (➲ see Chapter 39).
- Omenn syndrome (➲ see Chapter 6).
- Cystic fibrosis dermatosis (➲ see Chapter 6).
- Metabolic and nutritional diseases: zinc deficiency, free fatty acid deficiency, and amino acid disorders (➲ see Chapter 6).

Generalized redness with blisters or pustules

- See Box 22.6.

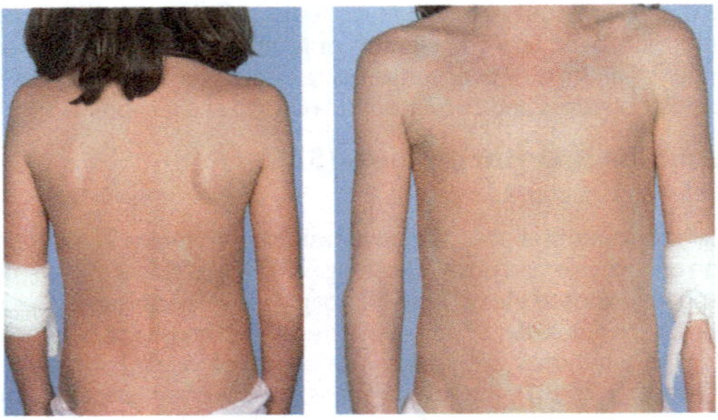

Fig. 22.17 Generalized erythrodermic psoriasis.
Reproduced courtesy of NHS Tayside Clinical Photography, Dundee, UK

Box 22.6 Likely causes of erythroderma and blisters

- Staphylococcal scalded skin syndrome (SSSS) (➲ see Infections causing erythroderma, p. 345)
- Epidermolysis bullosa (➲ see Genetic causes of blisters, p. 387)
- Toxic epidermal necrolysis (➲ see Blistering drugs reactions, pp. 352–7)
- Bullous ichthyosiform erythroderma (➲ see Rare genetic ichthyoses, p. 408)
- Generalized pustular psoriasis (➲ see Features of specific causes of erythroderma, pp. 343–5)
- Generalized congenital candidiasis (➲ see Infections causing erythroderma, p. 345)
- Diffuse cutaneous mastocytosis (➲ see Other dermatological investigations, pp. 24–6 and Inflammatory skin diseases, pp. 384–5)

Emergency investigations

Establish degree of dehydration with the usual markers: heart rate, blood pressure, skin turgor, and urine output. Check temperature with a low reading thermometer. Ask for urgent dermatological opinion.

Basic laboratory tests

- Bacterial and viral swabs of any broken skin, as appropriate.
- Full blood count.
- Biochemistry.
- Blood cultures if sepsis likely.
- Skin snip (➲ see Height, habitus, and skin changes, pp. 20–1) for blistering conditions.
- Skin biopsy may be required (➲ see Skin biopsy, p. 21).

Management

This depends on the specific diagnosis.

General measures include:

- Monitoring fluid balance and rehydration.

- Correcting severe biochemical imbalance such as hypernatraemia (common in Netherton syndrome; ➲ see Syndromes with marked ichthyosis, pp. 411–12).
- Monitor for hypothermia.
- Vigilance for sepsis and give appropriate treatment.
- In children with no blisters or crust, a bland emollient helps to reduce transepidermal water loss.

Features of specific causes of erythroderma

Once the patient is haemodynamically stable, treatment is of the underlying cause. When a child is generally red it can be difficult to determine the cause by visual inspection alone. The following highlight features in the history and examination, which may provide a clue:

Inflammatory dermatoses

Eczema

- *Atopic eczema*: intensely itchy with excoriations, redness, and dry skin often with crusted areas. Look for a previous history of eczema or other atopic disease, or a family history of atopy.
- *Seborrhoeic eczema*: in infants it typically involves the flexures and may be very extensive with yellowish scalp scales and is non-itchy (➲ see also Chapter 7 and Fig. 17.13).

Psoriasis

Generalized psoriasis can be preceded by a history of chronic plaque psoriasis (Figs. 22.1 and 22.2). Check the nails for features of psoriasis (➲ see Fig. 15.7). A family history may be supportive.

If there are pustules and the child has a swinging fever, consider generalized pustular psoriasis (Fig. 22.18; ➲ see also Psoriasis—clinical variants, pp. 322–4), a potentially lethal condition—*ask for urgent dermatological opinion.*

Pityriasis rubra pilaris

A very rare chronic disorder of unknown aetiology, characterized by reddish-orange scaly plaques, keratotic follicular papules, and palmoplantar keratoderma. Initially localized but there may be progression to erythroderma with distinct islands of spared normal skin (Fig. 22.19). Itching is variable but can be severe. It is often confused with psoriasis but is unresponsive to all treatments. Five types with differing patterns are described. Types 3–5 affect children (juvenile onset) classical (3), circumscribed (4), and atypical (5). A sixth HIV associated type is still debated. Children often have a better prognosis but it may persist for longer than in adults.

Congenital ichthyosiform erythroderma

Generalized redness from birth, usually with a shiny tight membrane (collodion baby; ➲ see Fig. 27.8).

Graft-versus-host disease (GvHD)

Seen in bone marrow transplant patients, particularly in association with other features of transplant rejection. Different morphologies of rash are recognized. GvHD may also occur when newborns with primary

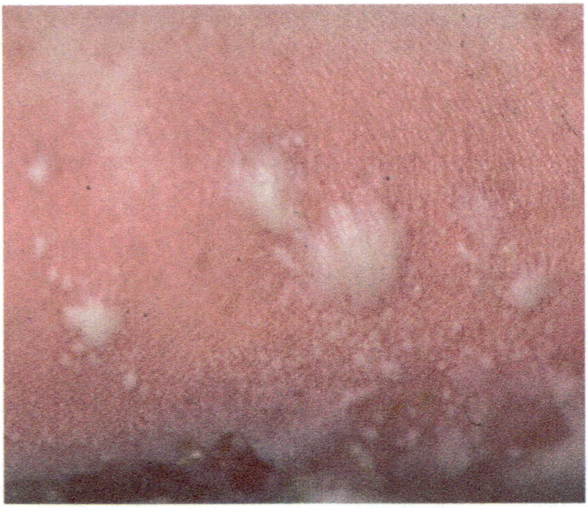

Fig. 22.18 Close-up of generalized pustular psoriasis showing flaccid pustules.
Reproduced courtesy of Susan Lewis-Jones, Hon Consultant Dermatologist, Ninewells Hospital and Medical School, Dundee, UK

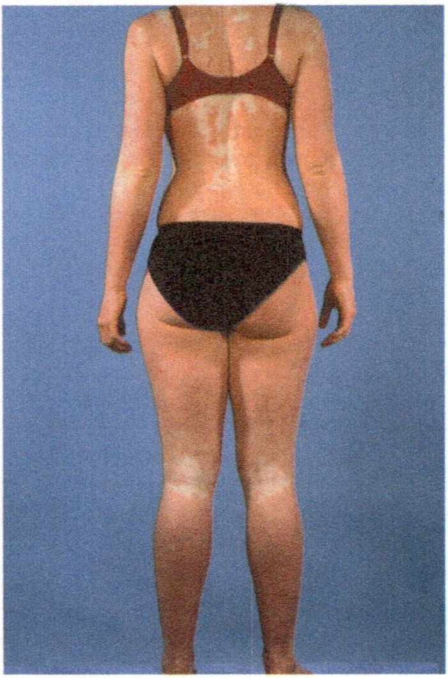

Fig. 22.19 Pityriasis rubra pilaris.
Reproduced courtesy of Sivakumar Natarajan, Consultant Dermatologist, The James Cook University Hospital, Middleborough, UK

immunodeficiency are transfused with non-irradiated blood. A biopsy is helpful to confirm the diagnosis (➲ see Chapter 39).

Cutaneous T-cell lymphoma

Mycosis fungoides and Sézary syndrome are very rare in childhood (➲ see also Rare skin diseases causing red rashes, pp. 339–40).

Infections causing erythroderma

Bacterial toxins

Staphylococcal scalded skin syndrome

Usually affects neonates, often with a history of fever and redness followed by peeling, predominantly umbilical stump in newborn or in flexures so check the nappy area (➲ see Fig. 7.6).

Clinical clue: extreme skin tenderness on handling.

Cause: *Staphylococcus aureus* is often only found at one site but produces systemic exfoliative toxins (A and B) with haematogenous spread:

- erythrogenic toxin (causes redness).
- epidermolytic toxin (causes blistering or superficial peeling).

Investigations: skin swab several sites for culture (negative swabs possible).

Skin snip test: ➲ see Dermatological procedures: skin surgery, pp. 21–23—avoids need for invasive skin biopsy.

Treatment: systemic antibiotics (for management, ➲ see Neonatal erythroderma, p. 87–8).

Streptococcal infections

Can produce a similar picture of erythroderma but less likely to blister. They cause toxic shock syndrome.

Scarlet fever (syn. scarlatina): a toxin-mediated disease, following some streptococcal infections, often of the throat. Bright red erythema with blanching on fingertip pressure, perioral pallor, and red lips with strawberry tongue (➲ see Fig. 10.10) is common. Previously rare but becoming more common again—risk of poststreptococcal nephritis with some strains.

Treatment: supportive with suitable early systemic antibiotics which may attenuate the disease.

Viral rashes (exanthems)

Often morbilliform (measles-like) and usually blanching. May cause an acute urticaria which can last for several weeks (➲ see Chapter 21 and Red viral exanthems, pp. 326–30).

- *Herpes simplex*: can result in widespread erythema multiforme (➲ see p. 191).
- *Infectious mononucleosis*: often causes a widespread morbilliform red rash following amoxicillin (administered for an accompanying sore throat) (➲ see pp. 326–7).

Erythrodermic drug rashes

Consider this possibility if there is a recent history of a new drug and ask about non-prescription medication (➲ see Chapter 23).

Generalized redness with blistering (rare)

Toxic epidermal necrolysis (TEN)

Usually drug-related (particularly anticonvulsants or antibiotics), rarely viral, but sometimes no cause is found (see Blistering drug reactions, pp. 352–7).

Epidermolysis bullosa (EB)

Neonates may be very red in addition to blisters and erosions (see Genetic causes of blisters, p. 387).

Generalized congenital candidiasis

May present with a widespread maculo-papular rash followed by pustule formation and scaling (see Congenital infection, pp. 88–9).

Bullous ichthyosiform erythroderma

Widespread redness at birth associated with blisters (see Rare genetic ichthyoses, p. 408).

Erythroderma, faltering growth, and recurrent infection

Rare (see Chapter 6 and Table 6.2). It is particularly associated with:

- Netherton syndrome.
- Omenn syndrome.
- Severe combined immunodeficiency.

Eczema, erythroderma, and severe recurrent infection (usually sinopulmonary and skin) is seen in the *Hyperimmunoglobulin-E syndrome* (Job's syndrome) with severe eczema, coarse facies, and very high levels of serum IgE >2000IU/ml (see Cold/red/purple lumps, p. 433).

References

1. Harnden, A., *et al.* (2014). Kawasaki disease. *BMJ* 17 (349):G5336. DOI: https://doi.org/10.1136/bmj.g5336
2. Newburger, J.W., *et al.* (2004). Diagnosis, treatment, and long-term management of Kawasaki disease: a statement for health professionals from the Committee on Rheumatic Fever, Endocarditis, and Kawasaki Disease, Council on Cardiovascular Disease in the Young, American Heart Association. *Circulation* **110**(17):2747–71.

Further reading

British Association of Dermatologists. *Patient Information Leaflets (PILS): Treatment of Psoriasis and Specific Drugs* [for adults but much is relevant to children], http://www.bad.org.uk

Centers for Disease Control and Prevention (CDC), *Lyme Disease*, https://www.cdc.gov/lyme/index.html

National Organization for Rare Disorders, https://rarediseases.org

Regional Office for South-East Asia, World Health Organization (2016). *Global Leprosy Strategy 2016–2020: Accelerating Towards a Leprosy-Free World.* WHO Regional Office for South-East Asia, http://www.who.int/iris/handle/10665/208824

Walker, S.L. and Lockwood, D.N. (2006). The clinical and immunological features of leprosy. *Br Med Bull* **77–8**(1);103–21.

Acknowledgement

We would like to thank Neil Rajan for his contribution to the first edition chapter.

Chapter 23

Cutaneous adverse drug reactions

Introduction

Drugs may be responsible for a great number of cutaneous reactions, which vary from mild to life-threatening (Box 23.1). In most cases the underlying mechanisms are incompletely understood and there are few tests that are helpful in confirming causality. The majority of reactions will arise within the first 2–3 weeks of therapy but there are rare exceptions occurring as late as 2–3y into therapy.

Always consider drugs as a possible cause of a skin reaction no matter how long established the therapy and ask about non-prescription medication and herbal or alternative/complementary therapies.

Types of cutaneous adverse drug reactions

Reactions may be due to toxicity or allergy and can be predictable, e.g. amiodarone pigmentation, but can be idiosyncratic and unpredictable, e.g. toxic epidermal necrolysis (Box 23.1).

Box 23.1 Types of cutaneous adverse drug reactions

Rashes
- Exanthematous (maculopapular eruptions).
- Erythema multiforme (EM).
- Lichenoid reactions.
- Purpuric rashes (➲ see Chapter 31). ⚑
- DRESS syndrome (Drug Rash with Eosinophilia and Systemic Symptoms).

Blistering reactions
- Bullous erythema multiforme (EM) (➲ see Fig. 4.12).
- Drug-induced pseudoporphyria.
- Stevens–Johnson syndrome (SJS). ⚑
- Toxic epidermal necrolysis (TEN). ⚑
- Fixed drug reactions.
- Vasculitis. ⚑

Pustular drug rashes
- Acneiform drug eruptions.
- Acute generalized exanthematous pustulosis (AGEP).
  Pigmentation (➲ see Chapters 32–33 and 35–37)

Fixed drug reactions

Nail changes (➲ see Chapter 15)

Hair changes (➲ see Chapter 14)

Oral problems (➲ see Chapter 10)

Photosensitive drug rashes (➲ see Chapter 16)

Urticarial drug rashes (➲ see Chapter 21)

Rashes

Exanthematous (morbilliform, maculopapular) reactions

This is the most common type of cutaneous drug reaction and presents with a characteristic maculopapular rash (Figs. 23.1 and 23.2), usually symmetrical and more severe on trunk and limbs but sparing mucous membranes. There may be large confluent areas or sometimes, urticarial lesions. It is often associated with low-grade pyrexia and pruritus.

Investigations: full blood count may show eosinophilia. Skin biopsy may show an eosinophilic infiltrate but often has non-specific features.

Treatment: mainly supportive:
- Discontinue suspected culprit drug but if no drug is clearly implicated then stop all possible drugs.
- Topical corticosteroids and antihistamines may help itching. Most rashes will resolve without problems over 7–14 days, often with caudal progression.

Warning signs of possible progression to a severe drug eruption (e.g. toxic epidermal necrolysis) are skin pain, facial oedema, blistering, and mucosal involvement.

Cause: the precise underlying mechanism is unknown although many appear to be due to a type IV hypersensitivity reaction. It usually occurs 7–14 days following first exposure to the drug and may commence after the drug has been discontinued. A wide range of drugs are implicated, particularly antimicrobials (e.g. penicillins, cephalosporins and sulphonamides) and anticonvulsants. Re-exposure may cause a more severe reaction, which can occur sooner.

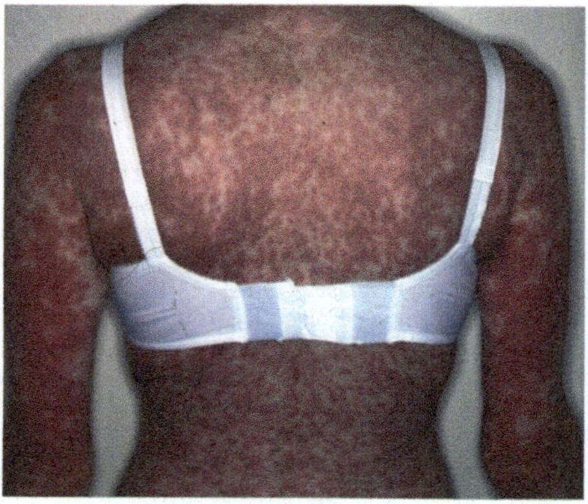

Fig. 23.1 Maculopapular rash due to penicillin allergy.

Reproduced courtesy of Susan Lewis-Jones, Hon Consultant Dermatologist, Ninewells Hospital and Medical School, Dundee, UK

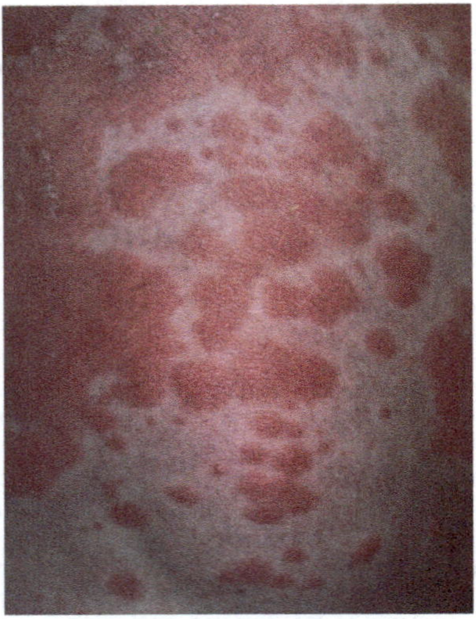

Fig. 23.2 Florid urticated maculopapular rash due to penicillin allergy.

Reproduced courtesy of Susan Lewis-Jones, Hon Consultant Dermatologist, Ninewells Hospital and Medical School, Dundee, UK

Erythema multiforme (EM)

This may present as a localized recurrent disorder or be part of a more severe skin reaction extending to more than 10% of the body surface area with systemic symptoms. In this context patient care may need to be escalated.

Clinical picture

- Sudden onset of erythematous papules and target lesions (Fig. 23.3 and ➲ see Fig. 4.11). These have a central dusky purple area, often crusted or blistered, which is surrounded by alternating pale and red ring(s). These are often confused with urticarial lesions, which are transient, unlike EM lesions which may last 7–14 days.
- The distribution is acral, predominantly on distal extremities and sometimes face or neck.
- Oral lesions and blistering and crusting of the lips are quite common.
- No prodrome and little associated malaise.
- Self-limiting, resolving in two or so weeks but can recur.

Treatment: oral antihistamines to ease skin discomfort. Treat any underlying infective triggers. Topical corticosteroids may also be helpful but there is no role for oral corticosteroids.

Cause: most cases are linked to preceding herpes simplex or mycoplasma infections. A wide range of drugs have been implicated but evidence for them is generally poor.

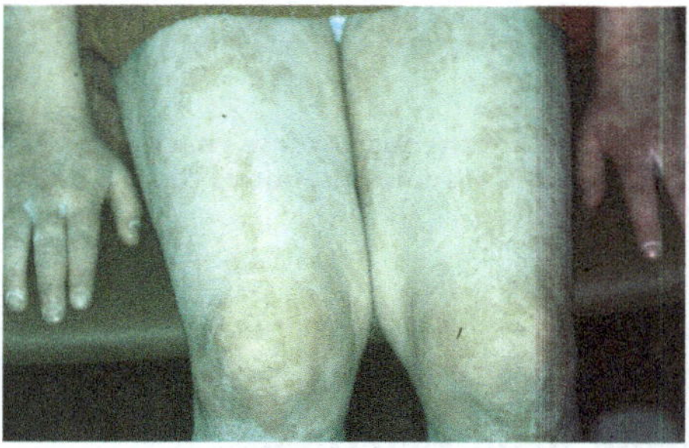

Fig. 23.3 Erythema muliforme-like rash due to ampicillin. Calamine had been applied by mother.

Reproduced courtesy of Susan Lewis-Jones, Hon Consultant Dermatologist, Ninewells Hospital and Medical School, Dundee, UK

Lichenoid reactions

Lichenoid drug eruptions are rare in children because the majority of causative drugs are used for treating adults. These eruptions clinically resemble lichen planus (see Fig. 19.6) presenting with purplish, flat topped, polygonal papules that may show an overlying white lacy pattern (Wickham's striae) or sometimes larger purplish patches with slight scaling. Oral involvement is less common in drug-related lichen planus. Eruptions generally resolve upon cessation of the suspect drug but this may take months. A large number of drugs have been implicated and gold and B-blockers are the most common.

DRESS syndrome (drug rash with eosinophilia and systemic symptoms) *Syn.* drug hypersensitivity syndrome

A serious reaction that usually appears 2–6 weeks after starting the causative drug. Clinical features are:

- Fever, facial oedema, and a morbilliform rash.
- Associated arthralgia and lymphadenopathy in some.
- Oedema of the skin, blisters, or pustules.
- Follicular accentuation of the rash (common).
- Erythroderma rarely, which can progress to toxic epidermal necrolysis (TEN) see Blistering drug reactions, pp. 352–7.

It is potentially life-threatening with multiorgan involvement, most commonly hepatitis that may be fulminant in around 10%; interstitial nephritis; myocarditis, or interstitial pneumonitis. Other life-threatening cutaneous drug reactions are listed in Box 23.2.

Investigations: Prominent eosinophilia is common. A skin biopsy may be helpful.

Treatment

- Stop offending drug.
- Topical corticosteroids may give relief for mild cutaneous symptoms.
- Systemic corticosteroids are required for visceral involvement and may be required for months.

Causes: the most important of the implicated drugs are anticonvulsants, sulphonamides, minocycline, allopurinol, and terbinafine.

Box 23.2 Severe cutaneous adverse reactions (SCARs)—potentially life-threatening cutaneous drug reactions

- DRESS syndrome
- SJS
- TEN

Note: always ask for urgent (immediate) dermatological opinion.

Blistering drug reactions

Many systemic drugs cause blistering reactions, e.g. antibiotics (particularly penicillins, sulphonamides, and erythromycin; see ➲ Fig. 23.4).
Blistering may be part of:

- Fixed drug eruption.
- Erythema multiforme.
- Stevens–Johnson syndrome or toxic epidermal necrolysis.
- Cutaneous vasculitis (➲ see Blistering drug reactions, pp. 352–7).
- Drug-induced bullous pemphigoid or pemphigus (both very rare in children).

Topical drugs may result in blistering as a result of contact dermatitis or chemical irritation.

Drug-induced pseudoporphyria

This may mimic porphyria cutanea tarda (very rare in childhood) with skin fragility, blister formation on photo-exposed sites (classically back of the hands), scarring, and milia formation. It may also resemble erythropoietic

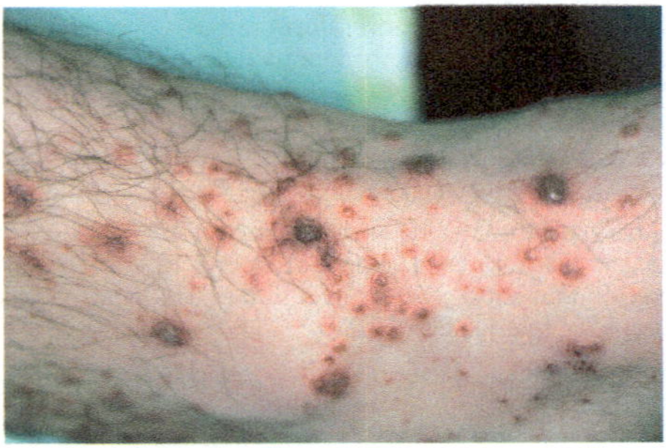

Fig. 23.4 Blisters and purpura suggesting a cutaneous vasculitis caused by erythromycin.

Reproduced courtesy of Susan Lewis-Jones, Hon Consultant Dermatologist, Ninewells Hospital and Medical School, Dundee, UK

protoporphyria (EPP), presenting with burning pain in the skin, erythema, chicken-pox-like scarring and thickening of the skin (➲ see Immediate photosensitive rashes, pp. 230–1). Some non-steroidal anti-inflammatory drugs (NSAIDs) have been implicated especially naproxen used for juvenile chronic arthritis.

Stevens–Johnson syndrome and toxic epidermal necrolysis

Severe life-threatening cutaneous drug reactions are fortunately rare. Among these reactions, Stevens–Johnson syndrome (SJS) and toxic epidermal necrolysis (TEN), along with DRESS are the most significant (Box 23.2). SJS and TEN are generally thought to be variants of the same disease with TEN carrying a poorer prognosis. Differentiation between SJS and TEN depends on extent of skin involvement (Box 23.3).

SJS and TEN are dermatological emergencies and urgent (same day) dermatological advice should be sought if either is suspected.

Clinical presentation

- *Prodrome*: with fever, malaise, and frequently cough, often associated with pain on swallowing and in the eyes. It may occur up to 14 days prior to the development of a rash in SJS but is usually 1–3 days before the rash in TEN.
- *Rash*: develops abruptly with symmetrical erythematous macules, some of which may be target-like (but lack the concentric rings of EM targets) often with central blistering. *In severe cases* the lesions become confluent with rapid extension of a dusky red/purple rash with flaccid superficial blistering (Fig. 23.5). The blisters exhibit a positive Nikolsky sign (superficial skin sloughs away with minimal sideways pressure) except on palmoplantar surfaces where the skin is thicker. Large areas of epidermal necrosis can occur in TEN.
- *Oral mucosa*: this is always involved in SJS and characteristic haemorrhagic crusting develops on the lips often with severe peri-oral blistering. Two or more mucosal surfaces are usually involved, including the eyes with associated purulent discharge; or genital and internal mucosal surfaces (gastrointestinal and respiratory tract).

These patients may be severely ill as a consequence of skin failure and suffer from severe fluid loss and electrolyte imbalance, especially those with TEN. Skin and mucosa are usually very fragile and extremely painful. Recovery can be very slow with the acute episode lasting 4–6 weeks, particularly in TEN and there may be significant sequelae: SEEK EXPERT HELP; IF >10% BSA skin detachment transfer to burns unit or ITU for specialized dressing support

- *Ocular* problems, e.g. corneal ulcers, synechiae, and panophthalmitis and occasionally blindness.

Box 23.3 Body surface area involvement

- SJS is generally accepted as involving <10% body surface area.
- TEN classification is not as well defined but >30% is usually accepted as diagnostic.
- SJS/TEN overlap between 10% and 30%.

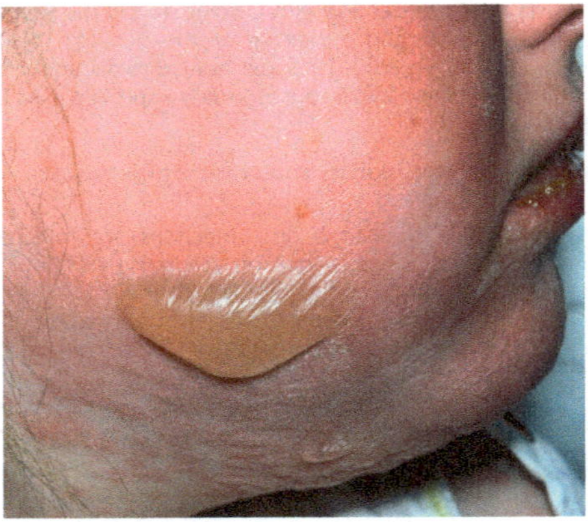

Fig. 23.5 Early TEN showing erythema with flaccid blisters.

Reproduced courtesy of Susan Lewis-Jones, Hon Consultant Dermatologist, Ninewells Hospital and Medical School, Dundee, UK

- *Skin and mucosal* sequelae include scarring, pigmentary changes, nail loss and urethral, anal, or vaginal strictures.
- *Death* often results from septicaemia through impaired barrier function, and multiorgan failure.

Investigations

There are no serological tests for SJS/TEN. Skin biopsy can be helpful in distinguishing from conditions such as EM, staphylococcal scalded skin syndrome (SSSS) (➲ see Infections causing erythroderma, p. 345) and acute generalized exanthematous pustulosis (AGEP) (➲ see Pustular drug rashes, p. 358). There have been attempts to predict severity and mortality, the most widely used of which is SCORTEN (Table 23.1), although this is mainly based on adult data.

Incidence

For SJS this is in the order of 1 per million per annum and for TEN 1–2 per million per annum, although in children SJS occurs more frequently than TEN.

Prognosis

Mortality rates for SJS vary between 5% and 30% but are up to 30–50% for TEN. Morbidity may be significant even upon recovery.

Cause

Infections such as herpes simplex virus and mycoplasma are implicated in the aetiology in children more than adults. Drug use is associated in over 80% of TEN cases (over 100 drugs are reported) and in SJS in over 50% (probably a significant underestimate). The main groups of drugs implicated are NSAIDs, anticonvulsants, and antibiotics (aminopenicillins and sulphonamides).

Table 23.1 Score for prognosis of TEN

SCORTEN-validated in adults	
Scoring: Yes = 1, No = 0	
Age >40	
Malignancy	
Tachycardia (>120/min)	
Initial surface area of epidermal detachment	
Serum urea (>10mmol/l)	
Serum glucose (>14mmol/l)	
Bicarbonate (<20mmol/l)	
Score	Predicted mortality (%)
0–1	3.2
2	12.1
3	35.8
4	58.3
≥5	90

Source: data from Bastuji-Garin S. *et al.* (2000). SCORTEN: a severity-of-illness score for toxic epidermal necrolysis. *J Invest Dermatol.* 115(2):149–53. DOI: https://doi.org/10.1046/j.1523-1747.2000.00061.x

Overview of management of SJS/TEN

- Stop causative drug **immediately**.
- Treat any identified underlying infection.
- **Urgent** dermatological review.
- Consider transfer to a **burns unit** (best prognosis).
- **IV access** and fluid replacement (Hartmann's or saline).
- Skin biopsy if there is uncertainty.
- Assessment of SCORTEN.
- Pressure-relieving mattress and a warm room.
- Analgesia: likely to require opiates and avoid NSAIDs.
- Early ophthalmology review.
- Thromboprophylaxis.
- Oral and nasal hygiene: soften and remove crusts, use analgesic and antibacterial mouth washes.
- Screen for sepsis.

The main treatment for these conditions is meticulous supportive care. Management is very similar to burns care. Initial assessment of body surface area can be carried out using the 'Rule of Nines' (Box 23.4)—be aware this is different in young children due to head size. All non-essential drugs should be stopped.

There is no clear consensus on medical management in SJS/TEN. Antibiotics should not be used prophylactically but should be used to treat sepsis.

The role of corticosteroids remains highly contentious and should not be used except under specialist supervision. Similarly, interventions such as IV immunoglobulin should only be considered with advice from a specialist with suitable expertise.

Box 23.4 Rule of Nines

- Head = 9%
- Chest (front) = 9%
- Abdomen (front) = 9%
- Upper/mid/lower back and buttocks = 18%
- Each arm = 9%
- Each palm = 1%
- Perineum = 1%
- Each leg = 18% total (front = 9%, back = 9%)

Fixed drug eruption

This reaction is characterized by ovoid brownish-red oedematous plaques that recur at the same site on re-administration of a culprit drug. The plaques may appear within hours following administration. The rash fades, often leaving a brown/greyish-blue discolouration in the affected area, which may last for a few weeks. There may be associated blistering which is occasionally extensive. Systemic symptoms are infrequent and usually mild. New areas may develop after subsequent rechallenge with the drug. The childhood frequency is estimated to be up to 20% of cutaneous drug eruptions. Commonly associated drugs include NSAIDs, anticonvulsants, paracetamol, and salicylates (Fig. 23.6).

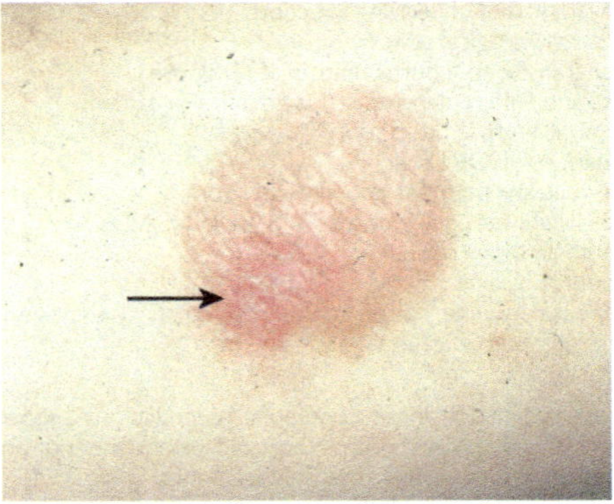

Fig. 23.6 Fixed drug eruption early erythematous stage, biopsy site is marked by an arrow.

Vasculitis

A wide range of drugs have been reported to cause vasculitis (e.g. penicillins, erythromycin, and phenytoin). Clinically vasculitis presents as palpable purpuric papules, which may blister or break down to form large areas of necrosis (Fig. 23.7). The main concern is of multiple system involvement, particularly renal, ocular, and gastrointestinal tract (GIT) with serious risk of high morbidity and death. This is more likely in extensive progressive disease.

Investigations: skin biopsy for histopathology and immunofluorescence can be helpful in aiding diagnosis. Urine testing for haematuria, red cell casts, and proteinuria (for investigation of vasculitis, ➲ see Cutaneous vasculitis, pp. 470–2). *Seek dermatological advice early.*

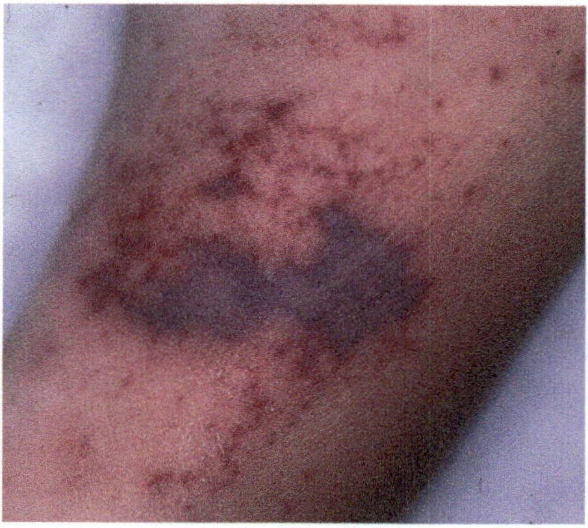

Fig. 23.7 Cutaneous vasculitis with early necrosis.

Reproduced courtesy of Susan Lewis-Jones, Hon Consultant Dermatologist, Ninewells Hospital and Medical School, Dundee, UK

Drug-induced nail changes

- ➲ See Chapter 15.

Drug-induced hair changes

- ➲ See Hair loss (alopecia), pp. 197–8 and Hypertrichosis, pp. 209–11.

Drug-induced oral changes

- ➲ See Chapter 10.

Drug-induced pigmentation

- ➲ See Chapters 31–33 and 35–37.

Drug-induced photosensitivity

- ➲ See Drug-related photosensitive rashes, p. 231.

Pustular drug rashes

- *Acneiform*: i.e. resemble acne with inflamed papules and pustules. Occur with systemic corticosteroids, potent topical corticosteroids on face (Betnovate® face), anabolic steroids, androgens (females), oral contraceptives, iodides, and bromides.
- *Acute generalized exanthematous pustulosis (AGEP)*: generalized pustules often within 24h of drug administration. Rare in children. May be associated fever, purpura, facial oedema, and transient renal failure. Commonest drugs implicated are antibiotics (80%), especially penicillins and erythromycin but many others are reported. Patch testing with the drug is sometimes positive. Main differential diagnosis is pustular psoriasis (➲ see Psoriasis—clinical variants, pp. 322–4).

Chapter 24

Abuse and self-inflicted disease

Introduction

Skin lesions from abuse can take many and bizarre forms or mimic skin problems like impetigo or vascular disorders, and sometimes distinction between the two can be difficult. Remember that although abuse is commonly perpetrated by adults, it can also be caused by siblings, as a part of peer-bullying, or may even be self-inflicted (➲ see Dermatitis artefacta (factitia), p. 371).

Cutaneous signs of child abuse

Common problems are:

- Bruising, purpura.
- Linear or patterned marks.
- Bite marks.
- Burns or scalds.
- Blisters.
- Ulcers.
- Hair or nail loss.
- Sexual abuse.

Always refer a child with suspected abuse to the local child protection team immediately and put the child in a place of safety.

Pointers on examination

Remember to undress the child and look in hidden sites such as the mouth, ear canals, and behind the ears (see Box 24.1).

Site: common, important sites for non-accidental bruising are:

- Buttocks and lower back (Fig. 24.1).
- Sides of face, scalp, and external ears.
- Eyes and mouth.
- Neck, lower jaw, and mastoid.
- Genital area—less common but very important to examine.

Accidental injuries predominantly affect bony prominences and the front of the body. No site is pathognomonic for abuse, and a careful history should be taken and recorded in detail in all cases together with suitable photographic documentation.

Box 24.1 Pointers in the history

- Age of child—majority are under 12y. Infants who are immobile rarely have accidental injuries.
- Vague and inconsistent story.
- Does not make sense (i.e. does not explain the injury or is inconsistent with child's development).
- Inappropriate parent or carer response (e.g. delay in presentation, lack of concern, or aggressive behaviour).
- Inappropriate child response (e.g. did not cry).
- History of other injury/repeated attendance to medical care.
- Known to children's social care or on Child Protection Register*.

* These registers vary between countries.

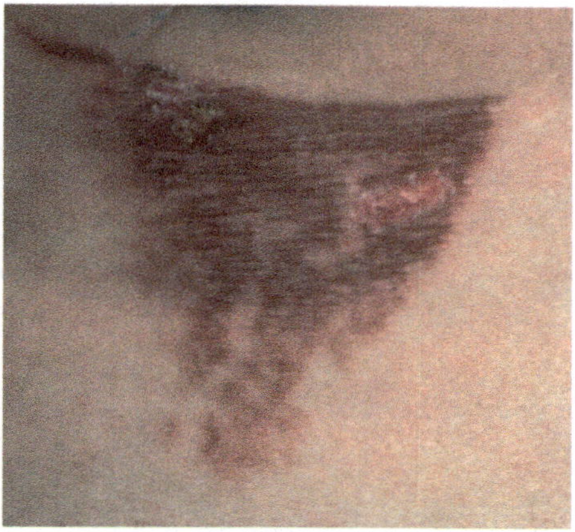

Fig. 24.1 Triangular mark on dorsal thigh with sharp edges. This is not a pattern associated with any skin disease. Consider abuse or dermatitis artefacta (see Dermatitis artefacta, this chapter).

Reproduced courtesy of Susan Lewis-Jones, Hon Consultant Dermatologist, Ninewells Hospital and Medical School, Dundee, UK

Bruising and purpura

Bruising, particularly in toddlers and very active children is normal but if it is excessive, unexplained, or in an odd pattern or site (e.g. finger-marks on jaw), then this should give cause for concern (see Box 24.1). Blunt injuries are often associated with bruising. Ears may be thickened from constant boxing (cauliflower ears).

Type of bruising: look at pattern, e.g. the mark of an implement is suggested by linear bruises or bizarre shapes (e.g. whips, belt buckle marks) or symmetrical 'grip marks', especially around the face and neck. Bruising of different colours and ages is very suggestive of repeated abuse. Biting may cause bruising or actual skin penetration.

Skin disease mimicking or causing bruises

Bruising (or the appearance of bruising) as a result of an underlying disorder is occasionally mistaken for child abuse, e.g.:

- Accidental bruising can be confused with abuse, especially in young children.
- Bruising following urticarial vasculitis (➲ see Chapter 21)—rare.
- Mongolian blue spots—common (Fig. 24.2).
- Café-au-lait macules (➲ see Fig. 33.3) may be mistaken for bruising.
- Deep haemangiomas appear blue (➲ see Fig. 8.6)—fairly common but other vascular anomalies such as venous malformations are much less common (➲ see Chapter 8).

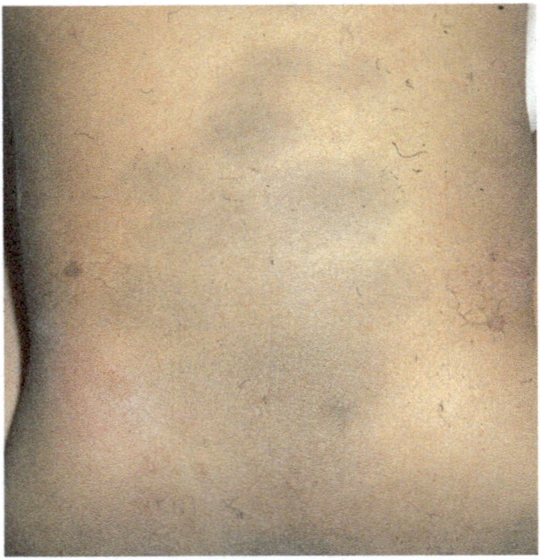

Fig. 24.2 Multiple Mongolian blue spots mistaken for bruises by healthcare professional.

Reproduced courtesy of Susan Lewis-Jones, Hon Consultant Dermatologist, Ninewells Hospital and Medical School, Dundee, UK

- Vasculitis of any cause, e.g. infective or hypersensitivity such as Henoch–Schönlein purpura (➲ see Fig. 31.4).
- Dermatitis artefacta, e.g. suction injuries or pinching (see Fig 24.12).
- Genetic skin disorders (rare) such as Ehlers–Danlos syndrome (Fig. 24.3; ➲ see also Chapter 29) or dominant dystrophic epidermolysis bullosa (➲ see Chapter 25).
- Connective tissue disorders such as morphoea (➲ see Fig. 29.1).
- Skin thinning, e.g. overuse of potent topical corticosteroids, Cushing's syndrome.

Systemic disease mimicking bruising

- Leukaemia cutis (➲ see Fig. 28.7).
- Blueberry muffin babies (➲ see Fig. 7.7).
- Clotting disorders.
- Secondary deposits, e.g. melanoma, neuroblastoma.
- Infections such as subacute bacterial endocarditis.

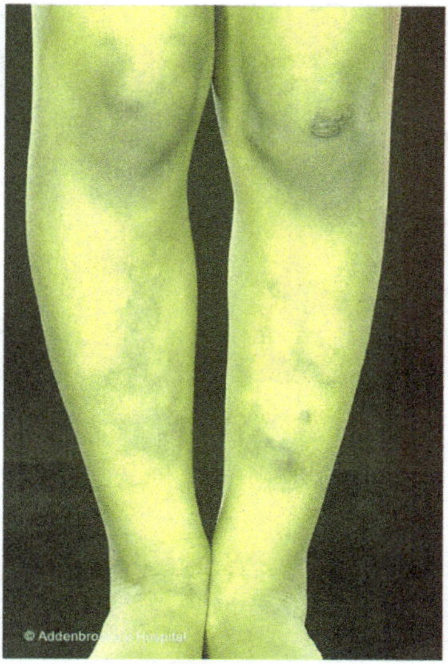

Fig. 24.3 Bruising on shins in Ehlers–Danlos syndrome. This is often mistaken for non-accidental injury.

Reproduced courtesy of Addenbrooke's Hospital, Cambridge, UK

Blisters

Blisters can be caused by thermal injuries, usually burns or scalds but also with prolonged cold exposure, usually to feet or hands.

Type of lesions: cigarette burns are circular and found particularly on the face, hands, and genitalia. Burns from hot instruments form linear or angular shapes (e.g. irons or pokers, Fig 24.1). Scalds are usually to hands, feet, and buttocks. Look for heel and buttock marks in a child dipped in scalding water. Typically the bony prominences (e.g. ischial tuberosities, central buttocks) are protected by pressure if the child is left sitting in scalding water.

Blistering disorders mimicking abuse

- ***Impetigo***: bullous form often mistaken for cigarette burns or scalds (Fig. 24.4).
- ***Ecthyma***: may present as deep crusts resembling cigarette burns (➲ see Fig. 26.3).
- ***Phytophotodermatitis***: e.g. from hogweed (➲ see Chapter 16 and Fig. 16.7).
- ***Jellyfish stings*** leave bizarre painful linear lesions, particularly on legs.
- ***Extreme photosensitivity*** presenting as sunburn (➲ see Xeroderma pigmentosum, p. 235.
- ***Inherited***: such as incontinentia pigmenti (➲ see Fig. 25.12).
- ***Acquired autoimmune***: e.g. pemphigoid (➲ see Chapter 25); very rare.

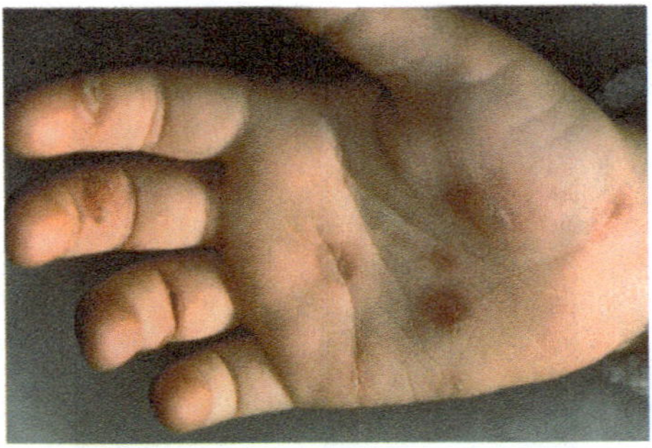

Fig. 24.4 Blisters from scabies and secondary impetigo, suspected to be cigarette burns by social workers.

Reproduced courtesy of Susan Lewis-Jones, Hon Consultant Dermatologist, Ninewells Hospital and Medical School, Dundee, UK

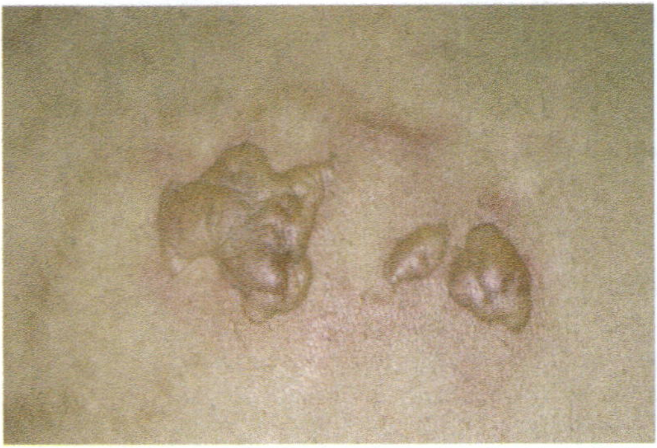

Fig. 24.5 Accidental blistering from hot water burn in young child with acute abdominal pain and peritonitis.

Reproduced courtesy of Susan Lewis-Jones, Hon Consultant Dermatologist, Ninewells Hospital and Medical School, Dundee, UK

- *Accidental thermal injuries*: e.g. hot water bottle burns (Fig. 24.5) or following cryotherapy (➲ see Fig. 25.6).
- *Fragility of the skin*: e.g. epidermolysis bullosa (➲ see Chapter 25).
- *Dermatitis artefacta*: e.g. by close prolonged spraying with deodorant or other sprays; or application of caustic substance such as ice, salt, bleach (➲ see Dermatitis artefacta, p. 371).

For other blistering skin diseases, ➲ see Chapter 25.

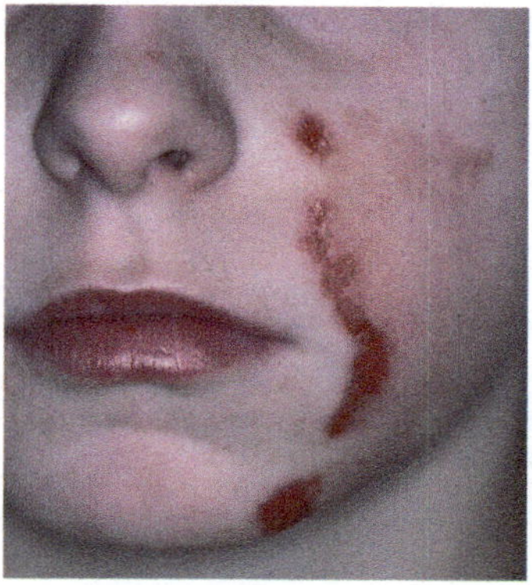

Fig. 24.6 Dermatitis artefacta (factitia)—linear marks.

Reproduced courtesy of Susan Lewis-Jones, Hon Consultant Dermatologist, Ninewells Hospital and Medical School, Dundee, UK

Linear marks

Usually from whips, cord, or belts that give distinctive patterns—look for impression of buckles, loops, etc.

Skin disorders which might cause confusion

- Phytophotodermatitis (➲ see Fig. 16.7).
- Jellyfish stings.
- Certain linear 'birthmarks', e.g. those following lines of Blaschko such as incontinentia pigmenti (➲ see Fig. 25.12) and flat epidermal naevi (➲ see Box 4.3 and Fig. 4.10).
- Dermatitis artefacta (Fig. 24.6; ➲ see also Dermatitis artefacta, p. 371).
- Linear skin diseases, e.g. psoriasis, lichen planus, lichen striatus (➲ Chapter 4).
- Adolescent striae may be mistaken for abuse (➲ see Fig. 29.6).

Scars

Scarring of the skin indicates full thickness damage of the epidermis or deeper layers.

Unexplained scarring should always raise alarm bells of abuse, especially in non-mobile infants.

Skin diseases causing poor healing and unusual scars

- Ehlers–Danlos syndrome (➲ see Fig. 29.9).
- Epidermolysis bullosa (➲ see Chapter 25).
- Porphyrias (➲ see Chapter 16).

- Connective tissue disorders such as morphoea (➲ see Fig. 29.1, Chapters 29 and 38).
- Dermatitis artefacta (factitia) (Fig. 24.1).
- Pyoderma gangrenosum (➲ Chapter 30).

Hair loss

Hair may be pulled out in clumps causing bald patches or may be burnt, causing frizziness and burns.

Hair problems mimicking abuse

- Most forms of alopecia (➲ see Chapter 14).
- Aplasia cutis: seen in infants at birth (➲ see Fig. 14.6).
- Self-pulling (➲ see Trichotillomania, pp. 368–9).
- Scalp ringworm (➲ see Figs. 14.7 and 14.8).

Nail loss

Nails are occasionally removed as a form of abuse. This has also been described in factitious or induced illness, ➲ see pp. 367–9.

Nail loss mimicking abuse

- Severe alopecia totalis with nail shedding.
- Severe destruction of nails, e.g. lichen planus (rare).
- Genetic disorders such as epidermolysis bullosa, pachyonychia congenita.
- Self-abuse.

Sexual abuse

Examination and investigation for sexual abuse requires specialist expertise. As soon as you become concerned that this may be an issue you should ensure:

1. The young person is in a place of safety. ⚑
2. The young person is clinically stable.
3. The young person should avoid bathing or discarding clothes until specialist advice obtained.

Before examining or taking the history any further, your local child protection policy should be followed. This will enable the process for assessment and examination to take place to maintain chain of evidence and quality of verbal statements that may be required for legal purposes.

The aim is for each child to be examined *just the once* by the most expert member of the team to minimize distress and discomfort while providing the most expert safeguarding advice.

Skin disorders that might cause confusion

- *Lichen sclerosus*: causes white areas and sometimes fusion of the labia (➲ see Chapter 13, Fig. 13.6). Purpura is common and indicates active disease. The area is usually sore, itchy, and may be painful, particularly on micturition or defecation. It classically extends in a figure of eight appearance around the vulva and anus. Prompt treatment with very potent topical corticosteroids is essential. It has been reported in association with sexual abuse. In boys it is known as balanitis xerotica obliterans and causes phimosis, but circumcision is usually curative.

- *Perianal and genital warts*: May be caused by innocent transfer during birth or from fingers at nappy changing, but can occur from sexual abuse. Look at the context in which they arise and if you are concerned, discuss with child protection. There should be a higher index of suspicion in children acquiring such warts for the first time over the age of 4y and in particular over the age of 8 when a positive predictive value of up to 80% is found (see also Fig. 13.7).
- *Bruising disorders*: see Bruising and purpura, pp. 361–2 and Chapter 31.
- *Self-inflicted injuries*: e.g. in Lesch–Nyhan syndrome.

Self-inflicted factitious diseases

These form a spectrum of disorders from simple habit disorders (tics) such as nail biting (onychophagia) or hair twiddling, common in 'normal' toddlers, to much more severe and intractable psychological problems such as neurotic excoriations (see p. 369) and hair-pulling (see Hair-pulling disorder (*syn. trichotillomania*), later in this chapter). A minority of children will have psychiatric disorders such as obsessive-compulsive disorders, dysmorphophobia, or phobias (Box 24.2). Terminology is often confusing and it is vital to record a good clinical description and photograph (especially if abuse is suspected).

Habit disorders

Some mild habit disorders often persist but may rarely develop into more serious psychiatric disease, e.g. habit scratching may evolve into the production of deep cutaneous scarring and ulceration later in life (Fig. 24.10).

Box 24.2 Types of factitious diseases

- Habit disorders (e.g. nail biting, hair twiddling).
- Hair-pulling disorder (trichotillomania).
- Neurotic excoriations.
- Dermatitis artefacta (factitia).
- Factitious and induced illness.
- Self-mutilation—cutting, ligatures, biting, needle insertion, etc.

Psychiatric disorders

- Obsessive-compulsive disorders.
- Phobias (e.g. parasitophobia).
- Mono-delusional parapsychosis (e.g. parasitosis, seen in adults).
- Dysmorphophobia.

- *Nail biting (onychophagia)*: common (➲ see Ingrowing nails, p. 215). Nail flicking produces horizontal ridges and disrupts normal growth.

  Note: similar changes occur in chronic eczema affecting the nail bed.
- *Knuckle pads*: thickened pads over the dorsum of hands/fingers due to constant biting and rubbing (Fig. 24.7).
- *Lichen simplex chronicus* (➲ see Fig. 29.3): thickening of the skin due to chronic scratching. Occurs in patches, particularly nape of neck, ankles, and genital areas. Usually adults but may be seen in teenagers.
- *Hair twiddling*: common in young children and may cause some alopecia but is usually a temporary event. Persistent severe forms may go on to *hair-pulling disorder (previously trichotillomania)*.
- *Finger sucking*: may cause paronychia and nail distortion (➲ see Fig. 15.2).

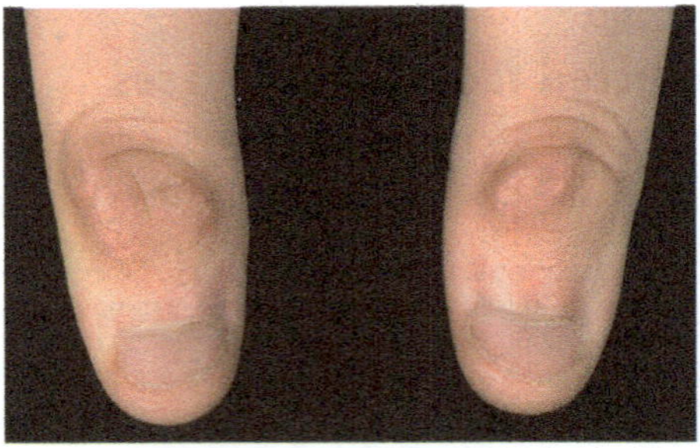

Fig. 24.7 Knuckle pads on fingers from constant biting and rubbing associated with nail biting (onychophagia).

Reproduced courtesy of NHS Tayside Clinical Photography, Dundee, UK

Hair-pulling disorder *(syn. Trichotillomania)*

A form of hair pulling causing alopecia (hair loss) of various patterns and severity. It is more often seen in girls and nail biting is commonly associated. The scalp hair may just appear thinner on the side of the dominant hand or both sides symmetrically, or on the crown (Fig. 24.8). In severe cases there may be almost total loss, although there is usually some short stubbly regrowth and smooth bald patches are not seen. In persistent cases, the alopecia may be permanent. The act of pulling (sometimes just cutting) is hidden from others and although parents may find clumps of hair, they often attribute this to dermatological disease.

It may be associated with:

- Other habit tics such as onychophagia.
- Iron deficiency—look for pica (including eating hair).
- Intellectual impairment or learning difficulties.

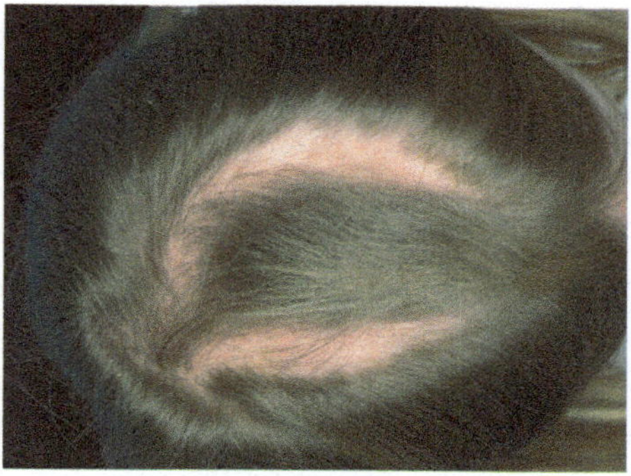

Fig. 24.8 Hair-pulling disorder. This has resulted in an oval patch of alopecia around the crown (known as 'Friar Tuck's' sign.)

Reproduced courtesy of Susan Lewis-Jones, Hon Consultant Dermatologist, Ninewells Hospital and Medical School, Dundee, UK

- Emotional problems (e.g. loss of parent, child abuse, peer rejection, poor self-esteem, depression).
- Substance misuse.

It is frequently self-limiting in infants but may develop into an obsessive-compulsive disorder and persist into adult life (mainly girls). Very rarely hair swallowing (trichophagia) and/or other fibres produces a hair ball (trichobezoar) causing abdominal mass, pain, and gastrointestinal symptoms, often requiring surgery.

Management: look for hairs of different lengths or cut ends. Examine the abdomen. Check for anaemia, iron deficiency, thyroid dysfunction and, if present, search for underlying cause. Obtain a full psychosocial history, and check for depression or schooling difficulties. Exclude abuse. Psychological support may be offered but is rarely accepted.

Neurotic excoriations

These are distinguished from dermatitis artefacta by the fact that the child admits to producing the lesions but finds it difficult to stop the habit. May be a response to stress.

- Minor forms of 'habit picking' (majority) may remit with time.
- Acne excoriée (Fig. 24.9) is a specific variant common in teenage girls (rarely boys) who often have little active acne. Can cause deep scars (➲ see also Chapter 18).

A minority (usually teenagers) may develop severe *obsessive-compulsive disorder* (Fig. 24.10) producing deep ulcerated scars on various body sites.

Differential diagnosis

Postherpetic neuralgia and other neuropathic conditions. Mid-face toddler excoriation syndrome (MITES)—very rare, some cases shown to be due to genetic mutations.

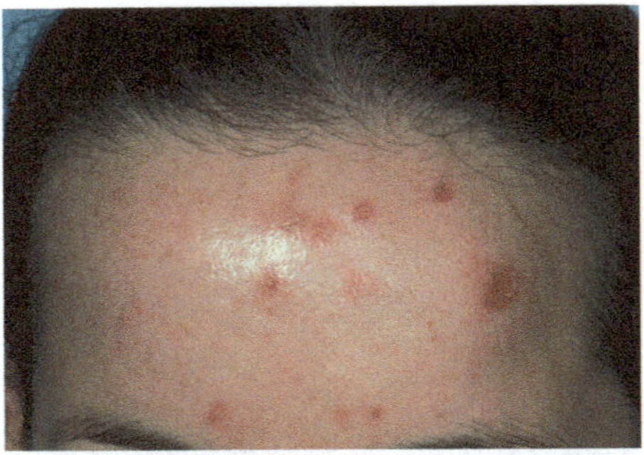

Fig. 24.9 Acne excoriée showing 'pick marks'. Very little active acne is present

Reproduced courtesy of Susan Lewis-Jones, Hon Consultant Dermatologist, Ninewells Hospital and Medical School, Dundee, UK

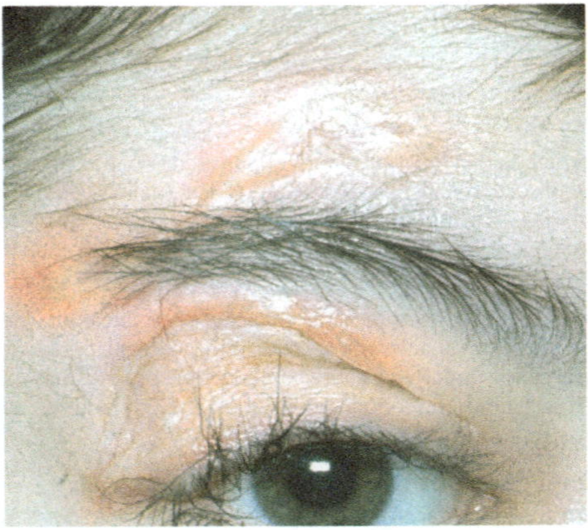

Fig. 24.10 Deep scars from long-standing picking, which was denied by child. This is a severe type of dermatitis artefacta/factitia. Exclude abuse.

Reproduced courtesy of Susan Lewis-Jones, Hon Consultant Dermatologist, Ninewells Hospital and Medical School, Dundee, UK

Dermatitis artefacta (factitia)

This is the action of consciously producing a skin lesion that is *hidden or denied* (in a child who is fully aware of their actions). In younger children it may be difficult to exclude abuse by others. Be aware of malingering from where skin lesions are produced for obvious benefit (e.g. missing school). The underlying reasons for dermatitis artefacta (DA) are not usually obvious but can include anxiety/depression, educational problems, attention seeking, bullying, or abuse. Most are young girls who may appear nonchalant ('La belle indifference'). Traumatic cheilitis (➲ see Fig. 10.5) and mild forms of hair-pulling disorder are generally accepted as forms of DA. Typically:

- The pattern of lesion(s) does not fit with any dermatological disease, e.g. they may be linear or a bizarre pattern, sharp edges, blisters, purpura, etc. (Figs. 24.1, 24.6 and 24.11).
- The commonest sites are face, hands, and arms. The central back is rarely affected (out of reach).
- Other habit tics such as onychophagia (nail biting) are commonly associated.

Minor forms usually have a good prognosis, especially in young children. Serious injury with marked scarring has a poor prognosis and is likely to persist (Fig. 24.10).

Management: seek a dermatological opinion. It is vital to exclude dermatological disease, abuse, or accidental causes. Do not challenge the child directly, although it may be possible to let them know what you suspect by indirect comments. Try to see parents and child independently at some point to discuss possible underlying factors. Many parents will not accept that it is factitious and it is helpful to build a good rapport before discussing causes. It can also be helpful to provide a 'label' such as 'dermatitis' and reassure that it may settle with time. Some children require admission and/or psychological help, although this is rarely accepted (Box 24.3).

Box 24.3 Methods of producing dermatitis artefacta

Physical: scratches, often in linear or bizarre shapes (Fig. 24.6); abrasions (Fig. 24.11), e.g. sandpaper, biting, tools. Pinching and suction cause purpura or bruises (Fig. 24.12).

Chemical: liquids cause caustic burns of any depth with tell-tale drip marks (Fig. 24.13). Sprays (e.g. hairspray) held close to skin produce blisters or burns. Biting, rubbing, or using glue on lips produces cheilitis (➲ see Fig. 10.5), with crusting and bleeding.

Plants: some cause toxic or allergic reactions, e.g. poison ivy sap causes severe allergic dermatitis, giant hogweed sap causes blisters on exposure to the sun (phytophotodermatitis; ➲ see Figs. 16.7 and 16.8). Usually these are accidental.

Thermal: hot or cold liquids or solids produce redness, blisters, and even full thickness loss with scabs or eschars.

Note: in the majority of cases the cause is not discovered.

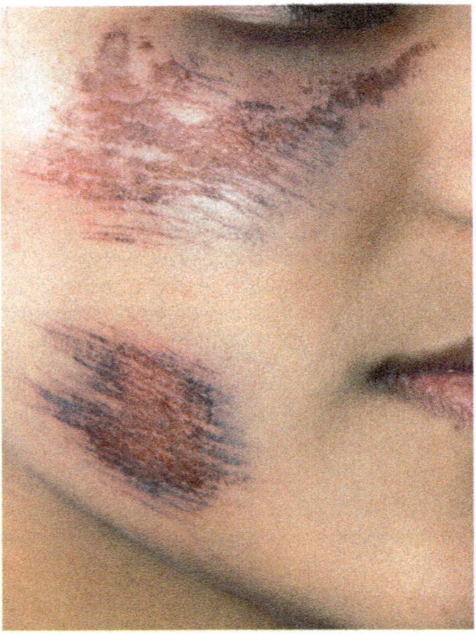

Fig. 24.11 Dermatitis artefacta—abrasions on the cheek probably produced by sandpaper.

Reproduced courtesy of Susan Lewis-Jones, Hon Consultant Dermatologist, Ninewells Hospital and Medical School, Dundee, UK

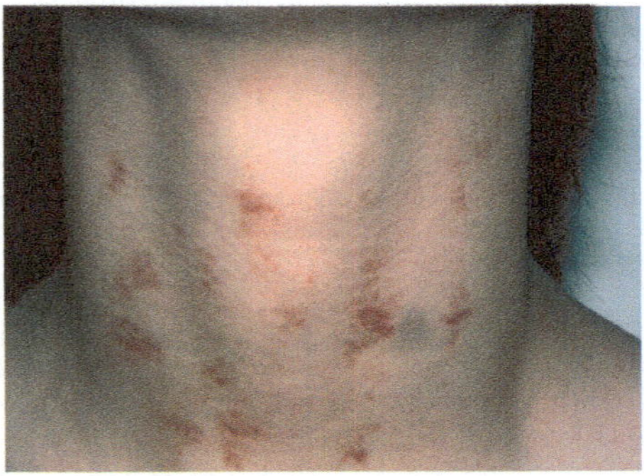

Fig. 24.12 Self-induced purpura caused by pinching—a manifestation of dermatitis artefacta/factitia.

Reproduced courtesy of Susan Lewis-Jones, Hon Consultant Dermatologist, Ninewells Hospital and Medical School, Dundee, UK

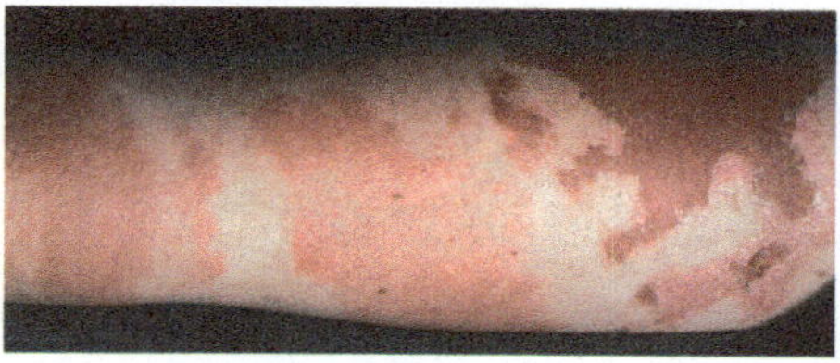

Fig. 24.13 Dermatitis artefacta/factitia with tell-tale drip marks from application of a caustic liquid.

Reproduced courtesy of Susan Lewis-Jones, Hon Consultant Dermatologist, Ninewells Hospital and Medical School, Dundee, UK

Psychiatric disorders and skin lesions

Children with severe psychiatric disorders should be referred for a formal psychiatric assessment.

Obsessive-compulsive disorders (OCD)

These include:

- Hair-pulling disorder (see Self-inflicted factitious diseases, earlier in this chapter).
- Persistent hand washing may cause hand dermatitis.
- Cutting, usually arms (occasionally genital area) leaves linear, often parallel white scars of various ages, depth, and length.
- Neurotic ulceration of skin (see Self-inflicted factitious diseases, earlier).

They are often associated with habit tics such as onychophagia.

Parasitosis

An unshakeable belief that a person is infested by insects (c.f. phobic states—'parasitophobia', a fear of insects/parasites). This is a mono-delusional parapsychosis usually seen in adults.

Dysmorphophobia

An altered perception of body image with an unshakeable belief in imagined or exaggerated signs. The skin appears normal or minimally affected.

It usually occurs in teenagers and adults. Face, scalp, and genital area are the commonest sites.

- *Face*: perception of redness; severe acne; enlarged pores or increased greasiness are commonest.
- *Scalp*: itching and hair thinning are commonest.
- *Genitals*: usually boys worried about normal features such as pearly penile papules (➲ see Lumps and bumps, pp. 187–9), or scrotal redness.

Management: needs time and sympathy. Suicidal ideation is common (affects approx. 30%). Enlist psychological help (rarely accepted). May be a feature of depression or mental illness or altered mental state (e.g. drugs).

Further reading

NICE (2009). *Child Maltreatment: When to Suspect Maltreatment in Under 18s: Clinical Guideline [CG89]*, https://www.nice.org.uk/guidance/cg89

RCPCH (2016). *Child Protection Evidence—Bruising*, https://www.rcpch.ac.uk/resources/child-protection-evidence-bruising

RCPCH (2015). *Physical Signs of Child Sexual Abuse*, https://www.rcpch.ac.uk/shop-publications/physical-signs-child-sexual-abuse-evidence-based-review

Section 5

Textural skin changes

Chapter 25

Blisters

Introduction

Vesiculobullous skin lesions include vesicles, bullae, or pustules. Vesicles are small fluid-filled blisters less than 0.5cm in diameter, whereas bullae are fluid-filled blisters more than 0.5cm diameter. Pustules are vesicles with a purulent exudate and can represent a primary lesion or a change in a bulla or vesicle. Erosions and ulcers are secondary lesions and occur after loss of part or all of the epidermis, respectively, when a blister ruptures.

Causes of blistering may be due to:

- Infection.
- Infestations.
- Physical or environmental factors.
- Adverse drug reactions.
- Inflammatory skin diseases.
- Autoimmune skin diseases.
- Genetic diseases.

For a list of the commonest causes of blisters in children, see Box 25.1.

Box 25.1 Commonest causes of blisters in children

Infections such as:

- *Scabies*—tiny blisters hands and feet (➲ see Fig. 24.4).
- *Impetigo*—usually large flaccid blisters or raw areas with peeling edges and golden crusts.
- *Chickenpox*—crops on face and upper trunk mainly.
- *Hand, foot, and mouth*—grey-coloured with narrow band of erythema (➲ see Fig. 12.2).
- *Herpes simplex*—crops of blisters quickly rupturing to form crusts (➲ see Fig. 12.1).

Others such as:

- *Insect bites*—usually small but can be large blisters with redness and sometimes pus filled (➲ see Fig. 20.5).
- *Burns and scalds* (➲ see Fig. 24.5).
- Acute eczemas such as contact allergy or pompholyx (➲ see Fig. 17.14).
- Phytophotodermatitis—bizarre linear patterns (➲ see Fig. 16.7).
- Erythema multiforme—usually secondary to *H. simplex* (➲ see Fig. 4.12).
- Cutaneous drug reactions—uncommon in children (➲ see Fig. 23.4)

Infections causing blisters

Bacterial

Bullous impetigo

Fragile superficial blisters which quickly rupture and usually present as patches of red skin with peeling edges that may be mistaken for cigarette burns. Golden crusts of dried serous exudate are usually present (Fig. 25.1; ➲ also see Fig. 26.1), especially on face, hands, and flexures. It is commoner

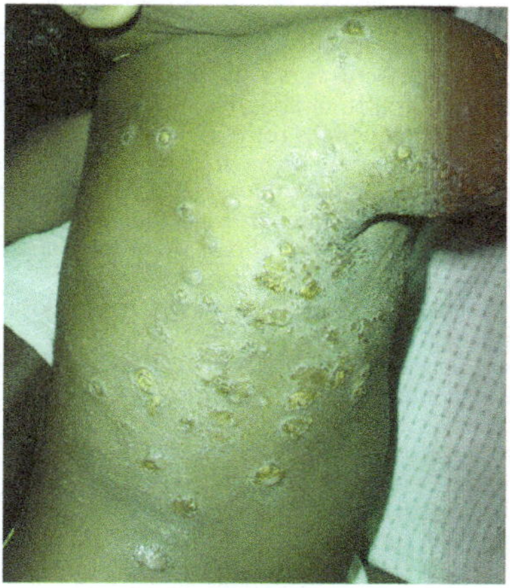

Fig. 25.1 Bullous impetigo.
Reproduced courtesy of NHS Tayside Clinical Photography, Dundee, UK

in children under 5y and may be an opportunistic infection in atopic eczema (➲ see Fig. 17.10) and in neonates especially around the umbilical stump.

Cause: *Staphylococcus aureus* and/or Group A β-haemolytic *Streptococcus pyogenes*.

Treatment: short-term topical antibiotics for localized infection. Systemic antibiotics; flucloxacillin (first choice), or erythromycin or clarithromycin if penicillin allergic.

Staphylococcal scalded skin syndrome

- ➲ See also Fig. 7.6 and Infection causing erythroderma, p. 345.

May develop from localized infection due to toxin producing *Staphylococcus aureus*. Signs are skin tenderness, redness, fever, large areas of skin peeling (blisters not always evident).

Viral

Herpes simplex virus (HSV)

Clusters of blisters on an erythematous background that recur in the same site (Fig. 25.2). Look for associated mouth lesions. Primary infection is often oral and may be severe (➲ see Infective, p. 138).
Treatment: aciclovir (systemic for severe cases).

- ***Eczema herpeticum*** (➲ see Fig. 17.11 and Specific treatments for eczema, pp. 255–9) is widespread HSV blisters/crusts in atopic children. This is a dermatological emergency.
- ***Erythema multiforme*** is a reaction to HSV (drugs are a less common cause in children, ➲ see Erythema multiforme (EM), p. 350). There are symmetrical, fixed, red lesions of various shapes some of which form target lesions (➲ see Fig. 4.12) and sometimes blisters. Child is usually well, although mouth lesions can be distressing (➲ see Fig. 10.3).

Varicella-zoster virus

- *Chickenpox* is a highly infectious disease caused by varicella virus, a member of the herpes virus family. It is transmitted by direct person-to-person contact, droplet, or airborne from an infected individual or indirectly from fomites. Lesions come in crops of small vesicles on a red background and predominate on the trunk and face (➲ see Figs. 9.1 and 25.3). Scabs are not usually infectious. Occult cases occur and infection can be very severe in immunosuppressed children. Onset is typically 14–16 days postexposure (up to 21 days). Generally, lifelong immunity results but virus can recur as shingles (herpes zoster).
  Treatment: if immunocompromised, give systemic aciclovir or valaciclovir and seek consultant advice.
- *Herpes zoster* ('shingles') follows skin dermatome(s). Shingles in infancy suggests previous intrauterine chickenpox (Fig. 25.4). It may be severe in the immunosuppressed (Fig. 25.5).
  Treatment: aciclovir or valaciclovir for early disease and immunocompromised patients.
- ***Hand, foot, and mouth disease***: small pearly-white round or crescent-shaped blisters with surrounding erythematous flare (➲ see Fig. 12.2). Characteristic acral distribution. May also be on buttocks. Lasts 3–10 days.
  Cause: Coxsackie usually A16.
  Treatment: supportive.

Poxvirus infections

- ➲ See Viral infections, pp. 398–401.

Most will start with blisters that later become scabs and eschars (e.g. orf, cowpox). Molluscum contagiosum is an exception with firm dome-shaped

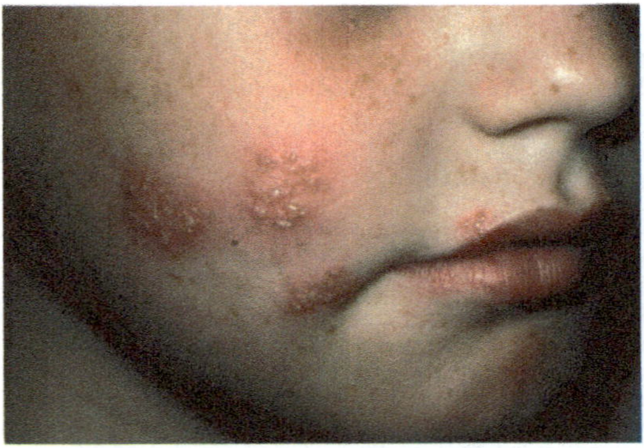

Fig. 25.2 Herpes simplex of face showing typical clusters of blisters on an erythematous base.

Reproduced courtesy of Susan Lewis-Jones, Hon Consultant Dermatologist, Ninewells Hospital and Medical School, Dundee, UK

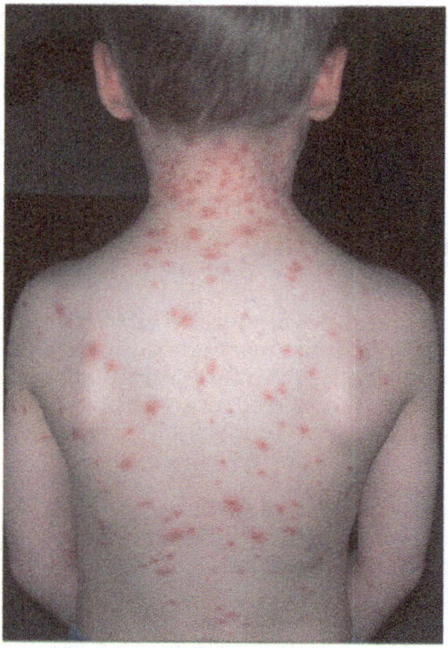

Fig. 25.3 Chickenpox. Blisters with characteristic erythematous flare.
Reproduced courtesy of Susan Lewis-Jones, Hon Consultant Dermatologist, Ninewells Hospital and Medical School, Dundee, UK

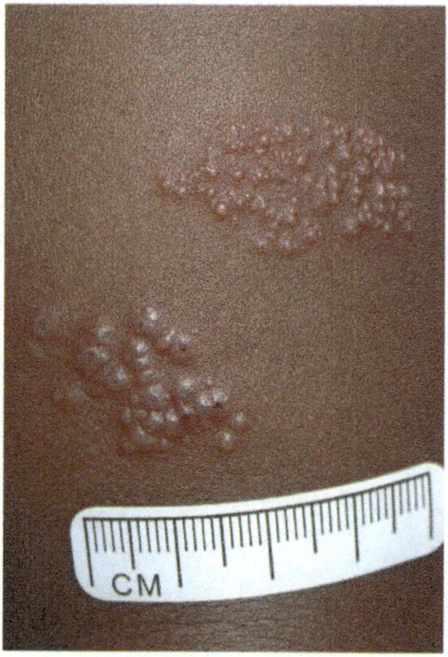

Fig. 25.4 Varicella-zoster in an infant following intrauterine chickenpox.
Reproduced courtesy of NHS Tayside Clinical Photography, Dundee, UK

papules with depressed centre that may be mistaken for blisters ('Water' warts) (➲ see Figs. 9.7 and 19.1).

Fungal causes

Tinea pedis

Small clear vesicles may be present but usually pustules.

Infestations causing blisters

Scabies

Itchy skin eruption due to *Sarcoptes scabiei* var. *humanis* (➲ see Figs. 22.13 and 22.14); Secondary impetigo may cause larger blisters (➲ see Fig. 24.4). *Note*: *infantile acropustulosis*—rare (➲ see Acral pustular rashes, pp. 297–8) occurs in infants with recurrent crops of acral blisters/pustules and possibly relates to scabies infestations.

Pediculosis

Scalp nits are often complicated by secondary impetigo, usually only as crusts but there may be occasional blisters (➲ see Figs. 2.3, 14.9, and 14.10). For body and crab lice, ➲ see Fig. 22.15.

Physical and environmental causes

- *Insect bites*: reactions may be urticarial, papular, vesicular or bullous, and often grouped and occasionally large (➲ see Fig. 20.5).
- *Papular urticaria*: usually itchy papules rather than blisters leaving purplish circular scars on lower legs (➲ see Infestations and parasites, pp. 283–5).
- *Trauma/friction*: from rubbing (e.g. wearing new shoes or splints). Consider non-accidental injury in differential diagnosis (➲ see Chapter 24).
- *Thermal*: from heat, frostbite, or following cryotherapy (Fig. 25.6).
- *Chemical*: look for drip marks. Also consider non-accidental cause or self-harm (➲ see Fig. 24.13).
- *Phytophotodermatitis*: from contact with plants and sun (➲ see Figs. 16.7 and 16.8).
- *Photosensitive reactions*: sunburn in exposed areas; polymorphic light reaction; porphyrias; hydroa vacciniforme and others (➲ see Chapter 16).

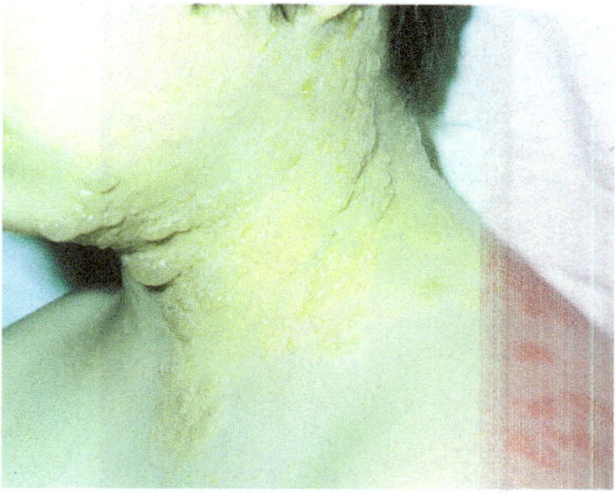

Fig. 25.5 Severe herpes zoster in immunosuppressed child.
Reproduced courtesy of NHS Tayside Clinical Photography, Dundee, UK

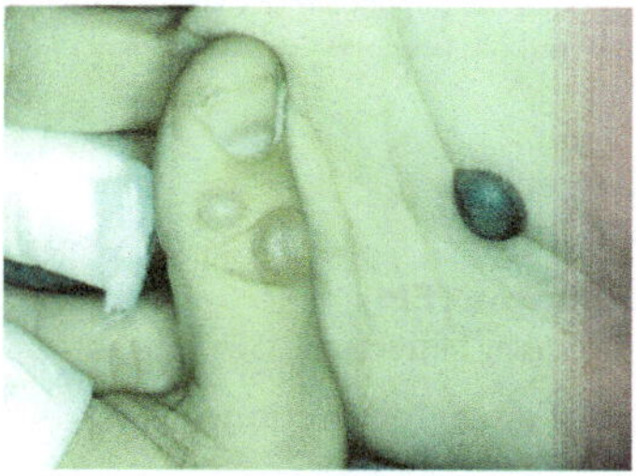

Fig. 25.6 Blisters following cryotherapy for viral warts.
Reproduced courtesy of Susan Lewis-Jones, Hon Consultant Dermatologist, Ninewells Hospital and Medical School, Dundee, UK

Drugs

- ➲ See also Chapter 23.

Topical agents

Blisters may occur from contact irritancy (Fig. 25.7) or contact allergic dermatitis (e.g. allergy to topical antibiotics).

Fixed drug eruptions

Lesions that may blister, recur at fixed sites when a culprit drug is taken and leave localized brown-purple plaques which are slow to disappear (➲ see Fig. 23.6).

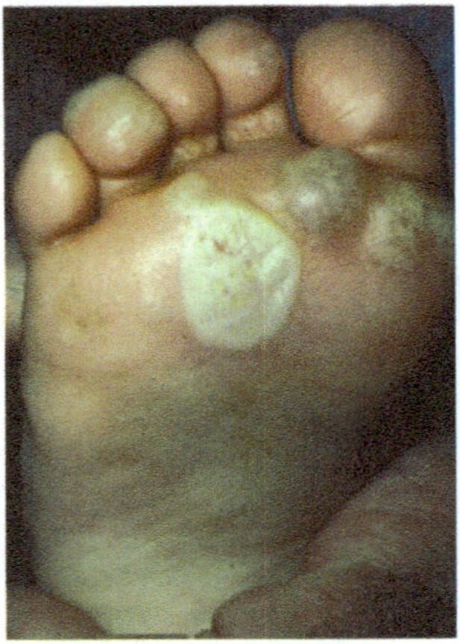

Fig. 25.7 Blisters following use of podophyllin wart paint.
Reproduced courtesy of Susan Lewis-Jones, Hon Consultant Dermatologist, Ninewells Hospital and Medical School, Dundee, UK

Photosensitizing drugs

- ➲ See Chapters 16 and 23.

Erythema multiforme (EM)

- ➲ See Infections causing blisters, pp. 352–7.

Severe cutaneous adverse reactions

- ➲ See Box 23.3.
- Both Stevens–Johnson syndrome (SJS) and toxic epidermal necrolysis (TEN) are severe mucocutaneous bullous disorders with involvement of ≥2 mucosal surfaces. In SJS <10% body surface area (BSA) is involved, 10–30% BSA is SJS/TEN overlap, and >30% BSA is TEN. Skin is tender with red macules that evolve to large flaccid blisters and denuded areas. Child is ill. In TEN there are extensive areas of skin necrosis. Skin changes tend to start more quickly after drug exposure and evolve more rapidly (➲ see Chapter 23 and Fig. 23.5).

Note: similar clinical presentations occur with EM and SJS, both of which are usually caused by infections in children (e.g. HSV) but children with EM are usually well. TEN is almost exclusively caused by drugs.

Inflammatory skin diseases

Allergic contact dermatitis

Consider if blisters appear in localized eczema (unusual to see blisters in atopic eczema which is less acute). Take a thorough history including exposure to plants (e.g. poison ivy, *primula obconica*) and sunlight. Diagnosis by patch testing (➲ see Patch testing, pp. 25–6).

Pompholyx

Vesicular eczema of palms, soles, and sides of digits. Small itchy blisters may coalesce to form large lesions which tend to be symmetrical (➲ see Fig. 17.14). Contact allergic eczema must be excluded by patch testing (➲ see Patch testing, pp. 25–6).

Pustular psoriasis

This may be acute and generalized with red skin and small pustules or localized including to the hands and feet. Rare in children (➲ see Psoriasis—clinical variants, pp. 322–4 and Fig. 22.18).

Bullous lichen planus

Very rare, pruritic papular eruption followed by blisters (➲ see Non-infective causes, pp. 285–8).

Mastocytosis

Cutaneous mastocytosis: caused by infiltration with mast cells (➲ see Fixed annual urticated rash, pp. 314–15).

- *Urticaria pigmentosa*: pigmented lesions from birth or early life, which urticate and often blister, especially on rubbing (Darier's sign). They may be generalized, particularly on the trunk (➲ see Fig. 19.8). It is rare to have systemic manifestations other than flushing and abdominal pain and the prognosis is good in children.
- *Mastocytoma*: oval skin coloured/yellowish brown lesions, which may be macular, nodular, or plaque-like (➲ see Fig. 28.6). They often blister on trauma and show a positive Darier's sign.
- *Diffuse cutaneous mastocytosis*: a very rare and potentially fatal variant presenting in neonates with large areas of diffusely thickened skin (Moroccan leather sign) and/or papules caused by infiltration with mast cells. Widespread blistering may occur, mimicking staphylococcal scalded skin syndrome. *Ask for an urgent specialist paediatric dermatological opinion.* 🚩

Autoimmune blistering diseases

A heterogenous group of rare diseases that are often difficult to manage. Skin biopsy for histopathological examination and direct immunofluorescence is required for diagnosis. Ask for specialist dermatological help.

Chronic bullous dermatosis of childhood

(*Syn.* Linear IgA disease). Usually occurs after aged 3y. Typically presents with perianal lesions that spread onto thighs and abdomen (Fig. 25.8) often with small tense blisters on a red background in rosettes ('string of pearls' sign). However, any skin site may be involved including mucosal lesions (genital, oral, and eye). It may persist for 3–5y, occasionally longer. Linear IgA immunofluorescence is seen at the dermoepidermal junction on skin biopsy.

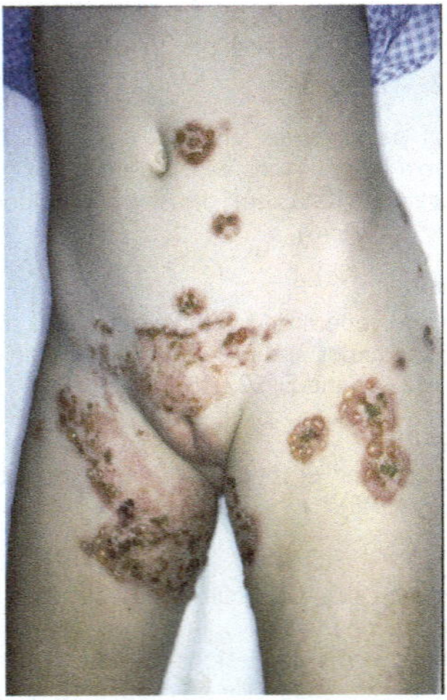

Fig. 25.8 Chronic bullous disease of childhood with typical annular pattern of blisters ('string of pearls' sign).

Reproduced courtesy of Susan Lewis-Jones, Hon Consultant Dermatologist, Ninewells Hospital and Medical School, Dundee, UK

Treatment: first line, usually dapsone; some require systemic immunosuppressants such as methotrexate or Mycophenolate mofetil.

Dermatitis herpetiformis

Typically presents as intensely itchy symmetrical small blisters on extensor aspects of elbows (Fig. 25.9), knees and buttocks, and often scalp. Scratching leads to excoriated papules. The oral mucosa is rarely affected.

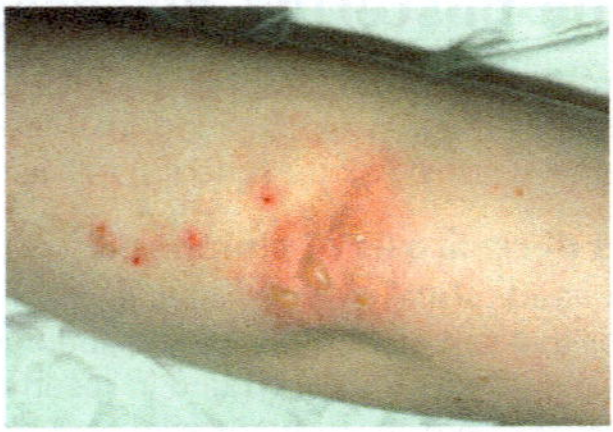

Fig. 25.9 Dermatitis herpetiformis elbow showing typical cluster of small blisters on an erythematous 'urticated' base, with older excoriated lesions.

Reproduced courtesy of Susan Lewis-Jones, Hon Consultant Dermatologist, Ninewells Hospital and Medical School, Dundee, UK

Skin biopsy shows granular IgA deposits at papillary tips on direct immunofluorescence. Screen for occult gluten sensitive enteropathy.

Treatment: dapsone or related drugs and gluten-free diet for life.

Pemphigus

A group of several, very rare superficial blistering disorders presenting as widespread, flaccid blisters and erosions. There is epidermal cell separation (acantholysis) caused by IgG autoantibodies which results in a positive Nikolsky's sign*. Skin and mucosal involvement occurs in 80% of those with pemphigus vulgaris, and stomatitis is the presenting feature in 50% of these. Pemphigus foliaceus presents on the scalp, trunk, and extremities.

Treatment: topical and systemic corticosteroids and/or other immunosuppressants may be required.

Prognosis: better in children than adults, especially for pemphigus foliaceus.

Bullous pemphigoid

Presents with large tense, sometimes haemorrhagic blisters at the dermoepidermal junction so Nikolsky's sign* is negative. Common sites are face, neck, groin, inner thighs, and genitalia. Oral lesions may be present. It may be localized to the vulva in children. It usually remits over time. IgG antibodies to target antigens are found in the basement membrane zone.

Treatment: similar to pemphigus but tends to respond better.

Acquired epidermolysis bullosa (EB aquisita)

Extremely rare, usually presenting as tense, itchy blisters on bony sites which are prone to trauma. The blisters occur due to antibodies targeting type VII collagen. Generalized and predominantly mucous membrane EB aquisita can also occur. There may be underlying conditions such as systemic lupus erythematosus and Crohn's disease.

Treatment: similar to pemphigus as well as treating any underlying disorder.

Genetic causes of blisters

Epidermolysis bullosa (EB)

A group of rare genetically determined disorders characterized by excessive susceptibility of skin and mucosae to separate from underlying tissues following mechanical trauma (Figs. 25.10 and 25.11). There are four broad categories, depending on the level of the split:

- *EB simplex*: split within the basal keratinocytes mainly caused by keratin gene mutations. May be localized or generalized (more severe).
- *Junctional EB*: generalized severe form with poor outlook and death within infancy and generalized intermediate form with milder course. Results from mutations in dermoepidermal junction components such as laminin 332.
- *Dystrophic EB*: due to mutations on the gene for collagen VII, the main component of skin anchoring fibrils. Dominant forms generally milder than generalized recessive forms that may be intermediate or severe.

**Nikolsky's sign* is deemed positive when, on lateral pressure, the superficial skin layers slip free from the underlying tissue—extending or producing a blister.

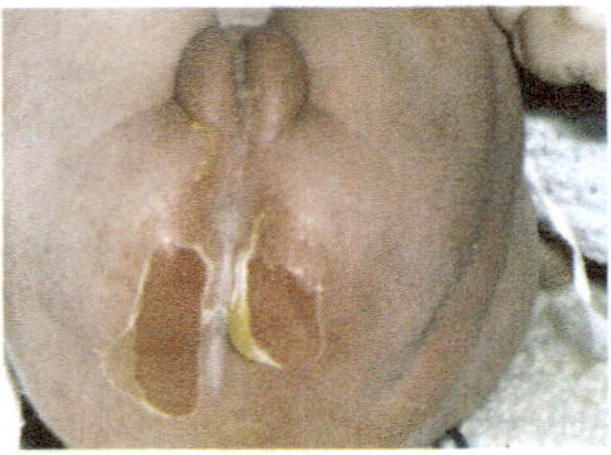

Fig. 25.10 EB in a newborn with typical blisters on pressure areas of buttocks. It is not usually possible to differentiate between some types clinically at this stage and it may be confused with early staphylococcal scalded skin syndrome.

Reproduced courtesy of Susan Lewis-Jones, Hon Consultant Dermatologist, Ninewells Hospital and Medical School, Dundee, UK

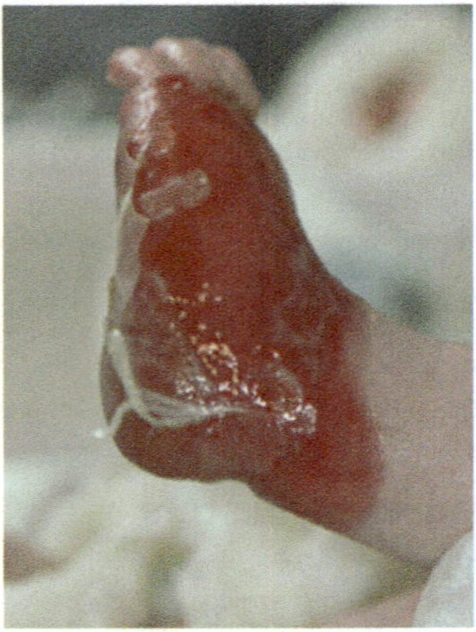

Fig. 25.11 Neonatal skin loss in recessive dystrophic EB.

Reproduced courtesy of Jemima Mellerio, Professor and Consultant Dermatologist, St John's Institute of Dermatology, Guy's and St Thomas' NHS Foundation Trust, London, UK

Severe type leads to widespread blistering, scarring, faltering growth, internal complications, and death in early adulthood from aggressive cutaneous squamous cell carcinoma.

- *Kindler syndrome*: very rare form with early onset blistering replaced later by poikiloderma.
- Differentiation of the different types clinically can be very difficult early in life. Blistering can occur at birth, shortly thereafter, or later depending on the type. It often presents with raw areas, particularly on the legs, and at sites of skin trauma. It may be difficult to distinguish from impetigo or staphylococcal scalded skin in neonates.

Management: handling of neonates with EB can result in severe denudation of skin (➲ see Fig. 29.11) and advice on management for suspected cases should be sought urgently. ⚑ England and Wales have a national paediatric service for EB based at Great Ormond Street and Birmingham Children's Hospital, where 24h advice is available for any infants and children with suspected EB. DEBRA (Dystrophic Epidermolysis Bullosa Research Association) provides a UK network of specialist nurses, available at http://www.debra.org.uk.

Hailey–Hailey disease (*syn.* benign familial pemphigus)

A rare autosomal dominant condition presenting from the second decade with blisters, erosions, pustules, and crusts to a varying degree. These build up as large wart-like plaques with offensive odour in neck, groin, perineum, and axillae. Treatment, aimed at reducing symptoms and preventing flares, includes antibiotics, topical steroids, and losing weight to avoid friction.

Porphyrias

A group of rare disorders, some with cutaneous manifestations of photosensitivity including skin fragility, blisters, and erosions (➲ see Immediate photosensitive rashes, pp. 230–1).

Hartnup disease

An autosomal recessive disorder of amino acid transport. Sun exposure leads to a pellagra-like rash (➲ see Vitamin deficiencies, p. 494) and sometimes blisters. Neurological symptoms occur in some. Check urine amino acids.

Treatment: nicotinamide.

Pachyonychia congenita

Autosomal dominant keratin disorders, some of which present in infants or young children with discolouration and thickened tented nails (➲ see Genodermatoses and the nail, pp. 223–4). Painful blistering, mainly of the feet may occur in some. The Pachyonychia Congenita Project provides support and information to those with the condition; see http://www.pachyonychia.org/.

Incontinentia pigmenti

A rare X-linked dominant, multisystem disorder with variable expression. Cutaneous lesions occur in the distribution of the lines of Blaschko (➲ see Fig. 4.6).

There are four stages occurring over time:

1. Blisters and erythema: variable numbers appear in patterns of streaks or whorls (Blaschko's lines), usually within the first 48h of life and lasting a few weeks (Fig. 25.12). They are often pus filled and rich in eosinophils.
2. Verrucous lesions: warty, scaling lesions lasting a month or so (Fig. 25.13). Sometimes blisters and verrucous lesions coexist.
3. Hyperpigmented flat linear lines and whorls: in site of verrucous lesions, which fade with time.
4. White linear atrophic streaks: lacking hair or sweat glands, particularly on the legs. Check mother for leg streaks, missing teeth, or patchy scarring alopecia.

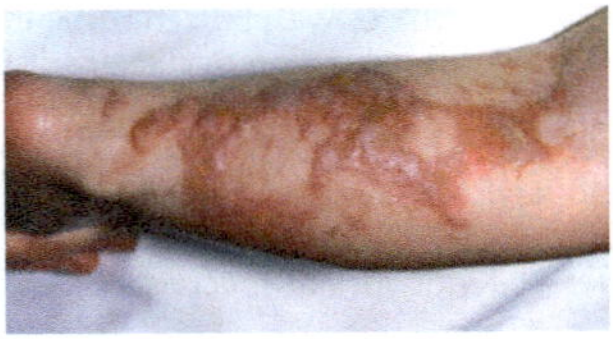

Fig. 25.12 Incontinentia pigmenti may present in the early stages with blisters.
Reproduced courtesy of Susan Lewis-Jones, Hon Consultant Dermatologist, Ninewells Hospital and Medical School, Dundee, UK

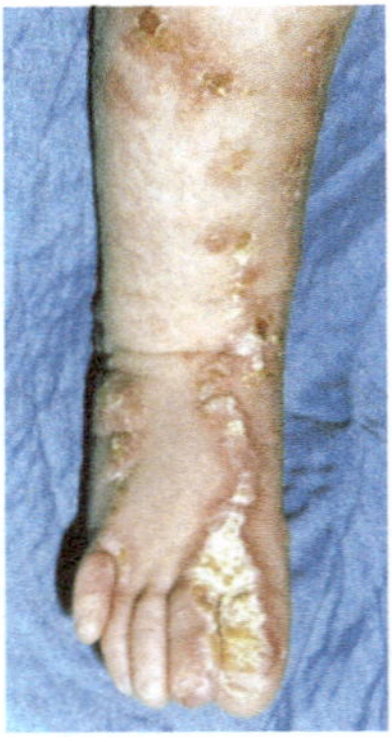

Fig. 25.13 Incontinentia pigmenti hyperkeratotic stage two.
Reproduced courtesy of Susan Lewis-Jones, Hon Consultant Dermatologist, Ninewells Hospital and Medical School, Dundee, UK

Cause: mutations in the *NEMO* gene, which cause apoptosis (cell death); usually lethal in males but females survive by mosaicism and there is skewed X-inactivation. The abnormal cells are gradually replaced as apoptosis occurs, hence the four stages.

Associated problems: varying degrees of ocular, dental, nail, hair (alopecia), and neurological involvement.

Note: neurological and other problems are not progressive, so if they are not present in early infancy then parents can be reassured (but watch for deafness, which can be missed).

Blisters and purpura

- See Box 25.2; ➲ see also Chapter 31.

Box 25.2 Causes of blisters and purpura

- *Infections*: e.g. meningococcal, haemorrhagic fevers.
- *Vasculitis*: many causes including autoimmune diseases.
- *Haematological disorders*: e.g. protein C deficiency.
- *Skin diseases*: e.g. pyoderma gangrenosum.
- *Adverse drug reactions*: e.g. antibiotics, anticonvulsants.
- *Allergy*: severe contact dermatitis (very rare).

Physical

- Severe trauma.
- Thermal damage.
- Chemical burns.
- Radiation damage.

Venom

- Stings, e.g. insects; poisonous fish and jellyfish, etc.
- Bites from snakes and spiders, etc.

Neonatal blisters

- ➲ See also Chapter 7 and Fig. 25.14.
- ***Sterile transient vesiculopustular conditions***, such as miliaria, erythema toxicum neonatorum, and transient neonatal pustulosis/melanosis (➲ see also Transient benign neonatal dermatoses, pp. 81–82).
- ***Sucking blisters*** are typically present at acral (peripheral) sites and may be present at birth as single lesions or ulcers.
- ***Infections*** including *Candida* and opportunistic infections.
- ***Genetic disorders***: a large number (all rare), including:
  - Epidermolysis bullosa: Figs. 25.10 and 25.11.
  - Incontinentia pigmenti: ➲ see pp. 389–90.
  - Epidermolytic ichthyosis (➲ see Fig. 27.6). Usually presents at birth with large areas of denuded skin, blisters, and varying degrees of erythroderma.
- ***Autoimmune***: due to passive transfer of maternal autoantibodies (e.g. pemphigoid gestationis, bullous pemphigoid, pemphigus vulgaris). All types are rare and maternal disease may not be active. Rash clears as the antibodies are destroyed.
- ***Physical***: from thermal, frictional (adhesive tape stripping), or other injury or chemical damage to the skin (e.g. surgical cleansers left in contact for long periods, especially in premature infants).

Further reading

BMJ Best Practice, *Epidermolysis Bullosa*, http://www.bestpractice.bmj.com/topics/en-gb/744/guidelines

British Association of Dermatologists Patient Information Leaflets (PILS), *Dystrophic Epidermolysis Bullosa*, https://www.bad.org.uk/shared/getfile.ashx?id=62&itemtype=document

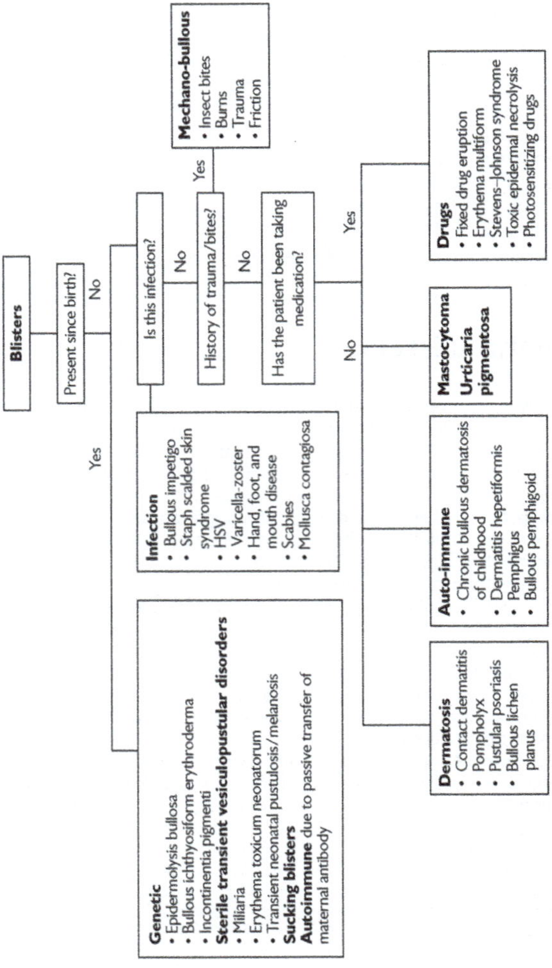

Fig. 25.14 Blisters algorithm.

Chapter 26

Crusts, scabs, and eschars

Introduction

Crusts and scabs are formed by dried serous exudate (Fig. 26.1). They are secondary skin lesions occurring as a result of blistering diseases or trauma (e.g. scratching or infection). It is important to differentiate them from scaling or dry skin, which consists of dead epidermal cells (corneocytes).

Eschars are large areas of firmly adherent crust, caused by local necrosis and involving the whole epidermis (sometimes including dermis) and can be of any size (Fig. 26.2). They may be solitary or multiple. Ulcers develop as the eschar separates and healing may be slow to leave scarring.

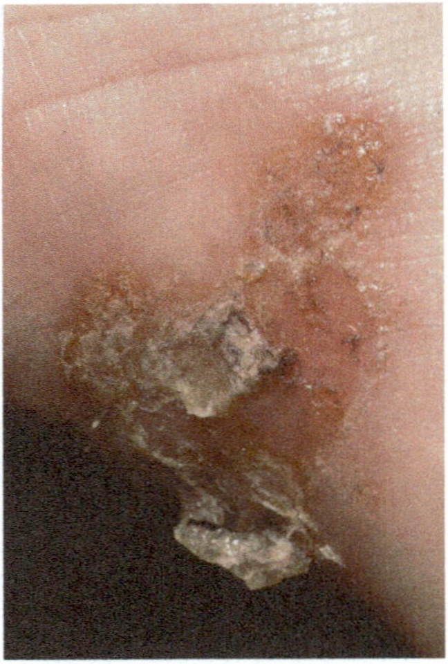

Fig. 26.1 Crusting in impetigo.
Reproduced courtesy of NHS Tayside Clinical Photography, Dundee, UK

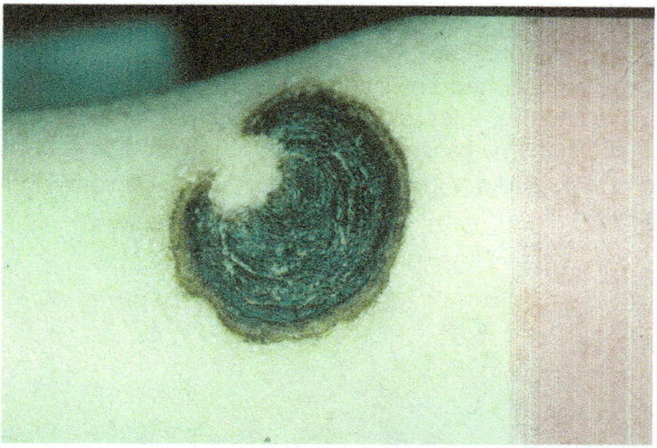

Fig. 26.2 Eschar.

Reproduced courtesy of Susan Lewis-Jones, Hon Consultant Dermatologist, Ninewells Hospital and Medical School, Dundee, UK

Crusts and scabs

Causes

Infections such as:

- *Bacterial*: e.g. impetigo (Fig. 26.1; ➲ see also Fig. 25.1), ecthyma (Fig. 26.3).
- *Viral*, such as:
  - Chickenpox (varicella-zoster; ➲ see Chapter 25).
  - Herpes infections (➲ see Chapter 25).
  - Some poxvirus infections (➲ see Viral infections, pp. 398–401).
  - Fungal infection of scalp (kerion) (➲ see Fig. 14.8).
- *Protozoal*: e.g. cutaneous leishmaniasis (common in endemic areas) (Fig. 26.4).

Skin diseases such as:

- Eczema and other itchy rashes, especially if infected (➲ see Chapter 17).
- Blistering disorders (➲ see Chapter 25).
- Rare conditions such as pityriasis lichenoides (➲ see Chapter 19).

Trauma such as:

- Scratches, cuts, grazes, lacerations, wounds.
- Thermal or photodamage damage.
- Chemical burns.

Treatment

Treat the underlying cause. Local antiseptic (e.g. 1% hydrogen peroxide cream) may be helpful but widespread infections may require appropriate systemic antibiotics. Large crusts can be soaked in either saline or dilute potassium permanganate solution (pale pink) or 1% hydrogen peroxide soaks for 15min or so, and then gently removed and covered with a sterile dressing. Silver impregnated dressings are useful to prevent infection but are expensive.

Ecthyma

Deep streptococcal infection, usually following insect bites. Commoner in tropics in malnourished children. Firmly adherent rings of crust occur (Fig. 26.3). Initially resembles impetigo and *Staphyloccus aureus* is commonly associated. For ecthyma gangrenosum, ➲ see Bacterial infections, p. 398.

Treatment: oral penicillin V (or erythromycin or clarithromycin in cases of penicillin allergy).

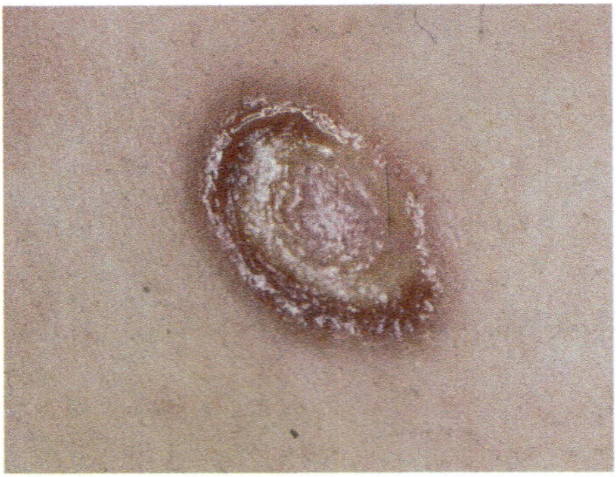

Fig. 26.3 Ecthyma following insect bite on neck. Concentric rings of adherent crusts.

Reproduced courtesy of Susan Lewis-Jones, Hon Consultant Dermatologist, Ninewells Hospital and Medical School, Dundee, UK

(a) (b)

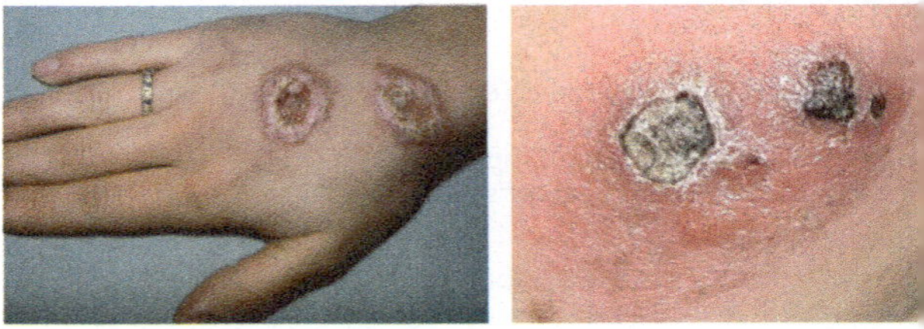

Fig. 26.4 (a) Old World cutaneous leishmaniasis of the hand. (b) Close-up of eschars (*Leishmania tropica*).

Reproduced courtesy of Ali Khamesipour, Center for Research and Training in Skin Diseases and Leprosy, Tehran, Iran

Eschars

- See Fig. 26.2.

Causes

Infections

- Bacteria:
  - Ecthyma (Fig. 26.3) and ecthyma gangrenosum (➲ see Bacterial infections, p. 398).
  - Anthrax (Fig. 26.6).
  - Meningococcal septicaemia (➲ see Chapter 31, Sepsis, pp. 467–70).
  - Papulonecrotic tuberculid (➲ see Chapter 22, Tuberculosis (TB)—skin diseases, pp. 333–5).
  - Syphilis and yaws (➲ see Chapter 22, Spirochete infections, pp. 336–7).
- Viruses:
  - Poxvirus infections (➲ see Viral infections, pp. 398–401).
  - Severe chickenpox (varicella-zoster) (➲ see Infections causing blisters, p. 378).
- Fungi:
  - Tinea capitis—kerion (➲ see Fig. 14.8; see also Scalp infections, pp. 203–4).
- Protozoa:
  - Cutaneous amoebiasis.
  - Leishmaniasis (Fig. 26.4; ➲ see also Infestation and parasites, pp. 283–5).

Skin diseases

- Pityriasis lichenoides—acute form (➲ see Non-infective causes, pp. 285–8).
- Vasculitic diseases with skin necrosis (➲ see Cutaneous vasculitis, pp. 470–2, and Fig. 38.3).
- Pyoderma gangrenosum: very rare in children. Usually sudden onset of painful red/purplish lesions which may go through a stage of eschar formation but eventually ulcerate (➲ see Causes of ulcers, pp. 456–9 and Fig. 30.3).

Systemic diseases

- Autoimmune vasculitis, e.g. systemic lupus erythematosus (➲ see Chapter 38).
- Calciphylaxis: found in terminal renal failure. Areas of black eschar, from ischaemic necrosis, usually on legs in older patients with end-stage renal failure. Skin biopsy shows vascular calcification and necrotic areas.

Toxins/allergens

- Insect bites and stings.
- Venomous bites, stings or puncture wounds from spiders, snakes, fish, and jellyfish, etc.

Other rare causes of eschars

- Haematological diseases such as protein C & S deficiency, purpura fulminans (➲ see Chapter 31).
- Tumours such as some rare lymphomas.

Bacterial infections

Ectyhma gangrenosum

Rare necrotic ulcers, that start as purpuric nodules.

Cause: *Pseudomonas aeruginosa* usually in association with neutropenia and immunosuppression.

Cutaneous anthrax

- Gram-positive bacillus (*Bacillus anthracis*) occurs on exposed sites following contact with spores from contaminated animals/animal products (e.g. hides or wool).
- One to five days' incubation. Itchy red papule then bulla with surrounding erythema similar to cowpox (➲ see Viral infections, pp. 398–401) and haemorrhagic crust/eschar (malignant pustule; Fig. 26.6). May be oedema and tender regional lymphadenopathy.
- Systemic symptoms (fever, toxaemia) usually mild.
- Healing in 2–3 weeks. Untreated cases occasionally severe with mortality of 5–20%.

Management: contact infectious disease physician. Take bacterial swabs for Gram stain and culture. Start treatment immediately with oral ciprofloxacin or amoxicillin (or doxycycline if over 12y) 7–10 days. If systemically ill, take blood cultures and start penicillin G IV (7–10 days).

Viral infections

Poxvirus infections

A group of viral infections, some of which start as blisters later evolving into crusted scabs or eschars; they heal slowly to leave depressed circular scars (varioliform scars). There are three main genera:

- ***Orthopoxviruses***—smallpox (extinct), monkeypox (Africa), cowpox (Europe), buffalopox (India), cattlepox (S. America).
- ***Parapoxviruses***—orf, sealpox, and deerpox.
- ***Molluscipoxvirus***—molluscum contagiosum, papular (➲ see Fig. 19.1 and Molluscum contagiosum, p. 281).

Management: take swabs or crusts for microbiological culture and electron microscopy.

Treatment: supportive with antipyretics, analgesics, and antibiotics for secondary bacterial infection. Seek dermatological and microbiological help and urgent ophthalmological opinion if the eyes are involved.

Orthopoxviruses

Smallpox (Variola major) (extinct)

Eradicated in 1980 but potential bioterrorist use makes knowledge of its presentation essential. It is very contagious; spread by droplet inhalation but is non-infectious during a 12-day (range 7–17) incubation.

Prodrome: severe flu-like illness with prostration, severe myalgia, headaches, abdominal pain, vomiting. Infants can develop fatal gastric dilatation.

Enanthem: lesions in the pharynx—saliva is very infectious.

Exanthem: 2–3 days later, red papules rapidly develop, predominately on face, hands, arms, and then lower extremities (centrifugal pattern). They evolve as large firm blisters, *all at the same stage of development* (see also chickenpox, ➲ see Infections causing blisters, p. 378, where lesions are central on face and chest with few on extremities). These later umbilicate and form scabs that separate around 3 weeks to leave deep pockmarks, mainly on the face. Long-term sequelae include osteomyelitis and encephalitis.

Mortality: 10–60% for Variola major the commoner severe form.

If smallpox is suspected, isolate patient and staff, and contact local smallpox team.

Vaccination against smallpox

Live *Vaccinia* virus is given to troops, laboratory workers, and specialist public health smallpox teams. Localized reactions may be severe, including eczema vaccinatum but cardiac and other complications are rare.

Avoid in infants under 2y and in those with immunosuppression or a history of eczema (high risk of eczema vaccinatum—widespread blisters with infantile mortality of 2–6%). In the immunosuppressed, slowly progressive ulcers and gangrenous lesions may occur.

For further information, see the Centers for Disease Control and Prevention website, https://www.cdc.gov/

Monkeypox

Similar to smallpox but less severe clinical presentation with marked adenopathy and lower mortality (11–15% in African series). Usually confined to tropical regions of West Africa but there were no fatalities in the 2003 USA outbreak, caused by imported African rodents.

Cowpox

Rare and confined to United Kingdom and Europe. Half give a history of animal contact, especially cats (rodents are the reservoir host). Incubation is about 7 days.

Prodrome: abrupt systemic flu-like malaise (may be severe) with fever, nausea, vomiting, and muscle aching.

Lesions: painful erythematous papules (resembles orf but more redness and swelling), usually solitary or just a few, on face or hands. Blisters and then eschars develop in about 7 days (Figs. 26.6 and 26.7). There is firm 'woody-hard' local swelling with marked regional adenopathy. Healing occurs over 4–6 weeks, leaving deeply pitted scars (Fig. 26.7). Treat symptomatically. The main differential diagnosis is anthrax (Fig. 26.5).

Parapoxviruses

Orf

Worldwide, common infection, contracted from sheep, goats, or rarely fomites.

Incubation: around 14 days.

Lesions: often multiple, usually hands, and localized with little or no surrounding erythema, swelling, adenopathy, or systemic malaise (see also cowpox and anthrax). Small red papules become blistered and may go through a granulomatous stage (very rarely giant-sized) before forming an eschar (Figs. 26.8 and 26.9).

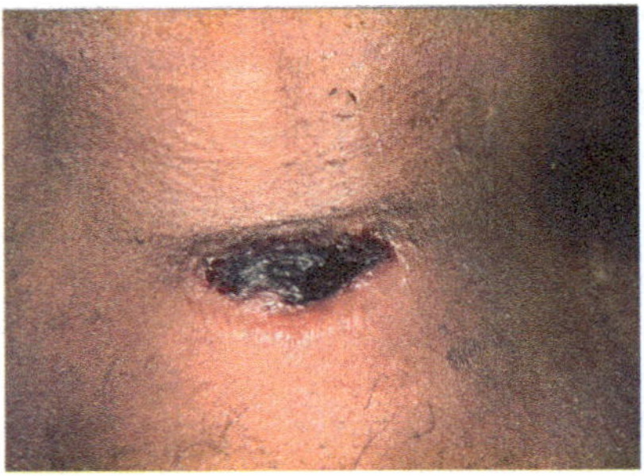

Fig. 26.5 Cutaneous anthrax with black eschar.

Reproduced courtesy of Stewart Douglas, Scotland, UK

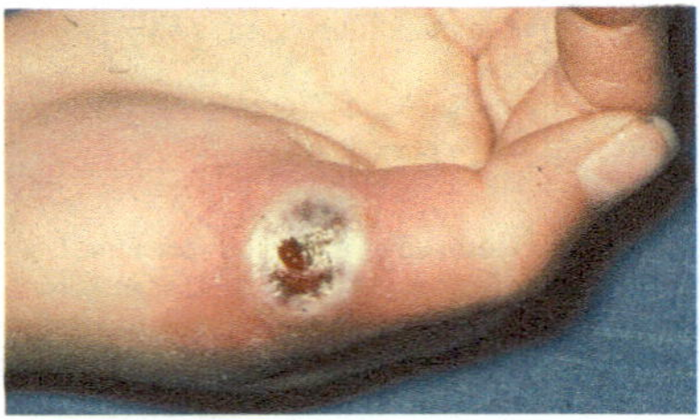

Fig. 26.6 Cowpox lesion at 11 days: haemorrhagic vesicular lesion with marked inflammation and oedema.

Reproduced with permission from Baxby D. *et al.* (1994). Human cowpox 1969–93: a review based on 54 cases. *Br J Dermatol.* 131(5): 598–607. https://doi.org/10.1111/j.1365-2133.1994.tb04969.x

(a) (b)

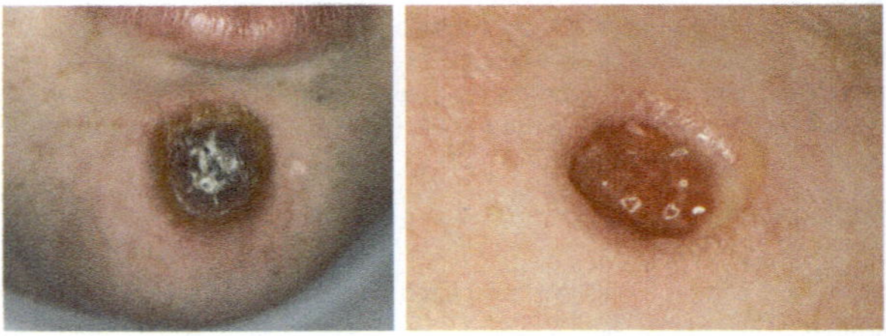

Fig. 26.7 (a) Cowpox eschar on chin in 15-year-old girl. (b) Cowpox– deep ulcer following separation of eschar.

(a) Reproduced with permission from Lewis-Jones M.S. *et al.* (1993). Cowpox can smimic anthrax. *Br. J. Dermatol.* 129: 625–7. https://doi.org/10.1111/j.1365-2133.1993.tb00499.x; (b) Reproduced courtesy of Susan Lewis-Jones, Hon Consultant Dermatologist, Ninewells Hospital and Medical School, Dundee, UK

Healing: 4–6 weeks—may leave some scarring.

Complications: erythema multiforme (see p. 190).

Others

Milker's nodules: contracted from cows and very similar to orf.
Rheindeerpox and sealpox: very rare occupational dermatoses resembling orf.

Tanapox (Yatapoxvirus virus): confined to tropical African flood plains. It presents with very few lesions similar to monkeypox but with little systemic malaise.

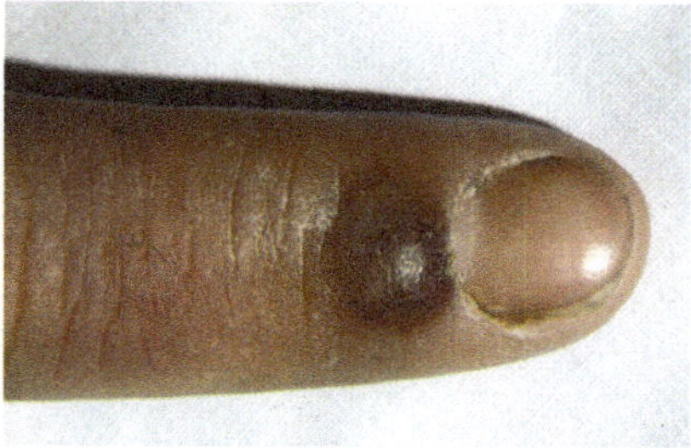

Fig. 26.8 Orf blister I typical site on hand.
Reproduced courtesy of NHS Tayside Clinical Photography, Dundee, UK

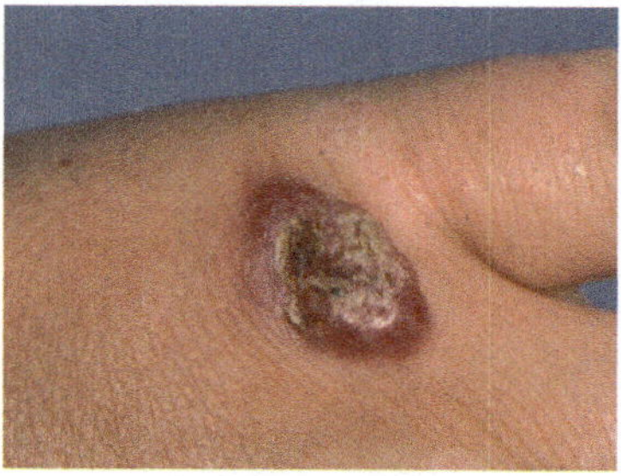

Fig. 26.9 Orf lesion showing crusting and early eschar formation.
Reproduced courtesy of NHS Tayside Clinical Photography, Dundee, UK

Dry skin disorders

Introduction

Dry or scaly skin may be an isolated finding or occur with erythema in skin conditions such as psoriasis and eczema (➲ see Chapters 22 and 17, respectively). Palmoplantar keratoderma, a localized hyperkeratosis of the palms and soles (➲ see Palmoplantar keratoderma, p. 164 and Fig. 12.4), may also occur in isolation or in conjunction with a more generalized ichthyosis or inflammatory skin disease. This chapter deals with:

- Dry, scaly skin.
- The ichthyoses.
- Collodion baby and Harlequin ichthyosis.

Dry scaly skin

Dry, scaly skin at any age is due to epidermal dryness (xerosis) for which there are many causes (Fig. 27.1). Dry skin reflects a loss of water from the skin due to low environmental humidity or faulty skin barrier function. In inflammatory skin disease such as atopic eczema, psoriasis, and erythroderma, the skin's natural upper epidermal barrier is damaged, resulting in increased transepidermal water loss.

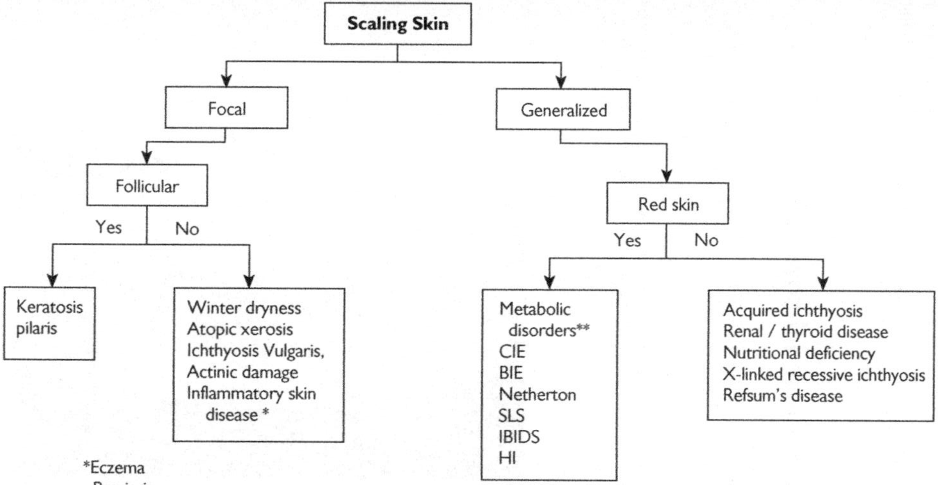

*Eczema
Psoriasis
Lichen planus
Fungal dermatosesetc.

**Zinc/biotin deficiency
Amino acid disorders etc.

Fig. 27.1 Dry skin algorithm.

The ichthyoses

If the epidermis is structurally abnormal due to genetic defects in differentiation or cornification, its function will also be defective. This occurs in a group of disorders known as the ichthyoses (literally 'fish-scale skin') whose hallmark sign is widespread persistent scaling. Additionally, in some ichthyoses there is deficient skin shedding (desquamation) or inflammation with increased epidermal cell turnover.

Common genetic ichthyoses

Ichthyosis vulgaris (IV)

Vulgar means common. IV affects 1 in 250 healthy people and causes fine, white scaling with surface fissures (like crazy paving), mainly on the lower limbs (Fig. 27.2). It presents in early childhood and improves in the summer months. It is often associated with keratosis pilaris (➲ see Chapter 9), a common follicular scaly disorder, which mainly affects the extensor limbs and which is a minor diagnostic feature of atopic eczema (➲ see Chapter 17). IV is due to an autosomal dominant genetic mutation in the filaggrin gene (➲ see Box 17.4).

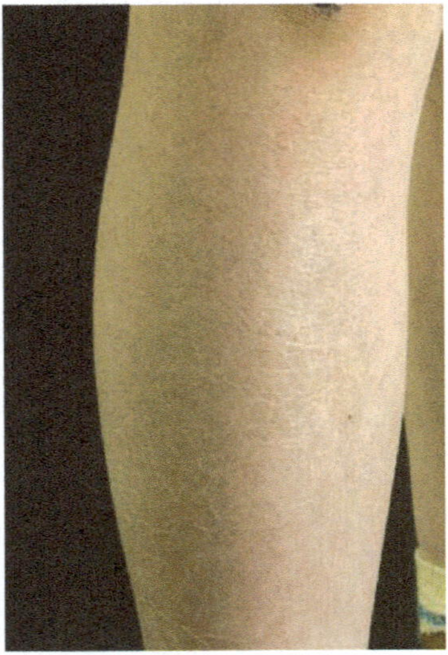

Fig. 27.2 Ichthyosis vulgaris.

Reproduced courtesy of NHS Tayside Clinical Photography, Dundee, UK

X-linked recessive ichthyosis (XLRI)

- Second most common genetic ichthyosis, affecting 1 in 5000 males.
- Female carriers have few signs.
- Characteristic brown or grey 'stuck on' scaling on the lower legs, upper arms, and flanks (Fig. 27.3).
- Improves in warmer weather and in adult life.

Other features

- Tiny corneal deposits (which generally do not affect vision).
- Prolonged labour (a perinatal risk: alert obstetricians and midwives).
- Higher than average incidence of testicular abnormalities.

Cause: a deficiency of aryl/cholesterol sulphatase C which controls cholesterol lipid metabolism, and therefore epidermal desquamation. A minority of patients with XLRI have more extensive X chromosome deletions (contiguous gene defects) which cause a variety of associated problems, including Kallmann syndrome (impaired sense of smell and hypogonadotropic hypogonadism, causing delayed/absent puberty).

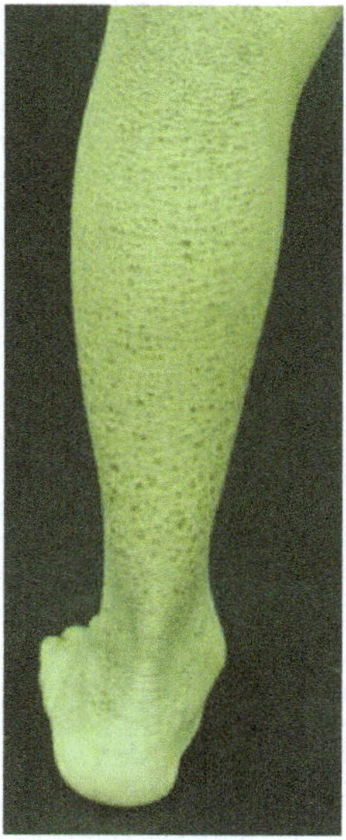

Fig. 27.3 X-linked recessive ichthyosis.

Reproduced with permission Griffiths C. *et al.* (Eds.) (2010). *Rook's Textbook of Dermatology, Eight edition*. Oxford, UK and New York, USA: Wiley-Blackwell.

Rare genetic ichthyoses

Congenital ichthyosiform erythroderma (CIE) affects 1 in 200,000 babies and causes generalized pink to red, taut skin with thin, grey, flaky scales (Fig. 27.4). Most are born with a collodion membrane (➲ see Collodion baby, p. 413).

The erythroderma leads to:
- High transepidermal water loss (TEWL).
- Temperature instability.
- Risk of cardiac or renal failure and infection, especially in the neonatal period.

Lamellar ichthyosis (LI)

Similar in incidence to CIE, LI usually presents as a collodion baby and causes plate-like, dark, adherent scale all over, often with thickening and fissuring of the palms and soles (Fig. 27.5). The underlying inflammation is mild but the taut, scaly skin causes constrictive effects on the digits (contractures), eyelids (ectropion) and ears, and variable functional and cosmetic impairment. Hair is lost from the margins of the scalp (scarring alopecia) and temperature dysregulation is a constant threat.

Children with CIE or LI are sometimes marginalized and teased at school and this can lead to psychosocial disability and isolation.

Bullous ichthyosiform erythroderma (BIE)

BIE is an autosomal dominant keratin (either keratin 1 or 10 mutation) disorder that causes both thick scaling (hyperkeratosis) with redness and skin fragility or blistering (epidermolysis).
- Occurs in 1 in 300,000 births and presents with friction-induced blisters leading to erosions and skin loss in the neonate, similar to staphylococcal scalded skin syndrome (➲ see Infections causing erythroderma, p. 345) or epidermolysis bullosa (➲ see Genetic causes of blisters, p. 387).
- Flexural hyperkeratosis, subtle in early infancy, gradually becomes generalized as the fragility improves. Bacterial infection, mainly staphylococcal, is a constant risk.
- Severely affected children and adults have widespread, ridged scaling (especially in flexures), episodic shedding and erosions, thickened palms, and soles (with keratin 1 mutations) and unpleasant body odour (Figs. 27.6 and 27.7).

Skin biopsy (which should be performed in any neonate with skin fragility or blisters) shows typical microscopic features termed epidermolytic hyperkeratosis. Immunohistochemistry and genetic studies will identify the underlying keratin mutation.

Prenatal diagnosis can be performed on a mid-trimester skin biopsy or with DNA-based testing of a first trimester chorionic villus sample (the index case keratin mutation must be known to do this).

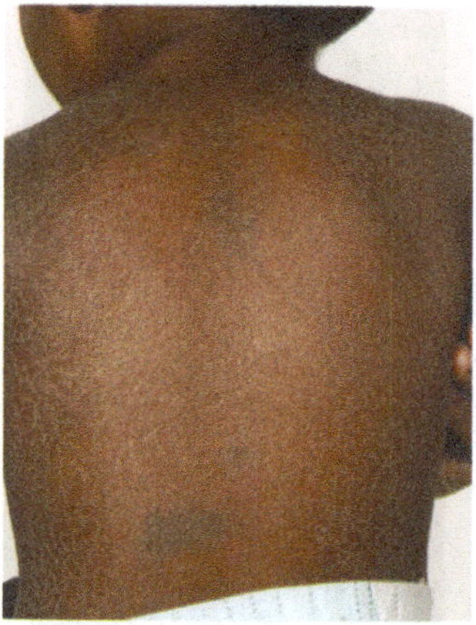

Fig. 27.4 Congenital ichthyosiform erythroderma.

Reproduced with permission Griffiths C. et *al.* (Eds.) (2010). *Rook's Textbook of Dermatology, Eight edition*. Oxford, UK and New York, USA: Wiley-Blackwell.

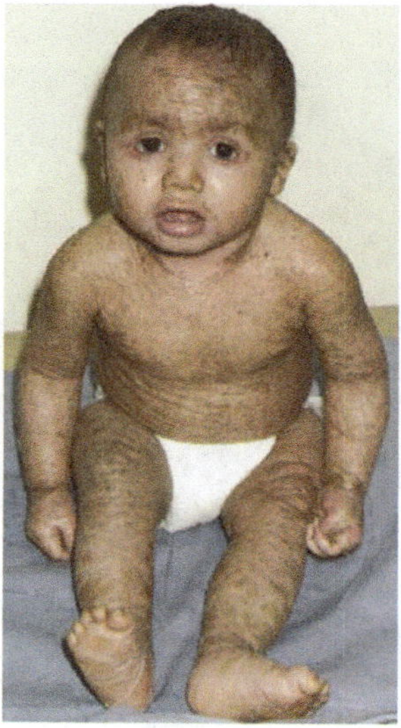

Fig. 27.5 Lamellar ichthyosis.

Reproduced with permission Griffiths C. et *al.* (Eds.) (2010). *Rook's Textbook of Dermatology, Eight edition*. Oxford, UK and New York, USA: Wiley-Blackwell.

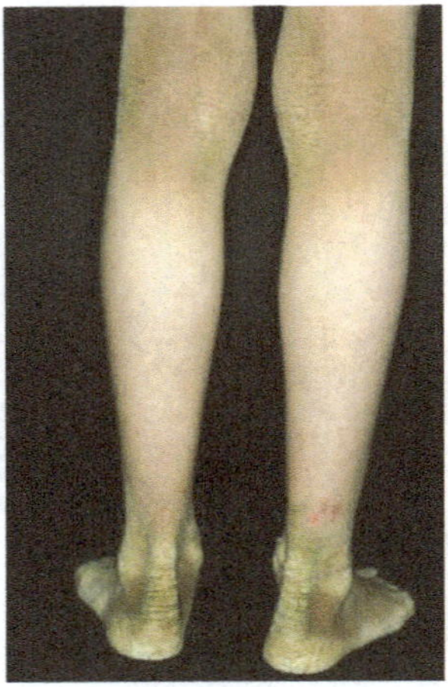

Fig. 27.6 Bullous ichthyosiform erythroderma in older child with ridged flexural hyperkeratosis, erythema, and erosions

Reproduced courtesy of Mary Judge, Consultant Dermatologist, Salford Royal NHS Foundation Trust, UK.

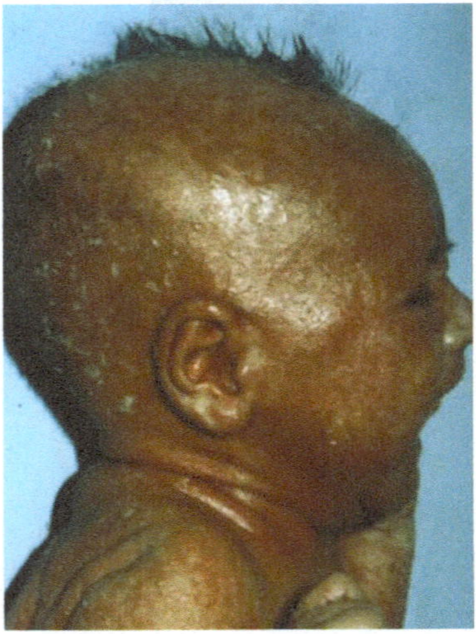

Fig. 27.7 Netherton syndrome with sparse hair, erythroderma, and scaly skin

Reproduced with permission Griffiths C. *et al.* (Eds.) (2010). *Rook's Textbook of Dermatology, Eight edition*. Oxford, UK and New York, USA: Wiley-Blackwell.

Syndromes associated with ichthyosis

Rarely, ichthyosis is associated with significant extracutaneous abnormalities that cause disability. These include:

- Netherton syndrome (➲ see Table 6.2).
- Sjögren Larsson syndrome.
- Refsum disease.
- IBIDS (trichothiodystrophy).
- Neutral lipid storage disease.

These are autosomal recessive disorders that are amenable to prenatal diagnosis.

Netherton syndrome

- See Fig. 27.7.
- An important cause of severe neonatal erythroderma (Fig. 27.10).
- Hypernatraemic dehydration is a particular risk in infancy.
- Associated with faltering growth in most cases (due to erythroderma and enteropathy), which improves in early childhood (➲ see Chapter 6).
- Sparse scalp and body hair due to a 'ball and socket' hair shaft defect (bamboo hair), visible on light microscopy of scalp or eyebrow hair (➲ see Chapters 6 and 14).
- IgE levels are usually raised and specific IgE reactions may develop, especially to food allergens such as fish. There may be associated eczema.

Cause: mutation of *SPINK5*, a gene controlling a serine protease inhibitor in skin and gut.

Treatment: prevention of hypernatraemic dehydration in early life. Manage erythroderma and infection risk. Consider nutritional support. Identify food allergies. For the skin, frequent application of greasy emollients will reduce dryness and water loss. Many patients require intensive care for weeks or months. Most will improve with age.

Caution: topical therapies such as corticosteroids, antiseptics, and calcineurin inhibitors are readily absorbed because of the erythroderma and reduced skin barrier function.

Sjögren Larsson syndrome

A rare neurocutaneous disorder consisting of a generalized, orange-tinged, lichenified scaling, spastic diplegia, and impaired neurological development. A specific retinopathy has also been described. An autosomal recessive disorder due to defective fatty alcohol metabolism in skin and neural (myelin) tissue.

Refsum disease

Classical Refsum's disease presents in early adult life with progressive neurosensory deafness and visual impairment (retinitis pigmentosa). Ataxia, polyneuropathy, and cardiomyopathy occur in some patients. Caused by abnormal metabolism of the long chain amino acid, phytanic acid. Consider screening of family members.

Note: *Infantile Refsum's disease* is an unrelated neurodegenerative disorder without ichthyosis.

IBIDS

An acronym for *i*chthyosis, *b*rittle hair, *i*mpaired intelligence, *d*ecreased fertility, and short stature. Reduced hair sulphur (trichothiodystrophy) is a hallmark and causes 'tiger tail' hair shaft defect. It is due to impaired DNA repair after ultraviolet (UV) exposure, similar to xeroderma pigmentosum type D. Neonates with IBIDS may present with collodion membrane or erythroderma which gives way to prominent ichthyosis, sparse hair, an elfin-face, and progeric features. Neurological deficits have been reported, while photosensitivity occurs in 50%.

Neutral lipid storage disease

Multisystem disorder due to triglyceride deposition (visible on microscopy) in the epidermis, white blood cells (except lymphocytes), liver, gut, and muscle. It may present with neonatal collodion membrane. Later a mild ichthyosis, hepatosplenomegaly, myopathy, and cataracts develop.

X-linked dominant ichthyosis (Conradi–Hünermann–Happle syndrome)

Distinctive skin, skeletal (chondrodysplasia punctata) and ocular syndrome occurring in female infants in a mosaic skin pattern (in Blaschko's lines; ➲ see Fig. 4.6). Presents at birth with a mosaic redness and scaling that improves. Later features include patchy scarring alopecia, atrophic and scaly areas of skin in Blaschko's lines (➲ see Fig. 4.6), cataracts, and bone defects such as scoliosis. It is a peroxisomal disorder, usually lethal *in utero* in affected males.

Treatment of ichthyosis

The aim is to hydrate, lubricate, and 'relax' the skin while enhancing its barrier function with topical agents.

- *Emollient moisturizers* can be regularly applied as creams or ointments and used for cleansing the skin as bath oils and soap substitute lotions. The benefits of emollients are enhanced by application after bathing, with the use of dressings or stretch garments, the addition of humectant agents or urea, and gentle abrasives such as a loofah.
- *Keratolytics* (to aid desquamation) such as alpha hydroxy acids, salicylic acid, or propylene glycol can be added to an emollient base. *Salicylic acid should not be used in infants and young children because of the risk of salicylate toxicity and acidosis, due to a large surface area and, when present, erythroderma* (➲ see Chapter 3).
- *Topical vitamin D compounds* (calcipotriol) and retinoids (tazarotene) are sometimes helpful in adults but may be irritant.
- *Oral retinoid therapy* (acitretin or isotretinoin) is beneficial in moderate to severe ichthyoses. Retinoids have side effects that are predictable (dry lips and skin, increased fragility in BIE) and unpredictable (musculoskeletal or liver dysfunction, raised serum lipids) and require careful monitoring (specialist prescription only).
- *Systemic retinoids are teratogenic.*

Although the gene mutations causing many of the inherited ichthyoses are known, gene replacement therapy or topical use of the gene products is still some way off.

Collodion baby

Neonates born with shiny, tight, yellow, membranous skin are called *collodion babies (Fig. 27.8; ➲ see Collodion baby, p. 88). They usually have everted eyelids and lips (ectropion and eclabium), reduced nasal airways, and tethered ears and digits. The membrane dries, cracks at the flexures and is shed within 2–6 weeks (Fig. 27.9).

Outcome: a small minority may go on to have normal skin (self-healing collodion baby) but in the majority, the membrane gives way to a generalized, inflamed ichthyosis of which there are two main types:

- Congenital ichthyosiform erythroderma (Fig. 27.4).
- Lamellar ichthyosis (Fig. 27.5).

A number of different gene mutations, including of transglutaminase 1, have been found in some of these patients.

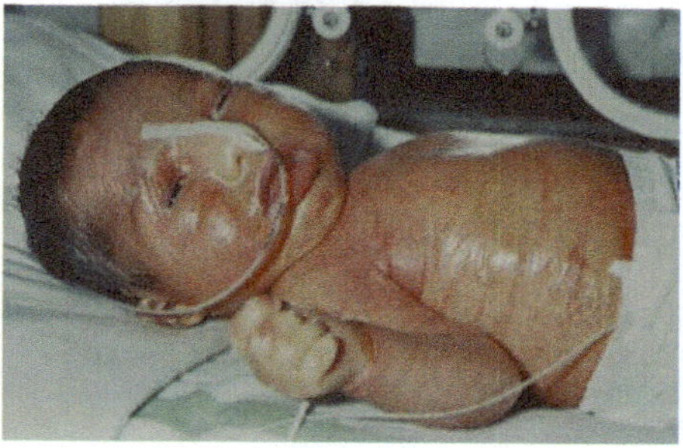

Fig. 27.8 Collodion baby

Reproduced with permission Griffiths C. *et al.* (Eds.) (2010). *Rook's Textbook of Dermatology, Eight edition*. Oxford, UK and New York, USA: Wiley-Blackwell.

*Collodion is a shiny, tacky, yellow substance which is used to seal and protect wounds, to apply wart paints, and in theatrical make-up).

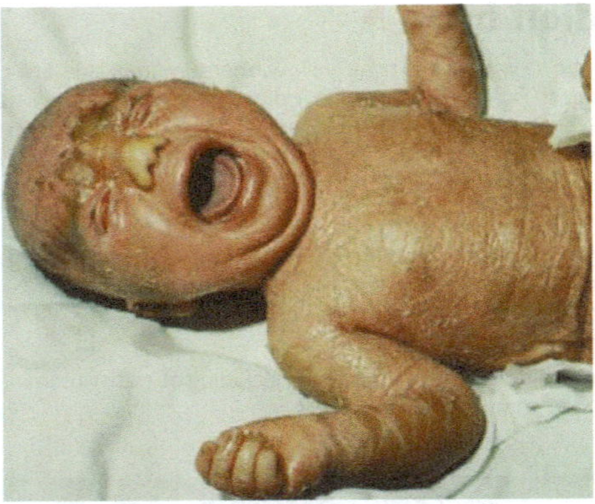

Fig. 27.9 Collodion baby in shedding phase (same baby as in Fig. 27.8 and Fig. 27.5)
Reproduced courtesy of Mary Judge, Consultant Dermatologist, Salford Royal NHS Foundation Trust, UK.

Harlequin ichthyosis (HI)

A very rare and severe congenital ichthyosis with a striking and distinctive neonatal presentation and high perinatal mortality.

- Causes generalized thickened, leathery, and taut skin encasing the newborn like a rigid coat of armour, restricting movement, breathing, and feeding, and affecting temperature control. There is marked ectropion, chemosis (conjunctival oedema), and eclabium (open mouth due to lip eversion).
- After birth, desiccation splitting of the thick, tight skin across the scalp, trunk, and flexures produces a pattern resembling a harlequin costume.
- HI is an autosomal recessive disorder due to mutations in an epidermal lipid transporter gene, *ABCA12*.

Outcome: many are either stillborn or quickly succumb to respiratory, metabolic, or infective complications. However, there are now several survivors (managed with specialized neonatal intensive care and oral retinoid therapy). They will usually have lifelong inflamed ichthyosis, similar to severe CIE.

Management of the collodion baby and Harlequin ichthyosis

Ask for an urgent dermatological opinion

Accurate clinical diagnosis is important, while skin biopsy is generally not helpful in the neonatal period.

- Admit to neonatal intensive care unit (NICU).
- Nurse in incubator with moderate humidity.
- Heated mat if in cot.
- Greasy emollients (e.g. emulsifying ointment, 50/50 paraffin mix) all over every 3–4h (new pot daily), cot-bath with an emollient antiseptic wash lotion.
- Lubricant for eyes (e.g. simple eye ointment, lacrilube, and tears). *Urgent ophthalmological consultation.*
- Regular skin and eye swabs. Watch for signs of infection and treat accordingly. Antibiotics only if clinically indicated.
- Baseline blood tests, monitor electrolytes, renal function, and albumen regularly. Adequate fluids, try modified teat if poor suck (➲ see also Chapter 25); use nasogastric feeding if unable to maintain intake; consider protein supplements.
- Consider early oral retinoid therapy for HI.
- Later on, genetics referral for DNA studies and counselling.

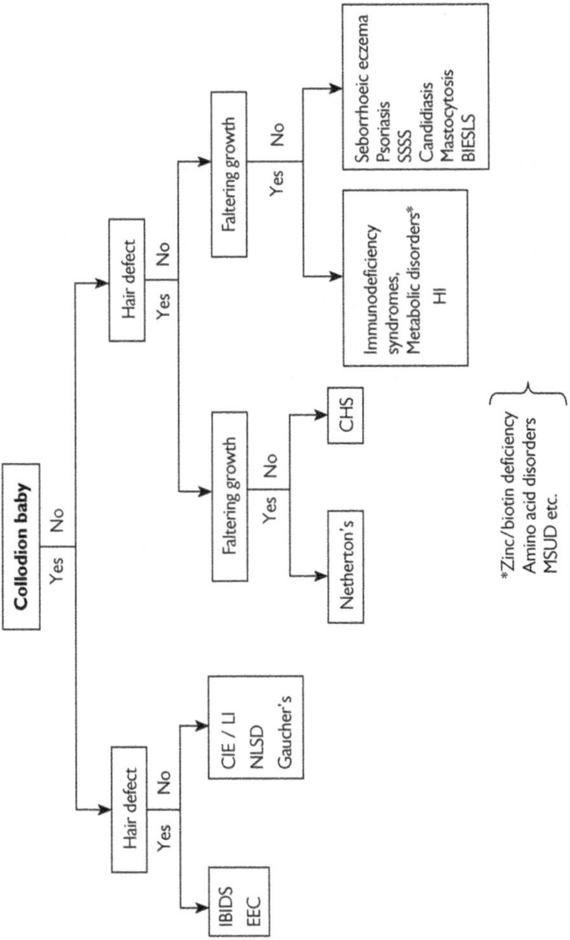

Fig. 27.10 Neonatal erythroderma algorithm.

Chapter 28

Lumps and bumps

Introduction

Lump and bump are non-medical terms of Nordic origin implying visible and/or palpable swellings, lump (technical term, nodule) meaning a deeper and larger entity than bump (papule). Many different processes can present as single or multiple papules and/or nodules, and a lump apparent at the skin surface may be due to deeper pathology (e.g. a lymph node or musculoskeletal structure). Some lumps and bumps may indicate underlying diseases or potential problems (Box 28.1). Only diseases that involve the skin and subcutaneous fat are considered in this chapter and some are also described elsewhere. There are a large number of skin tumours which are very rare in children and only the better known are discussed.

In children the *processes* that may cause lumps and bumps include:

- Hamartoma—an abnormal quantity or arrangement of cells or tissue.
- Neoplasm—a new growth, benign and malignant.
- Cyst—a walled structure with solid or fluid contents.
- Inflammation.
- Infection.

Box 28.1 Reasons that lumps and bumps may be important include:

- Malignancy, e.g. lymphoma, neuroblastoma.
- Infection, e.g. kerion.
- Sign of serious disease, e.g. Langerhans cell histiocytosis.
- Genetic implications, e.g. skin lesions of neurofibromatosis.
- Local disruption, e.g. massive facial haemangioma.
- Parental anxiety.

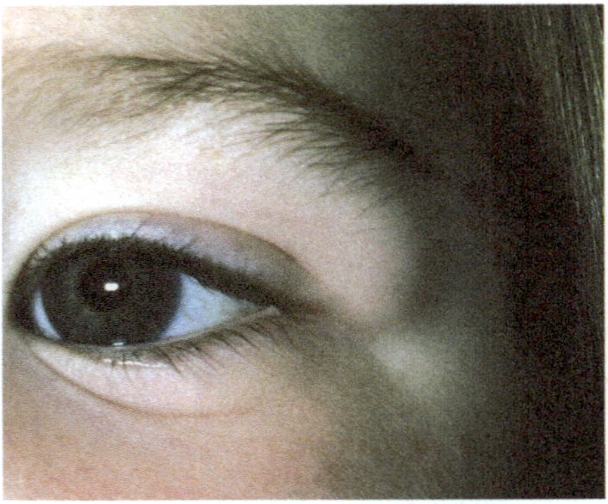

Fig. 28.1 Dermoid cyst.

Reproduced courtesy of Cameron Kennedy, Departments of Dermatology, Bristol Royal Infirmary and Paediatric Dermatology, Bristol Royal Hospital for Children, Bristol, UK

Assessment

A full history and examination in a good light with palpation and inspection are essential. To make a differential clinical diagnosis, the following information will be useful:

- Age at onset.
- Location on the body.
- Whether single or multiple.
- Characteristics of the lesion(s):
  - Size and colour.
  - Location within the skin/subcutis.
  - Surface and texture.
  - Symptoms (pain, tenderness, itch, etc.).

Notes

- Colour can vary in deeper lesions depending on local blood flow (e.g. panniculitis and nodular vasculitis may be skin-coloured, red, or bluish).
- It may be necessary to observe a lesion such as a mole over time with good-quality images incorporating a measurement scale.

Investigations

These depend on the clinical picture. Histology may be decisive for diagnosis and discussion with the pathologist before a biopsy can make the difference between diagnostic success and failure. Lesional swabs, blood tests, radiographs, etc. may be indicated when infection or neoplasia is suspected. Dermoscopy can assist in diagnosis of melanocytic, vascular and many other lesions (Box 28.1) (see also Chapter 2).

Diagnosis: take into account the colour, surface, texture, symptoms, and site of a lesion

Colour

- See also Section 6, Discolouration of the skin.

Skin-coloured lumps and bumps (lesions)

- ***Connective tissue naevi***: usually skin-coloured dermal plaques which can be single or multiple and can be associated with various syndromes, e.g. 'shagreen patch' of tuberous sclerosis complex (see Fig. 29.14 and Tuberous sclerosis complex, p. 483); Buschke–Ollendorff syndrome—an autosomal dominant condition with multiple small connective tissue naevi associated with osteopoikilosis (see also Connective tissue naevi, pp. 449–50).
- ***Molluscum contagiosum*** (see Infection, p. 281 and Fig. 9.7): usually multiple, with indented (umbilicated) centres. Sometimes lesions become inflamed (see Fig. 19.1).
  Cause: molluscipox virus.
- ***Closed comedo***: *syn*. Whitehead.
- ***Cysts***: especially dermoid (Fig. 28.1) a smooth cystic swelling, usually present at birth and fixed to periosteum. It is common around the eyes. Intracranial extension can occur so perform imaging prior to surgery. Other types of cyst, e.g. epidermoid cyst (see Neonatal/infantile lumps, p. 433) feel similar but are not present at birth and not fixed to bone.

- *Neurofibroma*: a softish, skin-coloured lump (Fig. 28.2) rare before adolescence. May be solitary but the presence of six or more café-au-lait macules is indicative of a diagnosis of neurofibromatosis type 1 (➲ see Localized forms of brown pigmentations, pp. 491–4).
- *Lipoma*: a benign tumour of fat cell origin. Feels soft, smooth, and is often large, and may be tender. Multiple lesions are occasionally associated with syndromes (➲ see Fat changes, pp. 452–3).
- *Granuloma annulare*: dermal papules and nodules usually in ring-shaped (annular) arrangement (Fig. 28.3; ➲ see also Fig. 5.1) in an acral distribution—may be red/bluish and there are rare variants (➲ see Fig. 9.9).
- *Keloid scars*: a firm/hard overgrowth of scar tissue, sometimes following injury, surgery (Fig. 28.4), in association with acne (acne keloids; ➲ see Fig. 18.8), or spontaneously. Unlike hypertrophic scars, they do not resolve spontaneously. They are red initially, slowly become skin-coloured with age and can be itchy and painful. Ear-ring keloids are common in young girls (➲ see Fig. 9.8).
- *Syringomas*: benign sweat gland tumours presenting as small papules around eyes and nose, usually in older children/teenagers. May be confused with milia.

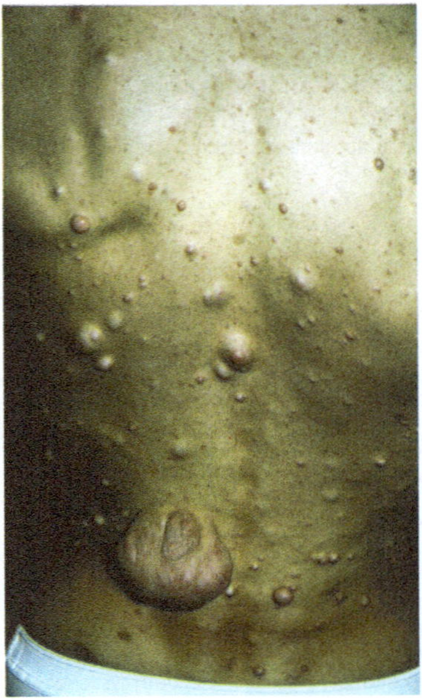

Fig. 28.2 Neurofibromata.

Reproduced courtesy of Cameron Kennedy, Consultant Dermatologist, Departments of Dermatology, Bristol Royal Infirmary and Paediatric Dermatology, Bristol Royal Hospital for Children, Bristol, UK

- *Milium(a)*: tiny skin-coloured or white papules common on the face (➲ see Fig. 9.6) especially in the newborn (➲ see Transient benign neonatal dermatoses, p. 81) and following some deeper blistering disorders or trauma. They contain layers of keratin.

Red lesions

- *Haemangioma of infancy*: superficial type (➲ see Vascular tumours, pp. 94–9 and Figs. 8.3 and 8.5).
- *Pyogenic granuloma*: a misnomer; actually a lobular capillary haemangioma, often following minor trauma. Bright red, often with rapid growth, and can bleed profusely (Fig. 28.5). May become crusted or superficially infected and thrombose (➲ see Black lesions, p. 426). *Treatment*: surgical excision or curettage.
- *Spitz naevus*: a melanocytic proliferation, benign, but has a distinctive histology that can resemble melanoma. Often red but can be brown or even black (➲ see Fig. 34.5). Rapid growth should prompt removal to exclude Spitzoid melanoma.
- *Mast cell naevus (syn. mastocytoma)*: dermal plaque usually appearing during infancy. The distinctive feature is acute swelling and sometimes blistering with pruritus when the lesion is rubbed. The colour varies from red to reddish brown or yellowish (Fig. 28.6); ➲ see Non-infective causes, pp. 285–8 and Differential diagnosis of urticarial rashes, pp. 313–16 for other types of mastocytosis.
- *Keloid*: ➲ see Colour, pp. 419–27 and Fig. 28.4.
- *Erythema nodosum*: subcutaneous/deep dermal nodules due to inflammation in the deep dermis and subcutaneous fat. It typically occurs as tender lumps on the shins (➲ see Fig. 12.10), often with arthralgia. Common causes include streptococcal infection and tuberculosis.
- *Leukaemia in skin*: subcutaneous/deep dermal, sometimes bluish (Fig. 28.7).

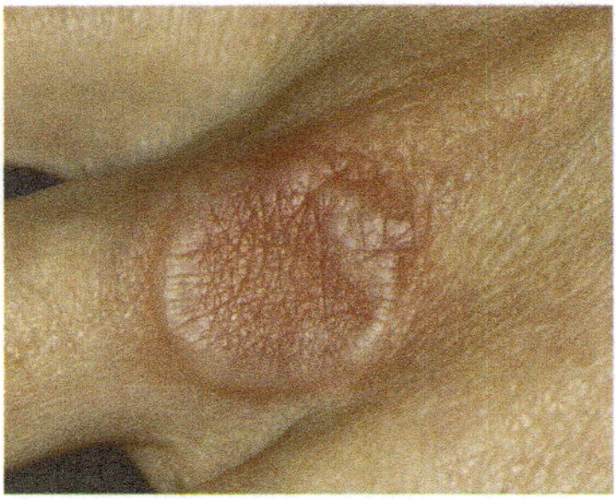

Fig. 28.3 Granuloma annulare.

Reproduced courtesy of Cameron Kennedy, Consultant Dermatologist, Departments of Dermatology, Bristol Royal Infirmary and Paediatric Dermatology, Bristol Royal Hospital for Children, Bristol, UK

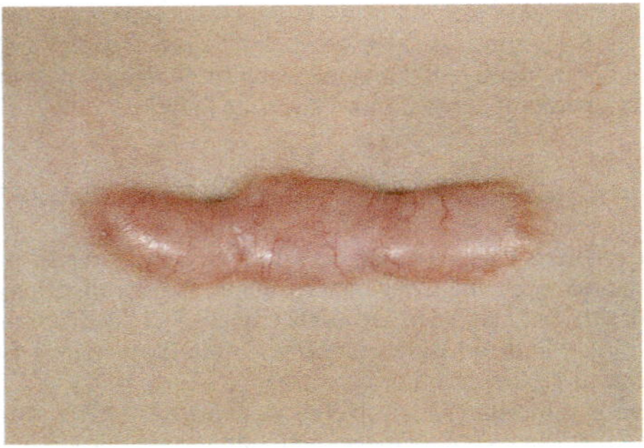

Fig. 28.4 Keloid on upper chest following surgery.
Reproduced courtesy of NHS Tayside Clinical Photography, Dundee, UK

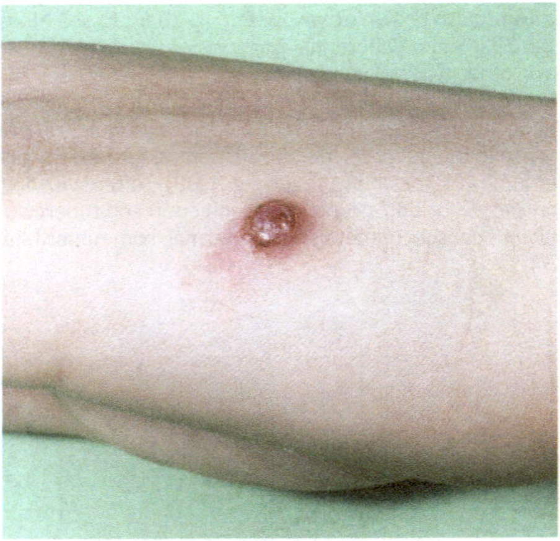

Fig. 28.5 Pyogenic granuloma.
Reproduced courtesy of Cameron Kennedy, Consultant Dermatologist, Departments of Dermatology, Bristol Royal Infirmary and Paediatric Dermatology, Bristol Royal Hospital for Children, Bristol, UK

- *Nasal glioma*: ➲ see Symptoms, pp. 427–9 and Some classical presentations, pp. 429–33.
- *Leiomyoma*: benign, smooth muscle tumours, often multiple on trunk, and painful to touch and in the cold.
- *Umbilical granuloma* or polyp: usually presents as recurrently infected, sometimes red nodule in umbilicus (Fig. 28.8). If there is persisting

discharge, it may represent persistence of the embryological connection to the gut or bladder. Therefore do not excise without imaging first.
- *Aseptic facial granuloma*: uncommon acne-like cysts on face in young children without evidence of true acne, commonly solitary, and may be a variant of rosacea. May respond to oral antibiotics.

Blue lesions

Common

- ***Haemangioma*** of infancy, deep type: often resemble a bruise
- ***Venous malformation***: soft, blue, partially compressible and can feel like spaghetti under the skin (➲ see Fig. 8.17).
- ***Pilomatrixoma***: benign hair follicle tumour; recognizable by the very hard texture, often multilobular (➲ see Surface and texture, p. 429). May see whitish centre from calcification (typically seen on histopathological examination).
- ***Blue naevus***: deep melanocytic naevus, usually benign. Often flat but can be raised papule/nodule (➲ see Fig. 35.1).
- ***Chilblains (perniosis)***: purplish blue-cold areas-usually toes where they may be nodular (➲ see Fig. 31.9).

Uncommon to rare

- ***Glomus tumour*** (glomangioma): tender/painful, often purplish, tumour of glomus apparatus (rare). Single or multiple and usually familial.
- ***Blue-rubber blebs***: multiple venous cutaneous anomalies associated with similar lesions in the bowel, leading to gastrointestinal haemorrhage and anaemia. Rare autosomal dominant.
- ***Secondary skin deposit from neuroblastoma***: typically blanch on gentle rubbing.
- ***Sweat gland cyst (e.g. hidrocystoma)***: uncommon in children, can be trans-illuminated (e.g. using an auroscope).

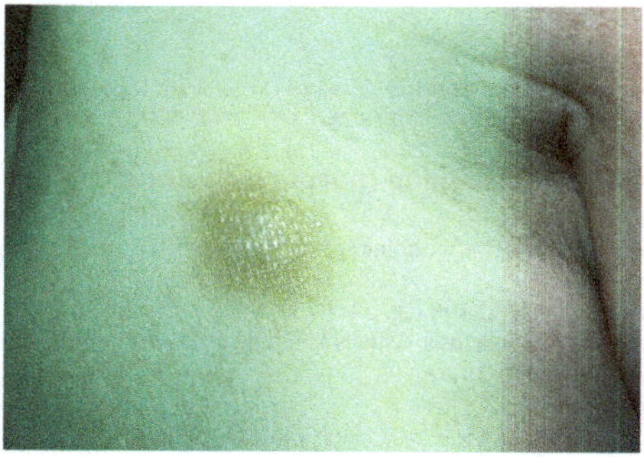

Fig. 28.6 Mastocytoma.

Reproduced courtesy of Cameron Kennedy, Consultant Dermatologist, Departments of Dermatology, Bristol Royal Infirmary and Paediatric Dermatology, Bristol Royal Hospital for Children, Bristol, UK

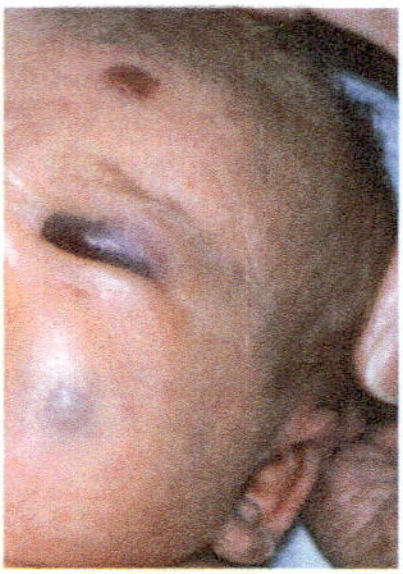

Fig. 28.7 Leukaemic deposit (blueberry muffin lesions).

Reproduced courtesy of Cameron Kennedy, Consultant Dermatologist, Departments of Dermatology, Bristol Royal Infirmary and Paediatric Dermatology, Bristol Royal Hospital for Children, Bristol, UK

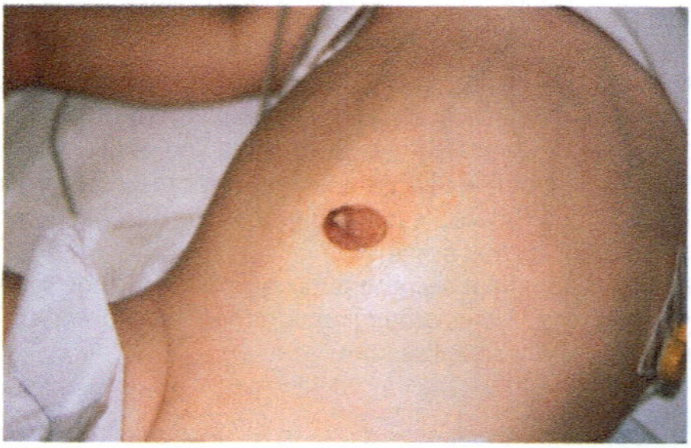

Fig. 28.8 Umbilical granuloma.

Reproduced courtesy of Cameron Kennedy, Consultant Dermatologist, Departments of Dermatology, Bristol Royal Infirmary and Paediatric Dermatology, Bristol Royal Hospital for Children, Bristol, UK

Purple and non-blanching (purpuric) lesions

- ➲ See also Chapter 31.
- *Vasculitis*: e.g. Henoch–Schönlein purpura (➲ see Fig. 31.4). May be nodular.
- *Perniosis* (chilblains; ➲ see Fig. 31.9).
- *Langerhans cell histiocytosis*: usually multiple small lesions that may be purpuric (➲ see Fig. 13.5).

Brown lesions

- ➲ See also Chapter 33.

Common

- *Melanocytic naevus (mole)*: ➲ see Fig. 34.1.
- *Dermatofibroma*: firm to hard dermal nodule, which feels attached to the skin surface, but mobile over deeper structures. May be skin-coloured, pink, or when pigmented often a rusty brown colour; usually more pronounced around the edges (Figs. 28.9 and 28.10). Uncommon before the second decade. Sometimes a secondary reaction to arthropod bites.

- *Epidermal naevus*: plaques of rough and bumpy brown papules (warty texture), in an arrangement determined by Blaschko's lines (➲ see Some classical presentations, p. 429 and Fig. 4.5). May be skin-coloured initially, becoming darker with age and sometimes increasing in numbers and distribution.
- *Viral warts*: ➲ see Some classical presentations, pp. 429–33 and Fig. 9.5; may be brown.

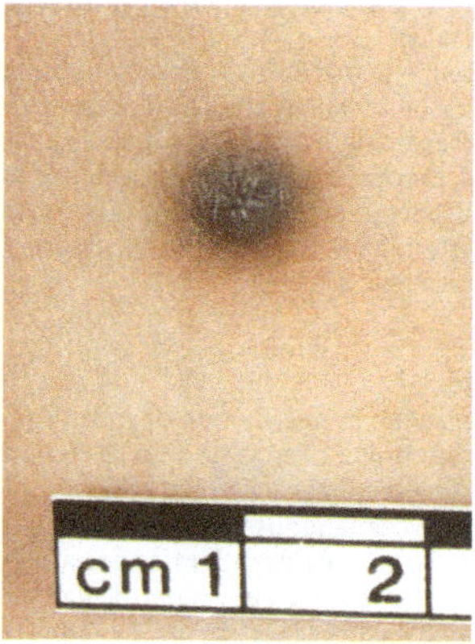

Fig. 28.9 Pigmented dermatofibroma.

Reproduced courtesy of Cameron Kennedy, Consultant Dermatologist, Departments of Dermatology, Bristol Royal Infirmary and Paediatric Dermatology, Bristol Royal Hospital for Children, Bristol, UK

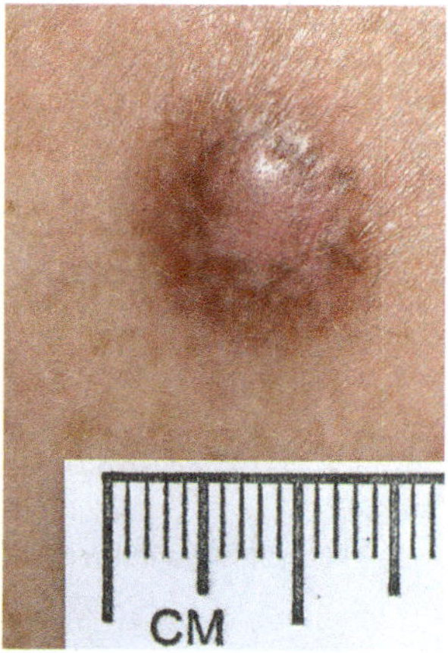

Fig. 28.10 Dermatofibroma with typical peripheral ring of pigmentation.

Reproduced courtesy of Susan Lewis-Jones, Hon Consultant Dermatologist, Ninewells Hospital and Medical School, Dundee, UK

Rare

- *Melanoma*: rare in children but should be suspected in a lesion with appropriate features (➲ see Malignant skin tumours, p. 435 and Fig. 34.8). May be dark brown or black or a mixture of colours including red.
- *Atypical mycobacterial infections*: may present as brownish or red, irregular nodules either on the neck (scrofuloderma; ➲ see Fig. 22.11), usually from bovine tuberculosis (common in endemic areas); or on the hands as fish-tank granulomas (➲ see Fig. 12.6), usually from *Mycobacterium marinum*.
- *Deep fungal infection*: e.g. mycetoma (tropics/subtropical regions). Caused by a variety of *Actinomycetes* and *Eumycetes*. Other rare fungal infections presenting with irregular papules and nodules are sporotrichosis, chromoblastomycosis, systemic mycosis (e.g. blastomycosis). Suspect in atypical nodular lesions, especially when associated with systemic malaise or immunosuppression, and in immigrants from endemic areas.

Yellowish lesions

- ➲ See also Chapter 37.
- *Juvenile xanthogranuloma*: classically one or more circular well-defined nodules varying from bright orange/yellow to reddish brown but can be highly variable in clinical appearance (Fig. 28.11; ➲ see also Fig. 37.3). They usually resolve spontaneously over years, but there is a rare association with more serious disorders, especially eye involvement so ask for an ophthalmological review for periocular lesions.
- *Cysts*: more frequently skin-coloured.
- *Mast cell naevus (mastocytoma)*: may be yellow, brown, or red (Fig. 28.6; see also Fixed annual urticated rash, pp. 314–15).
- *Xanthoma*: may also appear reddish, usually multiple, caused by deposits of histiocytic foam cells containing lipids. Several clinical types exist (➲ see Figs. 5.3 and 37.2).
- *Langerhans cell histiocytosis*: usually multiple small lesions which may be purpuric (➲ see Fig. 13.5).

Black lesions

- ➲ See also Chapter 35.

Common

- *Melanocytic naevus (mole)*: may be black (➲ see Chapter 34).
- *Thrombosed haemangioma*: e.g. pyogenic granuloma (Fig. 28.12).
- *Thrombosed vessels in warts* (➲ see Fig. 12.9).
- *Dermatofibroma*: very rarely dark brown/black (see brown lesions, earlier; Fig. 28.9).
- *Open comedo*: (blackhead; ➲ see Fig. 18.2).
- *Traumatic bleeding into skin*: talon noir (black heel) (➲ see Fig. 35.3).

Rare

- *Melanoma*: (➲ see Fig. 34.8 and Malignant skin tumours, p. 435).

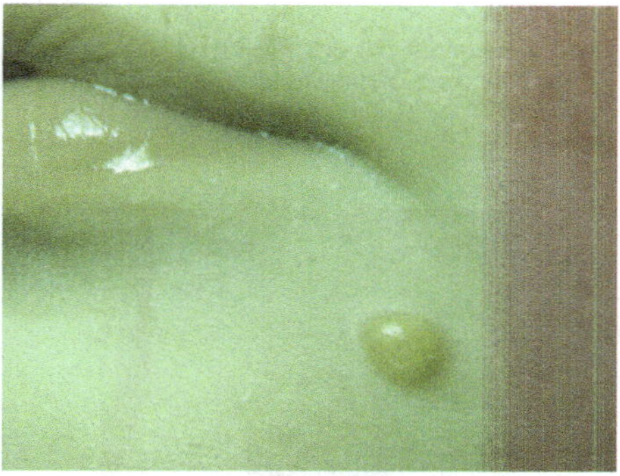

Fig. 28.11 Juvenile xanthogranuloma.

Reproduced courtesy of Cameron Kennedy, Consultant Dermatologist,Departments of Dermatology, Bristol Royal Infirmary and Paediatric Dermatology, Bristol Royal Hospital for Children, Bristol, UK

Translucent lesions

- ***Various adnexal tumours*** (e.g. sweat gland cyst): usually benign tumours (commonest type).
- ***Lymphangioma***: e.g. lymphangioma circumscriptum (*syn.* microcystic lymphatic malformation) often become blood-filled so there may be a mixture of translucent and red lesions (Fig. 28.13; see also Lymphatic malformations, pp. 112–16).

Symptoms

Painful or tender

- ***Corn***: yellowish hard skin, distinguished from warts by retention of dermatoglyphics (skin 'prints'), which are lost in warts.
- ***Plantar verrucae***: (warts; see Fig. 29.4).
- ***Foreign body granuloma***: e.g. on sole from stepping on glass, etc.
- ***Erythema nodosum***: tender red nodules on shins (see Fig. 12.10).
- ***Keloid scars***: often very painful or itchy (Fig. 28.4).
- ***Thrombosed or infected infantile haemangioma***: (see Fig. 8.6).
- ***Thrombosed pyogenic granuloma***: (Fig. 28.12).
- ***Neurofibroma***: (Fig. 28.2; see also Localized forms of brown pigmentation, pp. 491–4).
- ***Venous malformation***: (see Fig. 8.16).
- ***Glomus tumour***: (see earlier section in this chapter on Colour).
- ***Eccrine spiradenoma***: tumour of eccrine sweat glands.
- ***Leiomyoma***: benign smooth muscle tumours (several types). Small red papules/nodules, typically painful in response to touch and cold.
- ***Angiolipoma***: resemble lipomas but often bluish and have a marked capillary component. May be multiple and a rare infiltrative form occurs.

Itchy

- *Mast cell naevus (mastocytoma)*: urticates on rubbing (Fig. 28.6).
- Insect bite reaction: crops of itchy red papules, usually in exposed sites (➲ see Fig. 19.4).
- *Scabies nodules*: (Fig. 28.14; ➲ see also Chapters 20 and 22).

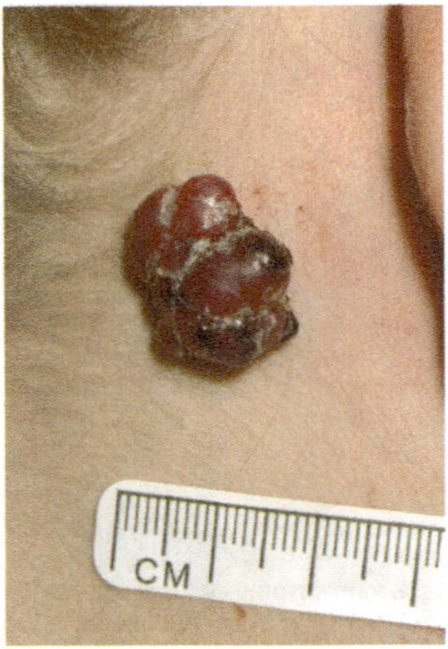

Fig. 28.12 Thrombosing pyogenic granuloma with early black necrotic areas.
Reproduced courtesy of NHS Tayside Clinical Photography, Dundee, UK

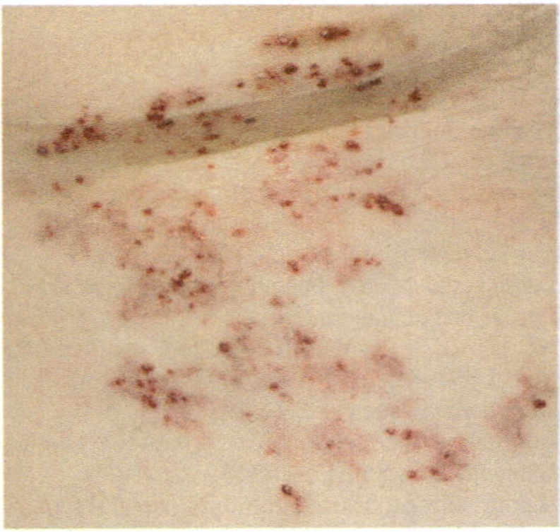

Fig. 28.13 Microcystic lymphatic malformation (Lymphangioma circumscriptum).
Reproduced courtesy of NHS Tayside Clinical Photography, Dundee, UK

- *Prurigo nodularis*: unusual in children (➲ see Other rashes sometimes confused with eczema, p. 262).
- *Keloid scars*: often very itchy or painful (Fig. 28.4).
- *Dermatofibromas*: occasionally mildly itchy (Figs. 28.9 and 28.10).

Surface and texture

Pay particular attention to the surface and feel; many lesions have a distinctive shape or surface, e.g. indented or ulcerated (see Box 28.2). There may be a particular texture, e.g. smooth, rough/warty, and they may feel soft, hard, or cystic (Box 28.3). Temperature is sometimes important, e.g. chilblains are cold, infective lesions are often hot (but not always).

Some classical presentations

Rapidly enlarging soft red lesions

- In a young infant this is likely to be an infantile haemangioma (IH)—soft and compressible (usually) and very common (➲ see Chapter 8).
- If small and bleeding, any age then pyogenic granuloma (Fig. 28.12) is most likely. It may be multilobulate and irregular.
- Consider sarcoma if reddish brown or purple firm tumour which may enlarge rapidly. Very rare but important not to miss. May be mistaken for haemangiomas.
- On glabellar area consider nasal glioma (rare). These are firmer than IH (Fig. 28.16).

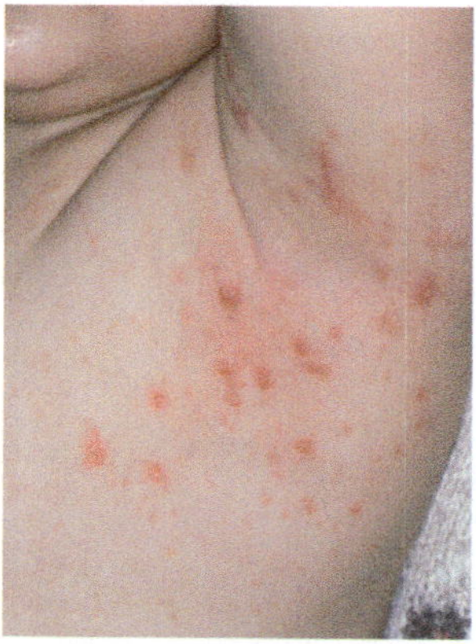

Fig. 28.14 Scabetic nodules, red-brown and very itchy.

Reproduced courtesy of Susan Lewis-Jones, Hon Consultant Dermatologist, Ninewells Hospital and Medical School, Dundee, UK

Firm red lesions

- *Erythema nodosum*: tender lesions, usually shins, last approx. 10 days or so, fading to leave temporary bruise (➲ see Fig. 12.10). Associated with streptococcal sore throats; tuberculosis (TB) (rare in the United Kingdom); inflammatory bowel disease; rheumatoid arthritis; sarcoidosis (rare in children); oral contraceptive pill. No cause found in many.

Box 28.2 Surface changes and shape of lesions

Indented (umbilicated)
- Molluscum contagiosum—lesions usually multiple.
- Giant comedo.
- Basal cell cancers (rare in children; ➲ see Malignant skin tumours, p. 435).

Exophytic (sticking out) or polypoid
- Filiform wart (➲ see Fig. 9.5).
- Pyogenic granuloma (Fig. 28.12).

Ulcerated (➲ see also Chapter 30).
- Superficial infantile haemangioma (➲ see Chapter 8).
- Pyogenic granuloma (➲ see Colour, pp. 419–27).
- Deep seated infection—fungal, pyogenic, mycobacterial.
- Poxvirus infections (➲ see Viral infections, pp. 398–401 and Fig. 26.7b).
- Leishmaniasis (➲ see Infections and parasites, pp. 283–5 and Fig. 30.2).
- Malignancy—primary, e.g. squamous cell cancer post-radiotherapy or secondary deposits (➲ see Malignant skin tumours, p. 435).

Hairy
- Melanocytic naevi (➲ see Chapter 34).
- Hairy naevus, e.g. Becker's naevus (➲ Fig. 33.2), faun-tail naevus (➲ Fig. 14.13).

See also Box 28.3 on textural changes.

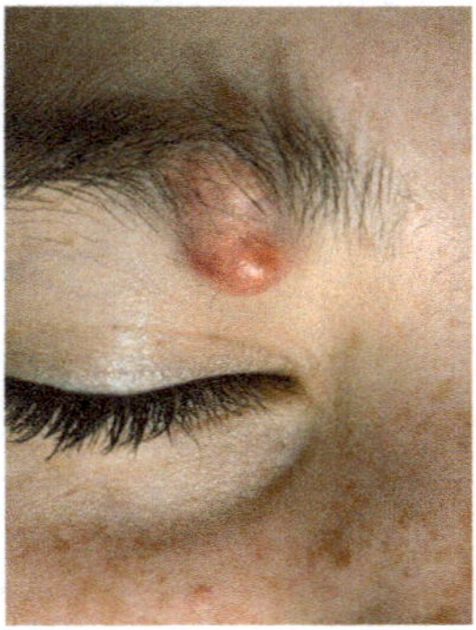

Fig. 28.15 Pilomatrixoma.

Reproduced courtesy of Cameron Kennedy, Consultant Dermatologist, Departments of Dermatology, Bristol Royal Infirmary and Paediatric Dermatology, Bristol Royal Hospital for Children, Bristol, UK

Box 28.3 Texture

Hard

- Pilomatrixoma (Fig. 28.15).
- Osteoma and exostosis.
- Calcinosis.
- Chondroma.

Soft

- Neurofibroma.
- Lipoma.
- Haemangioma.

Keratotic (warty)

- Wart.
- Angiokeratoma.

Smooth

- Lipoma.
- Pilomatrixoma.
- Dermoid.
- Keloid.

Firm

- Dermatofibroma.
- Keloid.
- Fibroma.
- Dermoid.
- Prurigo nodularis.
- Angiofibroma.
- Various malignancies.
- Accessory auricle, digit, nipple.

Cystic

- Acne (usually teens).
- Epidermoid (usually teens).
- Cystic hygroma—a macrocystic lymphatic malformation (➲ see Chapter 8).
- Dermoid.
- Steatocystoma.
- Eruptive vellus hair cysts.

- ***Spitz naevi***: quite common and very variable presentations—may also be brown or multicoloured (➔ see Fig. 34.5). Multiple grouped lesions (agminate spitz lesions) are rare.
- ***Scabetic nodules***: (Fig. 28.14).
- ***Sarcomas***: may be purplish brown (➔ see Rapidly enlarging soft red lesions, p. 429).

Firm brown lesions

- ***Dermatofibroma***; especially if skin-coloured with ring of pigment (commoner on legs). Feel smooth and may be itchy (Fig. 28.10).
- ***Moles (melanocytic naevi)***: ➔ see Chapter 34.
- ***Fibromas***, e.g. digital fibroma (➔ see Fig. 29.15).

Warty lesions

- ***Viral warts (verrucae vulgaris)***: small, usually multiple affecting almost every child and occurring anywhere on the body (➔ see Figs. 9.5, 12.9, and 29.4). Caused by human papilloma virus (HPV), which has many strains, some of which are linked to cutaneous and cervical cancer. May be a problem in the immunosuppressed (e.g. renal transplant recipients). All warts may koebnerize, i.e. appear in site of injury due to inoculation (➔ see Chapter 4).
  Treatment of warts: keratolytic agents (wart paints) and paring are usually effective in children and less painful than cryotherapy.
- ***Planar warts***: flat, small skin-coloured lesions usually multiple (➔ see Fig. 29.5).
- ***Epidermal naevus***: often in linear distribution. Do not resolve (Fig. 28.17; ➔ see also Figs. 4.5 and 4.10).
- ***Angiokeratomas***: rare warty vascular lesions—several types which may be single or multiple and the latter can be related to systemic disease (rare lysosomal disorders, e.g. Fabry's disease).

Smooth, umbilicated tumours

- ***Molluscum contagiosum***: usually multiple, small, and skin-coloured—often become inflamed when resolving (➔ see Figs. 19.1 and 9.7).

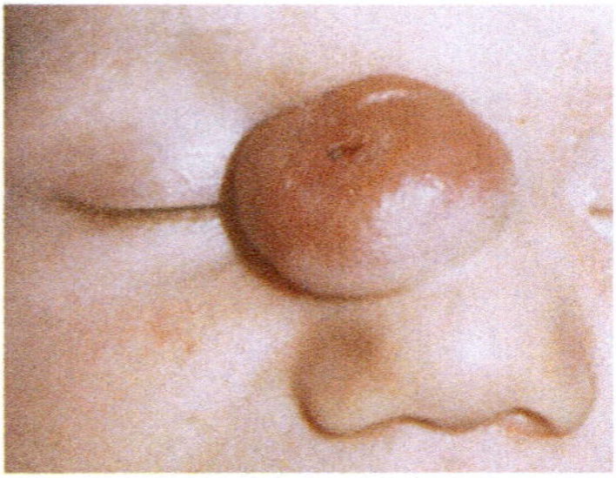

Fig. 28.16 Nasal glioma.

Reproduced courtesy of Cameron Kennedy, Consultant Dermatologist, Departments of Dermatology, Bristol Royal Infirmary and Paediatric Dermatology, Bristol Royal Hospital for Children, Bristol, UK

- *Epidermoid cysts* often have a central punctum sometimes causing an umbilicated appearance (Fig. 28.18).

Hot red lumps

- *Abscesses*: hidradenitis suppurativa (➲ see Flexural skin problems, pp. 155–8).
- *Erythema nodosum*: ➲ see Some classical presentations, pp. 429–33.
- *Idiopathic palmoplantar hidradenitis*: extremely rare.

Cold red/purple/blue lumps

- *Perniosis*: *syn.* chilblains (➲ see Fig. 31.9).
- *Job's syndrome*: *syn.* hyper IgE syndrome: recurrent respiratory and cutaneous infections, including cold abscesses; associated with severe eczema, high IgE levels, dental and skeletal problems. They have typical coarse facies with a broad nose. Very rare autosomal dominant.

Neonatal/infantile lumps

- ➲ See also Tumours in the newborn, p. 90.
- *Milia*: 1–2mm whitish papules on the face (➲ see also Colour, pp. 419–27).
- *Subcutaneous fat necrosis*: firm skin-coloured, red, or purplish nodules and plaques, often on buttocks, back, and cheeks; preceding hypoxia and/or trauma is common. They may become calcified (➲ see Other rashes in the newborn, pp. 82–3).
- *Bilateral congenital fatty heel pads*: smooth swellings.
- *Blueberry muffin lesions*: bluish solid lesions usually on the cheeks. Indicates extramedullary haemopoeisis (➲ see Fig. 7.7).
  Causes: include infection (check TORCH screen); haematological and neoplastic—leukaemia, neuroblastoma, and Langerhans cell histiocytosis.
- *Fibromatoses*: these firm deep lesions include:
  - *Infantile digital fibromatosis*—lumps on fingers/toes (➲ see Fig. 29.15).
  - *Fibrous hamartoma of infancy*.
  - *Myofibromatosis*—very rarely can be generalized.
- *Developmental anomalies*:
  - *Accessory tragus*—firm nodule(s) in front of ear (➲ see Ears, pp. 133–5).
  - *Wattles*—nodules or tags on the front of the neck (➲ see Fig. 7.8).
  - *Nasal glioma*—smooth mass usually at bridge of nose (Fig. 28.16)—may have evidence of hair.
  - *Dermoid cyst*—smooth subcutaneous swelling, often near lateral end of eyebrow (Fig. 28.1).
  - *Umbilical polyp (granuloma)*—red nodule, may discharge because of connection to gastrointestinal (GI) or genitourinary (GU) tract (Fig. 28.8 and ➲ see Red lesions, pp. 421–3).
  - *Median raphe cyst*—between urethral meatus and anus.
  - *Lipoma, hamartoma, or neoplasm* (including haemangioma) over lumbosacral region (may cause bifid natal cleft) often a sign of occult spinal dysraphism.
  - *Rudimentary meningocele*—a soft cystic mass usually over back of scalp, often with a ring of coarse black hair around it (hair collar sign) (➲ see Fig. 14.6).

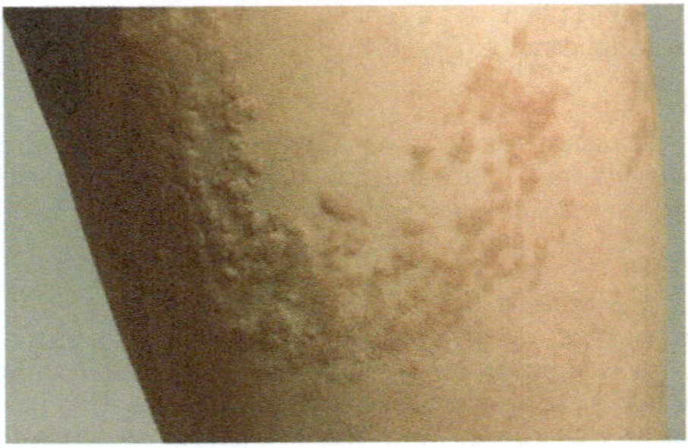

Fig. 28.17 Epidermal naevus with warty surface. Lesions distributed in the lines of Blaschko.

Reproduced courtesy of Cameron Kennedy, Consultant Dermatologist,Departments of Dermatology, Bristol Royal Infirmary and Paediatric Dermatology, Bristol Royal Hospital for Children, Bristol, UK

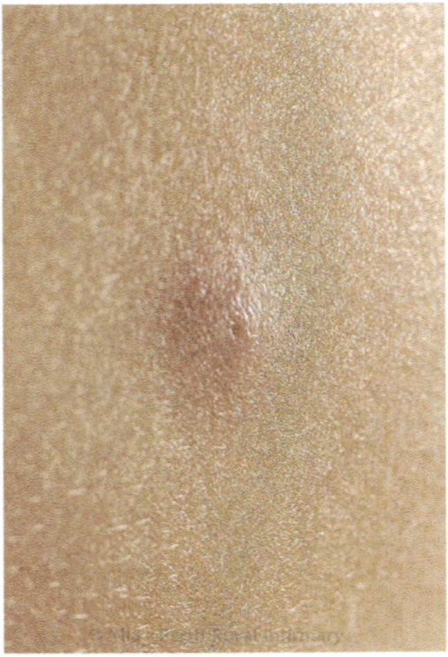

Fig. 28.18 Epidermoid cyst with central punctum.

Reproduced courtesy of Susan Lewis-Jones, Hon Consultant Dermatologist, Ninewells Hospital and Medical School, Dundee, UK

Malignant skin tumours

Rare in the paediatric age group. Some characteristics include:
- Rapid or progressive growth.
- Ulceration.
- Fixation to, or location deep to fascia.
- Firm mass >3cm diameter.

Examples include:
- ***Primary*** lesions such as rhabdomyosarcoma, basal cell carcinoma, squamous cell carcinoma and melanoma (➔ see Fig. 34.10), and primary lymphoma.
- ***Secondary*** lesions such as disseminated lymphoma, leukaemia (➔ Fig. 28.7), neuroblastomas, and internal cancers.

Further clues to the possibility of skin malignancy include:
- Faltering growth (➔ see Chapter 6).
- Haematological abnormalities.
- A cancer-prone background, such as:
  - Xeroderma pigmentosum (most autosomal recessive)—rare (➔ see Fig. 16.7) several complement types.
  - Gorlin's syndrome (*syn.* basal cell naevus syndrome), autosomal dominant—rare but tumours (basal cell cancers) can start in childhood.
  - Familial melanoma syndrome: associated with *CDKN2A* mutations.
- Post-irradiation field, e.g. basal cell cancers following treatment of Wilm's tumour.
- Immunodeficiency, e.g. Kaposi's sarcoma in AIDS patients.
- Immunosuppression, e.g. post-transplant squamous cell carcinoma from papilloma (wart) virus (usually adults) (➔ see also Chapter 39).
- Increased risk from some lesions, e.g. giant congenital melanocytic naevus (➔ see Fig. 34.9).
- Previous systemic cancer which commonly metastasizes to the skin, e.g. neuroblastoma.

Chapter 29

Changes in skin thickness and elasticity

Introduction

Abnormal texture (thickening, atrophy, and changes in extensibility and elasticity) of the skin arises due to alterations in the:

- Epidermis.
- Dermis and/or subcutaneous fat.

Palpation of skin lesions and rashes is important to help determine depth of involvement. Look for clues as to the cause by examining the whole skin. The following are the main changes considered in this section:

- Atrophy: a term used for thinning of the skin (or any body tissue) and can occur from thinning of any or all layers.
- Stretchy or baggy skin.
- Increase in thickness, firmness, or hardness.

Note: In some conditions, dependent on the stage of the disease there may be a mixture of the above, e.g. epidermal thinning occurs in morphoea (➲ see Epidermal texture change, pp. 438–41) but also a dermal thickening so that the skin feels thickened and firm on palpation. In linear morphoea and scleroderma there is gradual loss of underlying fat and muscle, often with subsequent atrophy from disuse causing an appearance of thinning of the affected site. Similarly, in dermatomyositis (➲ see Dermal thickening, pp. 448–50) there is localized dermal thickening in the form of calcinosis but eventual atrophy of the fat layer may occur (lipoatrophy).

For investigations of suspected skin texture, see Box 29.1.

Box 29.1 Investigations of suspected skin texture changes

- *Blood tests*: guided by history and examination.
- If diagnosis is uncertain, skin biopsy for:
  - *Histopathology*. If there is fat involvement a deep biopsy is required. Punch biopsy is usually insufficient.
  - *Direct immunofluorescence* for suspected connective tissue disorders, e.g. lupus erythematosus.
- *Ultrasound or MRI*: may be helpful to delineate deeper abnormalities.
- *Thermal imaging*: can be helpful in the sclerodermas but is not routinely available.

Epidermal texture change

Epidermal atrophy (thinning)

Skin may be shiny and have cigarette paper-like, fine wrinkling.

Causes:

- Prolonged application of topical corticosteroids (usually potent or super potent; ➲ see Anti-inflammatory treatments, pp. 30–6).
- Oral glucocorticoids (corticosteroids).
- Cutaneous scleroderma (morphoea). There is associated dermal thickening.
- Lichen sclerosus.
- Dermatomyositis.
- Inherited premature ageing disorders (progeria).
- Congenital: localized or widespread.

Cutaneous scleroderma (morphoea)

Presents with:

- ***Localized plaques (morphoea)***: lesions are inflamed initially with a characteristic red/purple border (Fig. 29.1) becoming fibrotic and indurated, finally atrophic, and pigmented. Usually only involves the skin and has a good prognosis.
- ***Linear scleroderma (linear morphoea)***: rare but particularly occurs in childhood. Skin feels firmer due to dermal thickening. A linear variety on the forehead/scalp is known as 'en coup de sabre' (Fig. 29.2). There may be significant morbidity with involvement of underlying tissues and progressive worsening can be rapid. Growth restriction, joint contractures, and progressive facial distortion with hemiatrophy (Parry–Romberg syndrome) are long-term sequelae and are indications for prompt systemic treatment.

Diagnosis: usually clinical although skin biopsy and histology can be helpful.

Treatment

- Topical options include potent topical corticosteroids, intralesional corticosteroids, calcipotriol under occlusion and imiquimod.
- Systemic treatment is required early in severe or rapidly progressive cases. Pulsed methylprednisolone with methotrexate, oral corticosteroids, ciclosporin, and other immunosuppressant agents have been tried.
- Physiotherapy and orthopaedic advice can be helpful in cases of limb involvement.

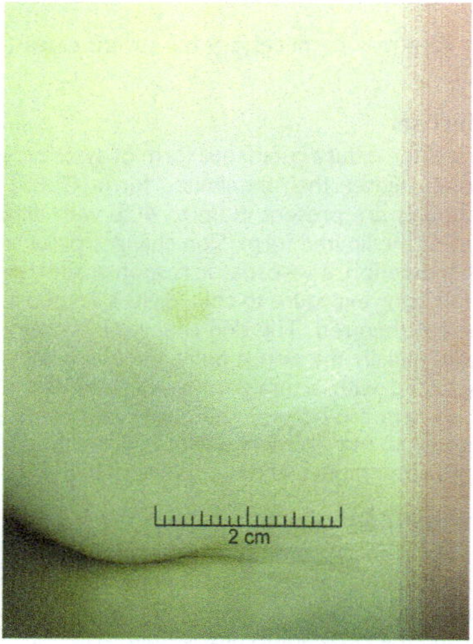

Fig. 29.1 Morphoea on the trunk—a typical site. Note violaceous border.

Reproduced courtesy of Susan Lewis-Jones, Hon Consultant Dermatologist, Ninewells Hospital and Medical School, Dundee, UK

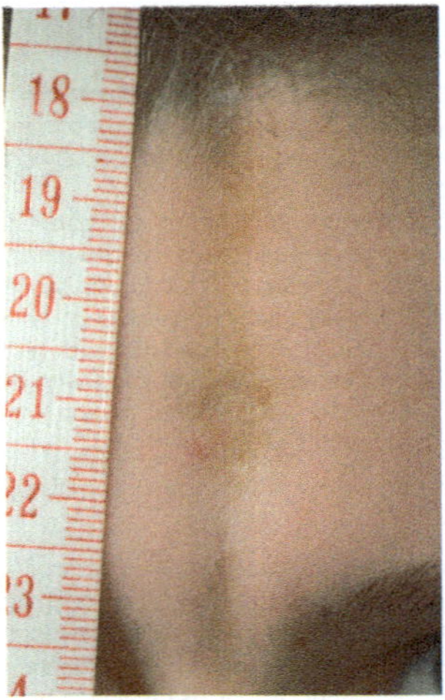

Fig. 29.2 Linear 'en coup de sabre' of the forehead and scalp.

Reproduced courtesy of Susan Lewis-Jones, Hon Consultant Dermatologist, Ninewells Hospital and Medical School, Dundee, UK

Multidisciplinary care may be necessary for severe cases (➲ see Systemic sclerosis, p. 440).

Systemic sclerosis

Although very rare, the diffuse cutaneous form of systemic sclerosis is more commonly seen in children than the limited form (CREST). Scl-70 (topoisomerase) antibodies are present in up to 40% with diffuse involvement and only 10–15% in the limited form. Skin changes occur at the same time as Raynaud's phenomenon, a vasospastic response affecting fingers and/or toes. Typically, following exposure to cold, digits go numb and white and on rewarming blue and then red. The skin changes in systemic sclerosis tend to be widespread. Initially the skin is puffy, becoming more taut and tethered, often associated with arthralgia, myalgia, and stiffness. Heart, lung and kidney involvement can occur within a few years of diagnosis. A multidisciplinary approach to management is essential, involving rheumatologists, paediatricians, physiotherapists, and occupational therapists.

Lichen sclerosus (LS)

Genital involvement is much commoner (➲ see Fig. 13.6) than extragenital skin involvement. In the latter lesions are white and feel thickened, sometimes with a rough slightly spiky surface (➲ see Fig. 32.5). It can be confused with morphoea and the two can occur together. Potent topical corticosteroids are helpful.

Congenital causes of epidermal atrophy

Localized

- *Scarring*: e.g. from intrauterine infections such as chickenpox; trauma.
- *Aplasia cutis*: loss of skin, usually full thickness, and may include loss of bone. Usually on scalp, often triangular in shape and commonly occurs in isolation but may be associated with other syndromic anomalies (➲ see Fig. 14.6).

Widespread

- *Epidermolysis bullosa*: a heterogenous group of inherited skin disorders characterized by mechanobullous skin lesions (➲ see Figs. 25.10, 25.11, and 25.12). It can present with localized areas of skin loss as well as blistering at birth.
- *Conradi–Hünermann–Happle syndrome*: (X-linked dominant chondrodysplasia punctata) (➲ see also X-linked dominant ichthyosis, p. 412). Very rare and lethal in males. Presents at birth as a collodion neonate (➲ see Fig. 27.8) with redness and overlapping scaling which clears but leaves linear atrophic, irregularly shaped depressed areas especially on the arms (following Blaschko's lines; ➲ see Fig. 4.6). The skin and hair are dry and patches of alopecia and hypopigmentation may occur. Associated abnormalities include eye (usually cataracts) and bony abnormalities.

Trauma/injury

Scarring from trauma or thermal/chemical injury will cause changes in skin thickness with both thinning (atrophy) or thickening (hypertrophy), which may be localized or generalized.

Epidermal thickening

The epidermal skin is thickened in conditions of friction such as chronic scratching. Localized thickening (hyperplasia) occurs in:

- *Lichenification*: commonly seen in eczema usually localized to wrists and flexures of elbows, knees, ankles, and neck (➲ see Fig. 17.6).
- *Lichen simplex chronicus*: an extreme form of habit scratching often seen in atopic eczema (Fig. 29.3). Commoner in adults. Sites include nape of neck, wrists, ankles, and genital area.
- *Prurigo nodularis* (*syn*. nodular prurigo): severely itchy nodules, commoner on limbs. It is probably a variant of lichen simplex chronicus.
- *Palmoplantar keratoderma*: a localized thickening of the palms and soles (➲ see Fig. 12.4 and Box 12.2). It is seen in:
  - Some rare forms of inherited ichthyosis (➲ see Chapter 27).
  - Some other genetic diseases such as pachyonychia congenita (➲ see Genodermatoses and the nail, pp. 223–4 and Pachyonychia congenita, p. 389).
  - Some dermatoses, e.g. psoriasis, pityriasis rubra pilaris. (➲ see Features of specific causes of erythroderma, pp. 343–5).
- *Epidermal tumours*: (➲ see Epidermal naevi, p. 444).

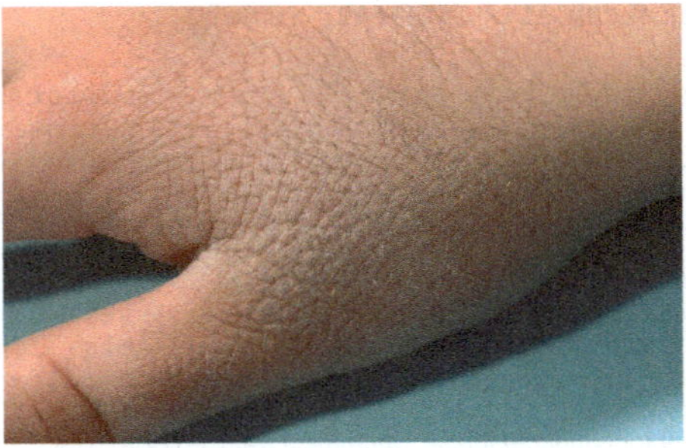

Fig. 29.3 Lichen simplex—close up to show epidermal thickening.
Reproduced courtesy of NHS Tayside Clinical Photography, Dundee, UK

Other epidermal textural changes

Skin may be rough (warty surface), show excessive scaling or rugosity. There may be tumours (lumps and bumps; ➲ see Chapter 28). Many inflammatory dermatoses show epidermal hyperplasia. Histologically this is characterized by acanthosis. Examples include chronic eczema with lichenification, psoriasis, lichen simplex chronicus (➲ see Epidermal thickening, p. 441), nodular prurigo (➲ see Other rashes sometimes confused with eczema, p. 262), and lichen planus (➲ see Non-infective causes, pp. 285–8).

Some common causes:

- Viral warts (➲ see Figs. 9.5, 12.9, and 29.4).
- Epidermal naevi (➲ see Figs. 4.5, 4.10, and 28.17).
- Congenital melanocytic naevi (➲ see Chapter 34).

Viral warts

Benign proliferation of the epidermis caused by human papilloma virus (HPV). If very extensive and persistent consider immunosuppressive causes such as transplants (➲ see Chapter 39) or HIV infection or epidermodysplasia verruciformis. All warts may koebnerize (➲ see Chapter 4).

- *Common warts* (verrucae vulgaris): vary from small papules to large fissured lesions, usually on the hands, knees, or elbows; to warty papillomas, often filiform on the face (➲ see Fig. 9.5). Plantar warts on the sole can be mosaic (Fig. 29.4). For genital warts, ➲ see Fig. 13.7.
- *Planar warts*: small, flat, often skin-coloured or of various shades of brown, usually seen on the face or the hands (Fig. 29.5).
  Treatment: keratolytic agents and paring are most effective. Cryotherapy for older children (over about 9y) but avoid on soles because of painful blisters.
- *Epidermodysplasia verruciformis*: rare autosomal recessive condition characterized by an increased susceptibility to infection with HPV, associated with decreased cell-mediated immunity. Extensive widespread wart-like lesions are evident from childhood. They resemble planar warts on face but more papillomatous lesions on limbs. *In adults, squamous cell carcinomas are common in sun exposed sites.*

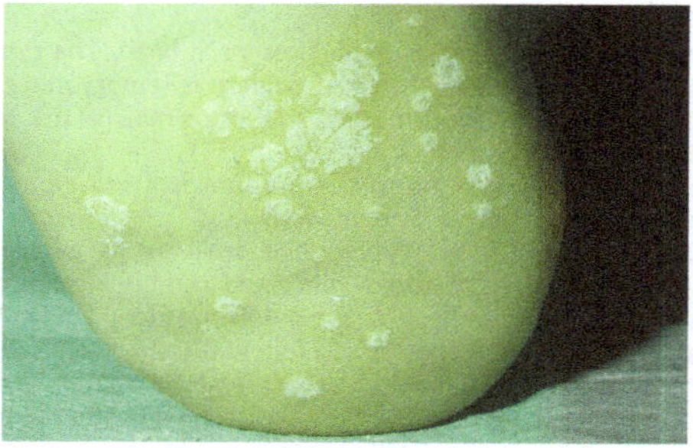

Fig. 29.4 Mosaic warts on sole.

Reproduced courtesy of Susan Lewis-Jones, Hon Consultant Dermatologist, Ninewells Hospital and Medical School, Dundee, UK

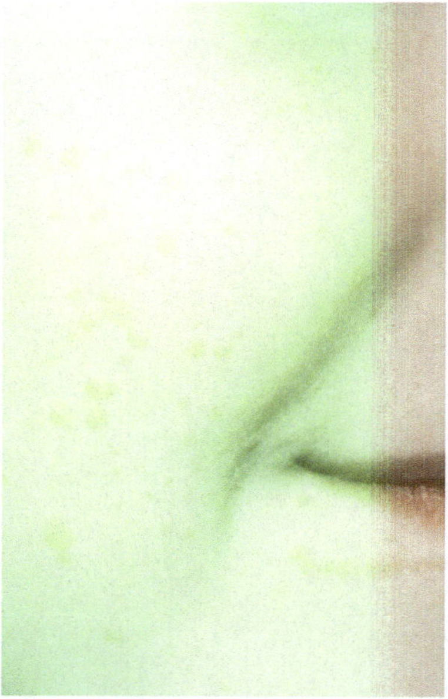

Fig. 29.5 Planar warts.

Reproduced courtesy of Dr Claire Benton, Consultant Dermatologist, Edinburgh Royal Infirmary, UK

Epidermal naevi

Common 'birthmarks', not necessarily present at birth. The term encompasses all hamartomas arising from the epidermis (embryonic ectoderm). These are developmental abnormalities, so there is minimal risk of a second child being affected.

They are classified according to the predominant cell type (e.g. sebaceous, keratinocytic, follicular, or comedonal).

Usually benign, ranging in size from single small warty papules to multiple and widespread 'systematized' types and can be linear (either localized, ➲ see Fig. 4.10, or widespread, e.g. Inflammatory Linear Verrucous Epidermal Nevi or ILVEN). They usually follow Blaschko's lines with streaks and whorls (➲ see Figs. 28.17 and 4.5), representing a cutaneous mosaicism. These more extensive lesions may be associated with other abnormalities (epidermal naevus syndrome, CHILD syndrome, and Proteus syndrome).

Treatment: none for small lesions. Surgery or ablative laser for cosmesis if required. This is very difficult in larger or systematized lesions. Which tend to recur and often require repeated treatments.

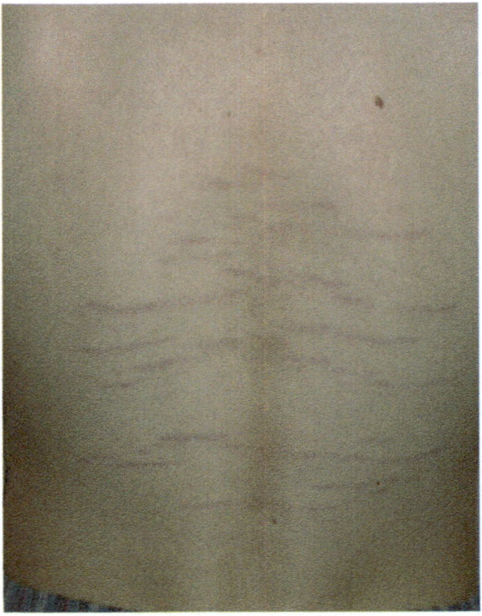

Fig. 29.6 Transverse adolescent striae on the back, ➲ see Dermal texture changes, p. 445–6.

Reproduced courtesy of Susan Lewis-Jones, Hon Consultant Dermatologist, Ninewells Hospital and Medical School, Dundee, UK

Dermal texture change

Dermal atrophy

Dermal atrophy is characterized by depression of the skin with increased visibility (translucency) of underlying venous network (Box 29.2).

Causes

- *Striae*: linear depressed scars that most commonly develop during puberty (adolescent striae; Fig. 29.6) and typically involve upper thighs, lower lumbar regions, and breasts in girls. Usually red initially and fade over years. Occasionally mistaken for child abuse. They can be a feature of Marfan's syndrome. Cushing's syndrome should also be considered if there is significant obesity or other signs such as hypertension. Most patients do not require any investigations and there is no definitive treatment.
- *Corticosteroids*: prolonged application of topical (or ingestion of oral) corticosteroids: More likely to occur with the potent topical corticosteroids and those applied to flexures or under occlusion, Dermal thinning follows epidermal thinning and may result in striae.
- *Anetoderma*: localized areas of flaccid or herniated sac-like skin which occur as a result of focal loss of dermal elastic tissue. May be primary or secondary to a pre-existing inflammatory condition (e.g. chickenpox scars).
- *Congenital causes*: aplasia cutis (➲ see Fig. 14.6).
- *Mycosis fungoides*: a rare T-cell lymphoma. Some lesions display marked dermal atrophy with cigarette paper wrinkling (➲ see Rare skin diseases causing red rashes, pp. 339–40).
- *Rare genetic causes*:
    - Vascular Ehlers–Danlos syndrome (type IV; ➲ see p. 448).
    - Focal dermal hypoplasia (Goltz syndrome; ➲ see Focal dermal hypoplasia, p. 446).
    - Cutis laxa (➲ see p. 446).
    - Restrictive dermopathy; a rare, lethal disorder presenting with tight, atrophic skin with erosions associated with contractures and fetal dyskinesia.

Ehlers–Danlos syndromes

A group of inherited disorders associated with stretchy* (hyperextensible), fragile skin (Fig. 29.7), bruising (➲ see Fig. 24.3), and lax joints (Fig. 29.8). Wide atrophic scars are common in sites of trauma (Fig. 29.9). The clinical

Box 29.2 Dermal texture change

Stretchy skin is seen in:

- Most types of Ehlers–Danlos syndrome to variable extent.

Loose skin is seen in:

- Cutis laxa (inherited or secondary causes).
- Pseudoxanthoma elasticum.
- Wrinkly skin syndrome.

*Stretchy skin is not the same as loose skin (see Box 29.2).

presentation varies between types and internal organ involvement and vascular fragility may occur in some subtypes. Different abnormalities of the extracellular matrix (mainly collagens) have been identified (see Table 29.1). Bruising and scarring on the shins (➲ see Fig. 24.3) and forehead (Fig 29.9) in Ehlers–Danlos syndrome is often mistaken for child abuse.

Vascular Ehlers–Danlos syndrome (type IV): thin translucent skin occurs, particularly at acral sites (acrogeria), in association with extensive bruising and modest skin fragility and joint hypermobility. There is a significant risk of arterial and intestinal rupture due to collagen III deficiency.

Focal dermal hypoplasia (Goltz syndrome)

Rare X-linked dominant disorder with congenital linear areas of erythematous depressed skin. Fat herniation through the skin may occur due to total loss of dermis. A wide variety of defects may also be seen in other tissues.

Cutis laxa

Although dermal atrophy is not seen dermal elastic fibres are reduced, leading to loose, redundant skin that hangs in folds. Congenital forms are more common than acquired. The autosomal recessive type is associated with severe emphysema and bowel and bladder diverticuli.

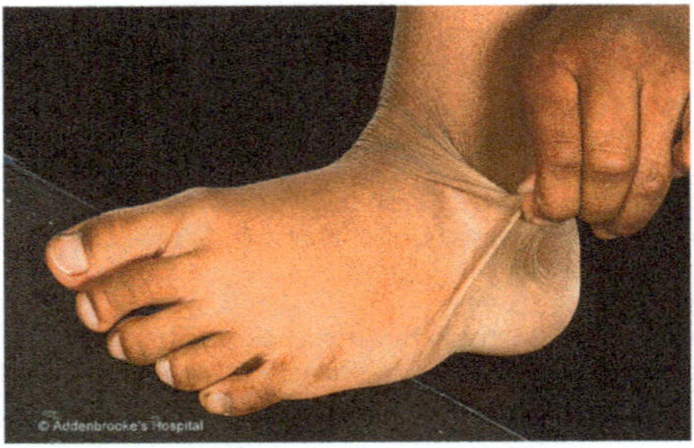

Fig. 29.7 Stretchy skin in classical Ehlers–Danlos syndrome.
Reproduced courtesy of Addenbrooke's Hospital, Cambridge, UK.

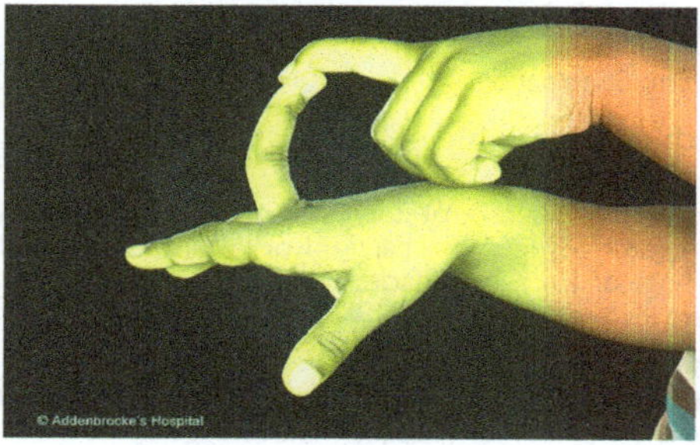

Fig. 29.8 Joint laxity in Ehlers–Danlos syndrome.
Reproduced courtesy of Addenbrooke's Hospital, Cambridge, UK.

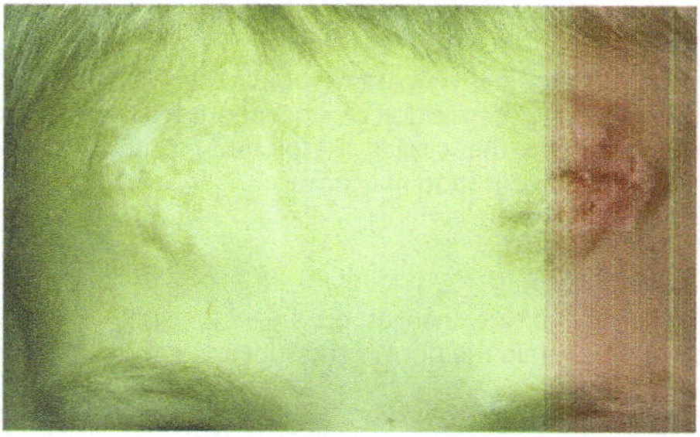

Fig. 29.9 Wide atrophic scars in Ehlers–Danlos syndrome.
Reproduced courtesy of NHS Tayside Clinical Photography, Dundee, UK

Table 29.1 Connective tissue disorders

Connective tissue	Syndrome with cutaneous manifestations
Collagen	Ehlers–Danlos syndrome (I, III, V) Epidermolysis bullosa (VII, XVII)
Elastic fibre	Cutis laxa (autosomal recessive, dominant, and x-linked recessive mutations) Pseudoxanthoma elasticum (ABCC6)
Microfibrillary protein	Marfan's syndrome (fibrillin-1)
Mucopolysaccharide	MPS I–VII (lysosomal enzyme defects)
Other	Buschke–Ollendorff syndrome (LEMD3) Lipoid proteinosis (ECM1)

Notes: Genetic defect in brackets. Collagen types in Roman numerals.

Dermal thickening

Skin feels firm on palpation.

Diffuse thickening

Mucopolysaccharidosis

A group of inherited lysosomal storage diseases, which include Hunter and Hurler syndromes. Symmetrical papular ivory-white lesions usually develop before the age of 10y. Coarse facies and mental retardation are common. Multisystem involvement occurs.

Pseudoxanthoma elasticum

Yellow papules are present at flexural sites; predominantly neck (Fig. 29.10) and axillae and they may form plaques. The average age of onset of skin lesions is 13y. It is important to look for retinal angioid streaks. Patients are at risk of visual loss, cardiovascular disease, and gastric bleeding.

Investigations: skin biopsy shows fragmentation and calcification of elastic fibres.

Lipoid proteinosis

Thickening of the skin and mucosa associated with hoarseness develops during childhood due to deposition of amorphous hyaline material. Beaded papules are typical on the eyelids. Respiratory, central nervous system (CNS), and ocular complication may occur.

Localized thickening

Scleroderma (morphoea)

- See Epidermal texture changes, pp. 438–41.

Deposition of collagen in the dermis and subcutis leads to thickening.

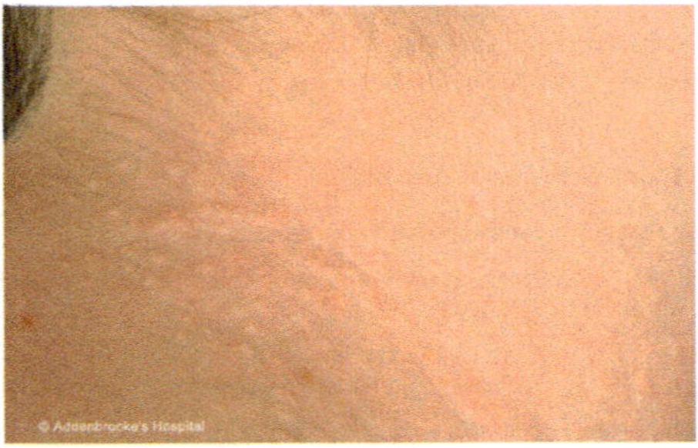

Fig. 29.10 Typical changes on the neck in pseudoxanthoma elasticum.
Reproduced courtesy of Addenbrooke's Hospital, Cambridge, UK.

Calcification (calcinosis cutis)

Extremely firm nodules or plaques that may perforate and/or ulcerate. Types:

- Idiopathic.
- Dystrophic, e.g. dermatomyositis.
- Metastatic, e.g. primary hyperparathyroidism.
- Iatrogenic.

Very rarely it can be very extensive in dermatomyositis (➲ see Dermatomyositis, Treatment, p. 449) encasing areas of the body in a rigid plate.

Dermatomyositis

Dermatomyositis is a multisystem condition involving skin and muscle. An inflammatory myopathy presents with muscle weakness and an elevated creatine kinase.

The cutaneous signs initially look atrophic with pinkish-violet erythema (heliotrope rash) and telangiectasia over the eyelids (Fig. 29.11) and also the nail folds. Violaceous papules occur over the knuckles (Fig. 29.12; Gottron's sign) and erythematous or urticated patches can occur on the trunk. *In children it is thought to follow a viral infection and is not related to systemic neoplasia.*

- ***Cutaneous calcinosis*** is more common in children and causes significant disability with pain, contracture formation, skin ulcers and muscle atrophy (Fig. 29.13).
- ***Lipoatrophy*** is a long-term consequence (➲ see Fat changes, pp. 452–3).

Treatment: early introduction of systemic treatment (corticosteroids—usually pulsed intravenous (IV) methylprednisolone and methotrexate) is usually effective and can reduce the incidence of cutaneous calcification—the most severe cutaneous feature of this condition (Fig. 29.13). Treatments are poorly effective for established calcinosis but include aluminium hydroxide, probenecid, diltiazem, and bisphosphonates. Localized problematic lesions can occasionally be excised.

Connective tissue naevi

Elastoma

These may be solitary patches with no obvious associated features (Fig. 29.14) or present at birth as multiple symmetrically distributed flesh- or yellow-white-coloured papules or plaques as part of Buschke–Ollendorff syndrome (associated with osteopoikilosis which may be misdiagnosed as metastatic disease on X-ray in the unwary).

Collagenoma

These also occur in Buschke–Ollendorff syndrome. The collagenomas in tuberous sclerosis complex are known as Shagreen patches and are commonly located on the lower back or posterior neck (➲ see Tuberous sclerosis complex, pp. 483–4).

Differential diagnosis: leiomyoma (often painful; ➲ see Red lesions, pp. 421–3), neurofibroma (➲ see Fig. 28.2, and Smooth muscle hamartoma, p. 490).

Fibromatoses

A number of types of spindle cell lesions (too numerous to list here) arise in the skin and soft tissues giving rise to firm masses. They may have an indolent course, e.g. myofibromatosis; or be locally aggressive, e.g. infantile fibromatosis. A local benign form of digital fibromatosis is sometimes seen (Fig. 29.15).

Cutis verticis gyrata

Thickened furrows of the scalp resembling a cerebriform pattern. Primary (idiopathic) cases usually develop after puberty and may reflect hormonal influences. If secondary to syndromic causes changes may be present at birth. It is sometimes seen in acromegaly (➲ see Pituitary dysfunction, p. 64).

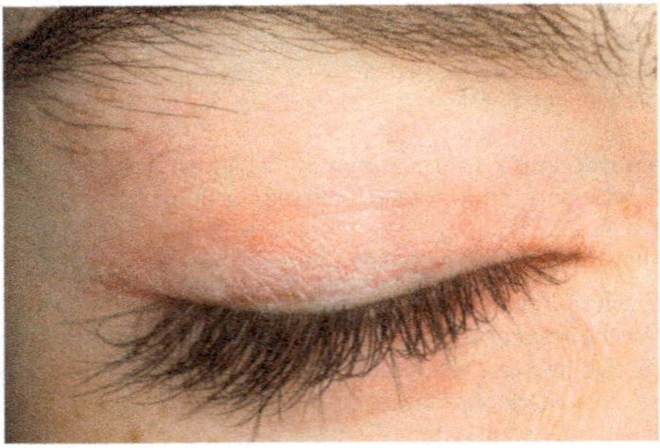

Fig. 29.11 Dermatomyositis showing purple heliotrope rash of upper eyelids.

Reproduced courtesy of Susan Lewis-Jones, Hon Consultant Dermatologist, Ninewells Hospital and Medical School, Dundee, UK

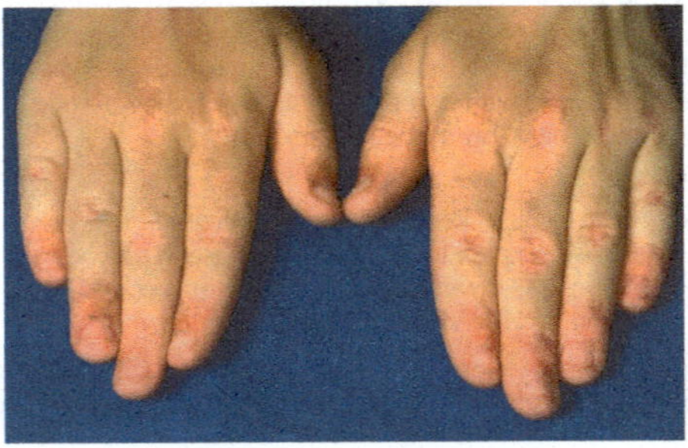

Fig. 29.12 Dermatomyositis of the hands showing erythema over joints and around nail folds with ragged cuticles.

Reproduced courtesy of Susan Lewis-Jones, Hon Consultant Dermatologist, Ninewells Hospital and Medical School, Dundee, UK

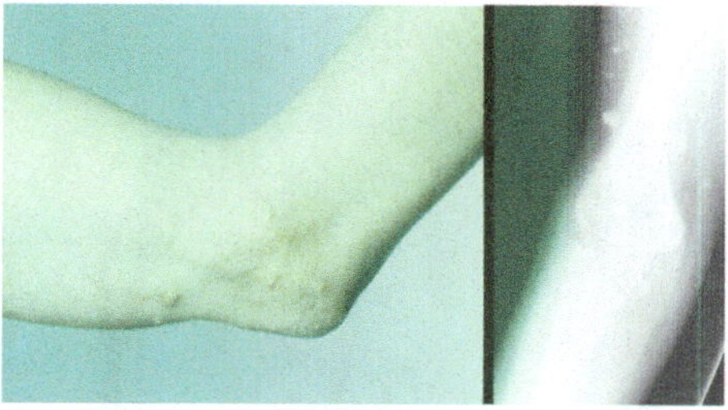

Fig. 29.13 Calcinosis cutis in dermatomyositis.

Reproduced courtesy of Gina Kavanagh, Department of Dermatology, Lothian NHS Trust, Edinburgh, UK

Fig. 29.14 Connective tissue naevus.

Reproduced courtesy of Addenbrooke's Hospital, Cambridge, UK.

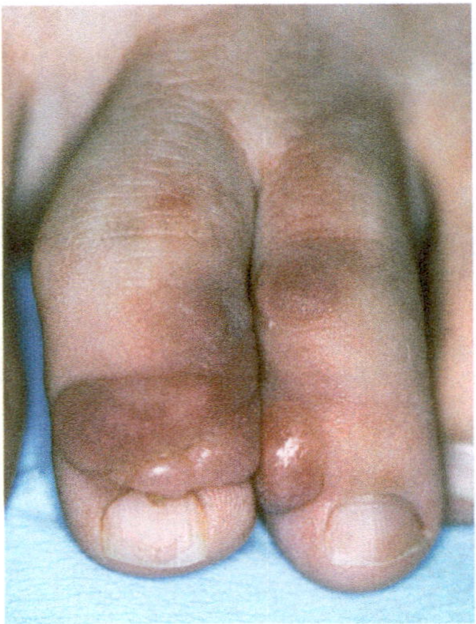

Fig. 29.15 Digital fibromatosis.

Reproduced courtesy of Susan Lewis-Jones, Hon Consultant Dermatologist, Ninewells Hospital and Medical School, Dundee, UK

Fat changes

Fat atrophy

Loss of substance but usually the overlying skin is normal. There are several causes:

Lipoatrophy

- Congenital, e.g. progeroid syndromes, familial partial lipodystrophy (autosomal dominant), congenital generalized lipodystrophy.
- Idiopathic.
- Inflammatory, e.g. lupus profundus (a rare form of lupus erythematosus) or following dermatomyositis (Fig. 29.16).
- Post-traumatic.
- Drugs, e.g. corticosteroids, insulin, protease inhibitors.
- Linear facial morphoea ('en coup de sabre'; Fig. 29.2) and progressive facial hemiatrophy (Parry–Romberg syndrome), both lead to lipoatrophy and loss of deeper tissue.

Inherited premature ageing disorders (progeria)

- *Hutchinson–Gilford syndrome (progeria)*: affected children are normal at birth but within 1–2y develop features resembling premature ageing with bird-like facies; alopecia; lipoatrophy; tight, translucent wrinkled skin with sclerodermatous changes over the trunk; short stature and skeletal abnormalities. It is an autosomal recessive condition due to a

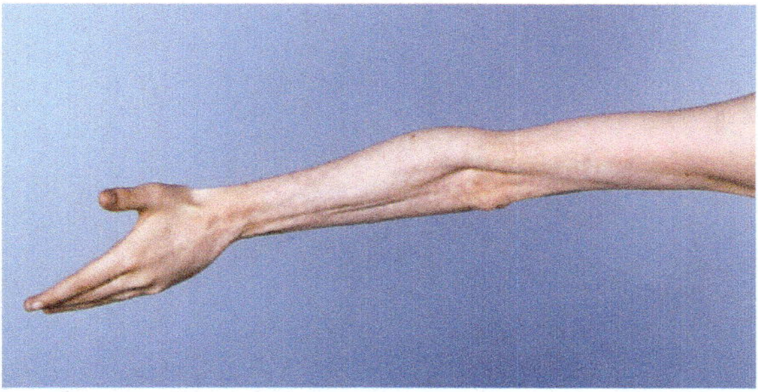

Fig. 29.16 Lipoatrophy of the arm following dermatomyositis.
Reproduced courtesy of Gina Kavanagh, Department of Dermatology, Lothian NHS Trust, Edinburgh, UK

defect in the *LMNA* gene. Cardiovascular abnormalities such as early atherosclerosis account for early death, usually in the second decade.
- *Werner's syndrome*: onset is later, with greying of the temples usually starting in teenage years.
- *Acrogeria*: cutaneous atrophy of the extremities occurs, which in some cases is associated with vascular EDS.
- *Xeroderma pigmentosum*: many subtypes exist but all are characterized by photosensitivity, malignancy risk and photodamage (hyper- and hypopigmentation, cutaneous atrophy, and telangiectasia— ➲ see Fig. 16.10). Eye and CNS changes may also be present.

Thickening of fat layer

Causes

Lipoma

Benign tumour of fat cell origin that feels soft and smooth, is often large, and may be tender. Solitary lesions are rare in childhood but may occur in Cowden's and Gardner's syndromes (rare inherited tumour-associated syndromes).

Panniculitis

Inflammation of the subcutaneous tissue is uncommon in childhood. Exclude drug and infective causes. Commonest presentation is tender, nodular lesions on the shins due to erythema nodosum (➲ see Fig. 12.10). In some countries panniculitis on the calves is seen (erythema induratum) caused by a cutaneous reaction to *Mycobacterium tuberculosis* (➲ see Tuberculosis (TB) skin diseases, pp. 333–5). In the later (burnt-out) stages of some types, fat atrophy can occur.

Subcutaneous fat necrosis of the newborn

Mobile nodule or plaque, usually on buttocks, posterior trunk, or cheeks. Most appear in first month of life possibly due to trauma and ischaemic injury. Self-resolving but hypercalcaemia may occur (➲ see also Other rashes in the newborn, pp. 82–3).

Chapter 30

Ulceration of the skin

Introduction

Ulcers are caused by complete loss of the epidermis, usually including some dermal loss. Partial loss is known as an erosion. There are many causes (➲ see also Arms and legs, pp. 170–3). Ulcers can be congenital or acquired and may follow trauma, infection, many skin diseases, severe drug eruptions (➲ see Chapter 23) or be due to abuse or rarely self-induced (➲ see Chapter 24). They are often preceded by crusts or eschars (➲ see Chapter 26), blisters (➲ see Chapter 25), cutaneous vasculitis (➲ see Chapters 31 and 38) and other causes of denudation of the skin including congenital causes.

Causes of ulcers

Congenital

- *Epidermolysis bullosa*: a group of inherited mechanobullous disorders leading to skin fragility with blistering and ulcers (Fig. 30.1; ➲ see also Figs. 25.10 and 25.11).
- *Aplasia cutis*: congenital absence of skin may present with ulceration at birth, most commonly on the scalp (➲ see Scalp lesions, pp. 201–2 and Fig. 14.6).
- *Goltz syndrome* (*syn*. focal dermal hypoplasia): rare X-linked dominant disorder caused by mutations in the *PORCN* gene. Lethal in non-mosaic hemizygous males, but postzygotic mutations or lionization in females may allow survival. A multisystem disease, which may present as congenital linear streaks of dermal atrophy and fat herniation in the lines of Blaschko (➲ see Fig. 4.6). Later papular lesions develop. Skeletal abnormalities are seen in 80%.

Infection

- *Bacterial infections*: *Streptococcus pyogenes* can cause crusted ulcers such as ecthyma (➲ see Fig. 26.3) or others causes of eschars (➲ see Eschars, p. 397), such as anthrax (➲ see Fig. 26.5), which separate to leave ulcers. Meningococcal disease (➲ see Sepsis, pp. 467–70) can cause extensive eschars and subsequent ulceration.

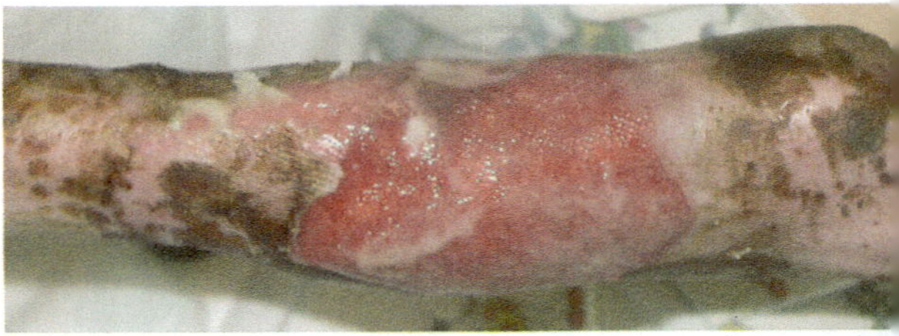

Fig. 30.1 Severe extensive skin ulceration in epidermolysis bullosa recessive dystrophic type.

Reproduced courtesy of Susan Lewis-Jones, Hon Consultant Dermatologist, Ninewells Hospital and Medical School, Dundee, UK

- *Viral*: e.g. herpes zoster (➲ see Infection causing blisters, p. 378); poxvirus infections, e.g. cowpox (➲ see Fig. 26.7).
- *Leishmaniasis*: usually starts with a pustule before ulceration (Figs. 30.2 and 26.4); ➲ see also Infestation and parasites, pp. 283–5.
- *Buruli ulcers*: deep and caused by *Mycobacterium ulcerans*. Start as a small nodule that may heal or ulcerate. Seen in children living in swampy areas. *Investigation*: acid-fast bacilli (Ziehl–Neelson stain) from base of wound smear.

  Treatment: early lesions—oral rifampicin, ulcers may need surgical treatment
- *Syphilis and yaws* (➲ see Spirochete infections, pp. 336–7).
- *Tuberculosis*: primary cutaneous inoculation by *Mycobacterium tuberculosis* and other types may result in ulceration (➲ see Bacterial infections, pp. 332–5).
- *Tropical phagedenic ulcers*: usually develop at a site of injury in malnourished children from tropical areas—grows rapidly. Caused by fusiform bacilli and treponemes.

  Treatment: oral erythromycin, phenoxymethylpenicillin, or metronidazole.

Trauma

- *Mechanical trauma*: e.g. pressure ulcers due to immobility, especially if malnourished or wearing of surgical appliances, such as leg braces; or primary irritant contact dermatitis, e.g. Jacquet's napkin dermatitis (➲ see Fig. 13.2).
- *Neuropathic ulcers*: particularly in diabetics, Hansen disease (leprosy) (➲ see Chapter 22), or neurological disorders including spina bifida.
- *Thermal damage* from heat or cold, e.g. full thickness burns; frost bite.

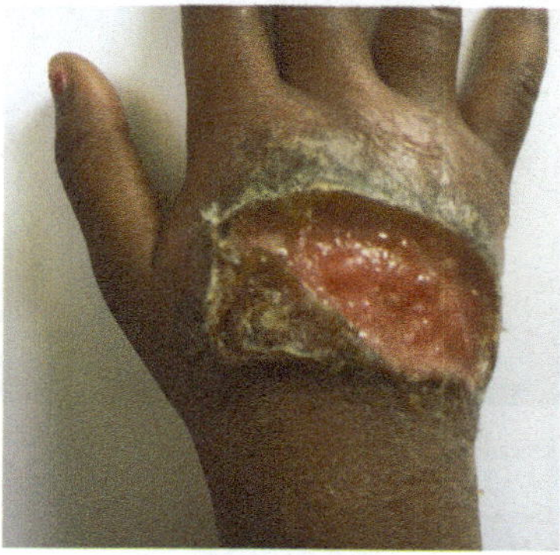

Fig. 30.2 Cutaneous leishmaniasis of 1y duration (untreated).

Reproduced courtesy of Susan Lewis-Jones, Hon Consultant Dermatologist, Ninewells Hospital and Medical School, Dundee, UK

- *Non-accidental causes*: especially if bizarre shapes or well-demarcated lesions are present. May be self-induced or by another (➲ see Chapter 24).

Inflammation

- *Tissue ischaemia*: due to increased plasma viscosity or vascular damage, e.g. vasculitis may lead to ulceration (➲ see also Cutaneous vasculitis, p. 470).
- *Pyoderma gangrenosum*: a rare ulcerative disorder of unknown cause although frequently associated with systemic disease, e.g. inflammatory bowel disease, blood dyscrasias, and rheumatoid arthritis. Ulcers form rapidly with a violaceous margin and undermined edges (Fig. 30.3). Around 80% appear first on the legs but buttocks and head are also involved in children.

Investigations: for underlying cause. Skin biopsy not usually diagnostic but can be helpful.
Treatment: systemic steroids and/or other immunosuppressive agents are usually required.
Ask for early dermatological opinion.

Drug reactions

Severe drug reactions: such as vasculitis, toxic epidermal necrolysis (➲ see Blistering drug reactions, pp. 352–7).

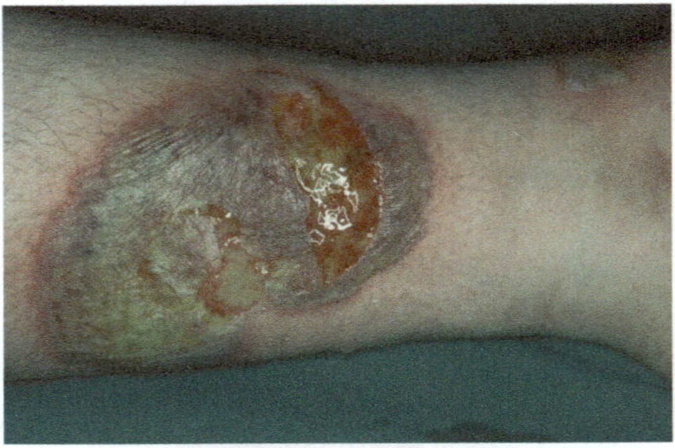

Fig. 30.3 Early ulceration of pyoderma gangrenosum.
Reproduced courtesy of Susan Lewis-Jones, Hon Consultant Dermatologist, Ninewells Hospital and Medical School, Dundee, UK

Toxicity

- Chemical burns.
- Bites from venomous snakes, spiders, etc.

Others

- *Beçhet's disease*: painful and recalcitrant. Scarring from oral and genital ulceration (➲ see Buccal and labial mucous and tongue mouth ulcers, pp. 143–4 and Ulcerations/erosions, p. 192–3).
- *Autoinflammatory diseases* such as DIRA (deficiency of Il-1 receptor antagonist) and periodic fever, adenitis, pharyngitis, aphthous ulcer (PFAPA) (➲ see Chapter 38, p. 531).
- *Infantile haemangiomas*: 5–10% have painful ulceration in the early stages, particularly lips and flexural sites (➲ see Chapter 8).
- *Scleroderma*: fingertip ulceration may occur on a background of sclerosis and telangiectasia (➲ see Epidermal texture changes, pp. 438–41).
- *Malnutrition*.
- *Haematological disease*: e.g. sickle cell anaemia. Confirm by haemoglobin electrophoresis.
- *Tumours*: especially if malignant.
- *Subcutaneous fat necrosis*: (➲ see Other rashes in newborns, pp. 82–3 and Fat changes, pp. 452–3).
- *Venous ulceration*: very rare in children (➲ see Chapter 8).

Oral ulceration

- ➲ See Buccal and labial mucous and tongue mouth ulcers, pp. 143–4 and Figs. 10.6 and 10.7.

Genital ulceration

- ➲ See Ulcerations/erosions, p. 192–3.

Section 6

Discolouration of the skin

Chapter 31

Purple colouration

Introduction

Purple lesions are usually related to a problem with the vasculature such as bruising, purpura, or deep vessels such as deep haemangiomas which can appear purple or blue (➲ see Chapter 8). Bruises change colour rapidly over a few days from purple to blue, yellow, and brown. Thin/atrophic skin or old scars, e.g. acne scars may look purple or bluish. This chapter covers causes of bruising, vasculitis, petechiae and purpura, and other causes of purple lesions.

Purpuric rashes

Purpura or petechiae do not blanch on pressure because blood has leaked out of vessels into the tissue. This is a useful distinguishing feature and forms the basis of the 'glass test' taught to the public to help in recognizing the rash of meningococcal septicaemia, which is the most important differential diagnosis (Box 31.1). This involves pressing on the skin with transparent glass to determine whether pressure makes the lesions fade away.

- *Purpura* is a sign of bleeding into the skin.
- *Petechiae* are tiny dot-sized purpura.

Diseases mimicking purpura

- Langerhans cell histiocytosis (➲ see Chapter 13).
- Pityriasis lichenoides acuta (➲ see Chapter 19).

Important causes of petechiae and purpura

- Trauma.
- Abnormality of clotting factors.
- Vessel fragility.
- Sepsis—meningitis (Box 31.1 ➲ and Sepsis, pp. 467–70).
- Vasculitis.
- Special considerations in the neonate.

Box 31.1 Purpura
The most important differential diagnosis is meningococcal sepsis and any systemically unwell child with petechiae or purpura should be treated promptly as for meningococcal septicaemia (➲ see Sepsis, pp. 467–70).

Trauma (bruising)

- *Non-accidental injury*: always consider it—if you don't, you will miss the diagnosis (➲ see Bruising and purpura, pp. 361–2).
- *Accidental injury* by child or another party.
- *Increased vascular pressure*: vomiting and vigorous coughing (e.g. from whooping cough), can produce petechiae in the distribution of the superior vena cava (i.e. above the nipple line or subconjunctival haemorrhage). Also suction injuries (e.g. 'love-bites' or suction toys applied to the skin).

- ***Bruising tendency***: accidental bruising that seems excessive may be due to a pathological cause of easy bruising. Think about:
  - *Abnormality of clotting factors*: e.g. thrombocytopaenia; clotting factor deficiency; thrombophilia.
  - *Vessel fragility*: e.g. vasculitis; scurvy (➲ see Vessel fragility, p. 466).
  - *Soft tissue fragility*: e.g. Ehlers–Danlos syndrome (➲ see Dermal textural changes, pp. 445–6). Bruising is a feature of all types (➲ see Fig. 24.3).
  - *Skin fragility*: e.g. dominant dystrophic epidermolysis bullosa often presents with bruising of the shins.

For diseases mimicking bruising, ➲ see Bruising and purpura, pp. 361–2.

Abnormality of clotting factors

Low platelets

Idiopathic thrombocytopaenic purpura (ITP)

The commonest cause of thrombocytopaenia in childhood, affecting 10–40 children per million per year. Usually occurs in an otherwise well child but may be due to a recent viral illness such as chickenpox.

- Bruising tends to be at normal sites on minor trauma.
- Spontaneous bleeding such as nosebleeds can occur when platelet count drops below 20.

Investigations: full blood count shows very low platelets but is otherwise normal.

Drugs

Drugs can cause thrombocytopaenia by inhibiting platelet production in bone marrow or by inducing platelet antibodies.

Commonly associated drugs: thiazides, sulphonamides, glibenclamide, ibuprofen, carbamazepine, phenytoin, vancomycin, piperacillin.

Acute leukaemia 🚩

The commonest of childhood tumours (➲ see Fig. 28.7). The blood count rarely shows an isolated low platelet count. The child may also have suffered from frequent infection, malaise, spontaneous bleeding, or bone pain. For other presentations ➲ see Causes of purple patches other than purpura, pp. 474–7.

Haemolytic uraemic syndrome (HUS) 🚩

Associated with *Shigella* or *E. coli 0157:H7* enteritis.

The presenting features are diarrhoeal illness, petechial, or purpuric rash. There may be fever and discolouration of urine due to endovascular haemolysis. Renal failure frequently occurs.

Thrombotic thrombocytopaenia purpura (TTP) 🚩

A rare, serious disorder due to platelet fragmentation, associated with renal dysfunction and neurological symptoms.

Autoimmune thrombocytopaenia 🚩

May occur following blood transfusion because of antibody production. Also occurs in neonates.

Abnormal platelets

Inherited platelet abnormalities

Rare diseases, e.g. Hermansky–Pudlak (associated with albinism), Glanzmann's, or Bernard–Soulier.

Acquired platelet abnormalities

Secondary to uraemia or drugs such as aspirin and non-steroidal anti-inflammatories. Clotting screen is normal but bleeding time is increased.

Inherited clotting factor deficiencies

Von Willebrand's disease

The commonest inherited clotting problem. Defective factor VIII with various types. Usually presents with bleeding after minor skin trauma or following tooth extraction.

Haemophilia

Typically presents with painful bleeding into a joint or following tooth extraction. Other clotting factor deficiencies are less common but may have similar presentation.

Prothrombotic disorders ⚑

These can present with purpura, less commonly with livedo reticularis or cutaneous infarction secondary to clotting and consumption of factors such as protein S or C deficiency, factor V Leiden deficiency, or antithrombin III deficiency. They often lead to deep vein thrombosis or pulmonary embolism.

Vessel fragility

Scurvy ⚑

Presents with purpura around follicles and in pressure sites particularly (Fig. 31.1). Bleeding occurs and if severe may cause haemarthrosis. There is angular cheilitis and gum enlargement. Corkscrew hairs are common on limbs and buttocks. Rare and potentially lethal.

Cause: vitamin C deficiency. Think about this when there is prolonged dietary insufficiency or evidence of malabsorption.

Inherited connective tissue diseases

Bruising is a feature of all types of Ehlers–Danlos syndrome (EDS). Look for skin fragility (easy scarring), cutaneous hyperextensibility, and joint laxity. Vascular EDS (type IV) patients have thinned skin, most noticeable at peripheral sites (acrogeria) and are at risk of internal artery/organ rupture (➲ see also Dermal texture changes, pp. 445–6).

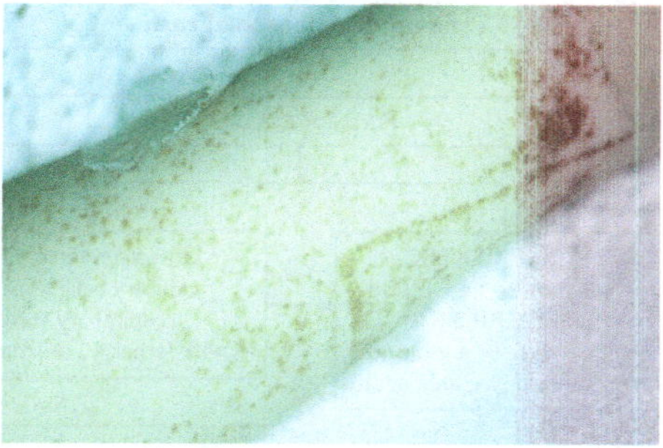

Fig. 31.1 Perifollicular purpura (with positive Hess's sign from dressing) in teenage vagrant with scurvy.

Reproduced courtesy of Susan Lewis-Jones, Hon Consultant Dermatologist, Ninewells Hospital and Medical School, Dundee, UK

Sepsis

Most febrile children with small petechiae will have a self-limiting viral infection. Any severe sepsis, e.g. *Escherichia coli, Streptococcus A, Pseudomonas*, rarely varicella, can cause purpura and disseminated intravascular coagulation (DIC) (Fig. 31.2).

The most important cause is meningococcal disease.

Meningococcal septicaemia

Background: meningococcal disease is the commonest infectious cause of death in children in developed countries. About 50% of UK cases occur in children under 4y of age and up to half the population may carry *Neisseria meningitidis* in the nasopharynx. The transfer of the organism into the bloodstream to cause invasive disease (septicaemia and/or meningitis) depends on a complex interplay of host, environmental, and virulence factors. An exotoxin produced by the bacterial cell wall causes activation of the inflammatory cascade, myocardial depression, and endothelial dysfunction with capillary leak and disseminated intravascular coagulation (DIC).

Presentation: the classic features of meningococcal disease are fever and a non-blanching rash in an ill child (Fig. 31.3). In this setting if the lesions are >2mm, then the diagnosis is very likely to be meningococcal disease. Some children present later with signs of meningism and their prognosis is better than those presenting early with septicaemia. A small proportion present with shock and no rash. Early features are vomiting, diarrhoea, and myalgia. Up to 30% have a non-specific maculopapular rash rather than a purpuric rash at presentation.

Progress: haematogenous spread occurs and the child may present at this stage with signs of shock: poor capillary refill; cool peripheries and

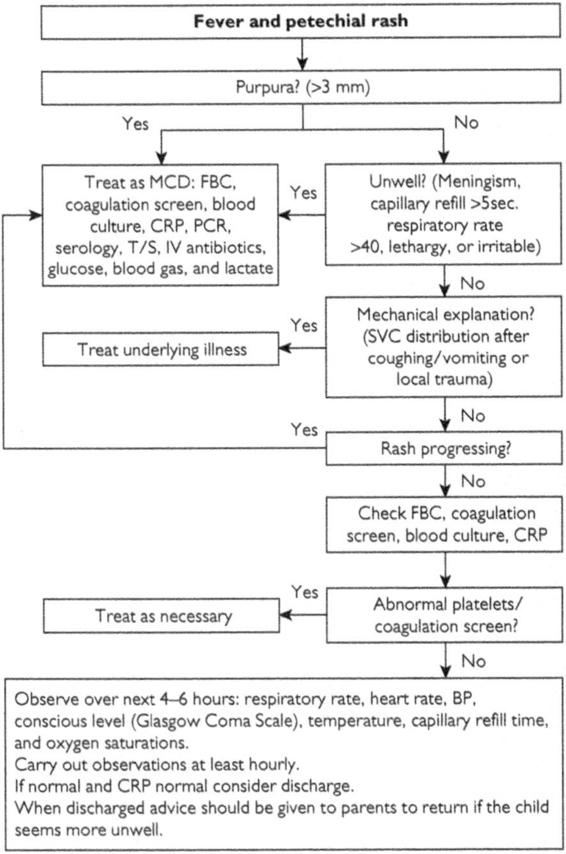

Fig. 31.2 Algorithm.

Adapted with permission from Hart C.A. and Thompson A.P.J. (2006). Meningococcal disease and its management in children. *BMJ*. 333(7570): 685–90. DOI: https://doi.org/10.1136/bmj.38968.683958.AE

a widening of peripheral and core temperature; tachycardia; oliguria and hypotension (a late and ominous sign). Pulmonary oedema may occur with tachypnoea and hypoxia.

- IV or IM penicillin (50mg/kg) should be given where possible and immediate transfer to hospital arranged when meningococcal disease is recognized in primary care (Box 31.2).

Box 31.2 Emergency treatment of meningococcal infection

Children with meningococcal septicaemia can become unwell very rapidly and die. If you suspect it, start treatment immediately with IV or IM penicillin (50mg/kg) if possible and arrange immediate transfer to hospital. IV ceftriaxone 100mg/kg (max dose 4g) should be given on arrival to hospital if no prior antibiotics have been administered.

- IV ceftriaxone should be given on arrival to hospital if no prior antibiotics administered (Box 31.2).
- High-flow oxygen.
- Shock should be vigorously treated with intravenous fluids (20ml/kg initially) followed by repeated boluses depending on response and early consideration of inotropes as necessary.
- The diagnosis should be confirmed with blood cultures and polymerase chain reaction (PCR) for *Neisseria meningitidis*. Also take blood for FBC, C-reactive protein (CRP), glucose, blood gases, and lactate.

Other infective causes of petechiae

TORCH infections

Infection in the third stage of pregnancy with pathogens such as toxoplasmosis, rubella, *Cytomegalovirus* (CMV), and herpes simplex can cause a low platelet count as part of a viraemic illness. The baby is usually jaundiced and small for age.

Papular-purpuric purpura (syn. Gloves and Socks purpura)

Uncommon, self-limiting sharply demarcated viral rash of the hands and feet (usually palms and soles) with oedema, erythema, and petechiae. Burning and itching occur and there is sometimes an associated vesicular oral enanthem and lymphadenopathy.

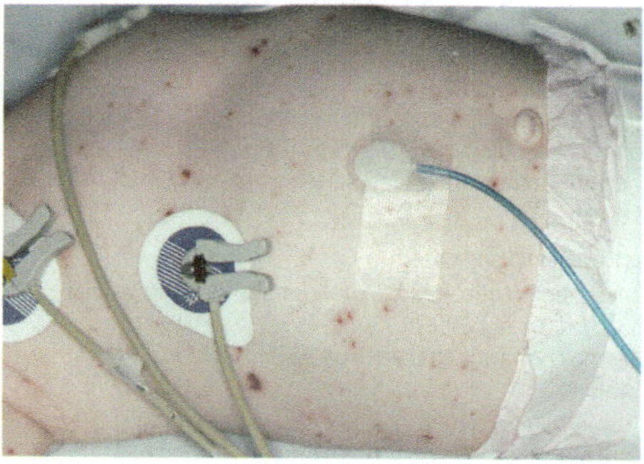

Fig. 31.3 Meningococcal septicaemia in a young infant with purpura. Management (see Fig. 31.2) Follow NICE meningococcal sepsis guidance.[1]

Reproduced courtesy of Susan Lewis-Jones, Hon Consultant Dermatologist, Ninewells Hospital and Medical School, Dundee, UK

Cause: viruses include parvovirus B19 and HHV6 and 7.

Ecthyma gangrenosum

Rare disorder of immunocompromised and neutropenic children. Starts as purplish, vasculitic lesions (➲ see Bacterial infections, p. 398).

Cause: Pseudomonas aeruginosa.

Cutaneous vasculitis

There are well-recognized clinical patterns such as Henoch–Schönlein purpura and acute haemorrhagic oedema of infancy (➲ see Cutaneous vasculitis, p. 471).

Cutaneous vasculitis can also occur as a result of:

- *Drug reactions*: such as antibiotics, thiazides, quinidine. Take a careful drug history including over-the-counter medications.
- *Infections*: such as *Streptococcus* and *Mycoplasma*.
- *Systemic vasculitis*: such as that associated with lupus erythematosus (➲ see Fig. 38.2), granulomatosis with polyangiitis (GPA), and polyarteritis nodosum.
- *Secondary*: a manifestation of underlying malignancy.

The most important clinical consideration is whether the vasculitis is limited to the skin or whether organs such as the kidneys, gut, or central nervous system (CNS) are involved.

In all cases of suspected vasculitis, blood pressure should be measured and urinary dipstix should be performed.

Investigation: see Box 31.3.

For vasculitis outside of the commonly recognized patterns mentioned next, investigation can be complex and should involve advice from a paediatric rheumatologist or dermatologist.

Box 31.3 Investigations for vasculitis

These include:

- Skin biopsy for histology and immunofluorescence.
- Blood tests: full blood count; urea and electrolytes; liver function; CRP; complements C3 and C4.
- Streptococcal serology: ASOT/anti-DNase B.
- Autoimmune profile: including ANA, ENA ds- DNA, ANCA.
- Throat swab.

Extra tests if clinically indicated

- Prothrombotic screen (anticardiolipin, lupus anticoagulant, protein S, protein C, factor V Leiden).
- Mycoplasma/hepatitis/parvovirus serology.
- Cryoglobulins.
- Immunoglobulins.
- Sinus X-ray.
- Renal ultrasound scan.
- Visceral angiography.

Henoch–Schönlein purpura (HSP)

The most common vasculitis of childhood.

- *Definition*: an immunologically mediated inflammation of small vessels which is probably a reaction to infection.
- *Clinical presentation*: usually presents in school-age children. The mean peak age range is 4–7y. Numerous 1–5mm palpable purple papules and associated petechiae are distributed on the backs of the legs and buttocks (Fig. 31.4). Low-grade pyrexia and malaise are present in 50%.
- *Complications/associations:*
  - Joint symptoms are common (60–90%). Flitting arthralgia or arthritis of large joints such as ankles and knees is typical. Joints of the upper limb are sometimes affected.
  - Gastrointestinal (GI) vasculitis occurs in 50–70% of patients. Rarely significant GI bleeding occurs—one of the potentially life-threatening complications.
  - Renal involvement is common (50–60%). Generally presents as microscopic haematuria but also proteinuria, frank haematuria, and hypertension. Approximately 5% of those with nephritis go on to develop end-stage renal failure.
  - Pulmonary and CNS involvement is rare.
- *Diagnosis*: the clinical findings are usually characteristic. In uncertain cases skin biopsy with direct immunofluorescence supports the diagnosis by showing a leukocytoclastic vasculitis with IgA deposition.
- *Management/follow-up*:
  - Most patients do not require hospital admission.
  - Pain relief (paracetamol and codeine are preferable to non-steroidal anti-inflammatory drugs).
  - Explanation of the likely prognosis and potential complications.
  - The use of systemic steroids to reduce renal complications is controversial. It is sometimes used in short courses of 1–2mg/kg/day to reduce joint or abdominal pain. Outpatient blood pressure monitoring and urine testing are necessary in all children with typical rash. This should be done weekly for 1 month and monthly for 6 months. Any child with haematuria should be followed up longer term.
- *Prognosis*: most children have a self-limiting illness which resolves in 4 weeks. Some have multiple recurrences over a period of a few months.
- *Mortality*: 1–2%. This is mainly related to end-stage renal failure but acute GI bleeding is occasionally fatal.

Acute haemorrhagic oedema of infancy

Once thought to be part of the spectrum of HSP this is now considered as a separate entity. It typically presents with bruise-like targetoid purpuric lesions on the limbs (Fig. 31.5) and face of an otherwise well preschool child. Oedema of the face and extremities is often a marked feature. Systemic involvement and long-term consequences are rare.

Capillaritis

A group of benign conditions, uncommon in children, in which small amounts of blood leak from superficial capillaries to produce lesions that

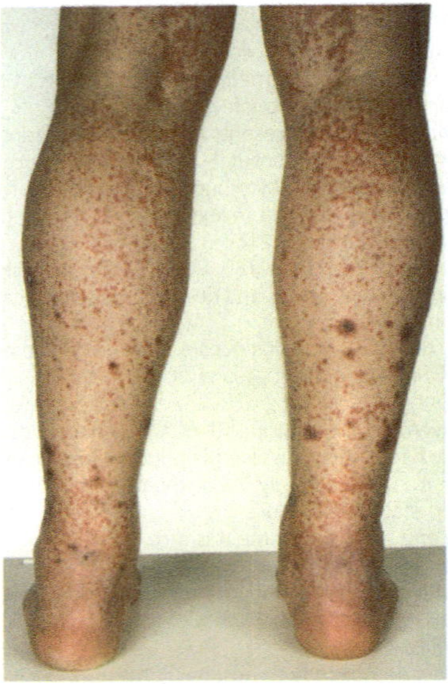

Fig. 31.4 Henoch–Schönlein purpura showing typical purpuric lesions on lower legs.
Reproduced courtesy of Cameron Kennedy, Consultant Dermatologist, Departments of Dermatology, Bristol Royal Infirmary, and Paediatric Dermatology, Bristol Royal Hospital for Children, Bristol, UK

fade through bruise-like colours (may worsen with exercise). Aberrant cell-mediated immunity leading to inflammation and fragility of capillaries may be the cause. They probably represent a spectrum of one disease but may be subdivided into separate clinical types:

- *Schamberg's disease*: a chronic condition with hyperpigmented (red/brown) macules usually distributed symmetrically on lower legs, containing tiny petechiae like sprinkles of 'Cayenne pepper'. Mildly itchy but often only a cosmetic concern.
- *Lichen aureus*: grouped papular golden/rust-coloured lesions which may coalesce into plaques (Fig. 31.6). Tends to persist. Sometimes mildly pruritic.
- *Majocchi's purpura*: annular purpuric lesions (initially pink) with telangiectasia, which spread slowly and may become atrophic centrally. Asymptomatic. Chronic recurrences over months to years.
- *Itching purpura*: similar to Schamberg's but intensely itchy and may be more papular and scaly. Tends to resolve spontaneously. Sometimes related to contact allergy to clothing dyes.

(a) (b)

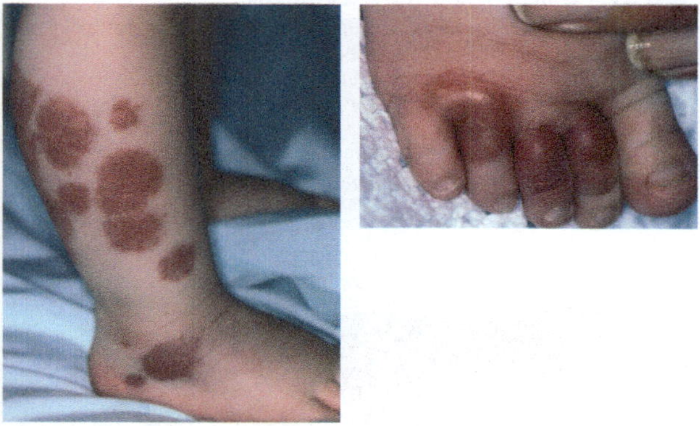

Fig. 31.5 (a) Acute haemorrhagic oedema of infancy with typical purpuric lesions on legs. (b) Acute haemorrhagic oedema, typical lesion on toes.

Reproduced courtesy of Susan Lewis-Jones, Hon Consultant Dermatologist, Ninewells Hospital and Medical School, Dundee, UK

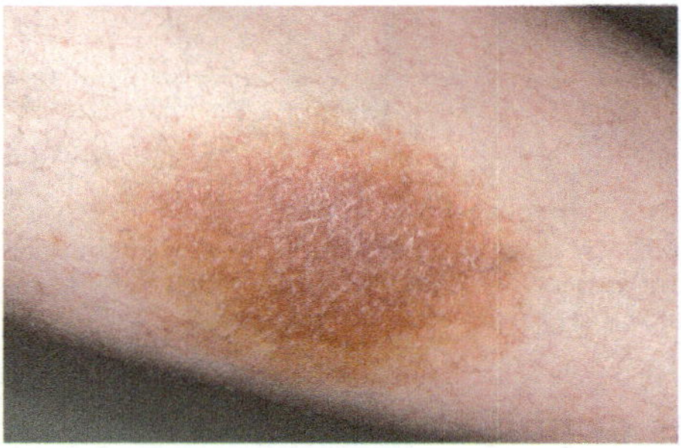

Fig. 31.6 Lichen aureus on lower leg.

Reproduced courtesy of Susan Lewis-Jones, Hon Consultant Dermatologist, Ninewells Hospital and Medical School, Dundee, UK

Special considerations in the neonate

Vitamin K deficiency

Acute haemorrhagic disease of the newborn is rare in the United Kingdom because of the use of prophylactic vitamin K. It may present with widespread bleeding into the skin 'purpura fulminans' (Box 31.4 and Fig. 31.7), although catastrophic intracranial haemorrhage or bleeding from the umbilical stump are more common presentations.

Box 31.4 Causes of purpura fulminans

Fulminating widespread purpura usually occurring in neonates or infants but sometimes older children. Caused by:

- Acute infections, e.g. *Neisseria meningitides, Staphylococcus, Streptococcus*, post varicella-zoster or rubella.
- Low vitamin K.
- Protein C or S deficiency—acquired or congenital.
- Low platelets, e.g. heparin toxicity.
- Toxins from bites, e.g. snakes or spiders (usually older children).

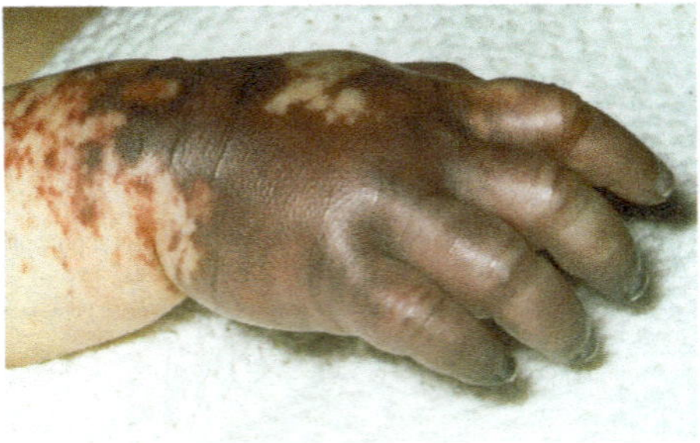

Fig. 31.7 Purpura fulminans.

Reproduced courtesy of Cameron Kennedy, Consultant Dermatologist, Departments of Dermatology, Bristol Royal Infirmary, and Paediatric Dermatology, Bristol Royal Hospital for Children, Bristol, UK

Autoimmune thrombocytopaenia

Low platelets may occur in the neonate because of incompatibility of parental platelet antigens. This is akin to rhesus incompatibility causing neonatal anaemia and can be confirmed by parental typing.

Causes of purple patches other than purpura

- ➲ See also Bruising and purpura, pp. 361–2 and Box 25.2.

Metabolic

Fabry' disease: rare lysosomal storage disorder with alpha-galactosidase A deficiency causing tiny cutaneous red, purple, or blue/black vascular lesions from age of 5y onwards. Mainly males, scrotal lesions common. Renal problems and hypertension in later life.

Livedo reticularis

A bluish-purple, mesh-like discolouration that occurs at sites of cutaneous arterial underperfusion. Physiological cutis marmorata (Fig. 31.8) is

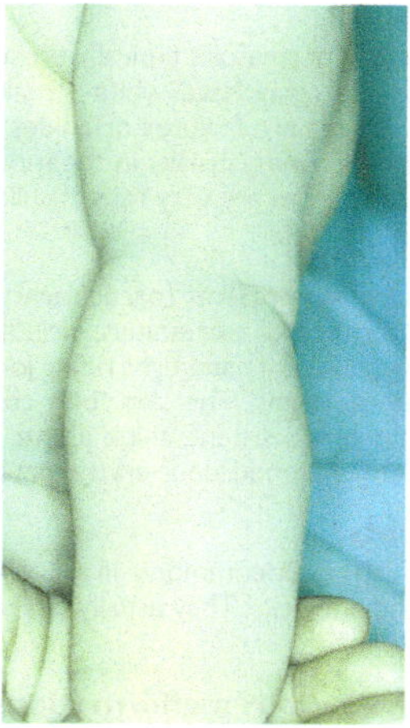

Fig. 31.8 Physiological cutis marmorata.

Reproduced courtesy of Susan Lewis-Jones, Hon Consultant Dermatologist, Ninewells Hospital and Medical School, Dundee, UK

common in infancy when it tends to be uniformly distributed. It is sometimes seen in thyroid disease.

Broken, patchy livedo is more likely to be pathological:

- ***Autoimmune connective tissue disease*** such as lupus erythematosus, antiphospholipid antibody syndrome, or polyarteritis nodosum (➲ see Chapter 38).
- ***Cutis marmorata telangiectatica congenita*** (➲ see Fig. 8.20), a congenital naevoid vascular malformation sometimes associated with other developmental abnormalities such as hemi-hypertrophy, aplasia cutis, and macrocephaly.
- ***Erythema ab igne*** from sitting close to a fire for long periods may be reddish purple initially but fades to reddish brown with time (➲ see Brown colouration, p. 488).

Dermatomyositis

Rash is classically purplish ('heliotrope' after a flower) and distributed in areas most exposed to sunlight, especially on cheeks and dorsum of the hands (➲ see Fig. 29.12) and also on upper eyelids (➲ see Fig. 29.11). There may be Gottron's papules over the knuckles and an associated proximal myopathy.

Morphoea

An inflammatory autoimmune skin condition which may present initially with bruise-like marks in patches or linear bands. Unlike bruising, it persists and may become sclerotic or atrophic with hyperpigmentation (➲ see Figs. 29.1 and 29.2 and Chapter 38).

Lichen planus

An idiopathic inflammatory dermatosis typically presenting with flat-topped polygonal purplish papules (may have white streaks—Wickham's striae; ➲ see Fig. 19.5). Typical sites are flexures of ankles and wrists but can be more generalized. Look for white streaks in the mouth and nail dystrophy (➲ see Fig. 15.8). Vulval changes are very rare in children.

Perniosis (*syn.* chilblains)

Caused by cold exposure and presents (particularly on warming) as painful purplish or blue discolouration of extremities, including the ears (Fig. 31.9). Mechanical factors may play a part and tight riding jodhpurs may contribute to perniosis of the lateral thighs. The skin feels colder than surrounding normal skin. If extreme or persistent, think about underlying connective tissue disease, particularly systemic lupus erythematosus (➲ Chapter 38).

Mongolian blue spots

Melanocytic lesions which occur commonly in racially pigmented skin, commonly over the back and buttocks. They usually fade over years (➲ see Figs. 7.5 and 24.2).

Haemangiomas and venous malformations

Some types are purple/bluish and mimic bruising (➲ see Vascular tumours, pp. 94–9).

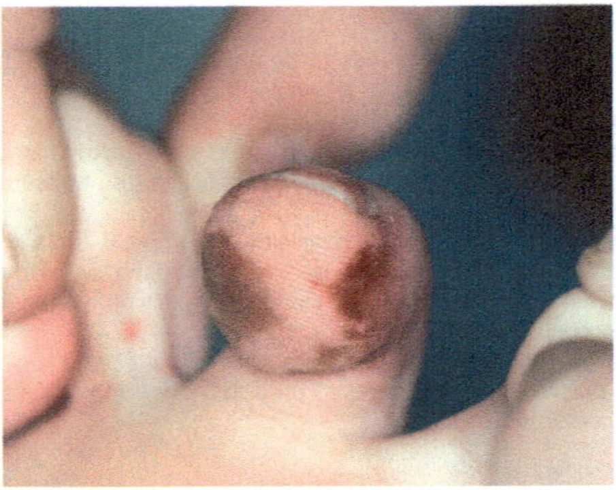

Fig. 31.9 Chilblains of the toes (perniosis).

Reproduced courtesy of Susan Lewis-Jones, Hon Consultant Dermatologist, Ninewells Hospital and Medical School, Dundee, UK

Tumours

- ➲ See also Chapter 28.
- ***Solid tumours*** such as sarcomas (rare).
- ***Vascular tumours*** such as haemangiomas (➲ see Vascular tumours, pp. 94–9).
- ***Acute leukaemia*** may present as:
  - 'Blueberry muffin' lesions (extramedullary haemopoeisis) in young infants (➲ see Figs. 7.7 and 28.7).
  - Petechial lesions from low platelets (➲ see Abnormality of clotting factors, pp. 465–6).
  - Primary or secondary cutaneous papules or nodules (➲ see Fig. 28.7). Small lesions may be mistaken for insect bites.
  - Rare associations with other skin disorders such as pyoderma gangrenosum (➲ see Causes of ulcers, pp. 456–9) or Sweet's syndrome (*syn.* acute neutrophilic dermatosis).

References

1. NICE (2010). *Meningitis (Bacterial) and Meningococcal Septicaemia in Under 16s: Recognition, Diagnosis and Management*, Clinical Guideline [CG102], https://www.nice.org.uk/guidance/CG102/chapter/1-Guidance#pre-hospital-management-of-suspected-bacterial-meningitis-and-meningococcal-septicaemia

Chapter 32

White colouration

Introduction

This chapter covers conditions that cause skin to appear white. This may be localized or generalized and it is sometimes associated with underlying disease.

Pigmentary changes

Normal skin colour is mainly determined by the melanin content (brown pigment).

- Eumelanin—black/brown (majority).
- Phaeomelanin—red/yellow—minority (except in redheads).

Other chromophores

Oxyhaemoglobin (red), deoxygenated haemoglobin (blue).
Rarely: carotene (yellow), haemosiderin (red/brown).

White skin (hypomelanosis)

Normal ethnic 'white' skin is not truly white but contains a small amount of pigment and the potential to tan with ultraviolet light exposure (➲ see Chapter 16 for skin types).

Commonest causes of abnormal white patches

- ***Vitiligo***: usually well-defined, symmetrical patches.
- ***Postinflammatory depigmentation***: follows many inflammatory dermatoses, e.g. eczema, psoriasis, pityriasis alba.
- ***Halo naevus***: melanocytic naevus with white halo around (➲ see Fig. 34.6).
- ***Ash leaf macules***: seen in tuberous sclerosis complex.
- ***Pityriasis versicolor***: rare prepuberty (➲ see Infections, p. 484).
- ***Extragenital lichen sclerosus***.
- ***Scars***.
- ***Infections***: secondary syphilis, yaws, pinta, leprosy, onchocerciasis, and post kala-azar (very rare in United Kingdom but common in some countries; ➲ see Chapter 22).
- ***Drugs and chemicals***: ➲ see p. 486.

Less common causes

- ***Birthmarks*** such as naevus depigmentosus, naevus anaemicus, hypomelanosis of Ito.
- ***Genetic disorders*** such as albinism, piebaldism, Waardenburg syndrome, homocystinuria, and Fanconi syndrome.
- ***Malnutrition***, e.g. kwashiorkor or selenium deficiency in total parenteral nutrition (➲ see Chapter 6).
- ***Tuberculoid leprosy***—pale anaesthetic patch (➲ see Fig. 22.9).
- ***Tumours***: such as hypopigmented mycosis fungoides (➲ see Chapter 22).

Vitiligo

- An autoimmune disease characterized by symmetrical (usually) well-defined ivory-white patches on sun-exposed areas: dorsa of hands, face (particularly perioral and periorbital), neck, and flexures (Fig. 32.1).

Pigmentation may be increased around follicles, and/or immediately around lesions.

- Generally quite subtle in Caucasians but a serious cosmetic and social problem in darker skin types and may be mistaken for leprosy.
- Common, affecting 2% of the population and is often familial. A quarter of cases start before 8y of age.
- Between 10% and 20% are associated with other autoimmune conditions, e.g. Hashimoto's thyroiditis, diabetes mellitus, alopecia areata, and polyendocrine deficiencies.
- There is a rare segmental variant.

Inheritance: autosomal dominant with incomplete penetrance.

Prognosis: variable course with remissions and exacerbations. Complete spontaneous repigmentation is unlikely to occur.

Treatment: sun-protection and cosmetic camouflage. Potent topical corticosteroids for up to 3 months (caution in large areas in young children). Phototherapy with PUVA (psoralen with UVA) can stimulate repigmentation in some cases but is inadvisable in younger children or skin type 1 or 2. Many other modalities have been advocated, reflecting the current lack of effective therapies. These include topical calcineurin inhibitors, short bursts of long-term, low-dose systemic corticosteroids, and surgical techniques. Most are not suitable for children. See also the National Institute for Health and Care Excellence (NICE) Guidelines for the diagnosis and management of vitiligo.[1]

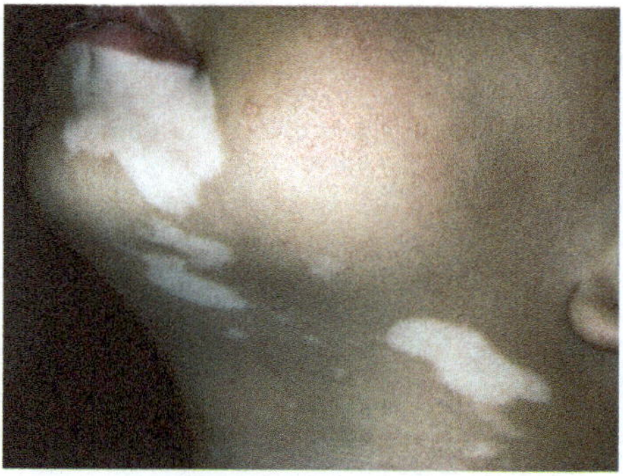

Fig. 32.1 Vitiligo on face and neck, with well-defined edges.
Reproduced courtesy of Patrick Yesudian, Consultant Dermatologist, Chennai, India

Postinflammatory depigmentation

Follows many inflammatory skin conditions, e.g. psoriasis or eczema (Fig. 32.2). Pale areas occur in sites of previous rash. It is temporary and non-scarring, fading with time. It is more obvious in darker skin types.

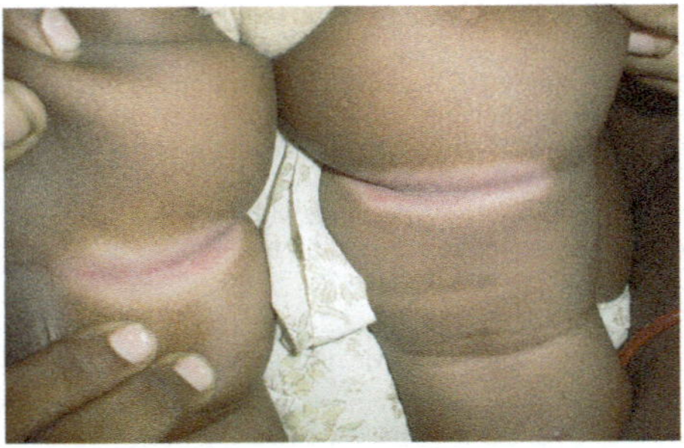

Fig. 32.2 Postinflammatory depigmentation in flexures in atopic eczema.
Reproduced courtesy of Susan Lewis-Jones, Hon Consultant Dermatologist, Ninewells Hospital and Medical School, Dundee, UK

Pityriasis alba

Usually asymptomatic but unsightly round to oval ill-defined patches with fine surface scale, mainly on face, neck, and trunk (Fig. 32.3). Caused by a low-grade postinflammatory eczematous process predominately in atopic children with dry skin. Extremely common and more obvious in darker skin types. Self-limiting and resolves within a few months but can rarely persist for years.

Treatment: Reassurance and emollients. Low-potency topical corticosteroid (hydrocortisone) if eczema is still active.

Note: A rare hypopigmented variant of mycosis fungoides can mimic pityriasis alba, so in extensive persistent disease a skin biopsy should be performed for histopathological examination.

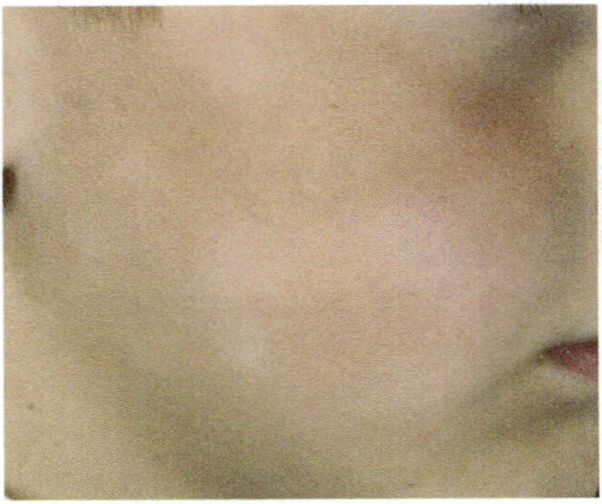

Fig. 32.3 Pityriasis alba showing poorly defined edges.
Reproduced courtesy of Susan Lewis-Jones, Hon Consultant Dermatologist, Ninewells Hospital and Medical School, Dundee, UK

Ash leaf macules and tuberous sclerosis complex (TSC)

- Seen in >80% of those with TSC (Fig. 32.4; also see next section).
- Irregular, roughly linear/leaf-shaped macules.
- May present at birth, preceding epilepsy, or postdate the fits.
- Seen best under Wood's lamp (see Examining the skin, pp. 18–19).

A confetti-like depigmentation is also seen, often most noticeable on the legs.

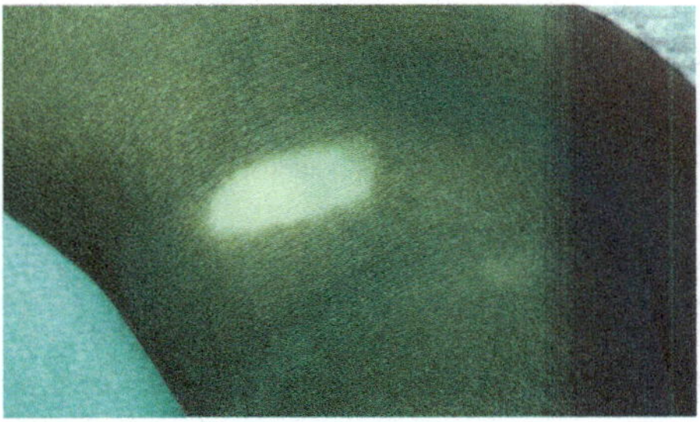

Fig. 32.4 Ash leaf macule.
Reproduced courtesy of Patrick Yesudian

Tuberous sclerosis complex (TSC)

Autosomal dominant, multigene, and multisystem disorder with variable penetrance (i.e. may not be obvious). Caused by an impairment of cell-cycling regulatory genes allowing development of tumours—typically hamartomas in skin, eyes and internally, including brain, heart, and kidneys. Renal failure is common in middle life. Epileptic fits are caused by cerebral tubers (hamartomas). Impaired intellectual development of varying degrees may occur and there may be significant psychological and behavioural problems. There are a number of cutaneous manifestations (Box 32.1).

Box 32.1 Cutaneous features of TSC

- *Ash leaf macules*: usually earliest sign and may precede fits.
- *Angiofibromas* (red papules) around mouth and nose (*syn.* adenoma sebaceum) from 3y but commonest in teens, worsen with age.
- *Shagreen patches*: irregular skin coloured papules on trunk in 50%.
- *Periungual fibromas*: hard irregular lesions around nail base causing nail distortion with longitudinal grooving (see Fig. 15.11). Most occur in teens onwards but can be earlier.
- *Fibrous forehead plaques*: firm irregular nodules.
- *Café-au-lait macules* (see Fig. 33.3 and Localized forms of brown pigmentation, p. 491–4) in 25% (usually just one or two). Not diagnostic
- *Enamel pits* on the teeth are common.

Box 32.2 Generalized hypopigmentation

- *Extensive vitiligo.*
- *Oculocutaneous albinism*: types I and II.
- *Phenylketonuria*: in those untreated.
- *Other rare genetic syndromes*: very pale skin, eyes and hair may be seen in Angelman, Prader–Willi, Apert, Menke's kinky hair, Chédiak–Higashi, Hermansky–Pudlak, Griscelli, and others.

Diagnosis: is clinical; always examine the parents carefully. Genetic testing is not always possible.

Management: multidisciplinary assessment and management with MRI and renal scans and genetic counselling and annual follow-up.

Extragenital lichen sclerosus (LS)

Uncommon. White patches, often rough or rugose (Fig. 32.5), and occasionally with hyperkeratotic follicular spicules. May occur in isolation or in association with genital LS (➲ see Fig. 13.6). Check genital area.

Treatment: may respond to potent/super potent topical corticosteroids.

Infections

Pityriasis versicolor

Seen occasionally in teenagers as fairly well-defined oval, pale, scaly patches (may be pink or pale pink/brown patches in pale skins—hence name), mainly on the upper trunk (➲ see Fig. 11.1). Usually asymptomatic.

Leprosy

Depigmented anaesthetic white macules occur in leprosy. Rare in UK but common worldwide. Consider in immigrants from endemic countries (➲ see Fig. 22.9).

Others: such as syphilis, pinta, and yaws, ➲ see Spirochete infections, pp. 336–7

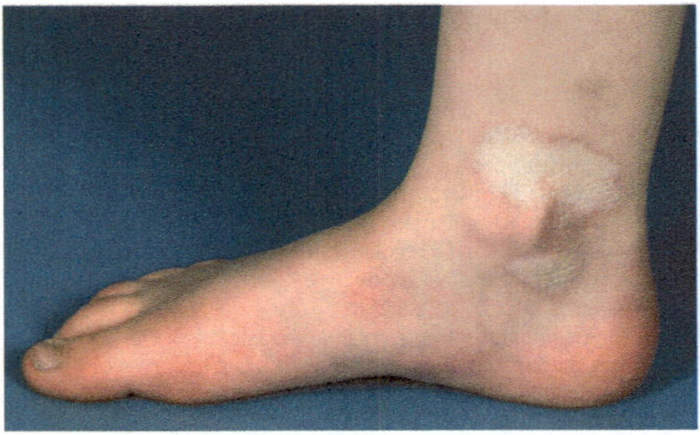

Fig. 32.5 Extragenital lichen sclerosus.

Reproduced courtesy of Susan Lewis-Jones, Hon Consultant Dermatologist, Ninewells Hospital and Medical School, Dundee, UK

Birthmarks

There are a number of rare congenital birthmarks presenting as hypomelanosis, some of which represent cutaneous mosaicism. The following are the better known:

- *Naevus anaemicus*: congenital patches of pale white skin with sharp edges produced by hypersensitivity of local vessels to circulating catecholamines. Edges disappear on application of glass (diascopy) or dermatoscope, and the surrounding skin, but not the patch itself. It will become red in response to local heat or rubbing.
- *Naevus depigmentosus*: unchanging, pale areas on trunk or proximal limbs caused by defective transfer of melanocyte pigment. It may be segmental but does not cross the midline.
- *Hypomelanosis of Ito*: often extensive lesions in whorls following lines of Blaschko (➔ see Fig. 4.6). It may be associated with systemic features, e.g. epilepsy, mental retardation, eye, or skeletal problems. It is seen as a result of mosaicism caused by several possible mechanisms.

Inherited diseases

There are a number of extremely rare genetic syndromes associated with generalized congenital hypopigmentation (Box 32.2).

Piebaldism

Autosomal dominant condition affecting melanocyte migration. Presents at birth with large areas of depigmentation, especially across anterior trunk (often diamond-shaped) and as a 'sleeve' around knees and elbows. Within the white areas there are usually oval areas of brown pigment that may enlarge with time and there is often a white forelock. Some types are associated with other anomalies, e.g. Waardenburg's syndrome (several types, often with deafness, heterochromia of the iris, and a broad nasal root).

Oculocutaneous albinism (OCA)

Several types exist with varying severity depending on the degree of tyrosinase deficiency. The two main types are OCA1 (tyrosinase negative—more severe) and OCA2 (some tyrosinase positivity). There is generalized hypopigmentation of hair and skin (with failure to tan), and ocular problems. These children are at risk of skin cancer in later life and need full sun protective measures (➔ see Photoprotective measures', p. 238). Different types look very similar at birth.

White hair

White hair may be acquired or inherited and may be generalized, e.g. in albinism, or localized, e.g. as a white forelock or in regrowth following alopecia areata, and sometimes in vitiligo (➔ see also Changes in hair colour, p. 208).

Xeroderma pigmentosum

Rare autosomal recessive disease of defective DNA repair. Freckling and hyperpigmentation occur initially, followed by white and atrophic spots as result of photosensitivity. It is associated with premature ageing and early death due to markedly increased risk of skin cancers from early childhood (see Fig. 32.6 and ➔ Exaggerated sunburn reactions, pp. 234–7).

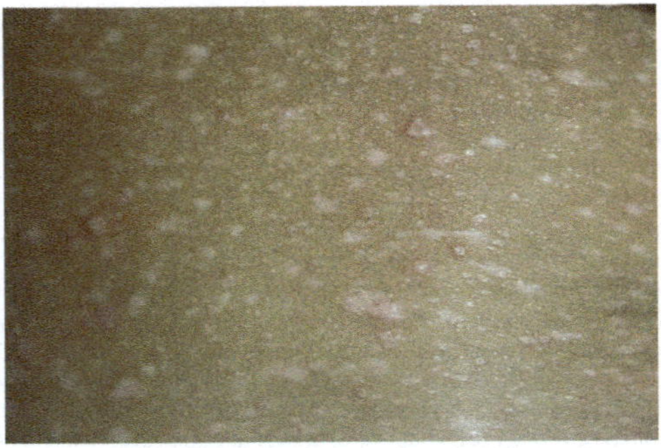

Fig. 32.6 Pigmentary changes of xeroderma pigmentosum (see Chapter 16).
Reproduced courtesy of Graham Sharpe, Consultant Dermatologist, Clatterbridge Hospital, UK

Drugs and chemicals

Unusual cause of hypopigmentation in childhood:

- Can occur with topical and intralesional corticosteroids. This resolves with time.
- Diphenylcyclopropenone used to treat alopecia areata (rarely).
- Phenols, catechols, and benzene derivatives used in industry as antiseptics and cleaning agents.
- Ingestion of arsenic can cause hypo- and hyperpigmentation (➲ see Drugs causing brown pigmentations, pp. 497–8).

References

1. NICE (2016). *Clinical Knowledge Summaries: Vitiligo*, https://cks.nice.org.uk/vitiligo

Chapter 33

Brown colouration

Introduction

This chapter describes brown skin lesions and rashes excluding moles (➲ for moles, see Chapter 34).

The brownish colouration of skin is attributable mainly to the melanin in the epidermal layer. It varies according to racial type (➲ see Table 16.1). It can be exaggerated in various genetic, inflammatory, metabolic, and nutritional conditions. Brown discolouration can also be caused by deposition of haemosiderin or the applications of chemicals or dyes.

Brown colouration

Pattern of distribution

Pigmentation may be diffuse and/or generalized or localized to body sites or appear as definite brown lesions, which may be flat or raised. There may be various patterns or shapes, e.g. linear or non-linear. Non-linear shapes include oval, round, or blocks of pigmented shapes that may represent various types of genetic mosaicism (➲ see Chapter 4).

Oval or round brown shapes

These may be macular (flat) or raised.

- Melanocytic naevi (moles)—usually raised (➲ Chapter 34).
- Café-au-lait macules—flat (➲ see Congenital/genetic brown pigmentation, p. 491).
- Naevus spilus—flat (Fig 34.7).
- Urticaria pigmentosa (➲ see Fig 19.8) or solitary mastocytomas (➲ see Fig. 28.6)—raised and urticate (red swelling) on rubbing (➲ see also Non-infective causes, pp. 285–8, Inflammatory skin, pp. 384–5, Systemic disease, p. 496, and Causes, p. 490).
- Postinflammatory, e.g. fixed drug eruption (➲ see Chapter 23 and Fig. 23.6), tuberculoid leprosy (➲ see Bacterial infection, pp. 332–5).

Shape may vary and all may present as birthmarks or be acquired.

Rippled pigmentation

- 'Dirty neck': common in chronic atopic eczema.
- Cutaneous amyloidosis (➲ see Localized forms of brown pigmentation, pp. 491–4).
- Acanthosis nigricans (➲ see Metabolic/endocrine, p. 495) may look rippled on the neck particularly (Fig. 33.1).

Reticulate pigmentation

- *Erythema ab igne*: postinflammatory usually from sitting close to the fire or prolonged use of hot water bottles or heat pads—uncommon in children so consider hypothyroidism.
- *Confluent and reticulated papillomatosis of Gougerot and Carteaud*: rare, seen in teenagers, usually in the flexures—may respond to oral minocycline.
- *Rare genetic disorders*: e.g. dyskeratosis congenita, Fanconi's anaemia, Dowling–Degos disease, reticulate acral pigmentation of Kitamura, acropigmentation of Dohi, and others.
- Macular amyloidosis and scleroderma can also cause reticulate pigmentation.

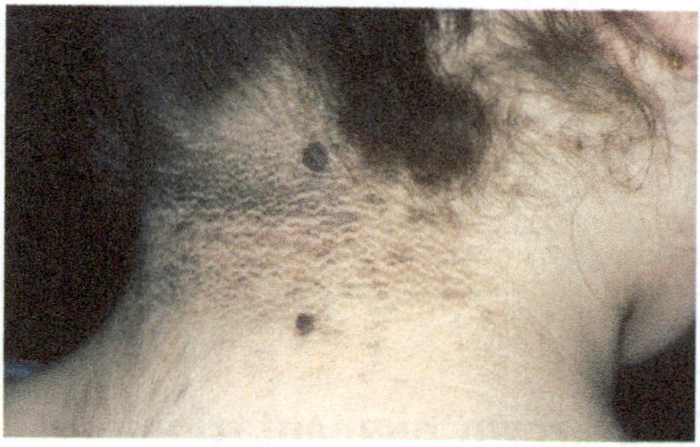

Fig. 33.1 Linear, rippled pattern of hyperpigmentation on the neck in acanthosis nigricans.

Reproduced courtesy of Susan Lewis-Jones, Hon Consultant Dermatologist, Ninewells Hospital and Medical School, Dundee, UK

Linear and whorled pigmentation

Following lines of Blaschko (➲ see Figs. 4.5. and 4.6), e.g. incontinentia pigmenti (➲ see Figs. 25.12, 25.13, and Genetic causes of blisters, pp. 387–90).

Linear brown shapes

- *Pigmentary demarcation lines*: these are non-palpable lines of apposition of two subtly different uniform skin tones in one individual. They are a normal finding, more common in darker skin types, and are most commonly seen on the upper limbs and chest.
- *Pigmentary mosaicism*: (➲ see also Congenital/genetic pigmentation, p. 491). A general term for a highly complex and rapidly expanding area of understanding. In essence, affected children have two clones of skin cells with different pigmentation. These develop along the embryonal Blaschko's lines (➲ see Fig. 4.6), producing either macular whorled pigmentation over the trunk (➲ see Fig. 4.5), and/or a streaky linear pattern on the limbs (➲ see Fig. 4.10). Other patterns such as segmental or phylloid shapes may occur. *Any patient suspected of having a mosaic disorder should be referred for a genetic opinion.*
- *Incontinentia pigmenti*: there is postinflammatory streaky macular hyperpigmentation in the third phase, which disappears with time. Seek a history of inflammatory blisters in the neonatal period (➲ see Fig. 25.12 and Genetic causes of blisters, pp. 387–90).

Box 33.1 Commonest causes of brown pigmentation

- Acquired.
- Congenital/genetic.
- Inflammatory.
- Metabolic/endocrine.
- Drugs.
- Moles (melanocytic naevi; ➲ see Chapter 34).

- *Epidermal naevi*: (➲ see Figs. 4.5, 4.10 and 28.17; see also Other epidermal textural changes, pp. 442–4).

Causes of brown lesions

Pigmented brown lesions are usually categorized as congenital, i.e. present at or soon after birth, or acquired (Box 33.1). They may be melanocytic (➲ see Chapter 34) or non-melanocytic and sometimes differentiation can be difficult. Lesions vary in colour from very light brown (often described as coffee-coloured) through any shade of brown to black (for black lesions, ➲ see Chapter 35).

Acquired brown pigmentation

Postinflammatory hyperpigmentation

Hypo- or hyperpigmentation occurs in skin previously affected by inflammation, friction, or burns. It can take up to 2y to resolve. It is more pronounced in darker skins, and commonly seen with childhood eczema from rubbing. Bizarre linear shapes may be seen as a result of phytophotodermatitis (➲ see Fig. 16.7 and Phytophotodermatitis, p. 233).

Freckles (ephelids)

- Tan-coloured macules in fair skins on sun-exposed sites, especially face, arms, and shoulders. They typically fade in winter unlike lentigines. Severe, heavy freckling in childhood may be a sign of xeroderma pigmentosum (➲ see Fig. 16.10 and Exaggerated sunburn reaction, pp. 234–7).
- Freckling in the axillae, groins, submammary region, and at the base of the neck are one of the features of neurofibromatosis type 1 (➲ see Localized forms of brown pigmentation, pp. 491–4).

Lentigines

Small (around 1–5mm), usually rounded and sharply defined macules of light to dark brown/black hyperpigmentation. They can appear anywhere on the body and are often multiple but rarely generalized. Can be related to ultraviolet exposure, but unlike freckles do not fade in winter. They have a characteristic histological appearance but can be difficult to differentiate clinically from freckles and/or junctional melanocytic naevi. They are also seen in certain rare genetic syndromes, e.g. Peutz–Jegher, LEOPARD syndrome, or Carney complex (➲ see Localized forms of brown pigmentation, pp. 491–4).

Becker's naevus

A unilateral hyperpigmented segmental patch on the shoulder or pectoral area (rarely in other body sites) appearing predominantly in teenage males (1 in 200). Lesions are usually large, often with associated hypertrichosis (Fig. 33.2).

Treatment: local shaving, depilatory creams, or laser epilation may help.

Smooth muscle hamartomas

Pigmented in 60% and may be confused with Becker's naevus.

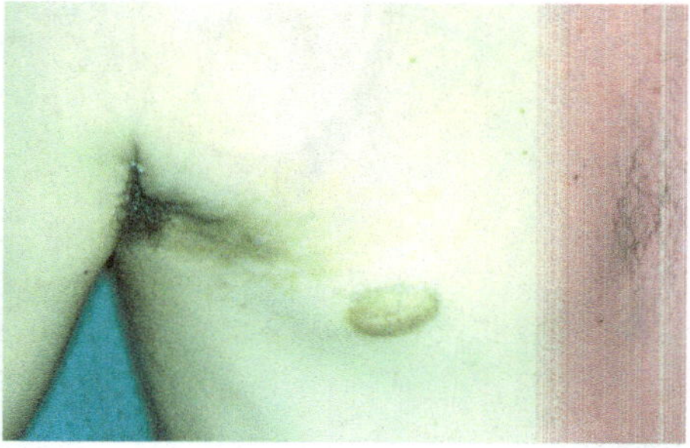

Fig. 33.2 Becker's naevus is often not hairy in adolescents.
Reproduced courtesy of NHS Tayside Clinical Photography, Dundee, UK

Congenital/genetic brown pigmentation

This may be generalized or localized patches and may be in a particular body site, e.g. flexural. There are several patterns of mosaicism described, such as naevoid, segmental, rippled, linear, or whorled (following Blaschko's lines, ➲ see Fig 4.6). This is often known as pigmentary mosaicism (➲ see Linear brown shapes, p. 489).

There are also various forms of dyschromatosis (exhibiting several different shades from white to brown patches), e.g. in dyskeratosis congenita (*syn.* Zinsser–Cole–Engman syndrome), a very rare X-linked dominant.

Localized forms of brown pigmentation

Café-au-lait macule (CALMs)

Congenital or acquired, flat, usually oval areas of increased pigmentation, varying from light to dark brown, and of any size, in any site (Fig. 33.3). Around 10–20% of normal people have one or two CALMs, but more than five is one of the cardinal features of neurofibromatosis type 1. Other syndromes associated with CALMs include tuberous sclerosis complex, Watson syndrome, ataxia telangiectasia, Bloom syndrome, Westerhof syndrome, and Silver–Russell syndrome. Large irregular CALMs are found in McCune–Albright syndrome (polyostotic fibrous dysplasia) with precocious puberty and bone lesions.

Neurofibromatosis type 1 (NF1)

NF1 is the commonest genodermatosis with a birth frequency of about 1 in 2500. It is an autosomal dominant mutation found on chromosome 17, with variable penetrance and expressivity. Around 50% are due to new mutations. Segmental NF is rare and usually without systemic problems. However, a child of a parent with segmental NF1 and gonadal involvement has an approximately 5% chance of developing 'full blown' NF1. Abnormal function of cell-cycle regulatory genes causes a neurocutaneous

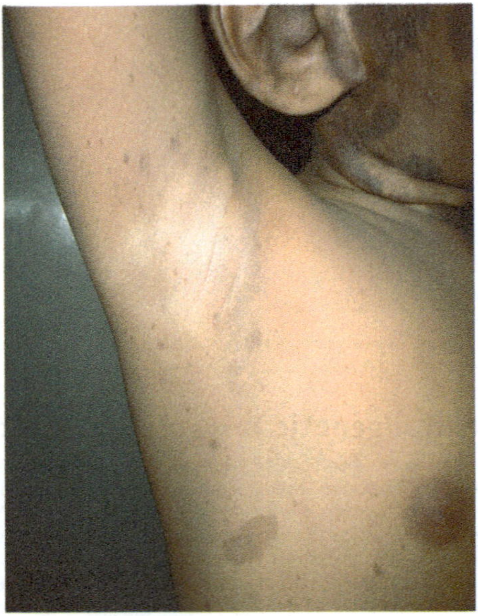

Fig. 33.3 CALM and axillary freckling.
Reproduced courtesy of Patrick Yesudian, Consultant Dermatologist, Chennai, India

multisystem disorder with skin tumours (neurofibromas; ➲ see Fig. 28.2), CALMs, macrocephaly (50%), skeletal, lung, ocular problems, and hypertension and there may be subtle learning difficulties. Rarely malignant or space-occupying tumours occur usually in adult life. *Legius syndrome is similar but lacks neurofibromas and Lisch nodules.*

Diagnosis: Clinical, see Box 33.2.

Children with NF1 and their families should be managed in a multidisciplinary setting with regular monitoring and provided with appropriate genetic counselling.

Naevus spilus (speckled lentiginous naevus)

Flat lesion that may be mistaken for a CALM but contains mottled areas of pigmentation (Figs. 33.3 and 34.4).

Syndromal lentigines

Multiple lentigines are found in:

- *LEOPARD syndrome* (*syn*. Moynahan): associated with multiple anomalies including eye, heart, and lungs with developmental delay.

Box 33.2 Diagnostic criteria for NF1

Two or more of the following criteria

- Five or more CALMS (90%) 1.5cm or 0.5cm prepuberty.
- Two or more neurofibromas (appear from end of first decade) or one plexiform neuroma (particularly on head and neck).
- Optic glioma—causes visual field defects usually before age 5y.
- Axillary or inguinal freckling in over 70% (Fig. 33.3).
- Two or more Lisch nodules (hamartomas of the iris seen on slit lamp examination).
- Skeletal abnormalities such as sphenoid dysplasia (causes large unsightly eye socket).
- Affected first-degree relative.

Note: in infants only CALMs may be visible.

Adapted from US Department of Health and Human Services. National Institutes of Health. *Neurofibromatosis*. NIH Consensus Statement Online 1987 Jul 13–15; 6(12):1–19. https://consensus.nih.gov/1987/1987Neurofibramatosis064html.htm

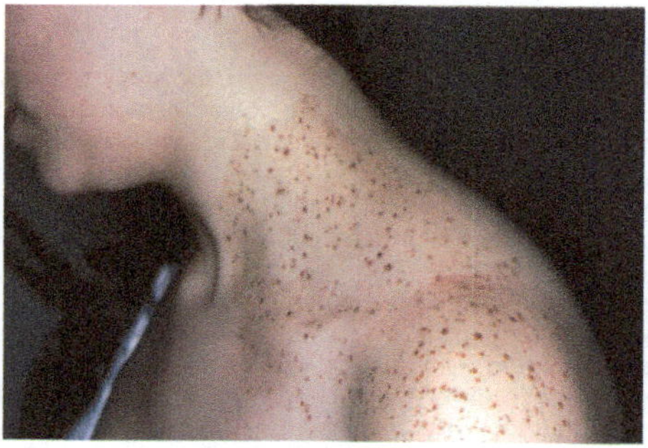

Fig. 33.4 Speckled lentiginous naevus.

Reproduced courtesy of NHS Tayside Clinical Photography, Dundee, UK

- *Carney complex (includes NAME and LAMB syndromes)*: associated with cutaneous and internal myxomas (especially cardiac) and sometimes endocrinopathies.
- *Peutz–Jegher syndrome*: autosomal dominant disorder characterized by pigmented macules on oral mucosa, lips and acral areas including nails, and associated with gastrointestinal polyps (Fig. 33.5). Complications include gastrointestinal tract (GIT) manifestations, e.g. intussusception, abdominal pain, vomiting, and bleeding. Malignancy within polyps in 2–3%. Other malignancies, breast, and gynaecological cancers—usually occur in adults.
- *Mucocutaneous lentigines* occur in Carney complex, Peutz–Jegher (Fig. 33.5), and Bannayan–Riley–Ruvalcaba syndrome.

Referral to the local Genetics service is essential if these are suspected.

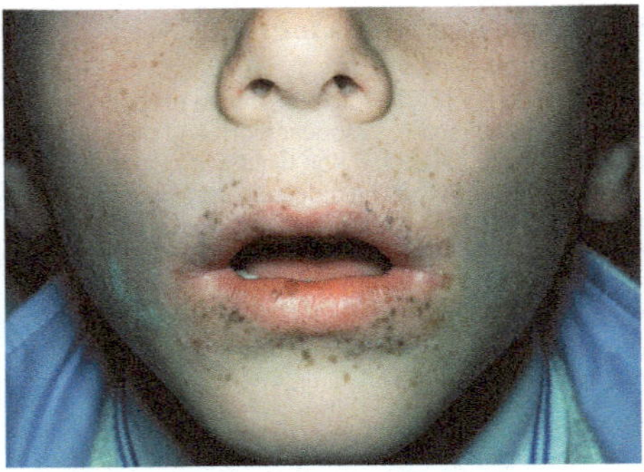

Fig. 33.5 Peutz–Jeghers syndrome with perioral lentigines.
Reproduced courtesy of Susan Lewis-Jones, Hon Consultant Dermatologist, Ninewells Hospital and Medical School, Dundee, UK

Postinflammatory

- *Following resolution of inflammatory skin rashes*: e.g. atopic eczema, lichen planus, following reactions to plants, e.g. contact dermatitis (e.g. poison ivy or primula) or ➲ Phytophotodermatitis, p. 233, and lupus erythematosus. The macular pigmentary changes have hazy margins corresponding to the primary eruption and can persist for months. A subset of lichen planus, lichen planus pigmentosus, presents primarily with pigmentation in the photo-exposed areas.
- *After dermatological procedures*: e.g. dermabrasion, chemical peels, or laser therapy.
- *From recurrent scratching or rubbing*, e.g.:
  - *Atopic eczema* (common): particularly on the neck (often rippled in this site), anterior wrists and flexures (➲ see Chapter 17).
  - *Macular amyloid*: a localized form of cutaneous amyloidosis producing a rippled brownish or bluish pigment of the involved skin.
  - *Capillaritis*: irregular brown staining from haemosiderin deposition due to capillary leakage. There may be purpuric lesions present (➲ see Cutaneous vasculitis, pp. 470–2).

Vitamin deficiencies

- *Pellagra*: caused by deficiency of nicotinic acid (niacin, vitamin B3) or its precursor amino acid, tryptophan (in diets based mainly on maize). *Signs*: thickened pigmented dry skin on bony prominences; a photosensitive eruption often with a sharply pigmented 'necklace'; perineal lesions and a seborrhoeic dermatitis-like eruption. Dizziness, anorexia, and numbness are common and severe cases have diarrhoea and dementia.
- *Vitamin B12 deficiency*: causes pigmentation accentuated on the knuckles. Can be associated with hair loss and glossitis.
- *Kwashiorkor*: due to protein malnutrition which can result in generalized pigmentation or dyschromatosis with pale and dark areas and desquamation (peeling). The hair may turn reddish.
  Signs: oedema (especially face, hands, and feet), diarrhoea, abdominal distention, and irritability. Potentially lethal if severe and untreated.

Metabolic/endocrine

Localized pigmentation

- *Melasma*: facial pigmentation especially around mouth and eyes, seen in some teenage girls, usually on hormonal contraception. Termed *chloasma* during pregnancy. Worsens with sun exposure, use of perfumed skin products, and paradoxically can occur with prolonged use of skin lightening products containing hydroquinone.
- *Acanthosis nigricans*: presents with increased flexural pigmentation (Fig. 33.6) especially axillae, neck, and groins but rarely causes a more generalized pigmentation. Associated with velvety thickening of the skin, exaggerated skin markings, and skin tags (Fig. 33.1). Can be a marker for diabetes mellitus or rarely inherited as an autosomal dominant, or syndromal with hirsutism, but is increasingly common in grossly overweight children. It is not associated with malignancy in children.

Generalized pigmentation

- ➲ See also Box 33.3.
- *Addison's disease*: caused by destruction of adrenal cortex, from autoimmune causes, tuberculosis, metastatic cancer, or amyloidosis. Pigmentation is most prominent in photo-exposed areas, mucosa, palmar creases, nipples, nails, and flexures. Systemic manifestations include hypotension, hyperkalaemia, hyponatraemia, shock—in extreme cases Addisonian crisis may be fatal. ACTH precursors known to contain peptide hormones with melanocyte-stimulating effects account for the pigmentation. ACTH-producing tumours can cause similar cutaneous changes (➲ see also Disorder of adrenal function, pp. 63–4).
- *Haemochromatosis*: characterized by brownish discolouration. Associated with diabetes mellitus, hepatomegaly, heart disease, cirrhosis of liver, and hypogonadism. Occurs from an inborn error of metabolism resulting in excessive iron absorption and subsequent deposition in organs, particularly liver. Excessive blood transfusions cause secondary haemochromatosis. Increased skin pigment is produced by iron and excess melanin.

Box 33.3 Causes of generalized brown pigmentation

- *Metabolic*: Addison's disease, haemochromatosis.
- *Systemic diseases*: liver and renal disease, Gaucher's disease, bronze baby syndrome, acanthosis nigricans.
- *Vitamin deficiencies*: vitamin A, kwashiorkor.
- *Drugs*: tetracyclines, beta-carotene, phototoxic drugs.
- *Heavy metal poisoning*: gold, silver, mercury, and arsenic (➲ see p. 498).
- *Rare acquired skin diseases*: e.g. universal acquired melanosis (Carbon baby).

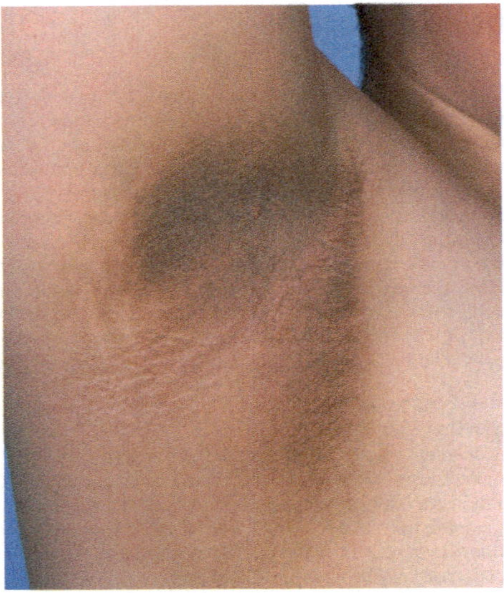

Fig. 33.6 Acanthosis nigricans due to obesity.
Reproduced courtesy of NHS Tayside Clinical Photography, Dundee, UK

Systemic diseases

- Diffuse hyperpigmentation is a feature of biliary cirrhosis, chronic renal failure, porphyria cutanea tarda, glycogen storage disease, and Gaucher's disease. Severe pruritus (➲ see Itching, pp. 262–4) is a prominent symptom of pigmentation associated with obstructive liver pathology and renal failure.
- ***Bronze baby syndrome***: in neonates who are hyperbilirubinaemic and treated with phototherapy. The pigment responsible is unclear.
- ***Urticaria pigmentosa***: oval and round pigmented (varying colours; may be red/brown) macules, papules, and nodules on the trunk and limbs due to deposition of mast cells in the dermis, which is variably extensive (Fig. 33.7; ➲ see also Fig. 19.8 and Differential diagnosis of urticarial rashes, pp. 313–16). Solitary lesions (mastocytomas; ➲ see Fig. 28.6) may be mistaken for melanocytic lesions. There is a positive Darier's sign *viz.* development of a wheal (oedema and erythema, rarely blistering) after firm stroking of a lesion.

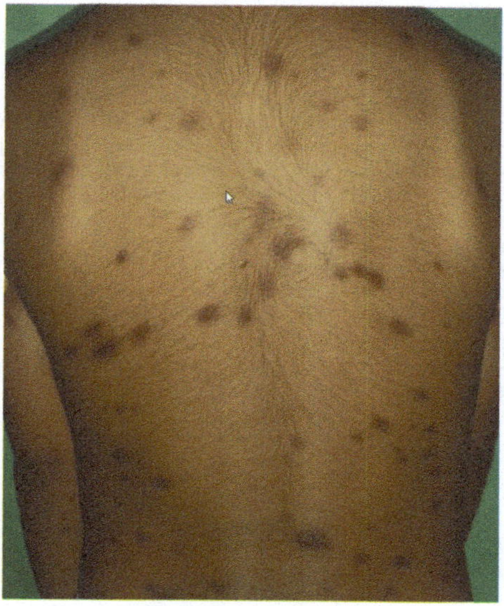

Fig. 33.7 Generalized urticaria pigmentosa.

Reproduced courtesy of Graham Sharpe, Consultant Dermatologist, Clatterbridge Hospital, UK

Drugs causing brown pigmentation

- *Tetracyclines*: usually avoided in children, but minocycline is sometimes used in pubertal acne. It can cause brown pigmentation or a slate-grey pigmentation (➲ see Fig. 35.2), that can be limited to photo-exposed areas, or sites of scarring, nails, teeth, and mucosal surfaces. The pigment is a complex of iron, the drug, and melanin, and the condition may only resolve partially after prolonged periods.
- *Fixed drug eruption*: usually from drugs taken intermittently (e.g. non-steroidal anti-inflammatory drugs (NSAIDs), sulphonamides, barbiturates, tetracyclines, laxatives). Occurs as a red patch evolving into a blister (➲ see Fig. 23.6). Prolonged or sometimes permanent hyperpigmentation occurs which may look blue or brown. Repeated ingestion causes more lesions to occur.
- *Beta-carotene*.
- *Laxatives*: those containing dithranol derivatives can cause postinflammatory brown hyperpigmentation around buttocks, genital area, and thighs from toxic reaction on skin (e.g. diarrhoea following laxative administration). Some laxatives can also cause fixed drug eruptions with pigmentation.

Other agents causing brown pigmentation

Heavy metals poisoning

- *Chronic arsenic ingestion*: is an emerging environmental epidemic unfolding in Southeast Asia due to contamination of drinking water. It is seen particularly in children from Bangladesh where deeply sunk wells are contaminated by arsenic. Guttate (raindrop-like) brown hyper- and hypopigmentation occurs particularly on trunk. On occasions, patchy pigmentation with accentuation in the inguinal folds, areola, and palmar creases is seen. Skin keratoses appear later, especially on palms, and there is a high risk of internal cancers.
- *Silver, gold, and mercury poisoning*: all cause pigmentation of skin and mucosa that may be bluish or brown (➲ see Localized and naevoid, pp. 510–13).
- *Henna*: and other staining agents applied to skin may give a brown, yellow-brown, or red colour that fades over several weeks (➲ see Chapter 36).

Chapter 34

Moles (melanocytic naevi)

Introduction

Melanocytic naevi are benign collections of melanin-producing naevus cells, thought to be immature melanocytes. They may be acquired or congenital. Acquired moles are very common and are seen in the majority of Caucasian children. They can cause anxiety when they appear and subsequently as they increase in size (see Boxes 34.1 and 34.2).

Box 34.1 Prepubertal acquired melanocytic naevi

It is important to remember that it is normal for moles to appear and mature (change) in early childhood, and to change at puberty, and that the incidence of melanoma (➔ see Malignant melanoma, p. 504–7) in prepubertal childhood is exceedingly low. In childhood, sometimes moles entirely regress. It is not usually necessary to remove benign moles unless they are causing symptoms or are very atypical.

Box 34.2 Congenital melanocytic naevi

The following groups of patients with congenital melanocytic naevi (CMN) should have a thorough neurological examination and referral to a paediatric dermatologist and/or neurologist:

- Any child with two or more CMN at birth.
- Any child with a CMN >20cm projected adult size.
- Any child with abnormal neurological signs.
- Any child with a lesion suspected of malignancy.

Acquired melanocytic naevi

Acquired melanocytic naevi (moles) are very common from the first year of life onwards (Fig. 34.1). They vary in colour from very pale brown to deep brown/black and some may contain various colours. They are increased in number in:

- White children with high ultraviolet (UV) light exposure, e.g. in north Australia.
- Children who are immunosuppressed, e.g. transplant patients.
- Various genetic syndromes, e.g. some of the RASopathies.

Benign moles

The majority of moles in prepubertal children are benign, even those of abnormal shape and colour but *refer for dermatological opinion in the following circumstances* (see Box 34.3 and Figs. 34.2 and 34.3):

- Asymmetrically shaped moles with irregular margins.
- Moles that have a lot of colour variation within them, especially if they are changing.
- A mole that is growing and changing when others are not.
- Moles that are inflamed and or bleeding (usually just due to infection and/or trauma).
- Children with over 100 moles.
- Children with moles from families with a history of malignant melanoma in close family relatives.

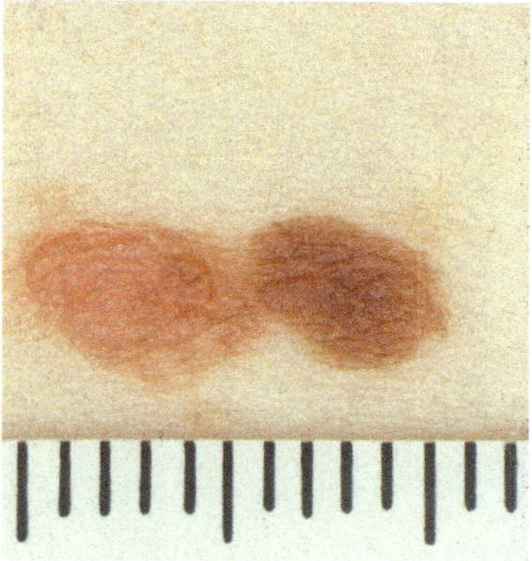

Fig. 34.1 Two adjacent benign acquired melanocytic naevi showing warty texture and different colours.

Reproduced courtesy of Susan Lewis-Jones, Hon Consultant Dermatologist, Ninewells Hospital and Medical School, Dundee, UK

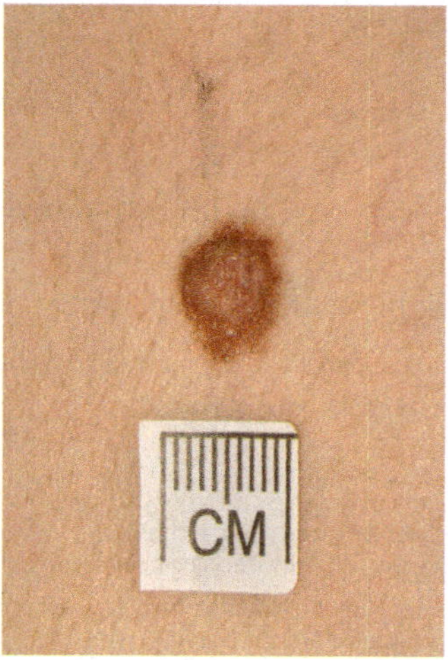

Fig. 34.2 Benign acquired melanocytic naevus: compound type. These typically have a central raised area with flat surrounding pigmentation.

Reproduced courtesy of Susan Lewis-Jones, Hon Consultant Dermatologist, Ninewells Hospital and Medical School, Dundee, UK

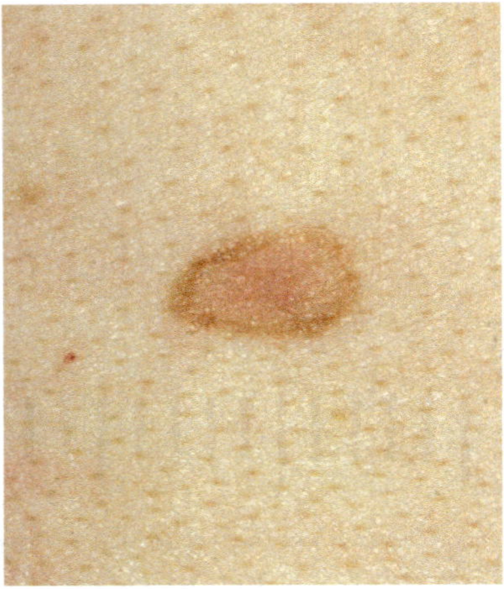

Fig. 34.3 Benign acquired melanocytic naevus. This variant with a darker halo is often referred to as a 'cockade' naevus.

Reproduced courtesy of Susan Lewis-Jones, Hon Consultant Dermatologist, Ninewells Hospital and Medical School, Dundee, UK

Box 34.3 Risk factors

Risk factors for childhood melanoma

- Multiple CMN.
- History of early and multiple cases of familial melanoma (especially possession of *CDKN2A* gene mutation).
- Maternal melanoma during pregnancy.
- Predisposing skin diseases, e.g. xeroderma pigmentosum (➲ see Chapter 16).
- Prolonged immunosuppression, e.g. transplants (➲ see Chapter 39).

Childhood risk factors for adult melanoma

All of the above plus:

- Frequent sunburn prepuberty.
- Excessive numbers of acquired melanocytic naevi >100.
- Possession of three or more atypical moles.
- Type 1 skin type and red hair/freckling phenotype.

See also Guidelines for melanoma: http://www.sign.ac.uk/ Clinical Guideline no 72, Quick Reference Guide.

Histology: melanocytic naevi may be situated at the dermoepidermal junction (junctional naevi), the dermis alone (dermal naevi), or both (compound naevi). There are many variants (e.g. spitz naevus, ➲ see Variants of melanocytic naevi, pp. 503–7) and interpretation of the histology of proliferative congenital or acquired melanocytic naevi in children can be very difficult, requiring a dermatopathologist specially trained in pigmented lesions who is part of a multidisciplinary team.

Variants of melanocytic naevi

Junctional naevi

Flat moles found on the palms or soles, which occasionally disappear with time (Fig. 34.4). Usually benign—especially in children.

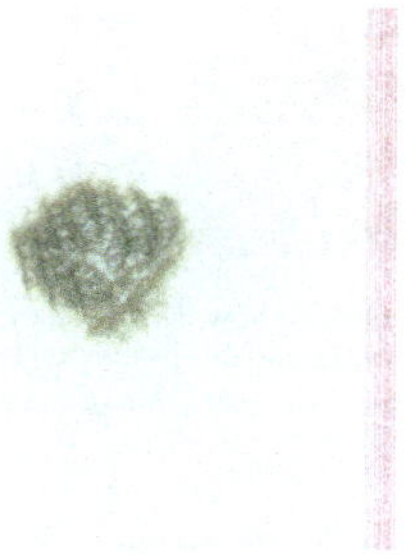

Fig. 34.4 Junctional melanocytic naevus.

Reproduced courtesy of Susan Lewis-Jones, Hon Consultant Dermatologist, Ninewells Hospital and Medical School, Dundee, UK

Blue naevi

Variant of melanocytic naevi that appear blue (➲ see Fig. 35.1).

Spitz naevi

Subset of acquired melanocytic naevi varying in colour from pink to deep brown and do not resemble ordinary moles (Fig. 34.5). Quite common and usually have a benign clinical course but often have a malignant-looking histology which can be difficult to interpret. *Referral for dermatological opinion is recommended for these and any atypical moles*. Spitz naevi increasingly are not excised, as where they are typical they can be diagnosed clinically, and can resolve spontaneously.

Halo naevus

Acquired white ring (sometimes pink initially) around a pre-existing mole (Fig. 34.6), which gradually disappears to leave a white area. This eventually regains normal skin colour. They may be multiple. Circulating antimelanocytic antibodies have been detected in some.

Naevus spilus

Benign speckled naevus, congenital or acquired, of any size or site. It usually has a café-au-lait macular background, with superimposed foci of increased pigmentation, which may be palpable (Fig. 34.7; ➲ see also Fig. 33.4). There are different types with different genetic bases and different clinical courses.

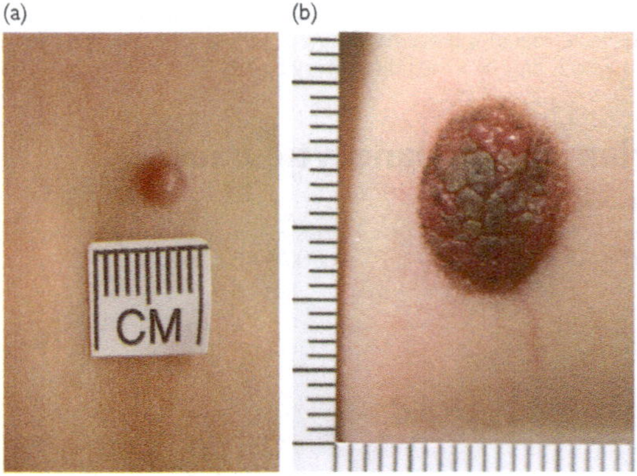

Fig. 34.5 Spitz naevi, showing how different they can look clinically from a pale pink smooth lesion (a) to a warty, variably pigmented lesion (b).

Reproduced courtesy of Susan Lewis-Jones, Hon Consultant Dermatologist, Ninewells Hospital and Medical School, Dundee, UK

Congenital melanocytic naevi

CMN are moles present at birth. They are brown or black or even red in appearance. They are permanent and grow with the child. Rarely they can appear after birth. The number is more important for clinical management than the size (Figs. 34.8 and 34.9):

- *Single small* (<2cm projected adult size) CMN are found in approximately 1% of newborns. They are not associated with other abnormalities and do not require routine follow-up or excision.
- *Multiple CMN* (two or more at birth) are rarer, and in 20% of cases can be associated with congenital neurological abnormalities (CMN syndrome), particularly where at least one of the naevi is very large.

Management: MRI scan of the brain and whole spine with contrast in the first 6 months of life.

Multiple CMN are usually seen in the context of one larger CMN and other small CMN (sometimes known as satellites—not to be confused with malignant satellites), and are often very heterogeneous, with variation in colour and texture between and within lesions (Fig. 34.10).

Melanoma

Sporadic melanoma remains *extremely rare* in childhood despite an increase in overall incidence over recent years. It does, however, occur and if in doubt refer to a dermatologist for an opinion (Box 34.3). Clinical signs of melanoma in a single mole in a prepubertal child include rapidly enlarging/changing shape, and frequently these lesions are amelanotic (lacking in pigment) so dermoscopy (➔ see Chapter 2) may not be helpful. Melanoma may arise from normal skin rather than from a mole.

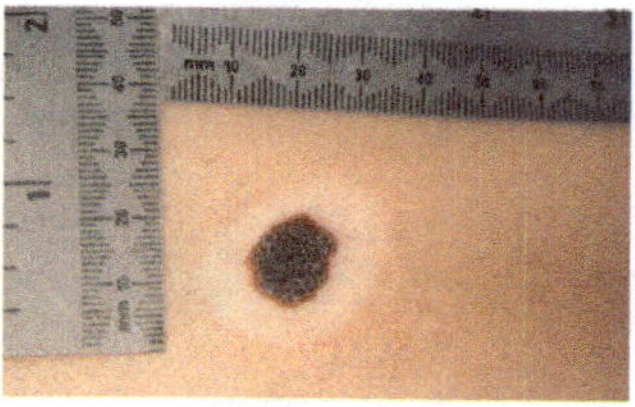

Fig. 34.6 Halo naevus.

Reproduced courtesy of Susan Lewis-Jones, Hon Consultant Dermatologist, Ninewells Hospital and Medical School, Dundee, UK

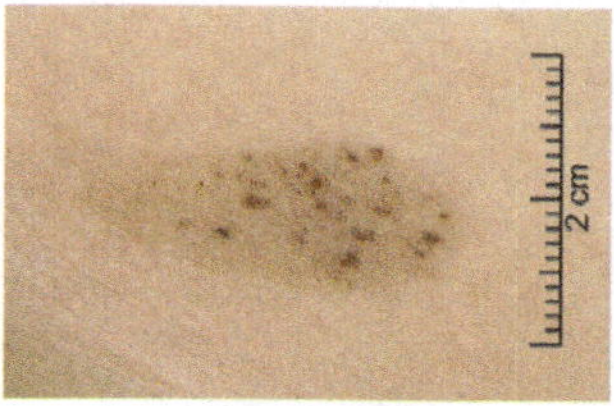

Fig. 34.7 Single small macular naevus spilus (speckled lentiginous naevus).

Reproduced courtesy of Susan Lewis-Jones, Hon Consultant Dermatologist, Ninewells Hospital and Medical School, Dundee, UK

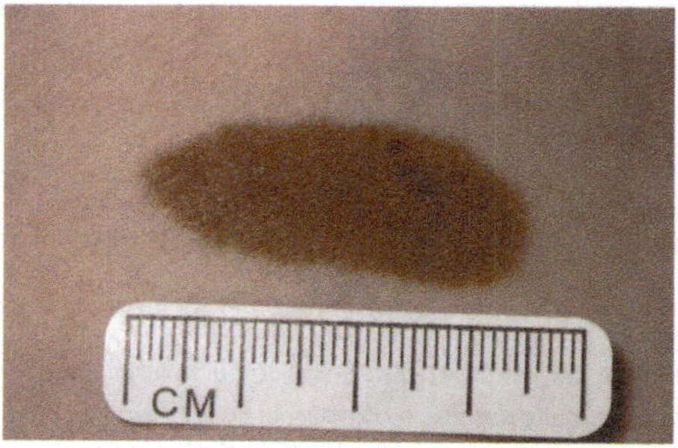

Fig. 34.8 Single congenital melanocytic naevus.

Reproduced courtesy of Susan Lewis-Jones, Hon Consultant Dermatologist, Ninewells Hospital and Medical School, Dundee, UK

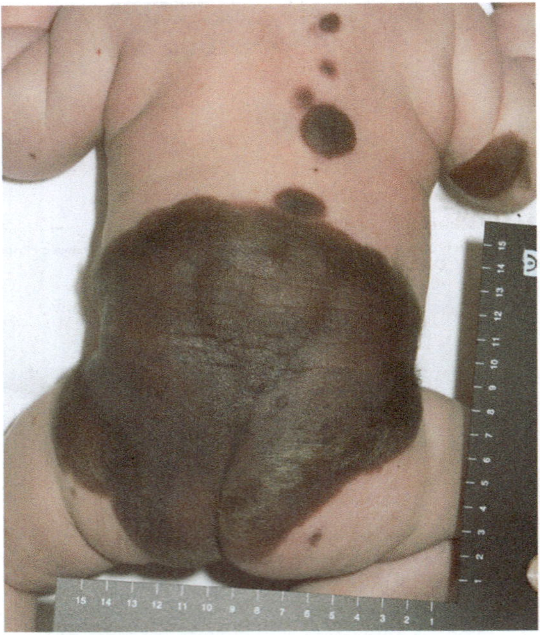

Fig. 34.9 Multiple congenital melanocytic naevi.

Reproduced courtesy of Veronica Kinsler, Professor of Paediatric Dermatology and Dermatogenetics, Great Ormond Street Hospital, London, UK

The clinical signs of melanoma in a single mole in a postpubertal child are the same as for adults (Fig. 34.10; ➲ see also Malignant skins tumours, p. 435):

- Rapidly enlarging mole (especially if no other moles are changing).
- Irregularly of shape (asymmetry) and borders.
- Irregularity of colour, especially several colours within one lesion.

Note: itching is usually not a sign of malignancy and many benign moles become itchy or inflamed in childhood. Bleeding is usually caused from trauma but any itchy bleeding mole should be examined by an expert in children's melanocytic lesions.

For children with multiple CMN (two or more at birth) the best predictor of melanoma risk is the outcome of a screening MRI scan of the central nervous system (CNS) in the first 6 months of life. Those with normal scans have a low risk (2% or less in childhood), whereas those with complex

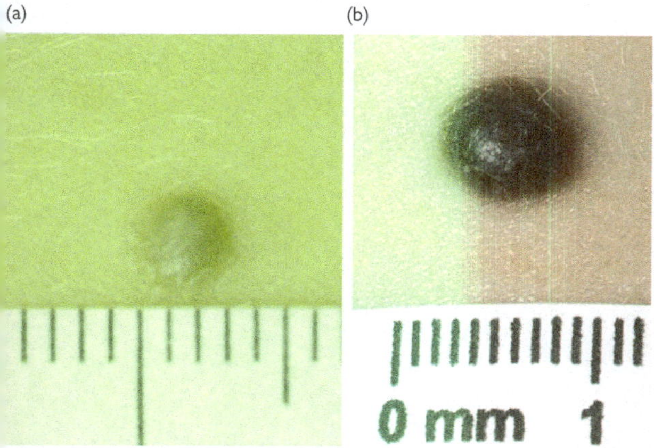

Fig. 34.10 Prepubertal melanoma. The lesion (a) grew and changed colour over 2 months (b). When excised it had already metastasized to the sentinel lymph node.
Reproduced courtesy of Cameron Kennedy, Departments of Dermatology, Bristol Royal Infirmary and Paediatric Dermatology, Bristol Royal Hospital for Children, Bristol, UK

congenital neurological abnormalities have approximately 10% risk. This risk is mainly from primary melanoma arising in the CNS, which presents with focal signs or symptoms or raised intracranial pressure.

Note: Sun protection in childhood (especially avoiding any sunburn before the age of 15 years) has been shown to reduce the risk of developing melanoma skin cancer in adulthood (➲ see also Chapter 16).

Chapter 35

Blue, grey, and black colouration

Introduction

This chapter describes the better-known causes of blue, grey, and black cutaneous discolouration and lesions. Melanin deposition deeper in the skin, in the dermis rather than the epidermis, gives a bluish hue to the skin due to light diffraction. Slate-grey pigmentation of the skin is also known as caeruloderma. It may be localized or generalized. Very deep blue pigmentation may appear black. Causes other than melanin include tattoos, blood disorders, vascular lesions, and ingestion of drugs or heavy metals.

Generalized forms

Changes in haemoglobin

- *Cyanosis* imparts a bluish discolouration and is due to excessive deoxyhaemoglobin in the cutaneous vasculature.
- *Methaemoglobinaemia* occurs after ingestion of dapsone or other sulphur-containing drugs, giving rise to a similar picture.

Drugs

- Can cause generalized blue/grey pigmentation (➲ see Rare skin disease causing red rashes, pp. 339–40).

Localized and naevoid

Mongolian blue spots

Normal in Black, Asian, and Chinese or Japanese neonates (approximately 90%). Uncommon in Caucasian races. Blue/black macular lesions with indistinct borders that can be single or multiple, and of any size. Commonest over the lumbosacral spine, although can occur anywhere but usually not the anterior trunk (➲ see Fig. 7.5). Will gradually fade during childhood. They should be noted at birth, as they can be confused with bruising and occasionally mistaken for abuse (➲ see Fig. 24.2). Very rarely, extensive dermal melanocytosis occurs, which can be associated with inborn errors of metabolism (mucopolysaccharide storage disorders, e.g. Hunter and Hurler syndromes) and neurocristopathies (e.g. cleft lips, neurofibromatosis).

Naevus of Ota (oculocutaneous melanocytosis)

Presents as a blue-black or slate-grey macule, very similar to Mongolian blue spots. Localized around the eyes (first and second branch of trigeminal nerve) and also conjunctiva, sclera, and/or retina. The area extends slowly and becomes darker with age. The colour is the result of the depth of excessive immature melanocytes in the dermis. Very rarely melanomas can arise.

Management: ophthalmological review. It may respond to laser therapy.

Naevus of Ito

Analogous to the naevus of Ota and may coexist within the same patient. Occurs in the distribution of the lateral supraclavicular and lateral brachial nerves.

Blue naevi

These are a benign variant of melanocytic naevi that appear blue rather than brown because the pigment cells are situated within the dermis (Fig. 35.1). Mixed types can occur (combined type naevus). They are occasionally multiple but malignant forms are exceedingly rare, particularly in children.

Metabolic (rare)

- *Alkaptonuria*: an autosomal recessive condition caused by lack of homogentisic acid oxidase which results in accumulation of homogentisic acid in the body deposited in the bone, cartilage, and skin. Bluish macules (ochronosis) appear, particularly on the fingers, ears, nose, genital regions, and buccal mucosa. The joints are also affected resulting in osteoarthritis. Urine stains black, an early clinical sign. *Management*: there is no current effective treatment but a carefully controlled diet may reduce the severity of the condition. Trials of the drug nitisinone are promising.
- *Macular amyloid*: usually more brownish rather than bluish and may be associated with lichenified skin (➲ see Localized forms of brown pigmentation, pp. 491–4).

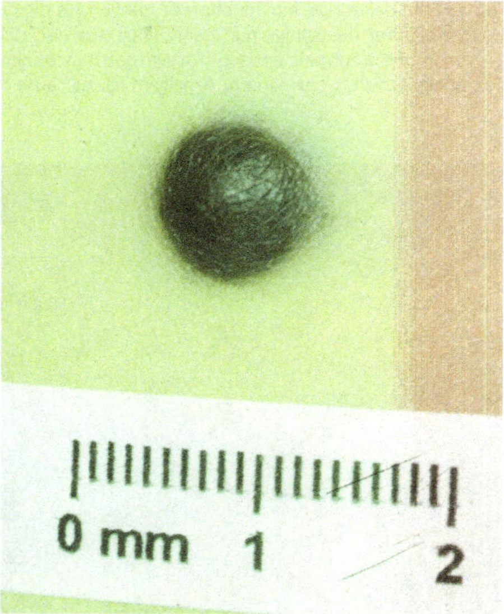

Fig. 35.1 Blue naevus. These usually have well-defined borders.

Reproduced courtesy of Susan Lewis-Jones, Hon Consultant Dermatologist, Ninewells Hospital and Medical School, Dundee, UK

Drugs and heavy metals

Mainly uncommon to rare reactions:

- *Drugs*: blue-grey discolouration (caeruloderma) can occur with phenothiazines (usually chlorpromazine), minocycline (Fig. 35.2), thiazides, and amiodarone. It is attributable to the deposits of the drug alone or chelation with melanin in the dermis. Chloroquine and hydroxycarbamide have a distribution mostly on the shins and back, respectively. Some fixed drug eruptions resolve, leaving slate-grey or bluish colouration (➲ see Fig. 23.6).
- *Exogenous ochronosis*: occurs predominantly in adults but has been reported in adolescent girls with racially pigmented skin using topical hydroquinones (cosmetic skin-lightening agents) in concentrations of about 6–10%. Rare and very resistant to any form of treatment.
- *Argyria*: deposition of silver in the skin giving a blue-grey colour, particularly in sun exposed areas. The degree of pigmentation depends more on the extent of silver exposure than the extent of sun exposure.
- *Chrysiasis*: similar to argyria but due to gold.
- *Lead poisoning*: causes a blue-grey pigmentation and a blue line along the gums.
- *Mercury*: long-term use of topical creams containing mercury (for psoriasis) has caused slate-grey pigmentation.
- *Tattoos*: usually the deliberate introduction of exogenous pigment or henna into the skin for decorative purposes. They may also occur accidentally from the traumatic entry of foreign substances like graphite from lead pencils, which is permanent. Amalgam fillings cause oral tattoos.

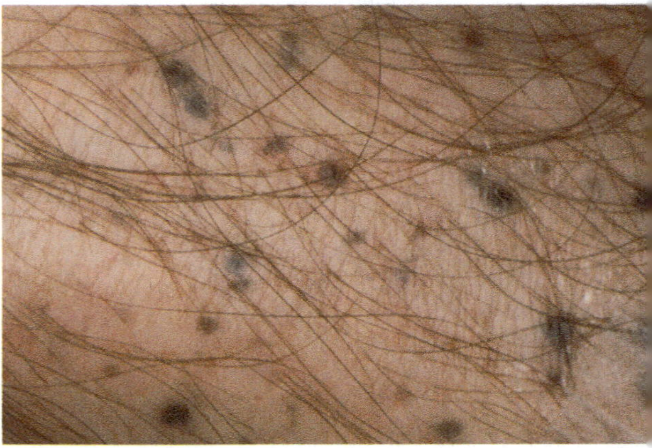

Fig. 35.2 Blue pigmentation caused by minocycline. It is often linear on the sides of fingers and in nails and may cause blue lunulae.

Reproduced courtesy of Susan Lewis-Jones, Hon Consultant Dermatologist, Ninewells Hospital and Medical School, Dundee, UK

Trauma

Vascular damage with bruises, either accidental or non-accidental. This may appear blue, purplish, or black but will fade in a few days to yellowish brown. If prolonged bluish discolouration is present on shins, consider Ehlers–Danlos syndrome (➲ see Fig. 24.3; and Dermal texture change, pp. 445–6) or epidermolysis bullosa (➲ see Genetic causes of blisters, pp. 387–90).

Genetic

Blue-rubber bleb naevi (➲ see Colour, pp. 419–27). Blue tumours (➲ see Colour, pp. 419–27).

Black colouration

Skin may appear black from:

- *Vascular changes*: e.g. extravasated blood products from bruising including 'black heel' (talon noir) from sporting injury (Fig. 35.3); thrombosed vessels in lesions such as pyogenic granuloma (➲ see Fig. 28.12), or in viral warts (➲ see Fig. 12.9).
- *Vascular lesions*: e.g. angiokeratomas are more usually dark red or purple. Arise without underlying problems or in Anderson–Fabry disease (very rare; ➲ see Causes of purple patches other than purpura, pp. 474–7).

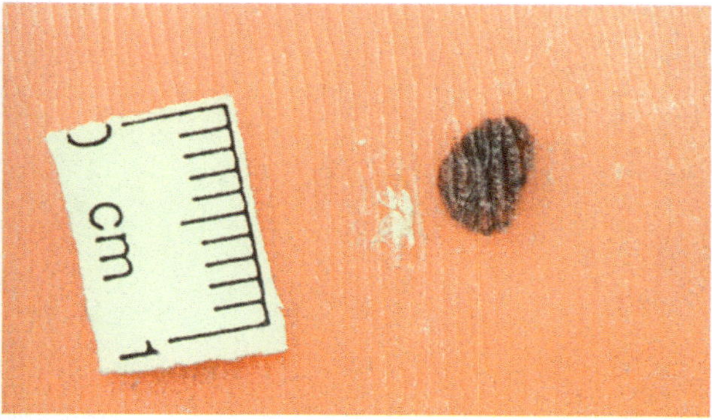

Fig. 35.3 Black heel (talon noir).

Reproduced courtesy of Susan Lewis-Jones, Hon Consultant Dermatologist, Ninewells Hospital and Medical School, Dundee, UK

- *Melanin deposition*: e.g. some melanocytic naevi (moles), melanoma, and lentigines (➲ see Chapter 34).
- *Drugs*: very deep blue deposition can look black, e.g. minocycline (Fig. 35.2), mepacrine.
- *Metabolic*: e.g. ochronosis (➲ see Localized and naevoid, pp. 510–13).
- *Necrosis* (eschar): many causes (➲ see Eschars, p. 397 and Fig. 26.2).
- *Infection*: tinea nigra (rare fungal infection); black hairy tongue (➲ see The tongue and gums, pp. 146–8).
- *Pigmentation*: e.g. epidermal naevi, particularly in black skin.

Nails may appear black from trauma (blood products) or melanin, e.g. melanocytic naevi, or melanomas (➲ see Chapter 15).

Chapter 36

Red colouration

Introduction

This chapter deals with red staining and marks on the skin other than red rashes and erythroderma (➲ see Chapter 22) and vascular birthmarks (➲ see Chapter 8). Skin may be temporarily stained red with plant juice such as beetroot.

Causes of redness of the skin

Localized redness (erythema)

Usually caused by:

- *Dilatation of the blood vessels*: common in inflammatory rashes (➲ see Chapters 17 and 22).
- *Postinflammatory staining*: (temporary) following skin infections such as impetigo, topical irritants (including chemicals), thermal burns, contact allergic reactions including to plants, fading skin diseases, e.g. eczema or psoriasis (although more common to see postinflammatory depigmentation with these).
- *Abnormal vasculature*: vascular birthmarks (➲ see Chapter 8).
- *Dyes*: accidental or deliberate.
- *Drugs and poisons*: may be localized or generalized.
- *Metabolic*: may be localized or generalized.

Abnormal vasculature

- *Vascular birthmarks* (➲ see Chapter 8): particularly port-wine stains and salmon patches, present at birth as pink to red flat stains. The term telangiectasia is used to describe abnormal small cutaneous vessels, which may look red or purple (➲ see Other vascular birthmarks, pp. 111–12). It can be acquired or congenital and is sometimes due to genetic causes.
- *Localized red tumours*: e.g. strawberry naevi start as flat lesions (➲ see Chapter 8, Vascular tumours, pp. 94–9), pyogenic granuloma (➲ see Fig. 28.5), and very rarely malignant tumours, e.g. sarcomas (several types).
- *Damage to vessels*: e.g. purpuric dermatoses (capillaritis) cause a reddish or purple discolouration due to inflammation of the capillaries with subsequent extravasation of blood into the skin. This often leaves brown or yellowish stains (haemosiderin; ➲ see Cutaneous vasculitis, pp. 470–2).

Dyes ⚑

- *Henna*: a vegetable dye which colours the skin red/brown, used extensively for skin decoration either painted topically or as a tattoo. Allergic contact dermatitis reactions may occur.
  Note: In children with glucose-6-phosphate dehydrogenase deficiency, topical application of henna can cause life-threatening haemolysis.
- *Paraphenylene diamine*: synthetic dye often used for 'holiday tattoos' because it gives a much darker colour. May cause a severe allergic reaction a week or two after the application, with severe redness and subsequent hyper or hypopigmentation.
  Management: potent topical corticosteroids are indicated for short-term use if allergic reactions occur.

Drugs and poisons

- *Clofazimine*: used in the treatment of leprosy, can cause a reddish colour to the skin (and bodily secretions, e.g. urine and tears). Frequently seen in children treated for lepra reactions (➲ Chapter 22).
- *'Red man syndrome'* (a form of erythroderma): classically attributed to intravenous vancomycin, but a variety of other drugs can cause widespread erythematous discolouration of the skin (rare in children).
- *Mercury (cinnabar)*: used in tattoos to impart a reddish colour and can cause an allergic reaction. Oral ingestion causes Pink's disease. Amalgam dental fillings can also cause contact allergy (➲ see Other oral changes, pp. 148–50).
- *Carbon monoxide* poisoning gives a cherry-red hue due to carboxyhaemoglobin.

Metabolic

Porphyrias: a group of rare inherited metabolic disorders involving the accumulation of abnormal porphyrins. Some impart a reddish colour to the teeth, most apparent in congenital erythropoietic porphyria (Günther's disease; ➲ see Immediate photosensitive rashes, pp. 230–1), which is associated with severe photosensitivity.

Chapter 37

Yellow or orange colouration

Introduction

Yellow or orange discolouration of the skin is most commonly seen in jaundice, carotenaemia, or fading bruises. There are a few skin lesions that may appear yellow or orange. Skin may be temporarily stained yellow with compounds such as nicotine, paints, dyes, etc.

Causes

Carotenaemia

Yellowish-orange hue, sometimes golden, due to deposition of beta-carotene in the skin, particularly on nose and palms (Fig. 37.1) Seen in:

- High intake from food, e.g.
  - Organic baby foods—those containing carrots and broccoli particularly. Mild cases very common.
  - Food faddism, e.g. excessive consumption of carrots; also reported with excessive consumption of a children's drink 'Sunny delight'.
- Anorexia nervosa.
- Drugs: beta-carotene—sometimes used to treat porphyrias.

Metabolic

- *Chronic renal failure*: severe anaemia and obstructive jaundice secondary to biliary pathology can give sallow complexion with yellowish discolouration.
- *Xanthomas*: usually caused by disturbed lipoprotein metabolism either inherited or associated with systemic diseases. All rare in children and tend to indicate severe disease. Can be confused with the histiocytoses (➲ see Non-infective causes, pp. 285–8). There are several types:
  - *Planar*: plaque-like yellowish areas on limbs, especially frictional sites. Can be associated with yellowish palms in severe cases.
  - *Generalized plane xanthomas*: widespread yellowish plaques on face and upper trunk often associated with IgA gammopathy. Rare, usually seen in adults.
  - *Tuberous*: deep lesions always associated with disorders of lipid metabolism (Fig. 37.2).
  - *Eruptive*: small yellow papules with reddish halo (➲ see Fig. 5.3).

(a) (b)

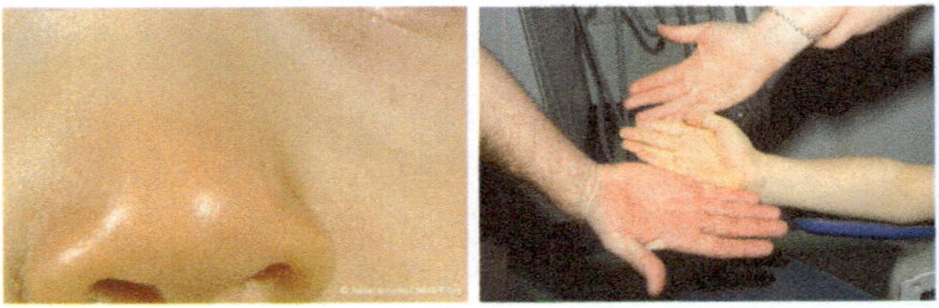

Fig. 37.1 (a) Carotenaemia nose. (b) Carotenaemia hand.

Reproduced with permission from Loo W.J. and Burrows N.P. (2006). An orange-tinted baby! *Clin Exp Dermatol* 31(3):495–6. https://doi.org/10.1111/j.1365-2230.2005.02057.x

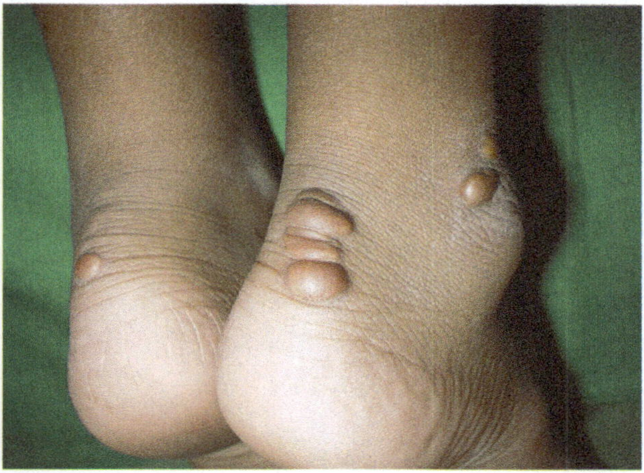

Fig. 37.2 Tuberous xanthomas over ankles.
Reproduced courtesy of Patrick Yesudian, Consultant Dermatologist, Chennai, India

Cause: familial; endocrine disorders such as hypothyroidism and diabetes mellitus; nephrotic syndrome; or can be induced by drugs or alcohol.

- Tendinous: overlying tendons (Fig. 37.2)
- Xanthelasma: yellowish deposits around the eyes.

Management: check for hyperlipidaemia and if present refer to metabolic specialist.

Genetic

- *Pseudoxanthoma elasticum*: yellowish papules in the neck are a classical feature. Screen for ocular and gastrointestinal problems (➲ see Fig. 29.10).
- *Palmoplantar keratoderma*: seen in a group of inherited disorders with hyperkeratosis of palms and soles which can look yellowish (➲ see Fig. 12.4 and Box 12.2).

Haemosiderin staining

Seen temporarily following bruising. In more persistent cases, consider capillaritis. Usually brown but can be golden yellow, e.g. *Lichen aureus*: patches of golden reddish-brown pigmentation found on legs, body, and even face (➲ see Fig. 31.6). Usually asymptomatic but can be very itchy. It may resemble bruising. Rare in children.

Tumours

- *Naevus sebaceous*: may be quite orange/yellow coloured (➲ see Fig. 14.5).
- *Juvenile xanthogranuloma*: a form of histiocytosis (➲ see Non-infective causes, pp. 285–8) and not a true tumour. Lesions can be strikingly orange or yellow (Fig. 37.3).

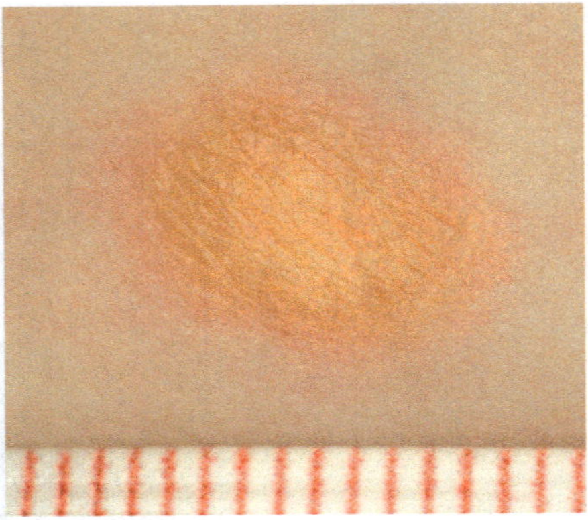

Fig. 37.3 Juvenile xanthogranuloma.

Reproduced courtesy of Susan Lewis-Jones, Hon Consultant Dermatologist, Ninewells Hospital and Medical School, Dundee, UK

Sporadic skin diseases

- *Mastocytomas and urticaria pigmentosa*: these can sometimes appear yellow or orange (➲ see Figs. 28.6 and 19.8; and Non-infective causes, pp. 285–8).
- *Pityriasis rubra pilaris*: yellow hyperkeratosis on palms and soles (➲ see Features of specific causes of erythroderma, pp. 343–5).
- *Xanthoma disseminatum*: a rare form of histiocytosis (➲ see Non-infective causes, pp. 285–8), which can involve the respiratory tract and brain (diabetes insipidus in 40%). May persist for years but can resolve. Usually affects young male adults.

Section 7

Rashes in rheumatology and transplant patients

Chapter 38

Skin changes associated with rheumatological disorders

Introduction

This chapter describes skin disorders found in the context of arthritis and arthralgia. When considered together, diagnoses can be made more rapidly to reduce risk of end organ damage, e.g.

- Skin lesions form part of the diagnostic criteria for systemic lupus erythematosus (SLE) (➲ see Chapter 38).
- Plaque psoriasis (➲ see Chapter 22) helps differentiate psoriatic arthritis from juvenile idiopathic arthritis.
- The heliotrope rash is pathognomic of dermatomyositis (➲ see Dermal thickening, pp. 448–50 and Fig. 29.11).
- Streptococcal disease may lead to arthralgias, annular erythema, and Henoch–Schönlein purpura (➲ see Chapter 31).
- Hypocomplementaemic urticarial vasculitis presents with urticaria and vasculitic changes.
- A palpable livedoid rash may indicate a medium vessel vasculitis such as found in polyarteritis nodosum.
- Aphthous ulcers affecting the mouth and/or genitalia and acneiform rashes are diagnostic features of Behçet's disease and other autoimmune conditions (➲ see Chapter 10).

Many rheumatological conditions evolve over time, so it is important to be aware of this to avoid labelling patients too soon.

Skin changes associated with connective tissue diseases

Neonatal lupus

This is a neonatal rash present from birth or shortly after. The face and trunk are often affected, with annular lesions, sometimes with atrophic scars. Periorbital lesions give the classical owl's eye appearance (➲ see Chapter 7 and Figs. 7.2 and 7.3).

Management: often resolves without therapy or using topical steroids or calcineurin inhibitors, but be aware of associated heart block, hepatitis, and thrombocytopaenias and treat accordingly.

Systemic lupus erythematosus (SLE)

- ➲ See also Chapter 22.

Diagnosis: currently still requires 4 out of the 11 diagnostic criteria summarized in Box 38.1. Skin disorders are the second commonest diagnostic criteria in children after haematological disease. Many of these rashes are triggered by ultraviolet light and may herald severe systemic inflammation.

Investigations: baseline tests include a full blood count (FBC), complement levels, U&E, LFT, ANA, CRP, anticardiolipin antibodies, echocardiogram, and respiratory function tests. Renal biopsy may be indicated if there is haematuria and proteinuria.

Management: ideally requires multidisciplinary input. In acute cases prompt treatment with intravenous methyl prednisolone, hydroxychloroquine, and methotrexate or mycophenolate mofetil reduces mortality risk. Use photoprotection for optimal disease control and to prevent disease flares once the condition is stabilized. Others such as topical corticosteroids,

Box 38.1 Diagnostic criteria for systemic lupus erythematosus

For diagnosis, 4 out of the 11 diagnostic criteria must be met:

1. Malar rash
2. Discoid rash
3. Photosensitivity
4. Oral ulcers
5. Arthritis
6. Serositis: pleuritis
7. Renal disorder
8. Neurological disorder
9. Haematological disorder
10. Immunological disorder
11. Antinuclear antibody in raised titre

Reproduced with permission from Ferraz M.B. et *al*. (1994). Valuation of the 1982 ARA lupus criteria data set in pediatric patients. Committees of Pediatric Rheumatology of the Brazilian Society of Pediatrics and the Brazilian Society of Rheumatology. *Clin Exp Rheumatol* 12(1):83–7.

hydroxychloroquine, methotrexate, or mycophenolate mofetil are often used in combination for long-term management.

Prognosis: depends on which systems are involved—renal and neurological disease are particularly serious.

Discoid lupus erythematosus

May affect the face, lips, hard palate, and trunk. Can be a cutaneous presentation of SLE or just occur without systemic features. The commonest sites are light-exposed areas of the face, scalp, and ears. May cause scarring and pigmentary changes.

Treatment: photoprotection (➲ see p. 238), potent topical corticosteroids +/– hydroxychloroquine.

Associated cutaneous findings in lupus

- *Malar rash*: this is the classical butterfly rash (➲ see Chapter 9, Fig. 9.3). It is more often associated with systemic disease than discoid lupus. It can blister and become secondarily infected with staphylococcal infection which may delay diagnosis. Consider SLE if associated with lethargy and weight loss.
- *Aphthous ulcers*: these are non-specific and occur in SLE on the oral and genital mucosae (➲ see Chapters 10 and 13).
- *Hair loss*: this can be diffuse, presenting as generalized hair thinning as part of SLE or a localized scarring alopecia due to discoid lupus (➲ see Chapter 14).
- *Urticarial lesions*: hypocomplementaemic urticarial vasculitis (HUVS) is a *non-itchy* urticarial eruption associated with SLE. It is diagnosed by urticarial and vasculitic lesions in the context of C1q antibodies which are usually at low levels or undetectable in the normal population (Figs. 38.1 and 38.2). The C1q antibodies are associated with lung and renal involvement.
- *Livedoid changes and infarcts*: anticardiolipin and/or antiphospholipid antibodies may be detected in systemic lupus. They can be associated with livedoid changes and/or small vessel occlusion (Fig. 38.3) and may be diagnostic of antiphospholipid syndrome.

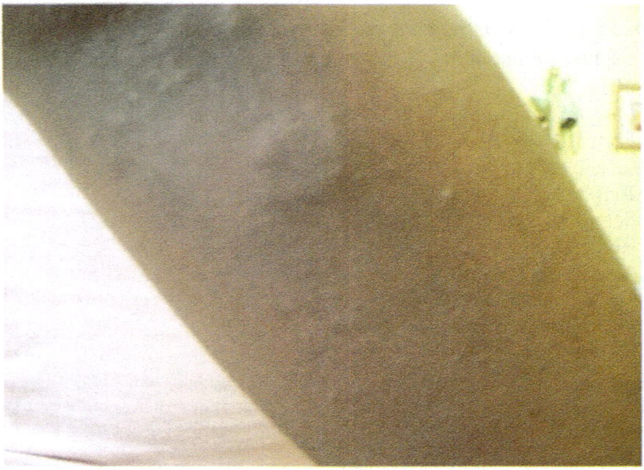

Fig. 38.1 Urticarial lesions associated with hypocomplementaemic urticarial vasculitis in a patient with systemic lupus erythematosus.

Reproduced courtesy of Ruth Murphy, Consultant Dermatologist, Royal Hallamshire Hospital, Sheffield, UK

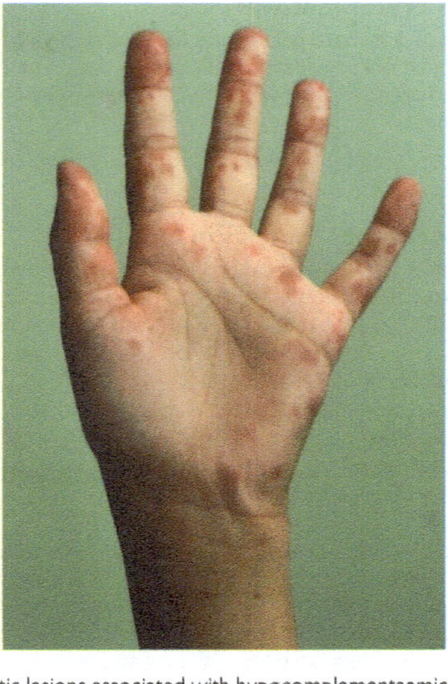

Fig. 38.2 Vasculitic lesions associated with hypocomplementaemic urticarial vasculitis in a patient with systemic lupus erythematosus.

Reproduced courtesy of Ruth Murphy, Consultant Dermatologist, Royal Hallamshire Hospital, Sheffield, UK

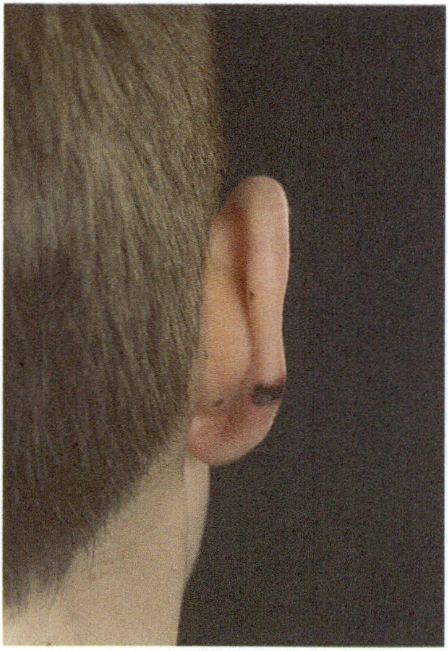

Fig. 38.3 Small vessel occlusion affecting the skin of the ear, triggered by cold weather in a patient with antiphospholipid syndrome.

Reproduced courtesy of Ruth Murphy, Consultant Dermatologist, Royal Hallamshire Hospital, Sheffield, UK

Lupus profundus

A deep nodular form of lupus erythematosus (LE), extremely rare in children. Disfiguring irregular purplish lesions, often progressive, which scar.

Skin changes associated with arthritis

Dermatomyositis

- *Violaceous rash* around the orbits (heliotrope rash); this may be subtle (➲ see Chapter 29, Fig. 29.11), a scaly erythema may sometimes be present elsewhere on the face which mimics psoriasis.
- *Erythematous rash* on the extensor aspect of the elbows, back (shawl sign), the erythema can occur in covered sites. Skin biopsy shows a lichenoid interface inflammation often very similar to SLE.
- *Cutaneous calcinosis*: this is very difficult to treat (➲ see Fig. 29.13) and frequently causes painful ulceration. It is not always a marker of poor disease control. It is more common and often more extensive in children, occasionally causing marked limitation of movement.

- *Poikiloderma* and *sclerodactyly* (Fig. 38.4) both occur as a result of poorly controlled chronic disease.
- *Periungual erythema and capillary dilatation* (➲ see Fig. 29.12) are pathognomic of active disease. Gottron's sign—violaceous papules on dorsal phalanges (➲ see Fig. 29.12).

Skin changes associated with autoinflammatory disease

Scleroderma

- *Localized scleroderma*: linear and localized plaques (➲ see Chapter 29). Treatment with immunosuppression such as methotrexate or mycophenolate mofetil is required for a minimum of 2y otherwise rebound inflammation leading to tissue damage is likely to recur.
- *Systemic scleroderma*: is rare (➲ see Epidermal texture change, pp. 438–41).

Antiphospholipid syndrome (APS)

- Rare in children.

Types: primary or secondary, the latter mainly associated with systemic lupus (SLE). Can present with livedoid changes or vessel occlusion (Fig. 38.3).

Treatment: aspirin or anticoagulants may be needed to prevent organ damage.

Other rheumatological conditions

Skin changes associated with juvenile idiopathic arthritis:
- Urticarial vasculitis (➲ see Chapter 21).
- Migratory erythemas (➲ see Chapters 21 and 22).
- Erythema marginatum (see Chapters 21 and 22).

Psoriatic arthritis

Any manifestation of psoriasis may present in the context of psoriatic arthritis (➲ Chapter 22), e.g. scaly patches on extensor aspects of limbs; guttate psoriasis following a sore throat; nail pits, subungual hyperkeratosis, or palmoplantar pustular lesions. Check hidden sites such as inguinal folds, natal cleft, or umbilicus.

(a) (b)

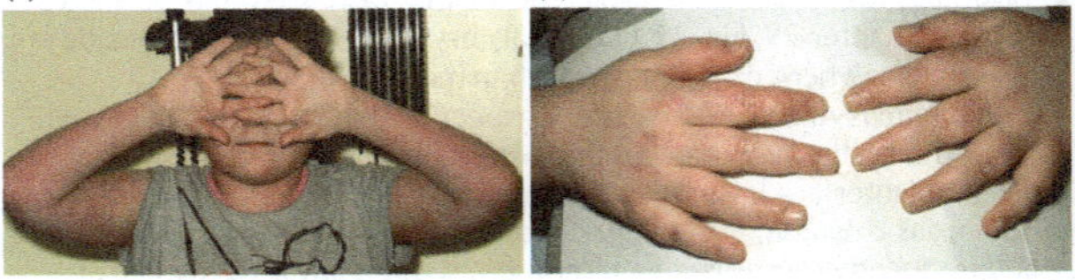

Fig. 38.4 Late skin changes associated with dermatomyositis: (a) poikiloderma; (b) sclerodactyly.

Reproduced courtesy of Ruth Murphy, Consultant Dermatologist, Royal Hallamshire Hospital, Sheffield, UK

Skin changes associated with vasculitis

Rare, may present with arthralgia and several types of skin lesions.

Pustular lesions

- *Deficiency of interleukin-1 receptor antagonist (DIRA)*: widespread pustular rash and mouth ulcers in neonates.
- *Majeed syndrome* (LPIN2): neonates to infancy. Neutrophilic dermatosis, lesions like *Sweet's syndrome, and intraepidermal pustules. Chronic recurrent multifocal osteomyelitis (CRMO).
- *Behçet's disease* with pseudofolliculitis (Figs. 38.5 and 38.6; ➲ also see Chapter 10).

Acneiform lesions

- *Chronic recurrent multifocal osteoarthritis* (SAPHO) synovitis, acne, pustulosis, hyperostosis, and osteitis (➲ see Chapter 18).
- *Pyogenic arthritis, pyoderma gangrenosum, and acne* (PAPA) (➲ see Chapter 18).
- *Pyoderma gangrenosum, acne, suppurative hidradenitis* (PASH) (Chapter 18).
- *Pyogenic arthritis, acne, pyoderma gangrenosum, suppurative hidradenitis* (PAPASH) (➲ see Chapter 18).

Urticarial lesions

- *Cryopyrin-associated periodic syndromes* (➲ see Chapter 21).
- *Familial cold autoinflammatory syndromes*, types 1 and 2 (➲ see Chapter 21).
- *Chronic infantile neurologic cutaneous and articular syndrome* (CINCA *syn.* CINCA-NOMID (➲ see Chapter 21).

Granulomatous lesions

- *Juvenile systemic granulomatosis* (*syn.* Blau syndrome); plaque-like lesions on face and torso. Skin biopsy: non-caseating granulomas.

Aphthous ulcers

- *Behçet's disease* (➲ see Fig. 10.7; Chapters 10, 13, and 38); aphthous ulcers may affect oral and genital regions.

Sarcoidosis

- This rarely presents in children.
- Skin lesions are well-demarcated erythematous, waxy plaques.

Skin biopsy: non-caseating granulomas. Arthritis of ankle joints is most common and may be self-limiting.

Monitor: renal and respiratory function.

Treatment: oral steroids and methotrexate.

Cutaneous vasculitis

- ➲ See also Chapter 31 and for investigations, Box 31.3.

* *Sweet's syndrome*: rare neutrophilic polymorphic dermatosis (tumid annular erythematous lesions), usually with fever +/– arthropathy.

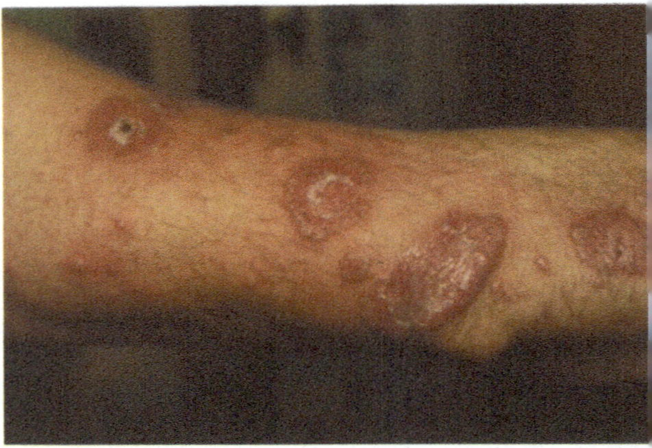

Fig. 38.5 Sweet-like lesions associated with Behçet's disease
Reproduced courtesy of Ruth Murphy, Consultant Dermatologist, Royal Hallamshire Hospital, Sheffield, UK

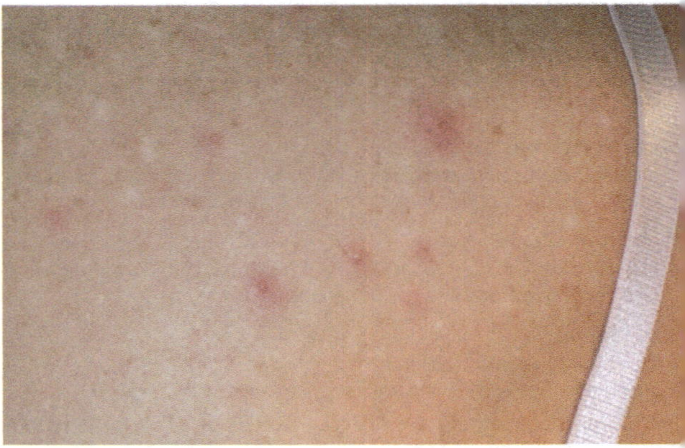

Fig. 38.6 Acneiform lesions associated with Behçet's disease.
Reproduced courtesy of Ruth Murphy, Consultant Dermatologist, Royal Hallamshire Hospital, Sheffield, UK

- *Small vessel vasculitis*: lesions disappear with adequate immunosuppression.
- *Henoch– Schönlein purpura* (➲ see Chapter 31 and Fig. 31.4).
- *Behçet's disease*: usually appears as acneiform lesions (➲ see Chapters 10 and 13) but may affect any type of vessel of any size at any body site. Look for neurological and ocular disease.
- *Systemic lupus erythematosus* (see Box 38.1).
- *Hypocomplementaemic urticarial vasculitis syndrome* (HUVS): vasculitis found in association with urticaria (Fig. 38.1).

Medium vessel vasculitis

- *Polyarteritis nodosa (PAN)*: this appears as a palpable livedoid, mesh-like rash mainly on the lower limbs. It can occur in conjunction with renal involvement and therefore renal angiography is essential, although the cutaneous variant is more common.
- *Kawasaki disease*: complications include coronary artery dissection and myocarditis (➲ see Chapter 22).

Chapter 39

Rashes associated with transplantations

Introduction

Haematological or solid organ transplantation may be associated with skin changes resulting from several different aetiologies. These include:

- Infections (bacterial, viral, and fungal).
- Adverse effects of immunosuppressive drugs.
- Graft versus host disease (GvHD).

Skin biopsy and appropriate microbiological tests are key to distinguish the cause of a rash in a child post-transplantation.

Infections

Infections are a very common complication as a result of the immunosuppression that is usually required, particularly in the first year or two following transplantation.

In general, the timeline for rashes following transplantation is:

- *Early* (within first few weeks): bacterial and mucocutaneous herpes simplex virus (HSV) infections.
- *Later* (within months): herpes zoster, viral warts, and fungal infections
- *Bacterial infections*: folliculitis, cellulitis, impetigo, and paronychia arising from *Staphylococcus aureus* or Group A *Streptococcus* are common following transplantation and can usually be managed with appropriate antibiotics, e.g. flucloxacillin or erythromycin. Necrotizing fasciitis can be rapidly progressing and potentially fatal. Oral mucositis predisposes patients to *S.viridans*, associated with antibiotic resistance.
- *Viral infections*: *varicella zoster virus (VZV)* can present as primary varicella or herpes zoster infection. Typical or atypical forms of HSV occur, with wider distribution, verrucous, pustular, crusted, necrotic, or exophytic character. Common warts, condylomata acuminate from *human papilloma virus* (HPV) infection (often very extensive). Cytomegalovirus (CMV) has cutaneous presentation of perianal ulceration, vesicles, purpura, or nodules.
- *Fungal*: *aspergillosis, cryptococcus, fusarium, and mucormycosis* are opportunistic mycoses in the immunosuppressed, with potential to cause deep fungal infections and disseminated disease.

Adverse effects of immunosuppressive drugs

- See also Chapter 23.
- *Systemic corticosteroids*: can cause cushingoid features, acne, and hypertrichosis.
- *Ciclosporin*: is associated with gingival hypertrophy.
- *Antibiotics, anticonvulsants, and others*: drug-induced lupus and drug reaction with eosinophilia and systemic signs (DRESS).

Photoprotection is recommended for immunosuppressed patients due to increased risk of future cutaneous malignancies.

Graft versus host disease (GvHD)

GvHD develops post-transplant when immunocompetent cells are transferred into the host, a disparity exists between tissue antigens of the host and donor, and the host is immunocompromised to not reject the graft. GvHD is broadly divided into acute and chronic presentations.

Acute GvHD

- *Chronology*: in haematological transplants, onset of symptoms is typically 10–14 days post-transplant, up to 99 days. In solid organ transplants, onset is 1–8 weeks post-transplant.
- *Cutaneous features*: erythematous, maculopapular, morbilliform eruptions. Severe manifestations include erythroderma, epidermal separation with bullae, toxic epidermal necrolysis (TEN) (➲ see Chapter 23).
- *Additional symptoms*: fever, diarrhoea, vomiting, abdominal pain, and ileus. In solid organ transplantations there can be haematological features (thrombocytopenia, neutropenia, haemolytic anaemia). Non-liver transplantations may have liver function derangement.
- *Histology*: skin biopsy can aid diagnosis and monitoring.
    - Grade I: basal cell vacuolation;
    - Grade II: cell necrosis;
    - Grade III: spongiosis and dyskeratosis;
    - Grade IV: epidermal loss. There is no correlation between histopathological grade and overall disease severity.

Management: first-line high dose corticosteroids and reduction/stopping immunosuppressants. Steroid-resistant cases may need addition of the following, e.g. mycophenolate mofetil (MMF), sirolimus, tacrolimus. *High multisystem disease burden carries a poor prognosis.*

Chronic GvHD

- *Chronology*: can occur with or without previous acute GvHD. Usually over 100 days after transplantation.
- *Cutaneous features*: lichen planus (LP)-like lesions (polygonal, violaceous, shiny papules with Wickham's striae) on dorsal hands, feet, forearms, and trunk. Follicular lesions early on. Diffuse/reticulate or follicular hyperpigmentation can become chronic. Sclerosis is a late manifestation and can progress to generalized scleroderma.
- *Additional symptoms*: buccal mucosal lesions (LP-like). Brittle, cracked nails. Alopecia, malabsorption, and chronic hepatitis can occur.
- *Histology*: epidermal atrophy with hyperkeratosis. Thickened basement membrane with condensed connective tissue in the upper dermis. Collagen bundles and adnexal structure destruction.

Management: topical steroids or tacrolimus for localized chronic lesions. Severe disease burden can be treated with prednisolone, ciclosporin, and other immunosuppressants. Extracorporeal photophoresis or PUVA ((psoralen with UVA) for scleroderma).

Index

D

O

P

Q

R

Medicine and Biomedical Sciences in Modern History

Series Editors

Carsten Timmermann
University of Manchester
Manchester, UK

Michael Worboys
University of Manchester
Manchester, UK

The aim of this series is to illuminate the development and impact of medicine and the biomedical sciences in the modern era. The series was founded by the late Professor John Pickstone, and its ambitions reflect his commitment to the integrated study of medicine, science and technology in their contexts. He repeatedly commented that it was a pity that the foundation discipline of the field, for which he popularized the acronym 'HSTM' (History of Science, Technology and Medicine) had been the history of science rather than the history of medicine. His point was that historians of science had too often focused just on scientific ideas and institutions, while historians of medicine always had to consider the understanding, management and meanings of diseases in their socio-economic, cultural, technological and political contexts. In the event, most of the books in the series dealt with medicine and the biomedical sciences, and the changed series title reflects this. However, as the new editors we share Professor Pickstone's enthusiasm for the integrated study of medicine, science and technology, encouraging studies on biomedical science, translational medicine, clinical practice, disease histories, medical technologies, medical specialisms and health policies.

The books in this series will present medicine and biomedical science as crucial features of modern culture, analysing their economic, social and political aspects, while not neglecting their expert content and context. Our authors investigate the uses and consequences of technical knowledge, and how it shaped, and was shaped by, particular economic, social and political structures. In re-launching the series, we hope to build on its strengths but extend its geographical range beyond Western Europe and North America.

Medicine and Biomedical Sciences in Modern History is intended to supply analysis and stimulate debate. All books are based on searching historical study of topics which are important, not least because they cut across conventional academic boundaries. They should appeal not just to historians, nor just to medical practitioners, scientists and engineers, but to all who are interested in the place of medicine and biomedical sciences in modern history.

This series continues the Science, Technology and Medicine in Modern History series.

William H. Schneider

Blood Groups and Human Heredity, 1900–1950

The First Genetic Marker

palgrave
macmillan

William H. Schneider
Department of History
Indiana University Indianapolis
Indianapolis, IN, USA

ISSN 2947-9142 ISSN 2947-9150 (electronic)
Medicine and Biomedical Sciences in Modern History
ISBN 978-3-031-69843-9 ISBN 978-3-031-69844-6 (eBook)
https://doi.org/10.1007/978-3-031-69844-6

Cover illustration: laboratory researcher at Polish National Institute of Public Health, circa 1930. “from the archives of the National Institute of Public Health (NIZP PZH), Scientific Library, Warsaw, Poland”

This Palgrave Macmillan imprint is published by the registered company Springer Nature Switzerland AG.
The registered company address is: Gewerbestrasse 11, 6330 Cham, Switzerland

If disposing of this product, please recycle the paper.

Preface

In the waning years of the First World War, Ludwik Hirszfeld directed a hospital laboratory at a large encampment of Allied soldiers north of the Greek port of Salonica. They were stationed there after the disastrous failure of the assault on the Dardanelles. Hirszfeld was a microbiologist who had left his native Warsaw for medical training in Germany, and when the war broke out, both he and his physician wife held positions at the prestigious University of Zurich. Despite the safety in neutral Switzerland, the Hirszfelds volunteered their services to the Allies.

The Hirszfelds established the hospital laboratory near Salonica, but with no military action for many months, they took advantage of the free time to do blood group testing of the soldiers who numbered over half a million and included many from the colonies and possessions of the Allied powers, as well as captives from the Central Powers. This was a project that followed from Ludwik Hirszfeld's earlier discovery of the Mendelian inheritance of the ABO blood groups. Securing agreement from the troops of such varied backgrounds, as described in Hirszfeld's memoir, required diplomatic as well as technical skill.[1] By the time the Hisrzfelds finished, they were able to report the results of 8000 tests for individuals from 16 different nationalities.[2]

The results of the Hirszfelds' work helped inspire an enormous amount of research on blood groups in subsequent decades, using much the same methodology. An example from the 1930s was the work of D.J. Buining, a naval health officer on the island of Java in the Dutch East Indies, who described his method of obtaining cooperation for one of his studies as follows:

> At a time fixed in advance, the chief of the "dessa" [village] assembled the families who seemed to him to be the most appropriate for our research. After having taken notes about the family which were related by the heads of the families during these meetings, we drew blood in a determined order. That same day the blood samples were tested.
>
> In the following days, the chief of the village, aided by his collaborators, established the lists wherein all the families were classified, and their particulars again mentioned. These details could only be obtained from long interviews and sufficient information. In general, these were done by the police or under their control. Often it took several weeks before such a report could be completed.[3]

Buining tested over 12,000 people, which added to the remarkable total of over a million subjects reported in more than one thousand articles published by 1939. The story of when, how, and why this research was done, as well as what it reveals about the history of science and society between the world wars, plus its impact thereafter, is the subject of the book that follows.

Part of the reason for the interest in this research is the crucial importance of blood, which is recognized by anyone who has been cut, every woman after the beginning of menstruation, and healers in all societies. Its importance in ceremonial rituals, as well as diagnostics and therapies, runs right through history down to present blood tests for AIDS and DNA identification. The additional links of blood to ancestry, inheritance, and descent have also made it a powerful and emotion-laden symbol of heredity in the language of most societies. There are six pages of definitions in the *Oxford English Dictionary* on blood and related words. For the French language, a 1959 edition of *Petit Littré* has 54 different uses of the word "*sang.*"

Jean Bernard, one of France's pre-eminent hematologists, published a popular book with the title *Le Sang et l'histoire*, in which he suggested three broad themes in popular folk knowledge, the first of which is that life depends on blood, the "vital fluid." Loss of large quantities will result in death. Records of this knowledge go back to prehistoric Altamira cave paintings, which show wounded and bleeding wooly mammoths. Modern science has not only confirmed but also explained the reasons for this phenomenon.

The subject of this book is the history of research following the discovery of blood groups and their inheritance, which quickly became enmeshed in two other long-standing themes identified by Bernard. One of these claims blood as the mark of inheritance, reflected in such common phrases as "blood does not lie," "blood line," "blood relations," "blood as kinship," "full-blood," and "half-blood." The other theme is that "all bloods are not equal." Hence, we talk about "blue blood," "royal blood," and "prince of the blood," to define the historical ruling classes, but also "new blood," "mixed blood," "bad blood," and "good blood" to distinguish between different qualities among commoners.

Researchers were aware of the novel historical nature of the discoveries about blood groups, especially their distribution and inheritance. As a result, they began almost immediately to record the cumulative results of the new line of research, starting with Leone Lattes in Italy, Louis Snyder and William Boyd in the U.S., and Michael Hesch in Germany. Following the Second World War, Arthur Mourant completed the best known of these efforts in three *magna opera*.[4] Beginning in the 1990s a new perspective on these developments was offered in studies by historians who placed the blood group research in its wider context, and recent scholarship has been more in depth, focusing on specific time periods, locations, and applications to the developing field of population genetics after 1950. They show the interconnections with and implications for other developments in science as well as society and politics.

This monograph presents a more complete description of the beginning and rapid establishment of blood group research in the first half of the twentieth century. It is meant to provide in-depth background that will serve as a base for further research. The main theme of this book is how blood groups were used as a scientific explanation of differences in race, health, and human behavior. The discovery of the inheritance of blood groups and their uneven distribution among various human populations quickly developed into a new field of scientific study in various countries around the world. Almost as quickly, the discoveries were studied as markers of race, disease, and behaviors such as crime, insanity, and temperament. The time period covered is the first half of the twentieth century, beginning with Karl Landsteiner's discovery and ending with the period following the Second World War when the research was picked up again just before the revolution in human genetics that began with the discovery of the double helix.

The first chapters look at the key developments in blood group discovery and the overall published record of research. Analysis of over 1100 articles published by 1939 reveals several features about the time, location, and motivation of researchers. For example, the number of publications grew rapidly in the 1920s, to over 120 per year, then declined in the 1930s. The number of people tested in studies grew, however, such that the numbers tested each year did not decline, with a cumulative total in these 20 years exceeding 1.3 million. Interest varied by country for reasons that reveal much about local scientific, political, and social circumstances. For example, studies in Germany and the Soviet Union far exceeded the numbers in other locations for a complex of reasons with some similarity (e.g., political revolutions that opened careers in medicine) but even more interesting differences (links to race in Germany as opposed to disease in the Soviet Union). The places of next largest interest included the U.S., Britain, and France, not surprising given their medical and scientific resources, but even greater was interest in Japan and Italy. These chapters also indicate different interests in the connections of blood groups to race, disease, and criminality, as well as the kinds of journals publishing these results in the new field.

Subsequent chapters use other primary and secondary sources to examine in greater detail the countries where the majority of blood group research was conducted as well as the circumstances producing similarities and differences. Germany and the Soviet Union warrant a separate chapter because research there was the most extensive. Another chapter compares France, Britain, and the U.S., where there was also considerable research, although for different reasons. Noteworthy research in other, sometimes surprising places (eastern Europe, Japan, the Netherlands, and colonial settings) is the subject of a chapter on the spread of blood group research around the world.

The next chapters analyze the record of blood group research for its impact on certain fields to which it was applied, such as anthropology, criminology, and medicine. The attempt to find a genetic determination of race was most extensive before the Second World War and Nazi atrocities, but the appeal of finding Mendelian markers indicating propensity for disease or criminality was part of a revival and growth of blood group studies in the postwar period. This beginnings and rapid establishment of this field of research on possible hereditary links of blood groups has been little studied and shows how deep-seated has been the interest in the genetic causes of these human conditions.

Anthropological and race studies linked to blood groups underwent the most interesting changes from the interwar to the post-1945 period. Initially, blood groups were taken as a new and potentially more precise way to define race, but by the end of the 1930s and especially after 1945, as is shown in the later chapters, blood group genetics undermined the very concept of race and became the foundation of population genetics. The latter focused on the distribution of genotypes rather than the definition of races as reflected by blood group phenotypes. A final chapter suggests broader conclusions that might be drawn from this study to provide perspective on the current role of genetics in science and society.

Indianapolis, IN William H. Schneider

Notes

1. Ludwik Hirszfeld, *The Story of One Life,* eds. Marta A. Balinska and William H. Schneider (Rochester: University of Rochester Press, 2005), 58.
2. Ludwik Hirszfeld and Hannah Hirszfeld, "Serological Differences Between the Blood of Different Races," *Lancet* 194 (1919): 675–9.
3. D. J. Buining, "Recherches sur les groupes sanguin au Indes neerlandaises," *Anthropologie* 43 (1933):301–2.
4. A. E. Mourant, *The Distribution of the Human Blood Groups* (Oxford: Blackwell, 1954, updated 1976); *The ABO Blood Groups* (Oxford: Blackwell, 1958); and *Blood Groups and* Diseases (Oxford: Oxford University Press, 1978).

Acknowledgments

This work has been long in preparation and grew out of a study of eugenics which revealed that researchers attempted to use the hereditary blood groups as a link to other desirable and undesirable inherited traits. The history of blood group serology has been viewed almost exclusively as a remarkable discovery in the growth of medical knowledge with unusually widespread uses. There has been less study of the broader social influences on research and applications which this book shows was a particularly rich and extensive subject of research.

Over the years I have been assisted by a large number of institutional and personal supporters. In fact, they are too numerous for all to be thanked, except for the following notable examples. Special thanks are due to Eric Juengst at the NIH Human Genome Project whose grant to study "Ethical, Legal, and Social Issues" supported the time for the extensive archival research plus a conference with international collaborators, notably Bernardino Fantini. Joe Christian of the Medical Genetics Department at Indiana University's School of Medicine provided encouragement, additional support, and technical expertise. Later support was provided by a Fulbright fellowship, and a grant from the National Library of Medicine for extensive research on the translation (with colleague Marta Balinska) of the autobiography of Ludwik Hirszfeld. The niece of Hirszfeld, Joanna Belin, provided crucial assistance for that work.

The librarians and archivists around the world whose collections I consulted were incredibly patient and helpful in identifying the enormous body of literature necessary for this study. Thanks to just two will have to suffice as examples: Tomas Allen at the World Health Organization and especially Brandon Pieczko at Indiana University School of Medicine library who has both assisted research and agreed to preserve many of the materials gathered in the course of this project.

Contents

List of Figures

List of Tables

CHAPTER 1

Background and Key Developments of Blood Group Research

The modern scientific study of blood and inheritance began at the end of the nineteenth century, following the rediscovery of Mendel's report of a new way to study the hereditary transmission of specific traits. This turned scientists' attention to the underlying genetic mechanism that produced these traits. From the turn of the twentieth century until the discovery of the molecular structure of DNA in mid-twentieth century, research on the workings of heredity generally followed one or both of the two methods used by Mendel: pedigree studies of phenotypic manifestations of presumed inherited conditions, and statistical analysis of possible links between phenotypic characteristics and their frequency of association. Key to the latter method was identifying traits that were inherited according to Mendelian laws, for they could be tested as markers linked to other possibly inherited traits.

The Scientific and Social Setting

This new approach was applied to the study of blood and inheritance in the first decade of the twentieth century when Karl Landsteiner discovered the ABO blood groups, as defined by four combinations of antigens on the blood cell surface and corresponding sera in humans. When these were soon shown to follow Mendel's rules of inheritance, the blood groups became one of the most studied features of human heredity until they

W. H. Schneider, *Blood Groups and Human Heredity, 1900–1950*, Medicine and Biomedical Sciences in Modern History,
https://doi.org/10.1007/978-3-031-69844-6_1

were superseded by genome studies after the middle half of the twentieth century. This gave the blood groups an importance beyond their practical use in transfusion. They were also of assistance in such matters of legal medicine as criminal identification and disputed parenthood. The most immediate and widespread subject of research, however, was the distribution of the blood types in different human populations, be they ethnic groups, criminals, or those afflicted with specific diseases. Underlying the motivations and presumptions of researchers was that blood types were a potential genetic marker for race, disease, criminality, and other human conditions.

In addition to inheritance, the other feature of blood groups that largely determined the nature and extent of research about them was the availability of populations that could easily be tested. The importance of the latter is evident from the start with Landsteiner's discovery of the blood groups in 1901, because he relied on a ready group of individuals to test: 22 patients and his laboratory personnel at the Vienna General Hospital. The interest in inheritance came shortly thereafter because of the new (simultaneous but independent) interest in blood transfusion which soon recognized the importance of using donors with matching blood type. The most readily available donors were family members, and doctors quickly recognized the greater chance of a match from relatives of patients. By 1908 this prompted Emil von Dungern and Ludwik Hirszfeld to study blood group inheritance more systematically, again using a convenient group of a much larger number of subjects (348): the families of faculty and staff at the University of Heidelberg where they worked.

The Mendelian pattern of inheritance they discovered greatly increased the potential interest in further study, but this took time to develop because testing was difficult (three hours for a test), and there were few populations available in large enough numbers as potential subjects. Hirszfeld later recalled his and von Dungern's interest in further testing but also the realization that it was "a project which under normal circumstances would have required dozens of years of work: a project of world exploration from the serological point of view. It is possible that the project would not have been realized in our lives."[1]

The First World War provided the unusual circumstances to overcome both these obstacles: subjects for study and more rapid tests. First was the mobilization of millions of soldiers and their stationing for long periods of time which made them potential subjects for testing. In addition, the recognition of possible transfusion needs, along with some technical discoveries, resulted in the development of much more rapid testing (a matter of minutes) that made it possible to test large numbers of troops, even in advance of stationing on the battlefront. In fact, these changes produced the conditions at the Salonica front in 1917–1918, where Hirszfeld and his wife were stationed and made their breakthrough discovery described below of the uneven geographical distribution of blood types.[2]

The Hirszfelds' 1919 article also applied their findings directly to the question of defining human races, which subsequently became the most important subject of interest in blood groups as a genetic marker. In fact, the interest in race had already prompted some independent studies, albeit on a much smaller scale, such as an article published in 1920 which reported earlier research that found differing blood group distribution in Hungarian, German, and Romanian populations living in Budapest.[3] A few other articles published in journals of limited circulation based on research independent of or before the Hirszfelds' *Lancet* article included reports of blood group distribution in China and Japan that differed from populations in other countries.[4]

Interest in blood groups as potential race markers was by no means the only line of inquiry for researchers. For example, two years after the Hirszfelds' article, a study was published showing a possible link between blood type and disease, and a few years after that another article suggested a link to criminality. The former was a 1921 article by a doctor in Scotland who reported a correlation between certain blood groups and cancer. W. Alexander of the Bacteriological Department of the University of St. Andrews in Dundee found a higher percentage of AB and B blood types among cancer patients (12 percent and 32 percent) compared to the normal population (4 percent and 12 percent), and although Alexander admitted the numbers involved (50 cases) were too small to justify conclusions, he compared his results to 125 patients with other diseases who showed no difference from the normal population.[5] Foreshadowing subsequent interest in the subject, Alexander's article prompted an immediate response from two other researchers who examined the records of thousands of patients at the Mayo Clinic, but they were unable to corroborate his findings for any disease. Nonetheless, Alexander's study established a methodology and opened a line of research and debate whose importance waxed and waned in subsequent decades but which left a voluminous record of publication.[6] Of note, these studies were possible because of the readily available population to test: hospital patients.

More controversial was the work of Max Gundel, a young German bacteriologist who in 1926 tested several thousand people in Schleswig-Holstein for distribution of blood types, including several hundred prisoners whom he found to have a higher percentage of type B blood than in the overall population. Gundel's findings were bolstered by the large sample of the population of the Schleswig-Holstein region that he tested, 8000 subjects which included 884 inmates at 5 prisons in the region. His findings immediately prompted studies that both supported and refuted his findings. The inconclusive results spurred additional research as did the readily available populations that could be easily tested, thanks to their confinement in prisons.[7] Gundel's methodology also provided a model for research on potential links to other inherited behavioral traits such as insanity, again made possible because of subjects accessible in asylums. But the number of these studies was significantly less than those testing for links to disease or race and nationality.

The availability of well-defined and accessible populations is an example of broader developments in science and society that stimulated the extensive research in blood group distribution. Others include the long-standing interest in differences between human populations, popularly labelled races, which was given scientific definition at the end of the eighteenth century, thanks to the classification system of Linnaeus. In addition, by the end of the nineteenth century, the expansion of European colonial rule brought increased interaction with new populations and ideas of hierarchy. At the same time, the successes of scientific discovery greatly increased confidence in the role of science to improve society, including improvement of humans. One quite revealing reflection of this was the new idea of eugenics which sought to apply discoveries about genetics to improve the hereditary qualities of the population. Racial hierarchy was an old idea, but genetics was seen by some as a new means to a better definition of populations with superior and inferior inherited qualities.

As mentioned, an important development that fed the great interest in blood group distribution was the growth of opportunities to do research. For example, the expansion of European empires at the end of the nineteenth century placed colonial doctors in previously remote lands inhabited by quite different populations. And the scientific discovery of blood groups, plus rapid improvements in ease of testing, made it possible for field research to be done all over the world. As a result, the research of the Hirszfelds was relatively easy to duplicate. Likewise, the dramatic growth in the nineteenth century of institutions to house and treat the sick (hospitals), abnormal (asylums), and criminals (prisons) collected large numbers of people who could be readily tested for blood type, and these numbers only increased in the first half of the twentieth century.

Another feature of the discoveries of Landsteiner and the Hirszfelds was their novel and unprecedented nature; hence, the research they inspired opened a new and extensive field of scientific research. As a result, the adoption and growth of the blood group research in different settings shows the interactions and influences that existed between this new scientific research and modern society. Perhaps most obvious is that because it was based on a previously unknown feature of human physiology, the history of research on blood group heredity offers a good example of the diffusion of a new scientific discovery. Like Landsteiner's initial discovery of blood groups in 1900, subsequent findings about their inheritance were equally sudden; hence, the pattern of diffusion is clearly discernable. At the other end of its history, the similarities of this research to work being done today with DNA—its sudden discovery, promises and disappointments, the social influences and impacts—offer historians as well as those concerned with contemporary scientific developments a historical framework of reference for judging future developments.

Key Scientific Discoveries

Modern science has confirmed some of the popular folk notions linking blood and heredity. Phenotypic markers of inheritance have been found in the blood, initially the blood groups, but of course now we know that DNA is found in the nucleus of every cell of the body. On the question of whether all bloods are equal, however, current science has come to a more mixed conclusion. Strictly speaking, the blood in the veins of all people is the same for most of its properties. But this makes even more striking the differences such as the blood groups which are numerous and varied enough so that the exact combinations of the hundreds of blood antigens are close to being unique for each individual.

To be sure, contemporary science has shown the error of considering blood as a symbol of hereditary differences in such things as intelligence, bravery, humor, or other physical or moral virtues or vices. But historically, this has come only after a very contentious first half of the twentieth century, during which both well-meaning scientists and calculating dictators using pseudo-scientific ideologies claimed that all bloods were not equal. Naturally, the broader social and political significance attached to blood had an impact on the blood group discoveries. Because of the age-old association of blood with inheritance, when Landsteiner discovered the

ABO antigens and within ten years they were found to be inherited, the discoveries attracted a great deal of public attention as well as scientific appreciation. Adding to the interest was the fact that the blood groups were also quickly recognized to have very practical applications in forensics and blood transfusions.

To understand the uses to which new knowledge about blood groups were applied, it is necessary to examine more closely the discoveries themselves. This is a fascinating and dramatic story, mainly because it is a rare example in the history of science of a discovery almost without precursor. Adding to that interest is the fact that these new ideas and medical discoveries were made by people living in a world of unprecedented change in science, medicine, war, and society. Moreover, the fact that many of the early pioneers in serology came from central Europe, added to the drama of the story because that is where the greatest upheavals occurred. This chapter serves the conventional purpose of providing background to the history of serology by describing some of the milestones in the history of blood group research. In addition, it provides biographical information about the main researchers themselves, thus providing important information about the times when they lived. In many ways the world was changing as rapidly as the new medical discoveries were made.

The discovery of blood groups was part of a wave of new scientific research that swept across Europe and America at the end of the nineteenth century. The giants who produced this work (the Curies and Roentgen, Einstein and Planck, Virchow and Ehrlich) benefited from a variety of new developments, ranging from increasing support for research from national, industrial, and university sources, to broader trends fostering wider dissemination of publications and such mundane advances as more powerful microscopes which made it possible to examine many hitherto undetectable phenomena. For medical researchers interested in serology, the spectacular achievements of Koch and Pasteur provided even more inspiration for further work in the last decades of the nineteenth century. In addition to hunting for microbes, researchers in Britain and on the continent examined the blood of patients for unusual conditions to be treated or for clues to future diagnosis. By the end of the nineteenth century, they had discovered some of the fundamental properties of sera and red corpuscles both in humans and animals. Ehrlich and Morgenroth in Germany, Maragliano in Italy, and Shattock in England were among those who made significant contributions to the beginnings of modern serology and immunology.[8]

Landsteiner's Discovery and the Naming of the Blood Groups

One of the researchers attracted to these questions was Karl Landsteiner, the son of an Austrian journalist who trained in medicine at the University of Vienna and spent five years studying with leading chemists in Switzerland and Germany.[9] In 1897 he was appointed an assistant at the University of Vienna Pathological-Anatomical Institute, where he remained for the next 11 years. Although his primary responsibility was autopsies (in all he performed 3639 postmortem examinations at the Institute), Landsteiner also took time to study the question that interested him most: the reaction of blood to foreign substances—immune reactions.

The phenomenon that attracted Landsteiner's attention was the clumping together (agglutination) of red blood cells and sometimes their actual breakup (lysis) with the subsequent release of hemoglobin. Previous researchers had produced this phenomenon by introducing blood from a different species. It was Landsteiner's combination of luck and genius to extend this research. In a footnote to a 1900 experiment involving bovine, swine, and human blood, he wrote,

> The serum of healthy humans not only has an agglutinating effect on animal corpuscles, but also on human blood corpuscles from different individuals. It remains to be decided whether this phenomenon is due to original individual differences or to the influence of injuries and possible bacterial infection.[10]

Landsteiner proceeded to test his idea on blood samples from 22 doctors, staff members and healthy patients at the Institute. He painstakingly separated the sera and red blood corpuscles from each individual, then systematically mixed them with the sera and corpuscles of the others. He found that sometimes the red cells clumped, but sometimes they did not. Most important, because of his methodical procedure, Landsteiner could recognize a pattern in the results as shown in Table 1.1.[11]

Overall, Landsteiner found first that the sera of almost half those tested (ten individuals, including Landsteiner) did not cause the red cells of the others in the group to clump, although it did for the rest. Likewise, the cells of this first group were caused to clump by the sera of the rest. Sera and red cells of another, smaller group (three) acted in similar fashion. Finally, sera from a group slightly smaller than the first (nine) caused

Table 1.1 Example of Landsteiner's results (1901) "Table I. Concerning the Blood of Six Apparently Healthy Males (plus sign designates agglutination)"

Serum from	*Blood cells from:*					
	Dr. St.	*Dr. Plecn.*	*Dr. Sturl.*	*Dr. Erdh.*	*Zar.*	*Landst.*
Dr. St.	–	+	+	+	+	–
Dr. Plecn.	–	–	+	+	–	–
Dr. Sturl.	–	+	–	–	+	–
Dr. Erdh	–	+	–	–	+	–
Zar.	–	–	+	+	–	–
Landst.	–	+	+	+	+	–

Source: Karl Landsteiner, "Ueber Agglutinationserscheinungen normalen menschlichen Blutes," *Wiener klinische Wochenschrift*, 14 (1901), 1134

clumping of all the others' red blood cells, but they were not clumped by any other sera. Landsteiner labeled the categories of individuals A, B, and C, depending on these clumping or "agglutinating" properties. This was later changed to A, B, Ø (zero) because the last group's cells had no agglutinating properties. When two of Landsteiner's students (Decastello and Sturli) confirmed his findings by testing more than one hundred subjects, they also found a small group whose cells were agglutinated by sera from both A and B. That category was labeled AB. Later the Ø was changed to O and the ABO nomenclature was worked out with its four types: A, B, O, and AB.[12]

Landsteiner's findings attracted the attention of other researchers interested in agglutination who were also able to observe this pattern among healthy humans. In fact, because of the general but sometimes isolated interest, as shown in Table 1.2, two other nomenclature systems arose which were a source of confusion for decades. One originated from research by Jan Jansky, a Czech psychiatrist who made no reference in his 1906 article to Landsteiner's 1901 results. The other was based on the work of the American William Moss who knew of Landsteiner's work but not Jansky's. In presenting their results, both Jansky and Moss used Roman numeral labels for their categories of individuals intended to be just that: headings for tables that showed the groups of individuals whose blood sera and cells had similar agglutinating properties. Although Jansky's use of different labels is understandable, one might ask why Moss used a new designation. The reason was that he did not know of Decastello and Sturli's discovery of the AB group. Hence, Moss thought his finding of a

Table 1.2 Three systems of blood type nomenclature, 1901–1910

Researcher	*Year*	*Blood type nomenclature*			
Landsteiner	1901	A	B	O	AB
Jansky	1907	II	III	I	IV
Moss	1910	II	III	IV	I

fourth group warranted a new nomenclature. Neither of these researchers gave much thought to their choice of Roman numerals or the fact that Landsteiner used Roman letters to identify the groups of individuals whose blood they tested for agglutination. Only later was the following possible confusion realized.

Jansky's work was published in a Czech language psychology journal; hence, it was lost in the large amount of undifferentiated medical research published at the beginning of the twentieth century. In contrast, Moss' research appeared in a 1910 article published in the much more widely read *Bulletin of the Johns Hopkins Hospital.*[13] Problems arose with subsequent researchers who confirmed and extended these findings but applied labels to their groups of individuals depending on whose previous work they cited. The three different nomenclatures continued to be used well into the 1930s, which is a testimony to the insularity and inertia of researchers in their own language and cultural areas.

American, British, and French blood group researchers generally adopted Moss' system, while other Europeans, especially German-speaking researchers, used either Jansky's or more often Landsteiner's. In 1921, a joint committee of immunological, bacteriological, and pathological associations in the U.S. recommended using the Jansky nomenclature so as to avoid "further confusion and the possibility of accident." This was despite Landsteiner's better claim to priority and the fact that Moss' nomenclature was much more widely used.[14] After many years of resistance to the recommendation—and with three-fourths of U.S. hospitals using Moss' system in 1927 while use of the Jansky system had risen to 20 percent—there was another recommendation by the American National Research Council to compromise by using the ABO nomenclature of Landsteiner who had emigrated to the U.S. in 1922.[15] The American Association of Immunologists agreed, and the suggestion was further bolstered by the recommendation in 1928 from a League of Nations Commission on Biological Standardization to adopt the ABO nomenclature.

Despite these good intentions, the author of a 1929 survey of blood group labelling in 552 North American hospitals said of the attempt to change to the ABO system: "the result will not be a compromise but a third classification ... [T]he new 'Landsteiner' classification bids fair to make matters worse, and it should be abandoned by the small number of institutions already employing it one way or another."[16] These fears were not realized, but they help explain why it took so many years for the confusion and double labelling of blood to subside and the ABO nomenclature eventually to become the universal practice.

The Heredity of the Blood Groups

The confusion in labeling the blood types was surprising, because the importance of the ABO blood group discovery was quickly apparent in both medical and non-medical fields. Landsteiner himself suggested two uses in his 1901 article: blood transfusion and legal medicine. The former he mentioned almost as an afterthought at the very end of the article, "Finally, it should be mentioned that the described observations permit the explanation of varying consequences resulting from therapeutical blood transfusions." Brief though it may have been, this comment was also farsighted because transfusion was a rarely practiced procedure at the time. In contrast, Landsteiner gave much more attention to the possible use of his discovery in criminal identification. In fact, two years later, he and Max Richter demonstrated that the agglutinating properties of blood cells and sera remained intact even after prolonged exposure to the environment.[17] Thus, within two years of their discovery, blood groups were recognized as useful for identifying blood stains in criminal investigations.

Despite Landsteiner's prediction, for a variety of reasons the use of his discovery for blood transfusions took longer than one might expect. Only at the end of the decade did practitioners begin testing for possible agglutination before transfusion.[18] In fact, it took the sharp increase in transfusions during the First World War (and much quicker methods of testing) before the discovery was applied routinely. In the process, some new and unexpected discoveries were also made about the blood groups, especially their inheritance and uneven distribution among peoples around the world.

The first published speculation about the possible inheritance of blood groups was by Reuben Ottenberg, one of the pioneers of blood transfusion at Mount Sinai Hospital in New York and a strong proponent of testing before selection of blood donors. It was in the course of checking family members for transfusion compatibility that he and a colleague, Albert Epstein, noticed that the blood types of parents and children were often the same. This led them to suggest in a 1908 article that the pattern of blood types in successive generations of two complete families indicated they might be inherited.[19] Moreover, because of what they noted to be, "the sharply opposed nature of the blood characteristics," they went on to suggest, "if they are inherited at all, they will form a very good example of the Mendelian law of heredity." Two years later Emil von Dungern and his assistant Ludwik Hirszfeld in Heidelberg published the results of a more extensive and systematic study along these lines.

Von Dungern and Hirszfeld examined the blood types of 72 families comprising 348 individuals and found that most of the time when both parents were A their children were A. The same was true for B, and always for O. The pattern was explainable by Mendelian inheritance, with A and B as dominant and O as recessive traits. Von Dungern and Hirszfeld also proposed that the underlying genetic mechanism was two pairs of alleles (A and non-A, B and non-B) which could occupy two loci on the chromosome with A and B dominant.[20] Even though they were mistaken about the underlying mechanism of inheritance (it was revised in the 1920s by Bernstein), von Dungern's and Hirszfeld's proof of Mendelian inheritance was convincing and suggested many applications.

Despite its potential, the discovery of the heredity of the blood types lay relatively unappreciated for several years. This was surprising because of the interest in human heritable traits that had developed at the end of the nineteenth century. For example, the founder of eugenics, Francis Galton, and the biometrical school of his successor Karl Pearson sought to prove inherited human qualities by statistical studies of height and stature as well as more general characteristics like intelligence.[21] After the turn of the century and the rediscovery of Mendel's work, a list grew of more specific human qualities that seemed to follow a pattern of inheritance similar to that found by the Augustinian monk, such as sex (1901), alkaptonuria (1902), and brachydactyly (1905). In Bateson's 1909 book *Mendel's Principles of Heredity*, he suggested other abnormal conditions such as cataracts, hemophilia, and color blindness which were likely to be inherited according to Mendelian{XE "Inheritance laws:Mendelian inheritance"} laws.[22] One persistent problem with most of these suggestions, however, was the difficulty in defining the traits, as well as recognizing the Mendelian pattern of inheritance in successive generations.

This problem, however, made human blood groups attractive as a hereditary trait for study. For one thing, the phenotypes were simply and clearly defined. Moreover, they were normal traits for all humans, unlike many of the other earlier discovered disorders such as brachydactyly or alkaptonuria. In addition, a person's blood soon could be tested relatively easily by mixing it with the sera of a known blood type to test for clumping. And finally, an individual's blood type was fixed at birth (or sooner) and was unaffected by environmental influence.

One problem at first with this line of research was that the blood type was not readily apparent. Landsteiner's procedure required mixing blood with the sera of a known blood type to test for clumping, but for a number of years the procedure was very time-consuming. In addition, given the human life span, with only two or three generations to study, it took time to recognize and prove even the invariability of the blood groups, let alone their exact pattern of inheritance. On this latter question, researchers eventually made up in breadth of testing what they were unable to do by longevity studies. Unlike the research of T.H. Morgan on drosophila flies at Columbia which was going on at the same time and depended on variations to appear in jars of rapidly breeding insects in successive generations, blood group research eventually went to the far corners of the earth to test human populations in every shape, form, and clime that researchers could find.[23] This did not occur, however, until after the First World War, and in large measure researchers were inspired by the remarkable findings of Ludwik and Hannah Hirszfeld who conducted blood tests of Allied soldiers on the Macedonian front during the war.

The Hirszfelds' Discovery of Distribution Frequency (1919)

The outbreak of war in Europe changed many areas of life including scientific investigations, with research disrupted unless it had obvious war applications. Thus, serologists turned to much more practical matters such as techniques of transfusion and preservation of stored blood. One of these practical developments had important consequences for subsequent discoveries about the genetics and distribution of blood groups: the discovery of more rapid and simpler blood group testing. Landsteiner's original method of determining blood type was lengthy and painstaking. In fact, one of the main reasons given by surgeons who ignored it in making the first transfusions was the possible loss of urgently ill patients because of the delay required for testing blood group compatibility. Ottenberg developed a more rapid test in 1909, but it still involved separating sera and washing cells which required special laboratory equipment and three hours time.

Then, in 1915, Peyton Rous and Joseph R. Turner of the Rockefeller Institute discovered a dramatic improvement. Using the recently discovered anticoagulant sodium citrate for dilution, the researchers could detect agglutination under a microscope in as little as 2–5 minutes and with certainty within 30 minutes.[24] The following year Moss suggested an even simpler procedure that involved use of standardized test sera of blood types A and B. If a drop of blood of an unknown type was added to a drop of known A and B sera, the unknown blood type could be determined based on agglutination (or lack thereof) visible to the naked eye. Beth Vincent and Roger I. Lee, two surgeons from Massachusetts General Hospital serving in the American army in France, independently and almost simultaneously discovered a method similar to that of Moss.[25]

The rapid test made it possible to determine the blood types of large numbers of people, which was the second prerequisite for the discoveries about blood group distribution. Of course, even more important was the world war that mobilized resources on an unprecedented scale, including the assembling of soldiers in groups numbering tens of thousands. By the end of the war there was sufficient need for transfusions of wounded to require doctors to test the blood types of large numbers of potential donors either as needed or in advance, especially once a simple and quick procedure was developed. For example, a U.S. army surgeon in France published an article in the spring of 1918 which reported the results of blood typing of one thousand soldiers using the method of Vincent and Lee. Similarly, in 1919 three doctors at Ft. McPherson, Georgia, reported the results of testing 1122 soldiers, which they had done toward the end of the war, including both a description of technique and the distribution of the four blood types.[26]

These numbers were much larger than prewar studies such as that done by Von Dungern and Hirszfeld which had proved the Mendelian inheritance of blood groups. In fact, following that study, Von Dungern and Hirszfeld realized that differences in blood type distribution might offer a new way of studying the hereditary definition of races, but as mentioned above because of the large numbers and travel required for testing, they assumed such an investigation would be a difficult undertaking and "would not have been realized in our lives."[27] As luck would have it, the war and other unforeseen developments provided the circuitous but much more rapid route which Hirszfeld and his wife Hannah followed to be able to undertake the project.

After finishing his medical studies in 1907, Hirszfeld went to Heidelberg University, where he became an assistant to von Dungern in the Institute for Experimental Cancer Research. They had great latitude in choice of work, which included the path-breaking demonstration of the Mendelian inheritance of ABO blood types. In 1911 Hirszfeld went to Switzerland in order to broaden his training at the Hygiene Institute of the University of Zurich, and his new wife Hannah, a pediatrician, took a position at the Zurich Children's Clinic. Thus, when the war broke out, the Jewish-born, Polish-Russian raised, and German-trained Hirszfeld was in a well-protected position in a neutral country. In his autobiography, Hirszfeld wrote of his conflicting sentiments as the war swirled around him.

> What was I to do?
>
> Great dramas, even the poor ones, draw into their whirlpool all who thirst for depth and are unable to remain standing at the edge of life.
>
> I went to the movies, where they showed the mobilization going on in all countries. I was often irresistibly attracted to the young enthusiasts shown on the screen who, with their fatherland in their hearts, went to their deaths. In the clinic, my wife was training nurses for the legions. I did not want to join the Russian army. Whom could I offer my help?[28]

Word of the outbreak of a typhus epidemic in Serbia at the beginning of 1915 finally provided the "call to combat." In Serbia, Hirszfeld could aid the cause of Slavic nationals while practicing his profession as a hygienist. He left Zurich in February and a few months later, his wife joined him. By the middle of 1915 the epidemic was under control, but a military offensive by the Central Powers broke through the Serb lines, forcing everyone to move south in retreat. In December 1915 the Hirszfelds reached Albania, where a ship took them to Italy, and they made their way overland back to Zurich.

Neither of the Hirszfelds was content to remain in neutral Switzerland after tasting the adventure and satisfaction of helping in the war. In an effort to continue studying tropical bacteriology, Ludwik wrote to London to offer his services to the Colonial Offices. Soon he received an invitation from the Serbian government to buy a laboratory of equipment in

Switzerland and accompany it to Corfu, where the Serb government had set itself up in exile. Shortly after arriving, Hirszfeld saw how much a bacteriologist was needed in Corfu, where a cholera epidemic had broken out and food was in short supply. But the ultimate destination for the laboratory was the more strategic location of Salonica, where a French-administered hospital was to be installed to support troops involved in the ongoing invasion of the Dardanelles. A British transport took Hirszfeld and his wife to the Greek port.

Meanwhile, the Central Powers offensive that forced the Serbs south did not stop until it reached the outskirts of Salonica. At the end of 1915, a new Franco-British expedition was also sent to Salonica where they were soon joined by many of the Allied forces retreating from the disastrous defeat at Gallipoli. Fate once again took an unforeseen turn when the entire contingent of Allies became bottled up in and around the Greek port for the next two years. The Germans thwarted any military advance, and Allied political leaders considered evacuation too embarrassing.[29]

Hirszfeld, thus, found himself as the head of a bacteriological laboratory of one of the largest Allied hospitals in Salonica. The significance of this turn of fortune for the history of blood group research was that the Allied forces included not just Serbian, French, British, and other troops drawn from eastern Europe but also soldiers from British and French colonies in Asia and Africa. Thus, in addition to permitting Hirszfeld to conduct research on typhus and other diseases, it was an ideal setting for him to undertake the study he and von Dungern had only theorized about before the war. In the next two years Hirszfeld and his wife conducted tests on 500–1000 individuals from 16 different ethnic groups, ranging from English and French to Greeks, Bulgarians, Senegalese, Malagasies, and Vietnamese. In all over 8000 tests were made.

It would be an understatement to say that the Hirszfelds welcomed the opportunity to do the research, even though as mentioned earlier, the problem of convincing so many troops of different backgrounds to submit to the tests was an anthropological challenge. As described in Hirszfeld's memoir,

> We had to speak in a different way to each nation. It was enough to tell the English that the objectives were scientific. We permitted ourselves to kid our French friends by telling them that we could find out with whom they could sin with impunity. We told the Negroes that the blood tests would show

> who deserved leave; immediately, they willingly stretched out their black hands to us.[30]

The researchers persevered, and the results of their tests showed not only differences in the proportion of the four ABO blood types for the populations tested but a pattern in the differences which was explainable by geography (see Fig. 1.1). In sum, they found a higher incidence of blood type A (and lower B) for peoples from northern and western Europe, with a corresponding lower percentage of A and higher B as one moved south and east into Asia. Above all, it was this link between geography and distribution that was to be the most enduring legacy of their discovery.

The methodology of the Hirszfelds and their conclusions will be discussed at greater length in the next chapter. They presented their findings first to the Salonica Medical Society in June 1918, but they had difficulty

TABLE IV.—*Showing the Percentage Frequency of A and B Serological Reactions in Various National Types*

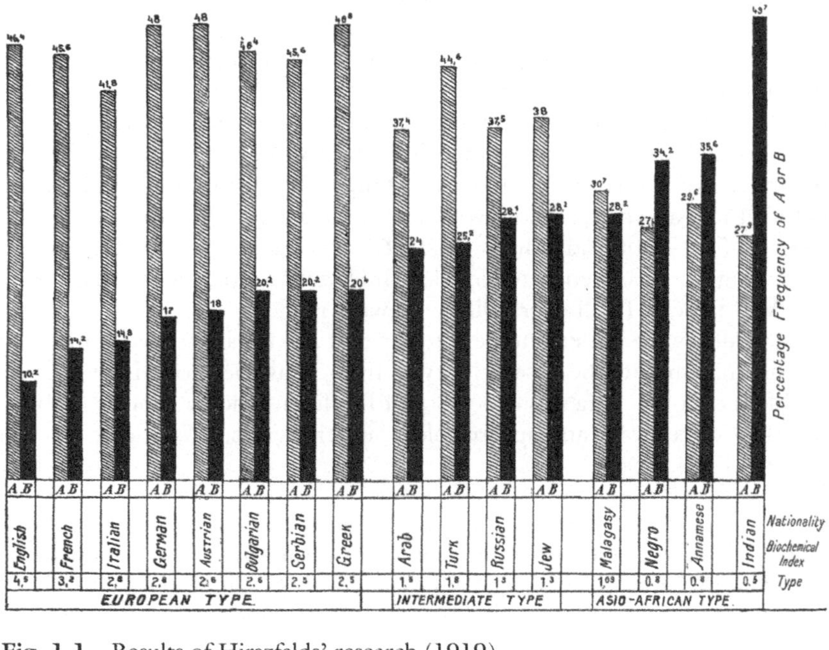

Fig. 1.1 Results of Hirszfelds' research (1919)

in finding a journal for publication. Part of the problem was typical of any study that breaks new ground or crosses fields of research. Thus, the *British Medical Journal* rejected the manuscript as not likely to be of interest to doctors. A French anthropological journal published their findings, but it was not until *Lancet* printed a summary in October 1919 that the results reached a broader medical audience.[31]

Landmark Blood Group Discoveries

The Hirszfelds' discovery about ABO blood group distribution, though remarkable, was slow to have an impact on other researchers. Nonetheless, within a few years, as indicated in Table 1.3, there were some surprising and dramatic confirmations of their findings which rapidly spread their notoriety and stimulated a great interest in the field during the 1920s and1930s.

This began in 1921 when Alexander in Scotland reported a correlation between certain blood groups and cancer, followed in 1923 when Arthur F. Coca reported his finding of a very high percentage of type O blood in American Indians. More controversial was the work of a German bacteriologist who tested a large selection of the population of Schleswig-Holstein and found a higher percentage of type B blood among prisoners than in the normal population. And in the mid-1930s serologists developed a technique for testing the dried and ancient remains of mummies to see if blood type had changed over long periods of time.

The first of these landmark papers was an independently inspired study of the blood types of cancer patients in Scotland by W. Alexander of the Bacteriological Department of the University of St. Andrews in Dundee. He reported a higher percentage of AB and B among cancer patients (12 percent and 32 percent compared to 4 percent and 12 percent in the normal population), and although Alexander admitted the numbers involved

Table 1.3 Landmark studies of blood group distribution, 1919–1940

Year	*Researcher*	*Study*
1919	Hirszfelds	Geographic distribution
1921	Alexander	Disease
1923	Coca & Diebert	Native Americans
1924	Bernstein	Genetic theory
1926	Gundel	Criminals
1933	Boyd & Boyd	Mummies

(50 cases) were too small to justify conclusions, he compared his results to 125 patients with other diseases, who showed no difference from the normal population.[32] More telling for the future, Alexander's article prompted an immediate response from two other researchers who examined the records of thousands of patients at the Mayo Clinic without being able to corroborate his findings for any disease. Nonetheless, Alexander's study established a methodology and opened up a line of research and debate whose importance waxed and waned in subsequent decades, but which left a voluminous record of publication.[33]

More in line with the anthropological findings of the Hirszfelds was an article on the blood types of Native Americans published in 1923 by Arthur F. Coca, and Olin Diebert. Coca is best known as the founder and editor-in-chief of the *Journal of Immunology* from 1916 to 1948. He studied medicine in his native Philadelphia at the University of Pennsylvania and remained after graduation in 1898 to work as an assistant under Simon Flexner. Coca studied immunology at Heidelberg with von Dungern from 1907 to 1909; hence, his work overlapped that of Hirszfeld. Then after two-years of service in the Philippines, Coca returned to a position at Cornell University Medical College, where he remained to the end of his career.

Coca had read the *Lancet* article of his former associate Hirszfeld, and during the study of almost one thousand students at American Indian schools in Kansas, Oklahoma, and New Mexico, he and Diebert found over 77 percent with blood type O.[34] This remarkable finding corroborated the Hirszfelds' broader contention that blood types offered "a new means of studying racial relationships." Specifically, they suggested the primordial existence of blood type O before Amerindians were separated from the Old World, with newer isoagglutinogens A and B appearing later in western Europe and Central Asia. Less theoretical but a more important practical result of this study was the opening of the pages of Coca's journal to articles on blood group research. The *Journal of Immunology* became one of the most important publications of the new field which added impetus to the worldwide study of all sorts of isolated populations for more clues about the origins of races.

The next important landmark in the study of populations for whom the blood types might be a marker of inheritance was a 1926 article published by a young German bacteriologist in Kiel, Max Gundel. His study included tests of criminals and the insane. Like many of his German colleagues, he began his career at one of the newly created Hygiene Institutes at the University of Kiel. He had recently completed his doctorate in bacteriology, but his interest in serology was kindled by the Hirszfelds' work and the subsequent writings on blood groups and race by Paul Steffan, a navy doctor at the Kiel Ostseestation, who as will be seen below did the first blood testing of populations in Germany.[35]

Gundel's approach was to test a large sample of the entire population of the Schleswig-Holstein region. Included in what would eventually be more than 8000 subjects were 884 inmates at 5 prisons in the region. When Gundel examined the results for the prisoners, he found what he described as "a significant increase" of blood type B of prisoners (19 percent) compared to the rest of the population (13.4 percent).[36] Gundel did further studies, dividing the prisoners into categories by crime committed and length of incarceration, in order to find an association of blood type with more specific criminal behavior. Despite (or perhaps because of) the fact that his number were limited and the differences relatively small, Gundel's findings sparked a lively debate and extended the blood group research into a new area of application. This was similar to the line of research started by Alexander on the link between blood groups and disease, with some studies corroborating and others refuting the initial results. Gundel also reported differences in the ABO blood type frequencies of populations in insane asylums, but his was not the first such research which had already emerged in previous years from the study of blood groups and disease. A subsequent chapter will discuss these and other more imaginative and far-fetched studies attempting to link blood groups with various conditions and behaviors presumed to be inherited.

The final example of landmark research extending the Hirszfelds' discovery to a new field was testing blood antigens in the mid-1930s of mummified remains. This was primarily the work of American researchers, an indication of the rising level of interest and technical expertise plus the luxury of being isolated from the dramatic political changes which were affecting central and eastern Europe. The technical basis for the work was first published by William C. Boyd in a 1933 article on testing preserved bone and muscle.[37] Boyd was the son of a midwestern farmer who went to Harvard, excelled in science, and then took up the study of immunology in 1930 at Boston University Medical School. Shortly after developing his new testing technique, Boyd and his wife published the results of tests on a handful of Egyptian and American Indian mummies in 1934.[38]

These articles quickly prompted further tests by G. Albin Matson, an immunologist at Washington University in Missouri, who studied native American mummies, and P. B. Candela, a practicing physician in Brooklyn who tested mummified Egyptian remains from the Brooklyn Museum.[39] These studies did not produce a large new body of research, but they do show how the extent of previous blood group research created and extended the demand for new approaches to resolving their problems. The mummy testing was aimed at determining the historical origin of type O blood among Amerindians and the appearance of type B in the Eurasian/African land mass.

Bernstein and the Genetic Theory of Blood Groups

In addition to extending the Hirszfelds' findings about distribution, the research on blood groups between the wars also helped produce more fundamental immunological discoveries. For example, the spread of work stimulated by the *Lancet* article very quickly permitted a better understanding of the genetics of blood groups. In fact, by 1924, enough additional test results had been reported to raise questions about the von Dungern/Hirszfeld explanation of the inheritance of the blood groups. These were answered brilliantly by the German mathematician Felix Bernstein whose revised theory used newly developed mathematical techniques of population genetics.[40]

Bernstein was the son of Julius Bernstein, a professor and head of the Institute of Physiology at the University of Halle. In fact, Felix studied physiology for three years while completing his graduate studies in mathematics. In 1907 he received his doctorate, and in 1911 he joined the Math faculty at the University of Göttingen.[41] Felix's daughter Marianne relates how Julius also played an indirect role in Felix's immediate interest in blood groups. After the First World War, Ludwig Hirszfeld mailed a reprint of his and von Dungern's prewar paper on the inheritance of blood groups, addressed to "Julius Bernstein, physiologist, Göttingen," not realizing that Julius had died in 1917. The package was delivered to Felix, who began reading the paper, "with great interest …, exclaiming 'Da stimmt doch was nicht [there is something wrong].'"[42]

Bernstein decided to confirm the agglutinating properties of blood and immediately ordered a microscope and centrifuge, despite the postwar shortages. He began with his own family. According to his daughter, "all four of us, father, mother, Ulrich and I had our ear lobes pierced by the assistant who was enjoying the warmth of the coal stove (there was little coal available for the Institute of Mathematical Statistics); and thus we learned with great delight that 'vatií' really was our father." Fortunately for subsequent researchers, Bernstein had enough sense to apply his considerable mathematical and statistical skills to the question of inheritance, rather than continue repeating the work of others.

To Bernstein the blood group tests could be most usefully interpreted in light of the work by the German pediatrician Wilhelm Weinberg, who was a pioneer in population genetics. Beginning at the turn of the century, Weinberg developed mathematical methods in order to make estimates of gene frequencies from observable phenotypic traits of rare disorders found in twins and some more frequent illnesses such as tuberculosis.[43] Bernstein became familiar with Weinberg's work shortly after the war in an effort to correct and refine some of his mathematical and statistical techniques. The small number of cases of obviously inherited diseases plus the complexity of the more common ones made it difficult to apply rigorous mathematical methods.

Human blood groups, on the other hand, were ideal for these methods since they were found in all humans yet were indistinguishable to the general populace (and of course unknown to anyone until 1901), thus assuring random mating, a key assumption in population genetics theory. After Landsteiner's discovery, the technique for determining blood type was known, and the results of tests on thousands of subjects had already been published by the time Bernstein learned of the work.

As a mathematician Bernstein first recognized a problem with the assumptions of von Dungern and Hirszfeld about the genetic basis of blood type. They had assumed the phenotype was determined by the inheritance of two pairs of alleles on two loci of the chromosome: A and non-A or B and non-B, with A and B dominant to either non-A or non-B but not each other. This theory explained the four blood types: A (either homo- or heterozygous), B (likewise), AB (if alleles of A and B were both present), or O (if any combination of non-a and non-B were present). It also explained some of the more readily observable Mendelian phenomena such as the fact that children with blood type B or A had to have at least one parent with that blood type. The problem was that as the results of more studies were published, small but significant discrepancies appeared between these results and what the Von Dungern and Hirszfeld theory predicted for blood types, especially less common ones in parents and their children.

In a 1924 article in the *Klinische Wochenschrift*, Bernstein analyzed data from American Indians, populations from Japan, Korea, Australia, the Philippines, Hungary, and Manchuria, as well as the 16 nationalities studied by the Hirszfelds during the First World War.[44] According to Bernstein, the results of these studies of blood type frequency could be explained far better mathematically if only three possible alleles were assumed for the two loci of the chromosome determining ABO blood type. As shown in Table 1.4, he labeled these factors A (the A genotype), B (B genotype), and R (O genotype). With A and B dominant to R but not each other, only six combinations of genotype would produce the four ABO blood types.

Since Weinberg's theory provided a way to calculate gene frequencies from phenotype frequencies in fairly large, randomly mating populations, Bernstein's proposal could be confirmed by using existing results of ABO distributions. Figure 1.2 illustrates how Bernstein predicted that his theory would be proven if the sum of the gene frequencies (p+q+r) would equal 100 percent.

The mathematics worked elegantly as indicated in Table 1.5 for the dozens of studies already published and provided added motivation for the dramatic rise in subsequent studies in the mid-1920s.[45]

Bernstein's theoretical discovery showed his brilliance as a mathematician. His suggestions about the larger anthropological implications of his work, however, show how far afield he was from his expertise in mathematics. For example, he agreed with the Hirszfelds' equally amateurish

Table 1.4 Hirszfeld (1910) and Bernstein(1924):theories of blood group inheritance

Hirszfeld's 2-allele (Aa, Bb) 2-loci theory		*Bernstein's 3-allele (A, B, R) 2-loci theory*	
Blood phenotype	*Blood genotype*	*Blood phenotype*	*Blood genotype*
A	AA, Aa, Ab	A	AA and AR
B	BB, Bb, Ba	B	BB and BR
AB	AB	AB	AB
O	aa, ab, bb	O	RR

$$(1-\sqrt{B + O})+(1-\sqrt{A + O})+(1-\sqrt{O}) = 1$$

\/ \/ \/

$$p \quad + \quad q \quad + \quad r = 1$$

Fig. 1.2 Bernstein's hypothesis. Source: Felix Bernstein, "Ergebnisse einer biostatistichen zusammenfassenden Betrachtung uber die erblichen Blutstrukturen des Menschen," *Klinische Wochenschrift* 3 (1924): 1497

Table 1.5 Examples of Bernstein's results "Race-Table" (selections)

Researchers	*Subjects*		*ABO blood type (%)*				*A-race*	*B-race*	*R-race*	
	No.	*Nationality*	*O*	*B*	*A*	*AB*	*p*	*q*	*r*	*p+q+r*
Hirschfelds	500	English	46.4	7.2	43.4	3.0	26.8	5.2	68.1	100.1
Hirschfelds	500	French	43.2	11.2	42.6	3.0	26.2	7.4	65.7	99.3
Hirschfelds	500	Italian	47.2	11.0	38.0	3.8	23.7	7.7	68.7	100.1
Hirschfelds	500	German	40.0	12.0	43.0	5.0	27.9	8.9	63.2	100.0
F. Verzar & O. Weszeczky	385	Gypsies	34.2	38.9	21.1	5.8	14.5	25.6	58.4	98.5
Liu & Wang	1000	Chinese	30.0	34.6	25.0	10.0	20.0	25.8	54.7	100.5
Coca & Diebert	862	Native Americans	77.7	2.1	20.2	–	10.7	1.1	88.0	99.8

Source: Felix Bernstein, "Ergebnisse einer biostatistichen zusammenfassenden Betrachtung uber die erblichen Blutstrukturen des Menschen,' *Klinische Wochenschrift* 3 (1924): 1496

theory of primordial races and even suggested that the high incidence of B blood type in central, south, and east Asia was connected to the rice diet of the populations there. Nonetheless, Bernstein's work had dramatic consequences not just for the recalculation of blood group genotypes but also for the whole view of what blood types represented. For physical anthropology, in retrospect, it signaled the beginning of the end of using blood types alone to determine race. In its place, Bernstein's work laid the groundwork for viewing blood group studies as a simple indication of gene frequency. According to this viewpoint, the concept of human races could be replaced by that of the gene pool now common in population genetics

The Discovery of New Blood Groups

Bernstein's work was elegant and brilliant, but in a sense, it was still a revision of Von Dungern's and Hirszfeld's earlier discovery. In the meantime, more fundamental research continued on the nature and properties of the ABO system, which eventually resulted in discoveries of new agglutinogens. For example, in 1911 von Dungern and Hirszfeld suggested the existence of sub-groups of blood type A. Their work was confirmed and extended after the war by Guthrie and Huck in the U.S., as well as others in Europe.[46] The discovery foreshadowed a much more important breakthrough in 1927 by Landsteiner working with Phillip Levine, his assistant at the Rockefeller Institute in New York, where Landsteiner had moved after the First World War.

By using sera from rabbits which had been injected with human red blood cells, Landsteiner and Levine were able to distinguish new agglutinins in human blood which acted independent of the ABO system. They labelled these M and N which were found to be complementary and analogous to the ABO system, and P which was an independent antigen. In addition to discovering new blood group antigens, their work shows how rapidly the level of serological sophistication was increasing. Also of note in their work—because it indicates the far-reaching impact of blood group distribution research—was one proof that they used to demonstrate that the MN system was the equivalent of the ABO. In 1928 they tested black, white, and American Indian populations in New York, finding differences in the percentages of the M and N antigens of each population.[47]

Despite this spectacular and well-publicized discovery (in 1930 Landsteiner received the Nobel Prize in medicine), it was over ten years before the next blood group system (Rh) was discovered. This landmark, which set the stage for the post-Second World War explosion of blood group research, was first suggested by Levine and Stetson only in 1939, then confirmed and defined by Landsteiner and Wiener the following year. This late date was even more surprising, since the condition which led to its discovery, maternal-fetal blood group incompatibility, had been a subject of interest to serologists for more than 20 years.[48] It is, thus, worth examining it as an example of a missed opportunity in scientific research, as well as a final landmark in the history of blood group genetics.

As early as 1920, William M. Happ of the Pediatrics Department of Johns Hopkins University reported on a study of "The Appearance of Isoagglutinins in infants and Children," begun in 1914, in which he compared the blood groups of mother and infants.[49] In subsequent years this line of research was picked up, especially in France and Poland, where Hirszfeld conducted sustained research on the permeability of placental blood. One French researcher, Nadia du Bouichet, reported in 1926 that in 2 of 24 cases, the blood of mother and newborn agglutinated despite being the same blood type. Her conclusion, however, was simply not to give transfusions from mother to newborn.[50]

In the meantime, as early as 1912, pathologists had given the name erythroblastosis fetalis (EF) to the disease process which produced anemia, jaundice, and other symptoms in stillborn and newborn infants.[51] In 1932 Louis K. Diamond, then a newly trained pediatrician at Harvard Medical School, co-authored an article surveying the literature reporting over one hundred cases of stillborn and newborn children manifesting edema, anemia, and jaundice, which he concluded were all attributable to EF.[52] Although Diamond was to become famous for his work on Rh antigens after the Second World War, he recounted how he missed an even earlier opportunity to diagnose that the cause of EF was from incompatibility in this as yet unknown blood group system.

In 1936 Diamond treated a newborn with anemia and jaundice by making a transfusion of a small quantity of the father's blood. After a brief improvement, the infant soon relapsed from destruction of red cells. Diamond rechecked his crossmatch and repeated the process three more times with similar results. He then tested the mother's O-type blood for compatibility and finding such, transfused a small quantity to the infant. The results produced an even worse reaction. Diamond double-checked the cross-matching by standard procedures, but when an additional test with a thicker suspension of red cells showed some agglutination, he brought in a blood grouping expert for consultation. According to Diamond,

> He too used [standard] 1–2% saline-diluted red cells and found no suspicious clumps. When shown my questionable agglutinates in a thicker smear, he criticized this as sloppy technique. He could not explain the infant's obvious transfusion reaction except to recall he had seen one before from the use of blood from a post-partum donor, and he said, "Women, especially during pregnancy, do queer things."

"Incidentally," Diamond added, "he was a confirmed bachelor." Even if Diamond exaggerated from hindsight, other evidence suggests it was not an isolated event. Diamond reported the incident to show how close he came to discovering the cause of Rh disease.

The actual discovery came in 1939 when Levine and his colleague Stetson were referred a case from Bellevue Hospital in New York with a similar set of circumstances, only this time it was a hemolytic reaction by the mother of a stillborn infant with EF. The mother had received a transfusion from her husband with the same blood type O. Retesting her serum against the husband's cells, the hospital found agglutination. Levine tested the mother's serum more systematically against blood samples of 104 otherwise compatible subjects and found agglutination in 83 cases. Because he suspected the cause might be the stillbirth, at the time Levine considered it a temporary phenomenon.[53]

The following year Landsteiner and Alexander Wiener published an article describing a new antigen they had found using immune sera from other mammals as had been done in the discovery of the M, N, and P antigens. They called the new antigen Rh since Rhesus monkeys were the source of test cells.[54] The fact that 85 percent of Caucasian subjects had a positive reaction (similar to the findings with Levine's serum), led Levine and his associates the following year to confirm that the new antibody was the cause of EF.[55] Although the Rh system proved to be quite complicated (in fact, this was one reason for the stimulus of so much new research after the war), the discovery not only explained the most common disease of blood group incompatibility, but it also identified yet another very important blood group system to be tested for transfusion as well as anthropological and legal purposes.

Conclusion

The story of the blood group discoveries is one of the noteworthy chapters in the remarkable biomedical advances of the first half of the twentieth century. Yet it has been overshadowed by the even more numerous discoveries made after 1945. The record of the pioneering work of the many researchers shows the role both of individual genius as well as the advantages of the worldwide network of publication which made new information available to other researchers far more rapidly than ever before. In addition, most of the methodology as well as the infrastructure was established before 1941, which was the basis for the expanded research after the war.

But the history of blood group research was not just one landmark breakthrough after another. It was much more the process of individuals in the medical and scientific infrastructure who recognized and worked on problems and questions judged of importance locally as well as internationally. As the following chapters will show, the conditions shaping the spread of the discoveries, let alone the nature of that research and its applications, varied considerably from country to country and between locales within given countries.

Notes

1. Ludwik Hirszfeld, *Les groupes sanguins: leurs applications à la biologie, à la medicine et au droit*, trans. by Hanna Hirszfeld (Paris: Masson, 1938), 130.
2. Ludwik Hirszfeld and Hannah Hirszfeld, "Serological Differences Between the Blood of Different Races," *Lancet* 194 (1919): 675–9.
3. Fritz Verzar and OskarWeszeczky, "Rassenbiologische Untersusuchungen mittels Isohamagglutininen," *Biochemische Zeitschrift* 126 (1921):33–9.
4. The 1916 Japanese article by Hara was cited in Shinichi Kirihara, "Uber die Isohämagglutination beim menschlichen Blute," *Zeitschrift für klinische Medizin* 99 (1924): 530. The Chinese study was by Alson R. Kilgore and J. Heng Liu, "Iso-agglutination Tests of Chinese Bloods for Transfusion Compatibility," *China Medical Journal* 32 (1918): 21. For more, see Chap. 2.
5. William Alexander, "An Inquiry into the Distribution of Blood Groups of Patients Suffering from Malignant Diseases," *British Journal of Experimental Pathology* 2 (1921): 66–9.
6. On the Mayo Clinic study, see J. Arthur Buchanan and Edith T. Higley, "Relationship of Blood Groups to Disease," *British Journal of Experimental*

Pathology 2 (1921): 247–55. Research on the relationship between blood groups and disease is examined in Chaps. 2 and 6.

7. Max Gundel, "Rassenbiologische Untersuchungen an Strafangefangenen," *Klinische Wochenschrift* 5 (1926): 2165–66. For more, see Chaps. 2 and 7.
8. For background, see Maxwell M. Wintrobe, ed. *Blood Pure and Eloquent* (N.Y: McGraw-Hill, 1980). On immunology, see Arthur M. Silverstein, *History of Immunology* (New York: Academic Press, 1989), and Anne-Marie Moulin, *Le dernier langage de la médecine: Histoire de l'immunologie de: Pasteur au Sida* (Paris: Presses Universitaires de France, 1991).
9. The best biography remains that of his co-worker at the Rockefeller Institute Peyton Rous, "Karl Landsteiner," *Obituary Notices of Fellows of the Royal Society* 5 (1947): 295–324. See also Paul Speiser, *Karl Landsteiner, Entdecker der Blutgruppen* (Vienna: Hollinek, 1961) and the more recent Pauline M.H. Mazumdar, *Species and Specificity: An Interpretation of the History of Immunology through the Work of Karl Landsteiner* (Cambridge: Cambridge University Press, 1995). An unpublished manuscript, complete with materials such as clippings and notes on interviews conducted shortly after Landsteiner's death, is in the MacKenzie Collection of the American Philosophical Society, B/L 23m.
10. Karl Landsteiner, "Zur Kenntnis der antifermentativen lytischen und aglutinierenden Wirkungen des Blutsera und der Lympho," *Centrallblatt für Bakteriologie* 27 (1900): 361.
11. Karl Landsteiner, "Ueber Agglutinationserscheinungen normalen menschlichen Blutes," *Wiener klinische Wochenschrift* 14 (1901): 1134.
12. Alfred von Decastello and Adriano Sturli, "Ueber die Isoagglutinine im Serum gesunder und kranker Menschen," *Münchener medizinische Wochenschrift* 49 (1902): 1990–95.
13. Jan Jansky, "Haematologicke studie u. psychotiku," *Sbornik Klinicky* 8 (1907): 85–139; William L. Moss, "Studies in Isoagglutinins and Isohemolysis," *Bulletin of the Johns Hopkins Hospital* 21 (1910): 63–70.
14. "Isoagglutination. Recommendation that the Jansky Classification be Adopted for Universal use," *JAMA* 76 (1921): 130.
15. "New Designation for Blood groups According to Iso-agglutinins," *JAMA* 88 (1927): 1421.
16. James A. Kennedy, "Blood Group Classifications Used in Hospitals in the United States and Canada," *JAMA* 92 (1929): 614–5. For background, see A.D. Farr, "Blood Group Serology -- The First Four Decades (1900–1939)," *Medical History* 23 (1973): 216–7; and William H. Schneider, "Chance and Social Setting in the Application of the Discovery of Blood Groups," Bulletin of the History of Medicine 57 (1983): 545. For the recommendations, see "Isohemagglutination. Recommendation that the Jansky Classification be Adopted for Universal

Use," I, 76 (1921), 130; "Current Comment," I, 88 (1927), 421–2; and League of Nations. Permanent Commission on Biological Standardisation, *Report of the Permanent Commission on Standardisation of Sera, Serological Reactions, and Biological Products (Frankfurt, April 25–28, 1928)* (Geneva, 1928).

17. Karl Landsteiner and Max Richter, "Ueber die Verwertbarkeit individueller Blutdifferenzen für die forenzische Praxis," *Zeitschrift für Medizinbeamten* 16 (1903): 85–9.
18. See William H. Schneider, "Blood Transfusion in Peace and War, 1900–1918," *Social History of Medicine* 10 (1997): 121–2.
19. Reuben Epstein and Albert E. Ottenberg, "A Simple Method of Performing Serum Reactions," *Transactions of the New York Pathological Society* 8(1908): 117–23.
20. The results were published in a series of articles in the same journal, Emil Von Dungern and Ludwik Hirszfeld, "Uber Nachweis und Vererbung biochemischer Strukturen. I," "Uber Vererbung gruppenspezifischer Strukturen des Blutes. II," "Uber gruppenspezifische Strukturen des Blutes. III," in *Zeitschrift für Immunitätsforschung* 4 (1910): 531–46; 6(1910): 284–92; and 8 (1911): 526–62.
21. Francis Galton, *Natural Inheritance* (London: Macmillan, 1889). For background, see Daniel J. Kevles, *In the Name of Eugenics* (Cambridge: Harvard University Press, 1985).
22. William Bateson, *Mendel's Principles of Heredity* (London: Constable & Co., 1929), 205–34.
23. On the unintended consequences of research subjects, see Robert E. Kohler, *Lords of the Fly* (Chicago: University of Chicago Press, 1994).
24. Peyton Rous and Joseph R. Turner, "A Rapid and Simple Method of Testing Donors for Transfusion," *JAMA* 64 (1915): 1980–2.
25. Agglutination of A sera and not B would indicate blood type B; B and not A would mean type A. Agglutination of both meant AB, and agglutination of neither meant the unknown blood type was O. See William L. Moss, "A Simplified Method for Determining the Isoagglutinin in Group in the Selection of Donors for Blood Transfusion," *JAMA* 68 (1917):1905–6; Roger I. Lee, "A Simple and Rapid Method for the Selection of Donors," *British Medical Journal* (1917): 683–84; and Beth Vincent, "A Rapid Macroscopic Agglutination Test for Blood Groups, and Its Value in Testing Donors for Transfusion," *JAMA* 70 (1918): 1219–20. The test was most commonly referred to as the Moss/Vincent test. All of these surgeons saw service in France during the First World War.
26. Howard T. Karsner, "Transfusion with Tested Bloods," *JAMA* 70 (1918): 769–71; George R. Moffitt, George F. Klugh and Chester E. Shepard,

"Blood Type Classification, with a Slight Modification of Technic: Report of the Results of More than a Thousand Tests," *JAMA* 73 (1919): 1821–2.
27. Hirszfeld, *Les groupes sanguins,* 130.
28. Ludwik Hirszfeld, *The Story of One Life,* eds. Marta A. Balinska and William H. Schneider (Rochester: University of Rochester Press, 2005), 30.
29. George B. Leon, *Greece and the Allied Powers, 1914–1917* (Thessaloniki: Institute for Balkan Studies, 1974), 256–69.
30. Hirszfeld, *The Story of One Life*, 58. The national/ethnic stereotypes were common at the time, although they have been taken by some as reflecting underlying racism of the Hirszfelds. For more on this, see Chap. 6.
31. See Schneider, "Chance and social setting," 557.
32. Alexander, "An Inquiry into the Distribution of Blood Groups of Patients," 66–9.
33. On the Mayo Clinic study, see Buchanan and Higley, "Relationship of Blood Groups to Disease." Research on the relationship between blood groups and disease is examined in a subsequent chapter.
34. Arthur F. Coca and Olin Diebert, "A Study of the Occurrence of the Blood Groups among American Indians," *Journal of Immunology* 8 (1923): 487–91.
35. For more on Steffan, see subsequent chapters.
36. In addition to Gundel's "Rassenbiologische Untersuchungen an Strafangefangenen," see "Einige Beobachtungen bei der rassenbiologischen Durchforschung Schleswig-Holsteins," *Klinische* Wochenschrift, 5 (1926): 1186.
37. William C. Boyd and Lyle G. Boyd, "Blood Grouping by Means of Preserved Muscle," *Science* 78 (1933): 578.
38. Boyd and Boyd, "An Attempt to Determine the Blood Groups of Mummies," *Proceedings of the Society for Experimental Biology* 31 (1934): 671–2.
39. G. Albin Matson, "A procedure for Determining Distribution of Blood Groups in Mummies," *Proceedings of the Society for Experimental Biology and Medicine* 31 (1934): 964–8; P. B. Candela, "Blood Group Reactions in Ancient Human Skeletons," *American Journal of Physical Anthropology* 21 (1936): 429–32.
40. For background and context, see Pauline M. H. Mazumdar, "Two Models for Human Genetics: Blood Grouping and Psychiatry in Germany between the Wars," *Bulletin of the History of Medicine* 70 (1996), 609–57.
41. In addition to Mazumdar's work, the most accessible biographical information on Bernstein is in the *Dictionary of Scientific Biography.* A doctoral thesis was written by Magdalene Frewer, "Das wissentschaftliche Werk Felix Bernsteins" (thesis, Göttingen University, 1977).

42. American Philosophical Society, Philadelphia, Curt Stern Papers, Ms coll 5, Bernstein folder, letter from Marianne Bernstein to H. Eldon Sutton, editor, American Society of Human Genetics, December 12, 1967. The story was confirmed in an interview with M. Bernstein September 1993.
43. On Weinberg, whose name is associated with the Englishman Hardy in the fundamental principle of population genetics, see "Bernstein" in the *Dictionary of Scientific Biography* and William A. Provine, *Origins of Population Genetics* (Chicago: University of Chicago Press, 1971).
44. Felix Bernstein, "Ergebnisse einem biostatistischen zusammenfassenden Betrachtung über die erblichen Blutstrukturen des Menschen," *Klinische Wochenschrift* 3 (1924):1495–7. For a more complete exposition, see his article the following year, "Zusammenfassende Betrachtungen über die erblichen Blutstrukturen des Menschen," *Zeitschrift für induktive-Abstammungs und Vererbungslehre* 37 (1925): 237–70.
45. There were some disagreements for a while, notably from such figures as the Japanese serologist Tanemoto Furuhata, the German geneticist Karl-Heinrich Bauer, and Englishman R.R. Gates. But with such authoritative figures as Landsteiner, Levine, and Laurence Snyder in the U.S., plus Fritz Schiff in Germany offering meticulous and irrefutable proof of Bernstein's hypothesis, it was quickly accepted. See Mazumdar, "Two Models," 624–8.
46. Charles G. Guthrie and John G. Huck, "On the Existence of More than Four Isoagglutinin Groups in Human Blood," *Bulletin of the Johns Hopkins Hospital*, 34 (1923): 37–48. See also V. Friedenreich and A. Zacho, "Die Differentialdiagnose zwischen den 'Unter'- Gruppen A1 und A2." *Zeitschrift für Rassenphysiologie* 4 (1931):164–91. For historical background, see Farr, "Blood Group Serology," 221–3.
47. Karl Landsteiner and Philip Levine, "A New Agglutinable Factor Differentiating Individual Human Bloods," *Proceedings of the Society for Experimental Biology and Medicine* 24 (1927): 600–2; Landsteiner and Levine, "Further Observations on Individual Differences of Human Blood," ibid., 941–2. See also Landsteiner and Levine, "On the Racial Distribution of Some Agglutinable Structures of Human Blood," *Journal of Immunology* 16 (1929): 123–31.
48. Among the researchers attesting to the importance of the Rh discovery, see R.A. Fisher, "The Rhesus Factor: A Study in Scientific Method," *American Scientist* 35 (1947): 95–102; Louis K. Diamond, "The Rh Problem: A Personalized History," *Turkish Journal of Pediatrics* 24 (1982): 35–47; and Walter F. Bodmer, "Early British Discoveries in Human Genetics: Contributions of R.A. Fisher and J.B.S. Haldane to the Development of Blood Groups," *American Journal of Human Genetics* 50 (1992): 671–6.

An unusual perspective is Doris T. Zallen, Daphne Christie, and Elizabeth M. Tansey, *The Rhesus Factor and Disease Prevention: Wellcome Trust Centre Witness Seminar* (London: Wellcome Trust Centre for the History of Medicine, 2004).

49. William M. Happ, "Appearance of Isoagglutinins in infants and Children" *Journal of Experimental Medicine* 31 (1920): 313–34.
50. Nadia du Bouchet, "Interagglutination positive malgré l'identité des groupes entre le sang de la mére et du nouveau-né," *Comptes-rendus de la Société de Biologie* (hereafter cited as *CRSB)* 94 (1926): 16–7. See also, Ludwik Hirszfeld and H. Zborowski, "Sur la permeabilité elective du placenta en rapport avec le groupe sanguin de la mére et la foetus," *CRSB* 92 (1925): 1253–5; and Laffont and Gaujoux, "Recherches sur l'agglutination des globules sanguins avec le maternal et foetal," *CRSB*, 88 (1923): 730–1.
51. The term was coined by H. Rautmann, "Über Blutbildung bei fötaler allgemeiner Wassersucht." Bei*träge zur pathologischen Anatomie* 54 (1912): 332–349, according to Louis K. Diamond, Kenneth D. Blackfan, and James M. Baty, "Erythroblastosis fetalis and its association with universal edema of the fetus, icterus gravis neonatorum and anemia of the newborn," *Journal of Pediatrics* 1 (1932): 269 - 309.
52. Ibid.
53. Philip Levine and Rufus E. Stetson, "An Unusual Case of Intra-Group Agglutination," *JAMA* 113 (1939): 126–7.
54. Karl Landsteiner and Alexander S. Wiener, "Studies on an Agglutinogen (Rh) in Human Blood Reacting with Anti-Rhesus Sera and with Human Isoantibodies," *Journal of Experimental Medicine* 74 (1941): 309–20.
55. Philip Levine, L. Burnham, E.M. Katzin, and P. Vogel, "The Role of Isoimmunization in the Pathogenesis of Erythroblastosis Fetalis," *American Journal of Obstetrics and Gynecology* 42 (1941): 925–37.

CHAPTER 2

The Pattern of Research About Blood Groups

In many ways research on blood groups was possible because of the scientific infrastructure that created a number of new fields of scientific and medical research in the first half of the twentieth century. For example, the new discoveries spread rapidly through an international network of publications that has become an essential part of contemporary science. In addition, new serological laboratories were created that served to train (or retrain) specialists in the field. In the process, an enormous amount of research was conducted, and the results were published and assimilated into the knowledge base of the new field. This included new journals, summary bibliographic publications, and ultimately worldwide reference laboratories.

Less well known about the history of this research is that there were many local and national differences in the speed, extent, and line of inquiry adopted in different parts of the world.[1] These were not only the result of the individual idiosyncrasies of the researchers but also local political, social, and historical traditions. The 1920s and 1930s were hardly times when scientists were able to remain detached and aloof from developments in the world. In fact, one of the features of twentieth-century science that became increasingly apparent between the wars was the growing interconnection between government, society, and scientific research, not just for funding but also the uses of research.

W. H. Schneider, *Blood Groups and Human Heredity, 1900–1950*, Medicine and Biomedical Sciences in Modern History,
https://doi.org/10.1007/978-3-031-69844-6_2

The previous chapter mentioned some of the most important discoveries in blood group research in the first half of the twentieth century. This chapter will survey that research from a global perspective in order to understand it as an example of the large-scale, worldwide scientific research that made the twentieth century different from previous periods in the history of science. This is not a simple task, because the interest in blood groups after their discovery in 1900 produced an enormous amount of scientific publication. Even excluding the application which generated the most interest—transfusion—by 1931 according to one bibliographer, almost 3000 articles had been published on blood group research.[2] Although it would be difficult to do an exhaustive analysis of all the literature published to 1940, the work on the distribution of the blood groups is of more manageable size. In fact, it was widespread enough to permit comparison and indicate patterns of research (over 1000 articles), while not being so overwhelming as to permit only superficial analysis.[3]

There is good reason to consider the interest in blood group distribution as typical of the interest in all blood group research. As the previous chapter showed, Landsteiner and Levine used frequency distribution in different populations as a way of confirming their discoveries of new antigens. Also, Bernstein's determination of the genetics of blood group inheritance was directly based on the results of distribution studies. The assumption that the research on blood group distribution reflected the general interest in blood groups for a given country may not be valid in every case, but a sample check of countries where there was significant research on the distribution of blood groups (such as Germany, Russia, or the U.S.), shows there was also a strong interest in the biochemistry, testing techniques, and legal applications (not to mention transfusion uses) of blood groups. Likewise, in places with little interest in distribution studies (such as Great Britain), there was relatively less or only later interest in these other aspects of blood group research. Whether it was typical or not, the research on blood group distribution mobilized extensive biomedical resources between the wars and ultimately led to important advances in immunology and human genetics.[4]

Besides the extent of blood group research, another major dilemma in studying its history concerns the national versus international perspective of researchers. On the one hand, the blood group researchers were consciously international, scientific, and universal in their goals and methodology, while, on the other, there were strong differences in the conduct of that research from country to country which make it necessary also to examine the national contexts. This chapter will first look at the overall publication record in order to see the pattern of research: that is, such things as broad differences in time and location, and motivation.[5] Subsequent chapters, using other secondary and primary sources, will examine and compare the major countries where the blood group research was conducted in an effort to understand the context producing these local differences. Then the blood group research will be analyzed for its impact in certain fields to which it was applied, such as anthropology, criminology, and medicine. A final chapter will suggest broader conclusions that might be drawn from this study.

Data Collected: Methodology

Two features of scientific bibliography between the world wars help in identifying the published research record of blood group testing from 1919 to 1939. First, it was the period after *Index Medicus* had been established as the most important reference work of medical research in the world. Growing out of the nineteenth-century *Index C atalog of the U.S. Army Surgeon General's Office*, the *Index Medicus* returned to Washington around 1900 after a brief time of being published in Paris. Shortly after the First World War it was firmly established in its role of collecting and disseminating medical research around the world.[6] Blood group testing began to be listed as a separate sub-heading in 1921, an appropriate reflection of the rising interest in that research. But *Index Medicus* was hardly exhaustive in collecting every article published on blood groups, even in medical journals. There were also many non-medical publications with articles on various applications of blood group research to anthropological or criminological questions.[7]

Fortunately, another aid in identifying these articles was the publication of several summary bibliographies compiled by blood group researchers themselves in the 1920s and 1930s. The practice of citing previous work was, of course, a well-established part of scientific methodology by the end of the nineteenth century, but the collection of and reference to previous publications on blood testing was not just a matter of paying homage or establishing legitimacy. Researchers interested in the distribution of the blood groups were aware from the start of the cumulative importance of their work, in which the whole of all research was worth more than the sum of the individual parts. To put it another way, the frequency of blood types in a given population meant far less in isolation than in comparison to frequencies in other populations. By definition, the results from any one study were only important in comparison to all other research.

The chronological record of these summaries is itself one indication of how the research spread, as shown in Table 2.1.

The first articles simply cited the results of previous blood testing, but very soon the amount of research was too large to cite. After 1923 Leone Lattes' *Individuality of Human Blood* became one of the most frequently cited reference standards because of its exhaustive bibliography plus the fact that it was often revised and translated (into German 1925, French 1929, and English 1932). In 1926 the American Laurence H. Snyder published an article in the *American Journal of Physical Anthropology* with an extensive bibliography, followed by a book in 1929 which became an English-language standard.[8] Then in 1932 the most extensive compilation to date (and in one sense ever) was published in Germany, entitled *Handbuch für Blutgruppenkunde* which listed 2927 articles on all aspects of blood group research. In fact, it was the last time anyone attempted to compile all research on blood groups, both because the field had grown too large and also as a result of the changes in political regime in Germany after 1933.

The German journal *Zeitschrift für Rassenphysiologie* published what amounted to an annual supplement to the handbook, but only for blood group research in the German language. In 1939 William C. Boyd published a compilation of all research on the distribution of blood groups, cross-referenced by geographical location of populations tested. This was the standard reference until Boyd gave his records to Arthur E. Mourant, who became director of the Serological Research Laboratory in London after the war. Mourant began publishing a series of books on human blood groups and other polymorphisms in 1954 whose second edition in 1976

Table 2.1 Bibliographies of blood group research

Researcher	*Country*	*Year*	*Note*
Lattes	Italy	1923	Translated into German, French, English (1925–1932)
Snyder	U.S.	1929	Expansion of 1926 article
Hesch	Germany	1932	Part of volume edited by Steffan
Boyd	U. S.	1939	On blood group distribution
Mourant	U.K.	1954	2nd edition published in 1976
Cavalli-Sforza	U.S.	1994	Incorporates DNA research

was over 1000 pages. Cavalli-Sforza et al. brought this work up to date in 1994 by including DNA research.[9]

Although these bibliographic tools reflect the increasing global interconnection of medical research in the twentieth century, even they contain significant omissions of research on blood groups. To identify these remaining works, a systematic search was done of the major medical and anthropological journals published in the U.S., Britain, France, and Germany. In addition, the citation trail was followed of most articles with significant bibliographies of blood group research. The following analysis is based on a reading of almost all articles, the most important exception being those published in Japan, where summaries in translation or secondary references provided the main source of information about research results.[10]

The results indicate that over 1150 articles were published between 1919 and 1939 on the distribution of blood groups. The main criterion for inclusion is that the authors reported the results of original research which tested the frequency of blood types in a given population. Summary or theoretical articles are not included. Numerous characteristics have been recorded for each of the articles (author's country, number of subjects, location of research, attempt to find correlations between blood type and other conditions such as disease or criminality), which form the framework of analysis from which the following conclusions are drawn. Before looking at the pattern of dissemination of research on blood group distribution, however, more needs to be said about the founding discovery of the Hirszfelds.

The Hirszfelds' Research as a Founding Discovery

The striking findings of the Hirszfelds' research during the First World War begged confirmation once the results were published in the French journal *Anthropologie* and the English medical review *Lancet* in 1919. Yet as striking as the results were, the Hirszfelds were not the only ones at the time to come across the phenomenon of differences in blood group distribution. The reasons why the Hirszfelds' work (and not one of several other studies appearing at the same time) became the standard reference is instructive of certain general influences on the diffusion of scientific discoveries.

The first researchers to report the distribution of blood groups were Jansky in 1907 and Moss in 1910. Their findings (and similar reports by others between 1910 and 1920) were typically incidental to other theoretical questions and were only recognized for their comparative importance at a later date. Even ignoring them, as Table 2.2 shows, between 1916 and 1921, there were at least seven other articles besides the work of the Hirszfelds' which were published independently and reported the distribution of ABO blood types in given populations.

It is obvious that this research was worldwide from the start. For example, two researchers in 1916 published results of 353 subjects tested in central Japan. In addition, the tests of 100 Chinese were published in 1918, and over 1000 U.S. army blood tests were reported in 1919.[11] A Hungarian doctor published his findings of tests on 550 inhabitants of central Hungary in 1920, and the following year Alexander reported on the blood types of 50 patients with "malignant" and infectious diseases in a Glasgow hospital.[12]

All of these articles reported results of distribution of blood types, yet none of them cited any of the other articles. For example, although the Hungarian Weszeczky's 1920 research was motivated by mass testing reported in the U.S., in fact, he did not even possess the original articles, just a citation from a Dutch book by van Leeuwen.[13] Weszeczky tested over 500 patients at his hospital, but his first attempt to divide them by

Table 2.2 First articles published independently on distribution of blood groups, 1916–1921

Year	*Author(s)*	*Journal*	*Subjects tested*
1916	Hara and Kobayashi	Iji-Shinbun	353 Japanese in Nagano
1918	Kilgore and Liu	China Med, Journal	100 Chinese tested after transfusion accident
1919	Hirszfeld & Hirszfeld	Lancet	7,900 tests, 16 diff. nationalities, also publ. in *Anthropologie*
1919	Moffitt, et al.	JAMA	1,122 tests at US army base
1920	Liu and Wang	Nat'l Med Jl of China	1,000 Chinese
1920	Weszeczky	Biochem. Zeitschr	550 Hungarians, Rumanians, & Germans in central Hungary
1921	Alexander	Br. Jl. of Exper Pathol	50 cases of "malignant" & infectious diseases
1921	Culpepper & Abelson	Jl. of Lab & Clin Med	5,000 tests at Parke Davis (Detroit)

disease did not reveal much difference in distribution of blood types. Only when he looked at the results by nationality (457 Hungarians, 81 Rumanians, and 2 Germans), did he find significant differences in the proportion of the different blood types. It was in Weszeczky's second study, co-authored with Verzar in 1922, that they had the benefit of the Hirszfelds' work. For this study, they deliberately sought for testing Germans from Budapest and Gypsies from another district of Hungary to build on previous work.[14]

Other features of the above articles, show why the Hirszfelds' work became the standard for subsequent research. In some cases, the other articles appeared in journals with limited circulation. For example, the Hara and Kobayashi study was not referenced in a Western language publication until an article by another Japanese researcher in the 1924 volume of the *Zeitschrift für klinische Medizin*.[15] Other authors were only interested in blood-typing technique and gave no references or any description about those tested. The article by Moffitt et al. simply reported the results of blood tests on soldiers at Ft. McPherson, Georgia. Rather than give a breakdown of those tested, the authors boasted about their efforts to obtain an average representation in the population tested. "The sera used were from adults of all ages, from all classes of society, white and negro races."[16] As late as the 1921 article by Culpepper and Abelson of Parke Davis Laboratory in Detroit, there was no mention of Moffitt, let alone the Hirszfelds' work of two years before. They simply described the distribution of the ABO types for 5000 blood tests they had made.[17]

The lack of comparative perspective in these articles points out another crucial reason why the Hirszfelds' work was so noteworthy. In addition to being published in *Lancet*, which had a circulation comparable to that of *JAMA*, they reported the results of tests on almost 8000 people which made it one of the largest studies for the next two decades, the Hirszfelds' article was comparative at its core. The scale and theoretical sophistication are not surprising since the idea was long in development, dating back to Ludwik Hirszfeld's prewar collaboration with Von Dungern.

Perhaps more important, the Hirszfelds also realized the potential significance of their research, and as a result, they made sure they had large enough samples from each nationality for comparison. For example, they noted (and controlled for) those who were sick and those who were healthy among the subjects tested. They sought out a Jewish community in Monastir because they appreciated the importance of that group in their comparative study. The Hirszfelds even recorded sub-categories of their 16 nationalities in a way that anticipated many of the future lines of research in the next two decades. For example, the Italians tested were divided into those from northern, central, and southern Italy because of the then-current ideas of racial difference between north and south (and they found differences in blood type distribution). The "English" soldiers tested were noted as including (and reported with a breakdown by) 29 Welsh, 52 Scots, and 16 Irish in origin. The tests of Greeks and Russians were sub-divided by geographical origins within those countries, as were the African and Asian populations tested, with designations of specific African and Asian peoples such as the Hovas, Bambaras, Toucouleurs, Cambodians, Tonkinois, and Hindus. The Hirszfelds even reported blood types for the French and English with correlation by hair color, a common feature of racial classification at the time.

In contrast, the other independent studies at the time were much less extensive than the Hirszfelds' work. Their existence, however, indicates that the knowledge about and interest in the distribution of blood types was widespread, a fact that helps explain why the Hirszfelds' discovery was so rapidly and widely noticed. This should not detract from the fact that in the end, the combination of the wide circulation of *Lancet* plus the remarkable nature of the Hirszfelds' research and their far-reaching conclusions are the most important reasons for the recognition given to their discovery. This was acknowledged in virtually all articles published on blood group distribution after 1922. The larger lesson about what determines a founding discovery article of reference is that it must, of course, present new and significantly different findings, but it should also contain substantial research to back up the findings, and the results should reach a sufficiently large audience.

One way to demonstrate how the Hirszfelds' discovery was diffused in time and space is to examine the speed and extent of the first appearance of articles reporting blood group distribution testing by researchers from different countries.

As Table 2.3 shows, from 1919 to 1929 researchers from 34 different countries published articles on the distribution of blood groups. Confirmation that this represents the diffusion of the Hirszfelds' discovery is that almost all of these researchers cited the Hirszfelds' work as the first discovery in the field, if not the direct inspiration for their research. Only the very earliest articles—Weszeczky in Hungary (1920) and Alexander in Scotland (1921)—did not acknowledge the Hirszfelds' work. As far away as India (Chaudhuri) and Brazil (Aben-Athar) or as close as Rumania and Bulgaria (Manuila and Seisov), the Macedonian

Table 2.3 First appearance of research on blood group distribution by country of author, 1919–1931

Year	*Country of author*
1919	Poland
1920	Hungary, China
1921	Gt. Britain, U.S. (3), Denmark, South Africa
1922	Holland, Japan, USSR, Australia
1923	Poland, Germany (2), Italy
1924	Rumania, Switzerland
1925	France, Belgium, Finland
1926	Sweden, Portugal, Austria, Argentina
1927	Brazil, Turkey
1928	Greece, Lithuania, Bulgaria, Egypt, Spain
1929	Yugoslavia, Czechoslovakia, Latvia, Norway, Peru, India

work was cited as the first discovery and in many cases a source for comparative data.[18]

Another indication of the manner of diffusion also can be found in a researcher's source of test sera. For these first studies, sera were most often locally prepared according to methods spelled out in articles by the Hirszfelds and others. Subsequent researchers used standardized sera supplied by Hirszfeld in Poland, Fritz Schiff in Berlin, or the Pasteur Institute in Paris. There are also a few other examples of diffusion links through travel or training. This includes Arthur Coca, the editor of the *Journal of Immunology* in the U.S. and discoverer of the high frequency of type O blood in American Indians in 1923, who studied at Heidelberg under von Dungern with Hirszfeld in the early 1900s. Likewise, Nicholas Kossovitch, who was most important in establishing blood group distribution studies in France, served on the Macedonian front during the First World War, where he was under the direction of Hirszfeld. Also, some of the early Japanese and Chinese researchers such as Furuhata and Liang were trained in Germany.

The Pattern of Research

To obtain an overview of the pattern of research on blood group distribution, it is necessary to step back from the close examination of these direct links in the immediate discovery and diffusion and look at the extent of research between 1919 and 1939.

Figure 2.1 shows that the number of articles and subjects tested each year rose steeply during the 1920s to a maximum of 126 articles published in 1928 and over 140,000 subjects tested in 1929. Frequency of publication then fell off in the 1930s to a level of 50–60 articles annually. The number of subjects tested, however, did not decline as rapidly, indicating that the size of the studies generally became larger. Information is not quite complete for all articles found (numbers tested are known for 945 or 82 percent of the 1158 articles), but the overall average size of the population tested per article is 1434. The total number of people whose blood was typed and reported in published articles between 1919 and 1939 was 1,354,806. Taken altogether, this was obviously a large-scale research effort, even by today's standards.

Not all countries exhibited the same amount of interest in blood group distribution. An indication of the geographical dimension of the research can be found in the country of origin of the authors of articles for the 1920s and 1930s. (For the sake of consistency, émigré authors are counted in their newly adopted country; authors in colonies are included with the colonial power except for Australia, South Africa, and Canada, which are considered as independent countries.)

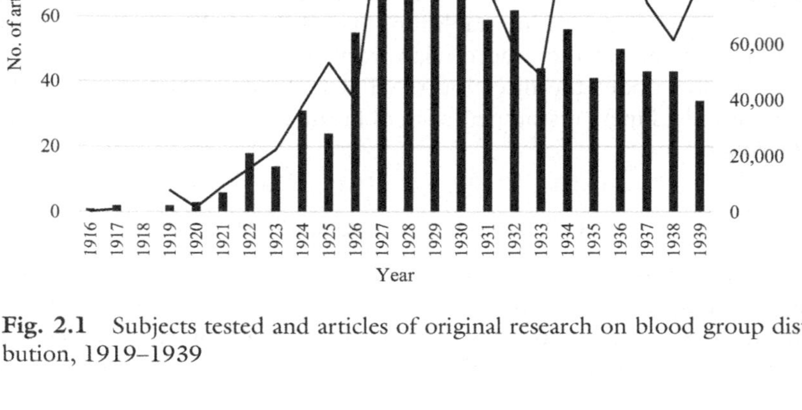

Fig. 2.1 Subjects tested and articles of original research on blood group distribution, 1919–1939

Most obviously of note in Fig. 2.2 was the large interest in Germany and the Soviet Union. There was much less in Great Britain but a surprisingly large interest in Italy and Japan. The amount and timing of work done by Soviet and German researchers is so large and concentrated, in fact, that it distorts the overall pattern of research over time. Without them, the peak in the late 1920s is much lower (about half the articles in 1927 and 1928), and the decline in the 1930s is much less pronounced. Indeed, if German and Soviet articles are removed, the resulting graph (see Fig. 2.3) is one of a gradual rise followed by a leveling off rather than a sharp rise and decline.

Looking more closely at the amount of research in Germany and the Soviet Union, Fig. 2.4 shows there was a strikingly similar pattern with a more rapid rise and decline of interest than elsewhere.

As will be seen in the next chapter, the similarity was for very different reasons. The decline in publications by Soviet authors coincided with Stalin's crackdown on scientists in the early 1930s. In contrast, the German decline had already begun before the Nazis took power, but there was at

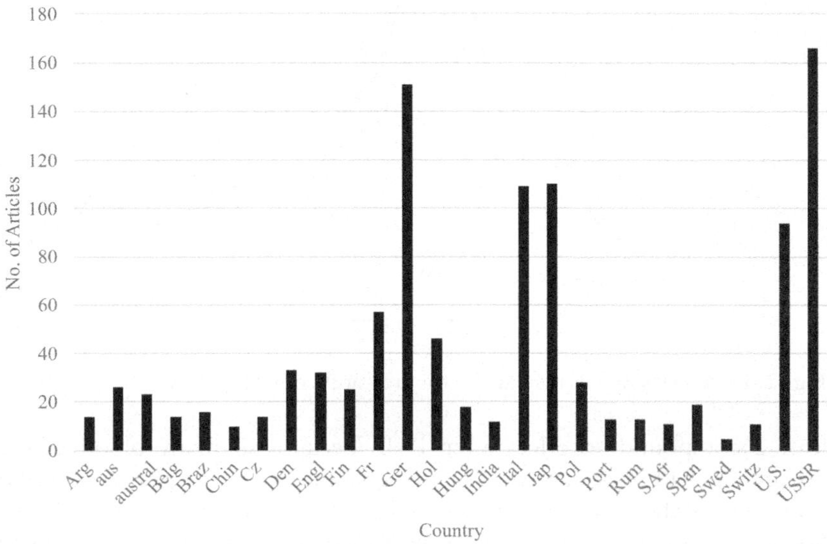

Fig. 2.2 Country of authors and number of blood group articles, 1921–1939

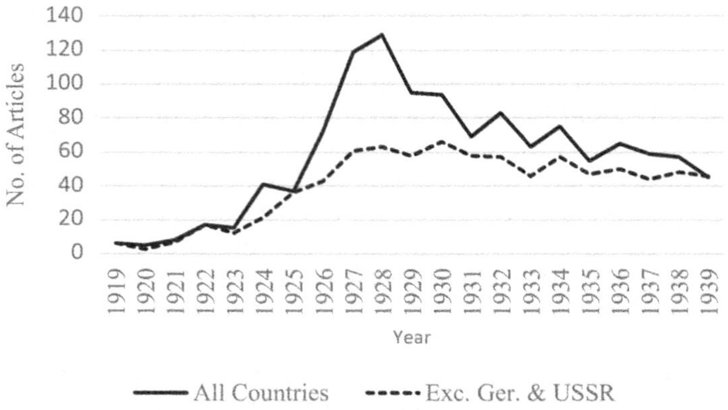

Fig. 2.3 Contribution of German and Soviet researchers to all articles of original research published on blood group distribution, 1919–1939

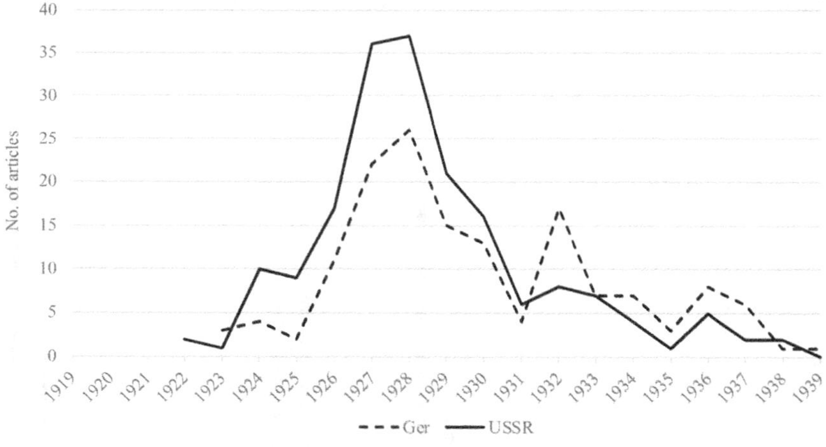

Fig. 2.4 Articles by German and Soviet researchers 1922–1939

least a compounding effect after 1933 because so many blood group researchers had been Jewish. Nonetheless, a number of right-wing blood group researchers continued to publish on blood groups through the Second World War. Hence, in absolute numbers, the German articles in the 1930s were comparable to the amount of publication in most other countries.

The pattern of publication of articles by researchers from some other countries, as found in Figs. 2.5 and 2.6, shows an overall increase of interest in the subject in the U.S. and France during the 1920s and 1930s, while Italian and Japanese interest followed the general pattern of a sharp rise and slow decline.

Summing up this overview of the pattern of all research on blood group distribution, there was first a rapid spread, the result of both the unusual findings and the general interest using blood groups as a marker for a number of possibly inherited traits. In other words, the ground was well prepared for reception of the Hirszfelds' extraordinary findings. Another reason for the large amount of research was that it could be conducted with relatively little difficulty. This was primarily because the importance of compatibility testing for blood transfusions during the First World War produced much simpler and faster techniques for determining blood types. In addition, the publication in *Lancet* of the Hirszfelds' research was a crucial step in speeding diffusion of their discovery.

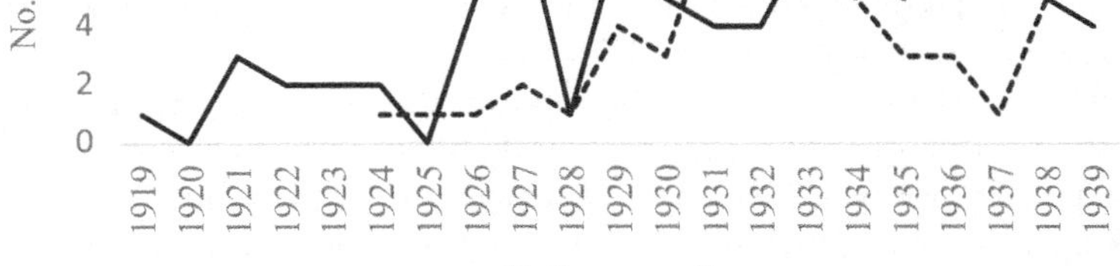

Fig. 2.5 Articles on blood group distribution by U.S. and French researchers, 1919–1939

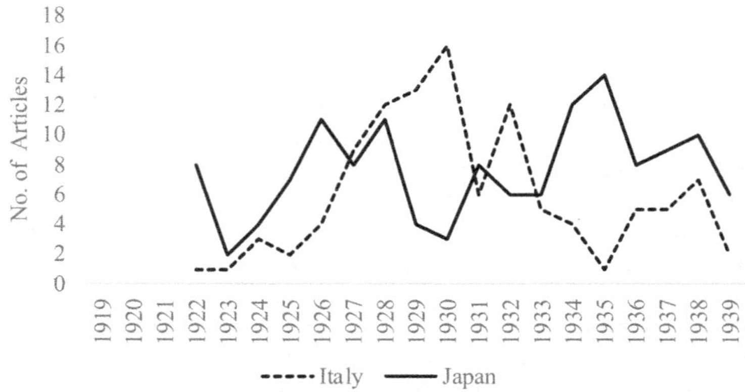

Fig. 2.6 Articles on blood group distribution by Italian and Japanese researchers, 1919–1939

The Journals of Record for Blood Group Research

An outline of the diffusion of this blood group research worldwide, as well as within given countries, can be seen in Table 2.4, which shows the publication record of the journals in which results of the research most frequently appeared.

The publication pattern reveals several features about the spread of research on blood group distribution and also raises some questions that warrant further examination. For example, there were two new journals created which were directly inspired by the new field of research: the *Zeitschrift für Rassenphysiologie* in Germany and the bilingual journal published in the Ukraine whose German title was *Ukrainische Zentralblatt für Blutgruppenforschung* (see Fig. 2.7).

Although these were two of the top four journals with the most articles on blood group distribution, significantly neither was the journal with the most articles, nor was their total (76 articles) as large as those published in a group of 4 journals which were devoted to experimental medicine and basic science: the *Comptes rendus de la Société de biologie* (Paris), *Journal of Immunology* (New York), *Zeitschrift für Immunitätsforschung* (Stuttgart), and *Proceedings of the Society for Experimental Biology and Medicine* (New York). Together these published 118 articles on the distribution of blood groups. This suggests that there was a strong enough interest in this discovery to create a legitimate new field of basic research.

Table 2.4 Journals with most articles on blood group distribution, 1919–1939

Journal	*Total*	*For. Auth.*	*Years*
Comptes rendus de la Société de biologie (Paris)	61	29	1923–1939
Zeitschrift für Rassenphysiologie (Munich)	43	22	1928–1938
Journal of Immunology (Baltimore)	33	10	1923–1939
Ukrainische Zentralblatt für Blutgruppenforschung (Kharkiv)	33	2	1927–1932
Klinische Wochenschrift (Berlin)	26	7	1923–1937
Geneeskundig Tijdschrift voor Nederlandsch-Indië (Batavia)	20	0	1924–1939
Acta Societatis Medicorum Fennicae Duodecim (Helsinki)	19	0	1925–1938
Taiwan Igakkai Zasshi (Formosa) [journal of the Taiwan Medical Assoc]	18	0	1925–1939
Münchener medizinische Wochenschrift (Munich)	17	2	1923–1932
American Journal of Physical Anthropology (NewYork)	14	2	1926–1939
Deutsche Zeitschrift für die gesamte gerichtliche Medizin (Berlin)	13	5	1927–1934
Zeitschrift für Immunitätsforschung (Stuttgart)	13	7	1925–1938
Medical Journal of Australia (Sydney)	12	0	1922–1939
Proceedings of the Society for Experimental Biology and Medicine (New York)	11	0	1927–1939
Ruskii Antropologicheskii Zhurnal (Moscow)	11	0	1924–1936

The findings of researchers, by contrast, had only a limited appeal to general/clinical medicine, as shown in Fig. 2.8. Of the 15 journals which published the most articles on blood group distribution, there were only 2 (which published a total of 43 articles) that were widely read publications devoted to general clinical medicine: the *Klinische* Wochenschrift and *Münchener medizinische Wochenschrift* published in Berlin and Munich. Although somewhat the result of local circumstances in Germany, the level of interest shown by these journals is indicative of a similar pattern of moderate but not leading interest found in other clinical/medical journals not among the top15. Indeed, of all articles published by journals with only a moderate interest (those with 5–10 articles on blood group distribution, or 30 journals with about 200 articles), slightly less than half (14 journals with 93 articles) appeared in these kinds of publications. As will be seen below, this indicates both an interest in and availability of the new discoveries to the general medical practitioner.

Three other journals reflected the interest in practical application of the discovery: two in anthropology (the *American Journal of Physical*

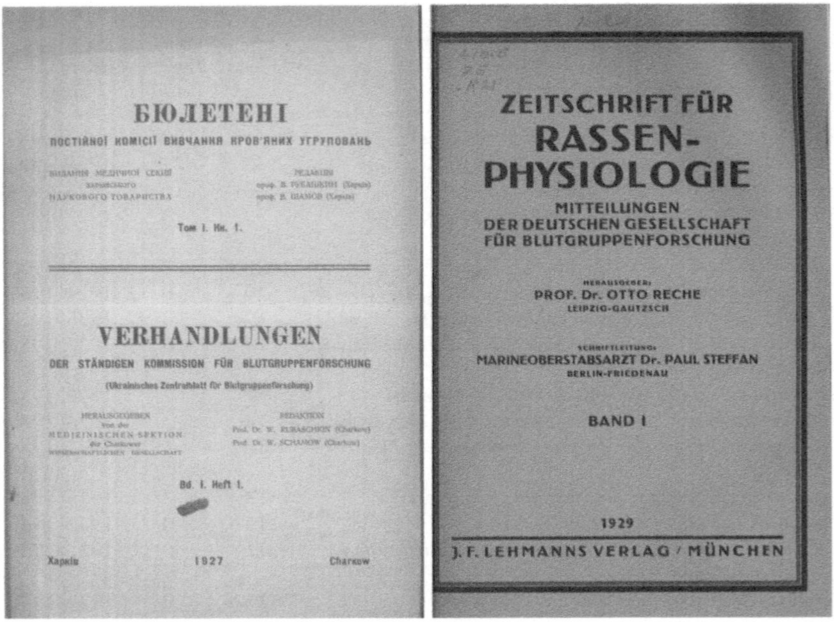

Fig. 2.7 New Soviet and German blood group research journals

Anthropology and *Ruskii Antropologicheskii Zhurnal*) and one in forensic medicine (*Deutsche Zeitschrift für die gesamte gerichtliche Medizin*). Together these journals published only 38 articles, and although it could be argued that legal medicine was a small field, that was not the case with anthropology. In fact, anthropologists were generally late in showing interest in the application of blood group distribution studies to their field.[19]

The remaining journals with the most articles on blood group distribution between the wars can be described as reaching smaller national or regional audiences: the *Medical Journal of Australia*, *Taiwan Igakkai Zasshi*, *Geneeskundig Tijdschrift voor Nederlandsch-Indië* (Batavia), and *Acta Societatis Medicorum Fennicae Duodecim* (Helsinki). Although they are also general interest journals of clinical medicine, the large number of articles stemmed mostly from local interest and the fact that researchers only had limited opportunities for publication elsewhere. Moreover, because of language, all but one were accessible to only a small readership.

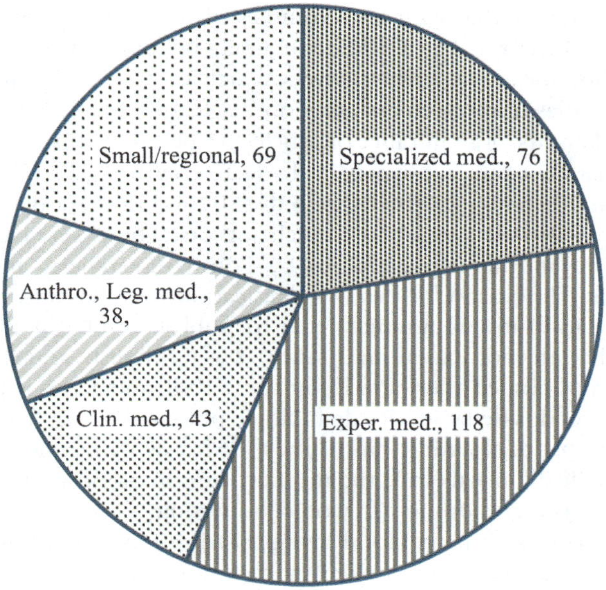

Fig. 2.8 Type of journal where articles on blood group distribution were published, 1919–1939

French and American Journals

Statistical summaries and general observations can only go so far in describing the establishment and spread of new scientific research. To understand better how blood group research came to be studied in a particular country or to make comparisons, it is necessary to look more closely at the specific publications where articles appeared. Perhaps the most surprising result of analyzing journals by frequency of publication is that the one with the most articles on blood group distribution (61) was the *Comptes rendus de la Société de biologie* (hereafter referred to as CRSB). This is unexpected because the journal was published in France, where there was relatively less research on blood groups compared to elsewhere. Five countries had researchers publishing more frequently than in France, in fact, as many as two to three times the number of articles.

The best explanation of this paradox is the nature of the journal and its place in French medical research between the wars. First, it was a large and comprehensive journal with four volumes of over 1000 pages published each year. Moreover, the CRSB contained no bibliographic or review information, nor any lengthy theoretical articles, only short two to three page summaries of research results. Another feature of the French journal which explains its large number of articles on blood groups was the international nature of its contributors. In fact, only half (32 of 61) of the articles published about blood group distribution in the journal between 1923 and 1939 were written by French authors. There were eight articles by Belgians, another eight articles by Polish researchers, and four by Rumanians. The reason for this was that learned societies in several countries made institutional arrangements to publish results in the journal. Thus, although not based in France, several Polish and Rumanians researchers published their articles in the CRSB under the rubric of the "Comptes rendus de la Société de biologie polonaise" and "roumane".

The international authorship of the CRSB was by no means unusual. Four of the five journals with the most articles on blood groups had over 25 percent foreign authors. It would be wrong, however, to conclude from this that research on blood group distribution was an international effort, where all scientists looked at common universal questions and wrote for a worldwide audience of colleagues. Systematic analysis of where authors published their research, shows in Table 2.5 that only in a few of the large countries was there any noticeable attempt by researchers to publish elsewhere.

Significant numbers of researchers in only two large countries published in foreign journals: Soviet authors (who published 23 of 167 articles outside the country) and Japanese researchers (19 of 110 articles). In fact, most authors who published in foreign journals were from smaller countries, especially those with a cultural affinity to a larger neighbor. These scientists (10 of 46 from Holland, 12 of 31 from Denmark, 13 of 26 from Austria, 13 of 14 from Belgium, and 11 of 13 from Rumania) were much more likely to publish in foreign journals. Whether from chauvinism, isolation, or self-sufficiency, the lack of publication in foreign journals by researchers from Germany, Italy, the U.S., and France is surprising. Only 5 of 143 articles by German authors were published outside Germany, 6 of 94 the U.S., and 3 of 57 French.[20] Regardless of reason, this fact helps explain why there were such differences between countries in the way research was conducted.

Returning to the analysis of publication in France, the 32 articles in *CRSB* by French authors accounted for over half of the 57 articles

Table 2.5 Authors publishing in foreign journals, 1919–1939

Country of author	*Total number of articles publ.*	*Articles publ. in foreign jls.*	*Notes*
Soviet	167	23	18 in German journals
Germany	143	5	3 in Austrian/Swiss journals
Japan	110	19	7 in U.S., 4 German, 5 int'l congresses and journals
Italy	109	4	
United States	94	6	4 in British journals
France	57	3	all in int'l congresses
Holland	46	10	Includes Dutch E. Ind
Denmark	31	12	6 in German, 5 French journals
Britain	30	6	
Poland	30	17	9 in French, 6 German journals
Austria	26	13	10 in German journals
Finland	24	1	
Australia	23	8	7 in British journals
Spain	19	4	
Hungary	18	13	all in German journals
Brazil	16	2	
Belgium	14	13	10 in French journals
Czechoslovakia	14	4	
Portugal	13	3	
Rumania	13	11	8 in French journals
South Africa	11	3	

published by all researchers in the country between the wars, which meant that their work did not appear with much frequency in many other French medical or anthropological journals. The only exception (not on the list) was the *Revue anthropologique* with nine articles. Most important for the broader question of diffusion is that because of the international nature *CRSB* authors, French researchers had access to a variety of research results from around the world and, thus, were well informed of the work being done in the field of blood group studies. In addition, French, along with English and German, can legitimately be regarded as one of the scientific languages of research in the field of blood groups.

The *Journal of Immunology* is one of three journals published in the U,S., which were among those with the most articles on the distribution of blood groups in the 1920s and 1930s. It was also the most international of these American journals, with 10 of its 33 articles authored by foreigners. (Only 2 articles were by foreigners among the 25 published in the

American Journal of Physical Anthropology and the *Proceedings of the Society for Experimental Biology and Medicine.*) The existence of these three publications among those with the most articles on blood group distribution research reflects the overall interest in the field by Americans, which included, unlike most other countries, an anthropological journal. However, the *JAMA* is not on the list, since it published only four articles of original research on the distribution of blood groups between 1919 and 1939. Despite not appearing in the broadest mainstream medical journal, these American articles included the pioneering, breakthrough discoveries of blood group researchers that were among the most significant in the interwar years. Thus, Landsteiner and Levine published their finding of the MN and P groups in the *Proceedings of the Society for Experimental Biology and Medicine*, as did Matson and Boyd for their work on blood groups from the remains of mummies. Earlier, Coca's discovery of a very high percentage of type O blood in American Indians was published in the *Journal of Immunology*.

German, Soviet, and Other Researchers

The journal with the second largest number of articles on blood group testing between the wars was the *Zeitschrift für Rassenphysiologie*, published in Germany by the Deutsche Gesellschaft für Blutgruppenforschung. It is not surprising to find a German journal with so many articles, given the high interest in the country. Indeed, there were 4 other German journals among the 15 with the most articles. This included two general interest medical journals—the *Klinische Wochenschrift* and the *Münchener medizinische Wochenschrift*—plus the more specialized *Zeitschrift für Immunitätsforschung*. The 13 articles in the *Deutsche Zeitschrift für die gesamte gerichtliche Medizin* were indicative of interest in blood group research in the field of legal medicine. Significantly, there were no German anthropological journals among these, although there was early interest shown by the *Archiv für Rassen-und Gesellschafts-Biologie* (six articles published from 1923 to 1930), and late interest in the *Zeitschrift für Rassenkunde* (six such articles between 1932 and 1939).[21] The majority of articles published in the German journals on the list were by German authors, although a significant number of foreign authors research (43 of 112) also appeared. Thus, from the standpoint of research done and availability of findings published, Germany rightfully deserves to be regarded as the country in the forefront of developments in the field of blood group studies in the 1920s and early 1930s.

The *Zeitschrift für Rassenphysiologie* was unusual in that it was especially created to publish the results of blood group research. As the name implied, it had a strong anthropological as well as a medical perspective. Also, despite the right-wing "*volkisch*" ideology of its editors, the journal was somewhat able to live up to its pretensions of being all-encompassing and international. Over half of its articles on blood group distribution (22 of 43) were by foreign researchers. On the other hand, although the editors of the *Zeitschrift für Rassenphysiologie* saw themselves as the center of a national and international effort to study blood group distribution, they were unable even to establish themselves as the predominant research center in Germany. For one thing, neither editor had an institutional medical research base. One of them, Otto Reche, eventually held the Chair in Anthropology and headed a museum of ethnology at Leipzig University beginning in 1926, but he had no ties to medical research faculties. Paul Steffan, the other editor, was trained as a doctor, but his institutional affiliation was with the German navy which moved him around too frequently to become well established with a hospital or university.[22]

A larger difficulty in attempting to guide German blood group research (besides the antisemitism of the editors) was the sheer volume of interest that developed in the subject which quickly became too widespread to control. Thus, Fritz Schiff in Berlin probably came to be recognized as the most important German serologist working on blood groups, but doctors and anthropologists all over the country (not to mention mathematicians such as Felix Bernstein) made significant contributions as well. In the end, Reche and Steffan had to lower their expectations of coordination and publication by using the *Zeitschrift für Rassenphysiologie* as an indirect means of influencing research. The data reveal they succeeded to an extent.

In the Soviet Union, a new publication, the *Ukrainische Zentralblatt für Blutgruppenforschung*, had been the inspiration for Reche and Steffans' journal. Its specific goals were to gather and disseminate results of large-scale blood group testing that was going on in the Soviet Union. The motivating force was W. J. Rubaschkin, an Emeritus Professor of Cytology in the Ukraine, who along with V. N. Schamov founded a "Standing Committee" of the Medical Section of the Kharkiv Scientific Society, which was part of the Ukrainian Academy of Sciences.[23] The 33 articles published in the journal in only six years indicate the strong interest that quickly developed in the USSR in the late 1920s. The fact that it was published bilingually (in Ukrainian and German) reflects the broader purpose of the journal to provide a way for Soviet researchers to make their findings known both to their countrymen and to the rest of the world.[24] Unlike the *Zeitschrift für Rassenphysiologie*, it was not intended to be a record of all research worldwide. Thus, only two of these blood group articles in the journal were by foreigners, although a number of prominent foreigner researchers, including Lattes, Hirszfeld, and Schiff, published theoretical and summary articles for readers of the journal.

This Ukrainian journal was begun as a result of peculiar local circumstances, but the large number of articles published also reflected a broad interest in the USSR. For example, the *Ruskii Antropologicheskii Zhurnal* had 11 articles on blood group distribution, indicating the strong anthropological interest in the country. This partly reflected another center of blood group research, headed by Boris Vishnevskii, at the Museum for Anthropology and Ethnography of the Soviet Academy of Sciences in Leningrad. The remaining 125 articles by Soviet researchers were published in 45 different journals, indicating the widespread interest that existed in the country. Most of these were medical publications, typically focused on a sub-specialty such as tuberculosis, anatomy, tropical medicine, eye and skin disease, but articles were also published in several regional medical journals (such as in Irkutsk and Kasan) and proceedings of national congresses. Moreover, several national medical journals published blood group distribution articles, including *Vrachebnoe Delo*. It should also be noted that in the 1920s and 1930s many Soviet researchers published in foreign journals (23 of all 167 articles by Soviet authors), with German journals (18) being the most frequent choice of authors.

The existence of a Japanese journal on the list of those with the most articles on blood group distribution research is indicative of the large number of articles published by Japanese authors between the wars. One particular publication, the *Journal of the Taiwan Medical Society*, is noteworthy in that it was in a setting of colonial occupation.[25] Fully half of the articles were published by researchers at the "Hygiene Section" of the "Government Institute for Scientific Study" in Taihoku who tested of over 15,000 of the island's indigenous population.[26]

Most of the remaining articles that appeared in the *Taiwan Igakkai* were by researchers at the Taihoku [Japanese name for Taipei] Medical School on a variety of subjects including Chinese and Japanese inhabitants, MNP blood groups, the relationship between blood groups and dental caries, and even a study of baseball players and blood types. This broad interest was typical of the wide range of articles on blood group distribution published during this period by researchers back on the Japanese home islands in many different journals. Some specialized in diseases such as cancer and tuberculosis, but a number of journals published in regional centers such as Kanazawa (six articles), home of Tanemoto Furuhata the most famous serologist of the period, Kyoto (four articles), and Nagasaki (three). Thus, the reason there are no other Japanese journals in the list of those with the most articles is that, similar to Soviet research, interest was widespread and no single, centralized journal of choice developed where researchers published their findings.[27]

To the extent that these articles reflect all research published in Japan from 1919 to 1939, a few observations can be made about the pattern. First is the lack of interest in anthropological journals. In fact, only two articles appeared in Japanese anthropological journals: one by Furuhata in 1927 and one by Grichi in 1928. Of more than 100 articles published by Japanese researchers, 4 appeared in publications of international anthropological congresses. Otherwise, the publication record in Japan primarily indicates the wide and continuing interest in blood group research by medical journals in Japan. In addition, the Japanese, like the Soviet researchers, published a significant number of articles in foreign journals: 19 of 110 articles spread among American (7) and German (4) journals, plus reports of international congresses (5). The publication of summaries and research results of blood group studies in the English-language *Japan Medical World* in the 1920s is similar to the *Ukrainische Zentralblatt für Blutgruppenforschung*, in that the Japanese publication was intended to make a broad range of Japanese medical research available to the rest of the world. Finally, in addition to the research center on Taiwan, Tanemoto Furuhata at Kanazawa University, whose work will be examined later in detail, was a main influence on blood group research and publication in Japan. He himself published 14 articles, and his students added significantly to that total. His bibliographies and travel to foreign conferences added to his role as the dominant researcher in the country.

The three remaining journals on the list are each the product of peculiar conditions in their country of publication. At the same time, they reflect certain common patterns of research on the distribution of blood groups between the wars. The twenty articles published in the *Geneeskundig Tijdschrift voor Nederlandsch-Indië* primarily reflect the Dutch interest in the great variety of peoples in their East Indian colonial holdings. In addition, this concentration of articles was also the result of the limited number of journals in which Dutch researchers could publish in their own language. Not evident in the list, however, is the strong interest back in the Dutch homeland where two other journals published a half dozen articles.[28] Among the most important blood group researchers in Holland was Marianne van Herwerden, Professor of Cytology at Utrecht, who was one of the few female directors of a blood group research laboratory. Overall, Dutch researchers authored 49 articles on blood group distribution between 1922 and 1939, 10 of which appeared in foreign publications.

The Australian journal on the list also reflects research in a setting of settlers and "natives" and the curiosity of researchers about the aboriginal population. In this case, however, it was probably not language but proximity and convenience that made authors prefer to publish in the *Medical Journal of Australia*. The existence of a Finnish journal on the list stems partly from subjects of interest in-country: the Lapps in the north and the mix of Swedes in the country's population in the south. Again, language restricted publication possibilities, but the relatively large number of articles was also the result of the centralized research program on blood group distribution organized by Oswald Streng and his students at the Sero- bacteriology laboratory of the University of Helsinki. The clearest indication of the in-country audience of these researchers is the fact that only one Finnish author published in a foreign journal.

One final question worth considering about the list of journals that published the most articles on blood group testing between the wars, is why some countries are not represented. Two in particular are noteworthy—Britain and Italy—but for opposite reasons. The lack of a journal published in the British Isles on the list was the result of the general lack of interest there in research on blood groups in the 1920s and early1930s.[29] Until 1932 a total of only ten articles were published on blood group distribution by all British researchers, at least those based in Great Britain. In fact, the only non-American, English-language journals anywhere with significant numbers of articles on the distribution of blood groups were those published in or about the empire. The *Journal of Tropical Medicine* had the most (eight articles) and all were published in the 1930s. Even by stretching definitions to include the whole Commonwealth, the *Medical Journal of Australia*'s 12 articles were more than any journal published in Britain, followed by the *Indian Medical Journal* with 5, but both were obviously in an overseas colonial setting. Significant by their absence were original articles on blood group research in British anthropological journals. Only four articles appeared in *Man* and those were from 1936 to 1938, thanks to R. R. Gates' editorial activity. Just three articles appeared in the *Journal of the Royal Anthropological Institute*, all after 1934. Also telling of the general lack of interest was that only five articles each appeared in *Lancet* and the *British Medical Journal* during the whole interwar period.[30]

The lack of interest in blood group studies in Britain, indicated by the lack of British researchers and relatively few articles appearing in British journals, produced a situation of relative ignorance of the new field in the country. As a result, when blood group studies finally began to appear in Britain, they were produced by a tight core of geneticists including J. B. S. Haldane, Lancelot Hogben, R. A. Fisher, R. R. Gates, and Lionel S. Penrose. Most significant, they quickly became leaders of a new understanding and application of blood group genetics, because in Britain through the end of the 1930s. Of note, Fisher's Galton Blood Group Laboratory developed in a very un-British, centralized French fashion.

The lack of an Italian journal among those with the most articles on blood group research is misleading, because unlike Britain there was a great deal of interest in the country. So much so that there were many research centers and no single publication of first choice; as a result articles appeared in many different Italian journals. Although no Italian journal published more than ten articles from 1919 to 1939, there were a dozen publications with three to nine articles on the distribution of blood groups, more than any country except Germany. These Italian journals included two each with an anthropological and colonial focus, as well as those in specialized medicine (gynecology, dermatology), general medicine (*Policlinico*), and regional journals, such as in Pavia the home of Leone Lattes, who became the acknowledged leader of Italian research.

Conclusion

This examination of the discovery and spread of research on human blood groups in the 1920s and 1930s has shown several features which were typical of scientific research in the twentieth century. First, it demonstrated the "democratization" of research, as laboratories and scientists from around the world became part of the scientific enterprise that previously had been limited to a very small circle. It is possible to locate the starting point of this large body of work (over 1000 articles) primarily to one source, but even without the Hirszfelds' work this research field would almost certainly have developed, as indicated by the fact that there were several independent discoveries at about the same time. This, in turn, partly explains why the Hirszfelds' discovery was so quickly and widely emulated. There were differences in individuals' approaches to that research, but because the Hirszfelds' work in Macedonia during the First World War was so extraordinary in its scope and conclusions, almost all others were guided by it.

Within two years of publication, the Hirszfelds' research began to be recognized for its importance. The fact that their research appeared in an English-language journal had consequences for its initial diffusion, but soon German superseded English as the most common language of publication. In addition, a French language journal had the most articles on blood group distribution during this period.

There is reason for viewing this blood group research as "international" in the sense of transcending national boundaries, another feature typical of twentieth-century science. Authors were very conscious of the importance of their cumulative effort, and there was significant publication in foreign journals. There is nonetheless strong evidence of differences in how research was conducted in the various countries, beginning with the fact that the discoveries spread more quickly and more thoroughly in some countries rather than others. Germany, the Soviet Union, and Japan saw early and rapid diffusion; Britain was most noticeable for the late and little interest of its researchers. Even in countries that showed moderate interest in blood group research, such as France and the U.S., there were very different developments and interests reflecting local circumstances and researchers. To fully appreciate these differences and similarities, it is necessary to look more closely at how the blood group research was conducted in individual countries.

Notes

1. Some examples of studies using this approach of national "styles" in science are Joseph S. Fruton, *Contrasts in Scientific Style: Research Groups in the Chemical and Biochemical Sciences* (Philadelphia: American Philosophical Society, 1990); Nathan Reingold, *Science, American Style: Selected Writings of Nathan Reingold* (New Brunswick: Rutgers University Press, 1991);

Jonathan Harwood, *Styles of Scientific Thought: The German Genetics Community, 1900–1933* (Chicago: University of Chicago Press, 1993).

2. Michael Hesch, "Die gesamte Schrifttum der Blutgruppenforschung in der drei ersten Jahrzehnten ihrer Entwicklung, 1901–1931," in Paul Steffan, ed., *Handbuch der Blutgruppenkunde* (Munich: Lehmans Verlag, 1932), 539–645. Hesch lists 2926 articles, to be exact. A Soviet researcher, E. Koenig, *Bibliography on Blood Transfusion* (Leningrad: Vestnik Chirurguii and Research Institute of Blood Transfusion in Leningrad, 1935), published a similar bibliography on blood transfusion to 1933 with over 4000 entries.
3. For more on methodology, see William H. Schneider, "Blood Group Research in Great Britain, France, and the United States between the World Wars," *American Journal of Physical Anthropology* 38 supplement 21 (1995): 88–90
4. See William H. Schneider, "Le rôle des groupes sanguins dans l'histoire de la génétique," in *Histoire de la génétique* (Paris: ARPEM, 1990), eds. Jean-Louis Fischer and William H. Schneider, 293–308.
5. For an early example of the extent to which bibliometrics developed in the field of information science, see Christine L. Borgman, ed. *Scholarly Communication and Bibliometrics* (Newbury Park, CA: Sage, 1990). For specific examples, one of the most important pioneers of this work was Derek J. de Solla Price, "Citation Measures of Hard Science, Soft Science, Technology, and Nonscience," in *Communicating among Scientists and Engineers*, eds. Carnot E, Nelson and Donald K. Pollock (Lexington, Ma: D.C. Heath, 1970), 3–22. For a historical introduction to this kind of research in the sociology of science, see Arnold Thackray, "Measurement in the Historiography of Science," in *Toward a Metric of Science*, eds. Yehuda Elkana, Joshua Lederberg, et al. (N.Y.: John Wiley, 1978), 11–30.

   Katherine W. McCain has applied these methods to modern genetics research in "The Paper Trails of Scholarship: Mapping the Literature of Genetics," *Library Quarterly* 56 (1986), 258–71 and "Mapping Authors in Intellectual Space: Population Genetics in the 1980s," in Borgman, *Scholarly Communications and Bibliometrics*, 194–216.
6. For background, see Frank B. Rogers, "Index Medicus in the Twentieth Century," in *Centenary of Index Medicus*, John B. Blake, ed. (Bethesda: U.S. Department of Health and Human Services, 1980), 53–61.
7. The index never listed even all the articles in journals collected by the Surgeon General's (later National) medical library. For more on what was contained in the index, as well as what was missing, see Leonard Karel, "Selection of Journals for *Index Medicus*. A Historical Review," *Medical Literature Association Bulletin*, 55 (1967), 259–78.

8. Laurence H. Snyder, "Human Blood Groups: Their Inheritance and Racial Significance," *American Journal of Physical Anthropology* 9 (1926), 233–63; and Snyder, *Blood Grouping in Relation to Clinical and Legal Medicine* (Baltimore: Williams and Wilkins, 1929).
9. Luigi Luca Cavalli-Sforza, Paolo Menozzi, and Alberto Piazza, *History and Geography of Human Genes* (Princeton: Princeton University Press, 1994). Mourant's first book in 1954, *Distribution of the Human Blood Groups* (Oxford: Blackwell, 1954), contained 1716 references that had appeared since or were not found in Boyd's 1939 article. The 1976 edition of *The Distribution of the Human Blood Groups and Other Polymorphisms*, 2nd ed. (London: Oxford University Press, 1976) had over 1000 pages concentrated on geographical completeness using the most recent studies. It had over 3100 citations, almost all dated after 1939.
10. In the analysis of Japanese research, slightly less than 20 percent of articles by Japanese researchers found in this manner appeared in foreign journals, the highest percentage for major countries. This means it is likely that enough articles have been identified in Japanese-language publications (80 percent) to be representative of all research, while the 20 percent available in foreign journals are sufficient to indicate the basic nature of Japanese research. At the least, enough Japanese scholarship has been found for general comparison to other countries, even if exact statistical comparisons cannot be made due to the lack of an exhaustive examination of all Japanese publications. While awaiting more study on Japanese blood group research, for recent scholarship on the Japanese fascination with blood, see Jennifer Robertson, 'Hemato-nationalism: The Past, Present, and Future of "Japanese Blood,"' *Medical Anthropology: Cross-Cultural Studies in Health and Illness* 31 (2012): 93–112.
11. Alson R. Kilgore and J. Hua Liu, "Isoagglutination Tests of Chinese Bloods for Transfusion Compatibility," *China Medical Journal* 32 (1918): 21–5; George R. Moffitt, George F. Klugh, and Chester E. Shepard, "Blood Type Classification, with a Slight Modification of Technic: Report of the Results of More than a Thousand Tests," *JAMA* 73 (1919): 1821–2.
12. Oskar Weszeczky, "Untersuchungen über die gruppenweise Hämagglutination beim Menschen," *Biochemische Zeitschrift* 107 (1920): 160; William Alexander, "An Inquiry into the Distribution of Blood Groups of Patients Suffering from Malignant Diseases," *British Journal of Experimental Pathology*, 2 (1921): 66–9.
13. Willem Storm van Leeuwen, *Indrukten van een statieris naar America* (1920), as cited in Weszeczky, "Untersuchungen über die gruppenweise Hämagglutination beim Menschen," 160.
14. Fritz Verzar and Oskar Weszeczky, "Rassenbiologische Untersuchungen mittels Isohamagglutinen," *Biochemische Zeitschrift* 126 (1922): 33–9.

15. The 1916 article was cited in Shinichi Kirihara, "Uber die Isohämagglutination beim menschlichen Blute," *Zeitschrift für klinische Medizin* 99 (1924): 530. The full citation can also be found in Tanemoto Furuhata, "Japanese Literature on Isohemagglutination," *Japan Medical World* 8 (1928): 321.
16. Moffitt et al., "Blood Type Classification," 1821–2.
17. William L. Culpepper and Marjorie Ableson, "Report on Five Thousand Bloods Typed using Moss's Grouping," *Journal of Laboratory and Clinical M*edicine 6 (1921), 276–83.
18. In fact, the Hirszfelds' tests of English, Italian, and even Indian soldiers were larger samples of the population than the first studies by researchers in these countries many years later.
19. Pauline M. H. Mazumdar, "Blood and Soil: The Serology of the Aryan Racial State," *Bulletin of the History of Medicine* 64 (1990): 187–219, comments on the lack of interest among anthropologists. See also later chapter.
20. This judgement should perhaps be qualified by the fact that these statistics are only for publication of research results. Summary and theoretical articles were often published in foreign journals. But a sample survey finds very few of 300 related articles were published in foreign journals.
21. It is somewhat arbitrary to consider the eugenics-inspired *Archiv für Rassen-und Gesellschafts-Biologie* to be an anthropological journal and not the *Zeitschrift für Rassenphysiologie*. In a sense, the latter could be considered a publication in the subfield of physical anthropology, but unlike the *American Journal of Physical Anthropology* it was created specifically as a result of the Hirszfelds' discoveries. Hence, the *Zeitschrift für Rassenphysiologie* did not reach the traditional anthropological community. More to the point, the German equivalent of the *American Journal of Physical Anthropology*, the *Zeitschrift für Morphologie und Anthropologie*, published only three articles on the distribution of blood groups during this time period. For more, see the next chapter.
22. See Mazumdar, "Blood and Soil," and the next chapter.
23. "Von der medizinischen Sektion der Charkower Wissentschaftlichen Gesellchaft," *Ukrainische Zentralblatt für Blutgruppenforschung* 1 (1927): 5–7; Boris Vishnevskii, "Professor Dr. W. J. Rubaschkin und seine Arbeiten auf dem Gebiete der Blutgruppenforschung," *Zeitschrift für Rassenphysiologie* 6 (1933).
24. It seems likely that the decision to use Ukrainian and not Russian language served nationalistic goals. Regardless of inspiration, the use of German made the results accessible to virtually all Soviet and foreign researchers.

25. This is similar to the French and Dutch journals which published many blood group articles from research done in colonies.
26. See, for example, Yoshito Maruyama and T. Wakeshima, "Blood Groups of Formosan Savages," *Taiwan Igakkai Zasshi* 30, (1931):35, the title of which reflects the colonial setting. Maryuma and Wakima published a six-part study of these populations from 1931 to 1936.
27. The reason may also be lack of complete bibliographic references for Japanese research. The two main sources which served as the starting point for this analysis were Furuhata's series of bibliographies published in *Japan Medical World* in the mid-1920s and *Index Medicus*, plus the bibliographies of Hesch, Boyd, and Mourant. It is, therefore, entirely possible that these sources did not exhaustively monitor all Japanese publications throughout the period.
28. Note: The *Geneeskundig Tijdschrift voor Nederlandsch-Indië* is considered for this analysis to be a Dutch publication, whereas South African and Australian journals are not considered British. See above for the rationale.
29. For background on research in England, see Jenny Bangham, *Blood Relations: Transfusion and the Making of Human Genetics* (University of Chicago Press, 2020), and for lack of interest, see Chap. 4.
30. For scholarship on British medical publications, see John C. Burnham, "The British Medical Journal in America," in *Medical Journals and Medical Knowledge*, eds. Stephen Lock and Roy Porter (London: Routledge, 1992), 165–87. P.W. Jartrip, *Mirror of medicine: The British Medical Journal* (Oxford: Clarendon Press, 1995): 216–7, indicates that the circulation of the *British Medical Journal* rose from 23,000 to 43,000 between the wars. See a later chapter for comparison to the German medical press.

CHAPTER 3

Blood Group Research in Germany and the Soviet Union

Germany and the Soviet Union stand out as the two countries where more research was done than anywhere else on blood group distribution between the world wars.[1] They were also the countries that underwent the most dramatic political and social upheavals in the 1920s and 1930s. Hence, one of the main questions to be examined is what common underlying features might explain the similarities. For example, the revolutionary circumstances brought tremendous changes to the whole infrastructure of science and medicine, including, of course, the conduct of research. At the least, the collapse of the German and Russian Empires after the First World War brought new political regimes that both permitted and encouraged research in new fields such as serology. Given the practical application plus the popular interest in the subjects of blood and inheritance, the research on blood groups was especially attractive to political leaders as well as scientists.

There was a rapid initial interest in the blood groups in Germany and the Soviet Union during the 1920s. Given this enthusiastic beginning, it is all the more striking that there was a precipitous decline in this research during the early 1930s in both countries. Much of the change was the result of political developments outside the scientific arena, but there were also certain internal scientific reasons for the sharp rise and decline of blood group research. Although the broad pattern of research in Germany

W. H. Schneider, *Blood Groups and Human Heredity, 1900–1950*, Medicine and Biomedical Sciences in Modern History,
https://doi.org/10.1007/978-3-031-69844-6_3

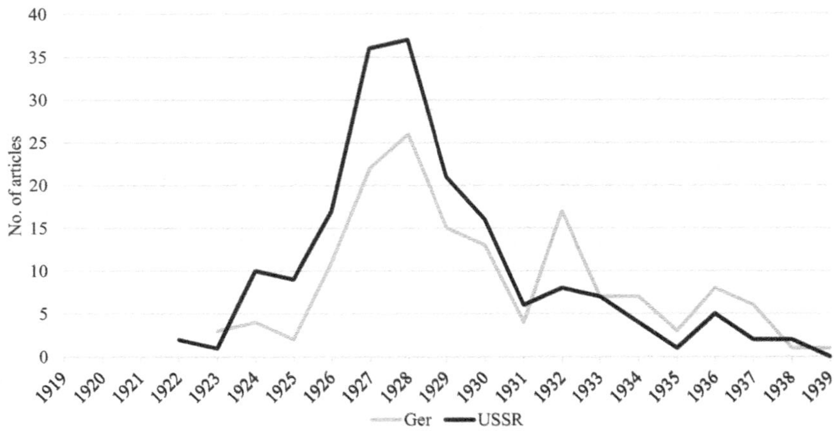

Fig. 3.1 Articles on blood group distribution by German and Soviet authors, 1919–1939

and the Soviet Union was generally similar, as indicated in Fig. 3.1, closer examination shows considerable differences in the specific reasons for them.

German and Russian Background: Blood Group Research Before 1920

German medicine, and in fact most scientific research in Germany, was the envy of the world at the beginning of the twentieth century. In the course of the 1800s private industries, the German states, and eventually the imperial government established research centers at universities and elsewhere, which by 1900 surpassed their counterparts in Britain and France, countries which had previously dominated basic scientific research. Although ardent French nationalists would never have admitted German superiority, after the defeat of 1871 it is clear from the actions of French educational and scientific reformers that they recognized and sought to emulate the achievements on the other side of the Rhine.[2] If science in the U.S. was also in the ascendant, it was still to Germany that young researchers went for their training. Another example of American recognition of German accomplishments were the reforms of medical schools in the

U.S. based on Flexner's 1912 report of European medical education which sang the praises of Germany.[3]

It is, therefore, no accident that German researchers led the way at the end of the nineteenth century in the new field of immunology, out of which the blood group discoveries emerged. Even if Austria is considered a separate cultural sphere, Landsteiner went to Germany to study before taking his post at the Pathological Institute in Vienna. Students from all over the world came to Germany to study medicine in the decades before 1914. As mentioned earlier, these included Arthur F. Coca from the U.S. and Ludwik Hirszfeld from Poland, who became future pioneers of serological research. Students came from as far away as Japan and China, and it was also a regular part of Russian medical training for the government to select for study abroad a few of the top students passing their medical examinations each year.[4] Germany was most frequently the country chosen.

Russian scientific and medical research also made great advances in the course of the nineteenth century. The biggest problem by 1900 remained the availability of medical care for the mass of the population, but the quality of treatment at the highest levels in Moscow and St. Petersburg was comparable to anywhere in western Europe. Indications of Russia's entry into the international scientific community by the beginning of the twentieth century include regular study by Russian students abroad and increasing state support for research institutes at the end of the nineteenth century. Hence, the specific accomplishments of scientists such as Mendeleev and Pavlov were not just a reflection of individual genius.[5]

Nonetheless, looking at the country as a whole, Russia was still on the margin of new and quickly changing fields such as blood group research in the early 1900s. There are no *Index Medicus* citations of Russian researchers' attempts at blood transfusion, let alone more fundamental blood group research before the First World War, although it is certain that the discoveries published in the German medical press were followed by Russians. The lack of many research centers lessened the chances that a Russian scientist would make a key discovery in these new fields.

Such was not the case in Germany where there was a steady stream of articles in the medical literature on questions about the newly discovered blood groups after Landsteiner's discovery, examining such features as the fixity of blood groups, their inheritance, and the relation of mother to newborn.[6] Moreover, at this peak of German predominance in world scientific research, there were noteworthy efforts to continue that dominance as shown by the creation of the Kaiser Wilhelm Gesellschaft in

1911. By the outbreak of war, a biological institute had been created as well as one devoted to the study of serotherapy.[7]

All wartime governments expanded funding for science, but unlike the case in France, Britain, and especially the U.S., the First World War was much more a disruption than a stimulus to medical research in Germany and Russia. The applied chemical research in Germany notwithstanding, German doctors were late in copying, let alone pioneering new serological discoveries even in such needed areas as shock and transfusion.[8] In Russia the government's resources were stretched to the limit just to conduct the war, and despite the example of N. K. Koltsov obtaining private funding for his Institute for Experimental Biology, the situation only got worse as the war progressed.[9]

German Blood Group Research in the 1920s

In the 1920s, research in Germany on blood group distribution started later than in other countries, but once begun it produced a flood of studies on all aspects of the subject. Most noticeable in this German research was an early and strong interest in the anthropology of blood groups. This was primarily the result of a research program connected to an ultra-nationalist *völkisch* group led by Otto Reche and Paul Steffan, who created a German Society for Blood Group Research. Among other things, they applied for government funding to conduct studies nationwide. Despite their concerted efforts to organize and direct the blood group research in Germany (including the founding of a new journal), the interest in the subject was so broad and diverse during this period that their efforts were unsuccessful. Ironically, it was the decline of interest by others in the 1930s which finally permitted the *völkisch* seroanthropologists to dominate blood group research in the Germany.

The First World War had taken its toll on the infrastructure as well as the conduct of German medical research. Yet even with the disruption of the war, it required a surprisingly long time for German researchers to reestablish an interest in the blood groups in the early 1920s.[10] For example, the first articles reporting original research on the distribution of the ABO blood types only appeared late in December of 1923 and early 1924, well after American and British, not to mention other European and Japanese researchers had begun to follow the lead of the Hirszfelds. Besides the effects of the war and the workings of chance, the only other broad influence that helps explain this delay was the relative lack of German experience with blood transfusion immediately before and during the war. Accidents in transfusion had been one of the most common reasons for the early blood group testing by Americans, in several cases even before they learned of the Hirszfelds' work. Whereas the Americans' response to transfusion accidents had been to test blood types in advance, the Germans relied much more heavily on an empirical procedure called the "biological probe," which consisted of transfusing a small quantity of donor's blood and waiting for signs of reaction before proceeding or stopping the transfusion.[11]

The first report of testing blood group distribution by a German researcher was a 1923 article in the *Archiv für Rassen-und Gesellschafts-Biologie* by Paul Steffan at Kiel. This was initially an isolated event, but it eventually led to a long line of research in Germany, scientifically inspired by the Hirszfelds but with strong political links to right-wing nationalists. This attempt to define races by blood type distribution eventually became the most persistent and coherent, if not the most influential, body of blood group research in the country.[12] It took a while, however, for Steffan and his collaborator Otto Reche to organize these efforts. In the meantime, a more general and widespread interest developed among German medical researchers about blood groups.

This interest was exemplified by four articles which were published in 1924: two in the *Klinische Wochenschrift* and two others in more specialized medical journals. It is telling that one of the main inspirations for these articles was the growing amount of work and publication by foreign researchers which was finally beginning to appear in German journals. For example, when *Index Medicus* began a separate heading for blood groups in 1921, it had seven entries. By 1923 the number had risen to 20, and the following year it cited 44 articles on blood group research. With the exception of a few articles on blood transfusion mentioning agglutination, the index rarely cited German authors on blood groups until 1923.

There were several publications on blood groups in 1923 by foreign authors in German journals, such as one on pseudo-agglutination by Leone Lattes that appeared in *Klinische Wochenschrift*, a report of blood type distribution in Hungary in the *Deutsche medizinische Wochenschrift*, and the results of tests on the effects of pregnancy on blood agglutination by Paul Schneider of the Gynecological Clinic of the University of Vienna published in the *Zeitschrift für die gesamte experimentelle Medizin*.[13] In 1924 when German researchers first reported the results of blood group testing in medical journals, readers were also presented articles about

Japanese and Chinese blood group research and a summary by Hirszfeld of his Macedonian research. In fact, it was in direct response to Hirszfeld's article that Felix Bernstein, a mathematician at the University of Göttingen, published his first suggestion of a fundamental revision in the Von Dungern-Hirszfeld genetic explanation of blood type inheritance.[14] This was the most important theoretical contribution to blood group and human population genetics by a German researcher between the wars.

One of the articles of original research on blood group distribution published in 1924 was by Fritz Schiff, who soon became one of the most important serologists in the world. He was the son of Emil Schiff, a Berlin journalist who was well known for his writing on science and medicine. In fact, when he was in his 40 s, Emil obtained a medical degree in order to understand better the developments in the field. Fritz was only ten when his father died, but the influence of father on son is manifest. Fritz received his medical degree from the University of Berlin in April 1914, with a thesis on heterogenic antibodies directed by the immunologist Ernst Friedberger.[15] Although the young Schiff first took a position in Switzerland as an assistant at Bern, he enlisted in the German army after the war broke out. He served on the front in Flanders until February 1916, when he joined Friedberger as part of the scientific staff of the German military mission to the Ottoman Empire. The assignment was not based simply on personal connections. Schiff had made two trips to the eastern Mediterranean before the war: one as part of an anthropological study tour to the Peloponnesus and Crete in 1912, and another to work at Hygiene Institutes in Alexandria and Jerusalem the following year.

Schiff had a variety of responsibilities while serving in Asia Minor until 1919, including care for German and Turkish military personnel, as well as direction of a laboratory and work at an Armenian orphanage in Aleppo. In the process, his attention shifted to public health problems of typhus, cholera, malaria, and other diseases, about which he published articles in the immediate postwar years. The blood group distribution studies of the early 1920s drew him back to his prewar research on immunology; in fact, before the war he had published an article on the inheritance of blood groups in twins. Schiff's 1924 article, co-authored with a colleague at the bacteriology laboratory which Schiff directed at the Berlin Friedrichshain City Hospital, was based on 1000 subjects of Wassermann tests.[16]

Although the article was entitled "Blood group distribution of the Berlin Population," most of it was devoted to a comparison between Jews and non-Jews. More will be said about this in a later chapter, but of note here is the fact that the authors found little difference between the two populations. When added to the finding that the blood group distribution of Jews in Berlin also differed significantly from Jews tested by Manuila in Rumania and those tested by the Hirszfelds in Macedonia, Schiff and Ziegler concluded with a warning about "drawing far-reaching anthropological conclusions" based on the results from isolated tests of different neighboring populations. This was a thinly veiled reference to the study by Verzar and Weczeckyof German, Hungarian, and Gypsy populations living in Hungary that had so impressed Paul Steffan. They agreed with Steffan, however, that a "systematic study of all parts of Germany and all Europe" would avoid accidents from different testing techniques and isolated studies.

The following year there were only two more articles of original research on blood group distribution by German authors: one in the *Archiv für Rassen-und Gesellschaftsbiologie* by two city health officials in the Ruhr who had been inspired by Steffan's earlier article in that journal, and the other by a doctor at the Frankfurt Women's Hospital who tested 500 competitors at the First International Workers' Olympics in Frankfurt.[17] Although relatively few, these half dozen articles in 1924 and 1925 were by a variety of researchers from all over Germany who published in a number of different journals. This breadth of interest helps explain the doubling of publications from 11 in 1926 to 22 in 1927. These included articles by new researchers following the lead of earlier authors such as Steffan and Schiff, who, in turn, also published the results of their subsequent research.

The increase was also the result of new findings which prompted others to enter the field, such as Max Gundel a young bacteriologist at Kiel who expanded upon Steffan's work by conducting large-scale tests on the whole population of Schleswig-Holstein. Included were inmates in the region's prisons who provided a large number of subjects that could be persuaded to participate. Gundel's finding of a higher percentage of blood type B among criminals (20 percent) compared to the surrounding population (12 percent) prompted several researchers in many countries besides Germany to attempt confirmation of his results.[18] In 1926 the first article was also published on tests of German patients in a mental home which had a similar effect of stimulating research on a possible link between insanity and blood type.[19]

More will be said about this line of research in a later chapter, but of note here was the methodology used in these linkage studies that compared the distribution of ABO types to that in the "normal" population. This was the same methodology used in another line of research that became even more significant than Gundel's criminal tests: the link between blood groups and disease. For example, in 1926 and 1927 alone, 16 articles appeared in national medical journals such as the *Münchener medizinische Wochenschrift* and the *Klinische Wochenschrift*, which compared the distribution of the ABO blood types among patients with such diseases as cancer, leukemia, and tuberculosis to the blood group distribution of the healthy populace. Most of the remaining articles for those years simply reported the distribution of blood types of an ethnic group or region of the country such as Schleswig-Holstein, Berlin, Cologne, Munich, Upper Silesia, and Hesse. In 1927 the first articles on blood group distribution appeared in the most important German journal of legal medicine, the *Deutsche Zeitschrift für die gesamte gerichtliche Medizin*.

There were 25 articles published on blood group distribution research by German authors in 1928, a figure that was never surpassed. They appeared in national medical journals as well as specialized and regional ones. Authors attempted both to find links between blood groups and disease as well as simply to record the ABO frequencies for a given population. That year also saw the appearance of the *Zeitschrift für Rassenphysiologie*, the journal co-edited by Paul Steffan and Otto Reche, which signaled a new phase in the persistent efforts of right-wing nationalists to direct and utilize the new blood group research in Germany for their own purposes.

Although *völkisch* race ideas had roots deep in the nineteenth century, their form in the 1920s was shaped overwhelmingly by the German defeat in the First World War, which brought the collapse of the Second Reich and the end of its conservative, aristocratic political order. More to the point, the Versailles Treaty which redrew the boundaries of eastern Europe, raised the question of racial or ethnic definition to the level of national and international political significance. German nationalist anthropologists sought any means of proving the identity and priority of Germans living beyond the frontiers of the new Weimar state, as well as a way to identify the biological threat of "foreigners" to German racial purity inside the state. Blood group anthropology was welcomed as a new "scientific" weapon in the battle.[20]

Reche was the senior member in the partnership that produced the *Zeitschrift für Rassenphysiologie*. He had already established his reputation as a researcher before the First World War when he was appointed a lecturer in anthropology at the Colonial Institute of Hamburg University in 1909. Reche participated in expeditions to New Guinea and German East Africa, the latter of which aroused his interest in the "race mixing" of Hamitic and Negro populations.[21] Reche was appointed a Professor of Anthropology at Hamburg after the war where Paul Steffan had come to study tropical medicine.

Steffan was only six younger than Reche, but he was not an academic. Instead, Steffan brought medical training and practice to the team. Although he had studied obstetrics in medical school, Steffan's service as a naval doctor during the First World War changed his interests. It was apparently while he studied after the war in Hamburg at Bernard Nocht's world-famous Institute of Naval and Tropical Medicine that Steffan made the acquaintance of Reche.[22] Steffan was first interested in trypanosoma, but after being stationed at Wilhelmshaven in 1921 and then the main German naval base in Kiel in 1922, Steffan turned his attention to blood groups. This was partly from his reading of the work of the Hirszfelds as well as contact with Verzar and Weszeczky, who had published findings on blood groups of mixed population regions in the new Hungarian state during and after the war. What gave Steffan the practical opportunity to do blood group testing was a circumstance similar to Schiff: his responsibilities for giving Wassermann tests to naval personnel.[23]

Steffan's first article was based on a paper he presented in March 1923 at the Naval Medical Society of Kiel, which summarized the work on blood group anthropology to date. He also gave the results of his own tests of 500 sailors at Kiel and called for systematic testing of the German population. Steffan stressed two points that became cornerstones of the German nationalists' subsequent view of blood groups. The first followed from the Hirszfelds' finding of a higher frequency of blood type A in northwestern Europe and higher occurrence of blood type B in central Asia, from which Steffan derived his "Atlantic" and "Gondwana" race markers. These he attributed to the existence of two aboriginal human races of the Eurasian and African land mass. The second point followed from Verzar's and Weszeczky's report in 1922 of testing German, Hungarian, and Gypsy blood group distributions in Transylvania, from which Steffan concluded that further study of blood groups could show "the manner and degree of race mixing of different peoples" that had taken place in Europe.[24]

The publication of this paper in Alfred Ploetz' *Archiv für Rassen-und Gesellschaftsbiologie* in December of that year was the first report of blood group distribution research in Germany. Although it was cited by Schiff and Sucker in their 1924 articles, Steffan's legitimacy was questionable from the start, as indicated by an editorial disclaimer which accompanied the article. After noting on the first page that the article was being published to show some other possible ways besides hair color and head form to identify races, the editors added, "the acceptance of this work naturally does not mean agreement with all the conclusions contained herein."[25]

Two years later, however, the editors of the *Archiv* had apparently changed their minds. The 1925 volume published the findings of two medical officials in the Ruhr who noticed Steffan's call for systematic blood group testing, and their results were but one of several articles to appear on the subject in the journal that year.[26] Steffan's influence through Gundel went even farther, because of the provocative findings of his tests of criminals and the fact that Gundel eventually published nine articles based on his study of several thousand subjects. Meanwhile, Steffan wrote an article in Nocht's *Archiv für Schiffs und Tropenhygiene*, which claimed that the new research on blood group distribution was being published worldwide.

Both he and Reche attempted to stimulate and lead German blood group anthropology research in the next few years by writing articles in the *Mitteilungen der anthropologische Gesellschaft in Wien* (Reche took a Chair in Anthropology at the University of Vienna in 1924 where Steffan joined him), as well as the new völkisch periodicals such as *Volk und Rasse* which Reche edited (subtitle: "Illustrated quarterly for German folkdom") and *Die Sonne* (subtitle: "monthly for Nordic world-view and life formation").[27] In these latter publications, the authors expressed much more openly their racist conclusions. For example, Reche explained in his article for the *Mitteilungen* of the Vienna Anthropological Society how he had been deeply struck by the maps of Steffan which showed lines connecting populations with similar percentages of type A and B blood.

Figure 3.2 shows a pattern which confirmed the Hirszfelds' discovery of a rise in frequency of B from west to east and a rise in frequency of A from east to west. The change was not uniform but showed an abrupt difference (represented by gradient lines being close together) which seemed, in the words of Reche, "as if a very strong wedge of type 3 [another term for blood type B] had forced itself almost brutally right into the middle of central and even northern Germany." Reche went on to conclude,

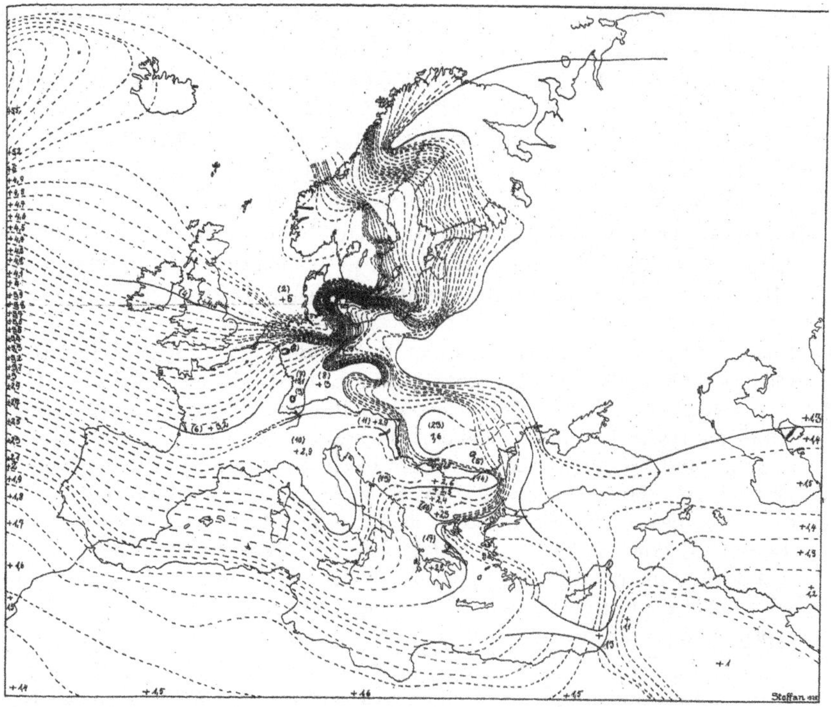

Fig. 3.2 Reche's map of blood group race indices in Europe. ("Kartographische Darstellung des biologischen Rassenindex von Europe," map from Steffan, "Weitere Ergebnisse der Rassenforschung," 83)

> The map of Russia gives the clue from whence this 3 [B] - wave comes: doubtless out of the East. One sees graphically on the map, the strong invasion of Asian masses who have broken through an obviously almost regular population which to the north and south has maintained itself.[28]

In addition to their effort to reach the broader general public about the new blood group research, Reche and Steffan also attempted to give their ideas scientific legitimacy in 1926 by creating an institutional base for their future projects: the German Society for Blood Group Research. Pauline Mazumdar has described in detail the work of this organization which had 49 founding members evenly divided between Germany and Austria, a reflection both of the *grossdeutsch* ideology as well as the fact that Reche was still in Vienna. (He moved to Leipzig the following year.)[29]

Reche and Steffan took out advertisements and made announcements in scholarly journals and magazines of general medical practitioners.[30] At first the society was small and did not include the most important serologists of the day, several of whom were of Jewish ancestry: e.g., Landsteiner, Hirszfeld, Schiff, and Bernstein. This was not entirely deliberate, as indicated by the fact that Steffan tried to recruit Schiff to join. When Steffan sent him an announcement of the society with a list of founding members, Schiff sent the following pointed reply in October 1926:

> I have read your announcement about the founding of the German Society for Blood Group Research and thank you for the friendly invitation to join.
>
> Reading through the announcement, I found it strange that the most important researchers in the field are missing, among them those who have done ground-breaking research. Absent in particular are Landsteiner, Von Dungern, and Hirszfeld, as well as Kruse, Sachs, Schütz, Bernstein, and others. The omission of these names is all the more striking since the circle of those who signed the invitation is otherwise broadly drawn.
>
> For the time being I cannot tell which criteria counted for making this selection. I could think about joining only if I were to receive satisfactory explanation on this point[31]

Hirszfeld reflected a more open disdain for Steffan and Reche's society in a letter to Bernstein the following year after an international anthropological conference in Amsterdam. He stated that they must be on guard "to insure the true international and scientific nature of research" on blood groups. As an encouraging example he noted, "It is a sign of healthy instincts that the laughable efforts of the German Society for Blood Group Research are not taken seriously."[32] Steffan and Reche were eventually more successful with Landsteiner whose adhesion to the society in 1928 prompted a special notice in the *Zeitschrift für Rassenphysiologie*. But as late as 1930, only Von Dungern's name from those mentioned by Schiff had been added to the membership list of the society which included 180 names.[33]

One practical reason for seeking wide publicity about the society's creation was to recruit help in its first and most ambitious undertaking: the serological mapping of Germany and Austria. Assistance was necessary because the plan called for systematic local testing based on a grid of the two countries which divided them into 900 districts. In each, local doctors were expected to test at least 500 subjects in order to determine the distribution of the blood groups. Although ambitious, it was not an impossible goal according to Steffan, "for an area as densely populated with doctors as Germany and Austria."[34] Reche suggested, "It would be especially appreciated if the medical societies for each region designated one man for the effort. But others could also learn the blood agglutination technique without difficulty."[35] Researchers were also encouraged to seek the cooperation of local school districts to permit testing of school children as a convenient source of the large numbers needed for the project.

Several researchers took up the idea and reported their findings in the German medical press. For example, the Frankfurt Anthropological Society sent members to seven school districts in the countryside around Frankfurt.[36] Meanwhile, the Blood Group Society submitted ambitious proposals between October 1926 and February 1927 in Württemberg, Mecklenburg, and Prussia for funding these studies. When the Prussian Health Council recommended against support for the project, however, plans were abandoned in Württemberg, and school authorities in Baden, Bavaria, and Saxony also declined to participate.[37]

Undaunted, Reche and Steffan attempted to enlist help for their survey from Eugen Fischer's new Institute for Anthropology, Human Heredity, and Genetics in Berlin for a scaled-down version of the survey.[38] More important in the long run, however, was their founding of a journal in June 1928, the *Zeitschrift für Rassenphysiologie* which was published by J. F. Lehmann, a major medical publisher and noted supporter of the *völkisch* movement.[39] This publication soon became the most important element in their effort to collect and disseminate new research on blood group anthropology. From 1928 to 1939, more than 40 articles of original research on blood group distribution were published in the journal, although only half by German authors. In addition, numerous summary and theoretical articles were published by Reche, Steffan, and others, and there were annual cumulative bibliographies of published blood group research compiled by Reche's assistant at Leipzig, Michael Hesch.

To what extent was Reche and Steffan's German Society for Blood Group Research, in the words of the founders, "a crystallization point for the numerous individual researchers," and was it successful in its goal "to make possible research into all problems and closer contact and mutual cooperation among all those scientists interested in blood group research"?[40] In this initial phase their success was limited. They were unsuccessful in obtaining government funding for their first priority project of a national blood testing program, but many researchers, whether inspired by *völkisch* ideology or not, conducted studies of blood group distribution in several regions of Germany. The society began publishing a journal, thanks to the help of the right-wing nationalist publisher Lehmann, but the most important researchers in the field failed to participate.

The overriding reason for the limited nature of their success in directing blood group research in Germany during the 1920s was that the field expanded too rapidly and too broadly for anyone to dominate it. Two graphic illustrations of the breadth and diversity of German blood group research during this extremely active initial period, as well as the relative importance of the Steffan/Reche group, are found in Fig. 3.3 showing the journals where blood group distribution articles were published and the subjects of researchers' interest.

In the initial period from 1923 through 1928 articles on blood group distribution by German authors appeared in a variety of journals, the most important single group of which were the large weekly medical journals (38 articles 1923–1939): *Deutsche medizinische Wochenschrift*, *Münchener*

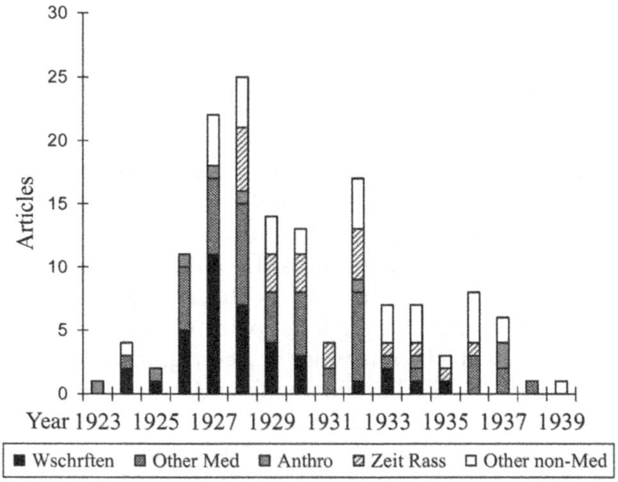

Fig. 3.3 Journals where German researchers published articles about blood group distribution, 1923–1939

medizinische Wochenschrift, *Klinische Wochenschrift*, and *Medizinische Welt*. Admittedly, one of these, the *Münchener medizinische Wochenschrift*, was a Lehmann publication, but it remained well respected and independent. Moreover, the *Klinische Wochenschrift*, owned by the Jewish publisher Springer, carried just as many articles on blood group distribution.[41] An even larger number of articles appeared in other medical periodicals (46 articles 1923–1939), some in a medical specialty (e.g., *Archiv für Dermatologie und Syphilographie*), and others which were more research oriented (e.g., *Zeitschrift für Immunitätsforschung*). Anthropological journals (nine articles) showed only a brief and intermittent interest in blood group distribution. Membership shows a few important members from German anthropology (Georg Buschan, Augustin Krämer, Martin Gusinde, Hans Plischke, Bernhard Struck, and Georg Thilenius), but most remained members for only few years.[42]

This analysis of journals illustrates the limited impact of the *Zeitschrift für Rassenphysiologie* after it appeared in 1928. There is no doubt that its articles immediately represented a sizeable part of the blood group distribution literature published by German researchers in subsequent years (21 articles 1928–1939). It is difficult to say, however, that the journal dominated the research. In no single year did more than 25 percent of German articles on blood group distribution appear in the journal. During its first few years of publication, the *Zeitschrift für Rassenphysiologie* carried 23 percent of such articles; between 1932 and 1936 it carried only 16 percent.

Taken together with Fig. 3.3, this publication record shows that the importance of the medical weeklies declined steadily after 1928, but this mirrored the overall decline in German articles after that peak year. The *Zeitschrift für Rassenphysiologie* maintained its level of interest through 1932, after which it also showed a drop in the number of articles published on blood group distribution by German researchers. The result was only a relatively small increase in the journal's overall importance as a publisher of results of blood group distribution testing.

Blood testing of populations in a given region or ethnic group was the single most frequent subject of German researchers' articles. In fact, this inward-looking research was to the exclusion of interest in foreign peoples or publications. Only 15 of the more than 150 articles by German researchers were on the distribution of blood groups of populations outside Germany. This was in marked contrast to the pattern in France, Britain, or the U.S. Moreover, these German researchers wrote primarily for a home audience. Only five of their articles of original research were published in foreign journals.

This serological focus on Germany was in keeping with the goals of the *Zeitschrift für Rassenphysiologie*, which did what it could to encourage this research. All but two of its articles by German researchers on blood group distribution were on race or region in Germany. But as the earlier graph indicates, many more articles were published in medical journals, not anthropological ones or the *Zeitschrift für Rassenphysiologie*. Thus, researchers, Jewish or self-described "Aryan," had many places to publish their findings.

Another indication why Steffan and Reche were thwarted in their early attempt to direct blood group research was the development of other subjects of interest besides race and region.

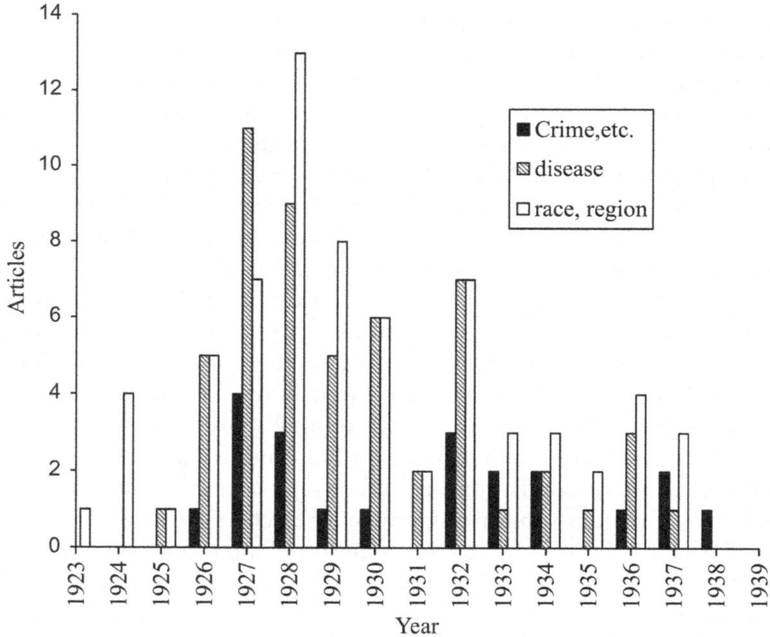

Fig. 3.4 Subjects of articles on blood group distribution by German researchers, 1924–1939

Excluding the initial and last years, Fig. 3.4 shows that from 1925 to 1938 the number of articles on race were more numerous than those on disease in seven years while those on disease were equal to or greater than those of race in four years. Overall, the numbers of race and non-race articles were the same. Other subjects also included articles on blood groups and criminality, insanity, and a handful of other human characteristics.

The history of researchers' interest in the possible link between blood groups and disease has been largely ignored by scholars. More will be said about this in a later chapter, but the overall goal was to find whether people with certain blood types had a greater incidence of specific diseases. The assumption was that this would be the result of selection for the type found least frequently because of greater survival of those genetically related of that blood type. Beginning in 1925 German researchers, like their counterparts around the world, tested the blood group distribution of patients suffering from a variety of illnesses. Of 50 such articles by Germans, 8 were on possible links between blood type and venereal disease, 7 on tuberculosis, and 6 on skin disorders, presumably because dermatology was the specialty of those treating venereal disease. There were three or fewer articles each on a dozen other diseases, such as cancer, scarlet fever, diphtheria, leprosy, and leukemia. This line of research partly explains the appearance of so many blood group articles in German medical journals. Of note, only one of these articles appeared in the *Zeitschrift für Rassenphysiologie*, reflecting its primary focus on race As for other subjects, despite Gundel's early association with Steffan in Kiel, none of his articles on the blood groups of criminals were published in Steffan's journal. In fact, only one article by a German researcher testing links between insanity or criminality and blood groups ever appeared in the *Zeitschrift für Rassenphysiologie*.

German blood group research, along with that in the USSR, was the most extensive of any country in the 1920s. Both the number of articles published on the distribution of blood types and the theoretical contributions of researchers such as Bernstein and Schiff were ample evidence of the importance of German research. In fact, the interest was so strong and varied that no one research center or group dominated it. The variety of subjects and venues for publication combined to limit the influence of Reche and Steffan's blood group research plans in Germany. That situation changed in the 1930s, but the reason was only partly the result of the friendly Nazi regime coming to power.

Soviet Blood Group Research in the 1920s

There is much to analyze in the extraordinary burst of research on blood group distribution in the Soviet Union during the 1920s. By the time the activity dropped off precipitously in the early 1930s, it was the largest body of research published on the subject in any country, with the most people tested by over 100 different researchers all over the Soviet Union. This new work was largely stimulated by the human and geographical diversity of the country, as well as the upheaval of the Russian Revolution which permitted the establishment of new institutions in both the medical and anthropological fields. In the process three research centers were established for the new field of seroanthropology in Moscow, Leningrad, and Kharkiv (Ukraine).

One common goal of all three centers was to coordinate and encourage blood group studies as a way of distinguishing between the ethnically diverse populations of the vast regions of the Soviet Union. This anthropological emphasis was much earlier than the recognition a decade later of the value of blood groups by anthropologists in western Europe and the U.S. Also setting Soviet researchers apart from their German counterparts who also had an early anthropological interest, was a fundamentally different motivation. Whereas most German researchers focused on attempting to define the differences between "foreign" minorities and the presumed ethnically homogeneous majority population, in the Soviet Union the goal can best be described as a scientific cataloging of the scores of different populations in the country. In addition to this anthropological interest, Soviet researchers had an equally strong interest in the study of possible links between blood groups and disease or other human conditions.[43]

Soviet interest in blood group research first developed at Nikolai Koltsov's Institute for Experimental Biology, one of the new research facilities growing out of the "hardships and opportunities" of the war and revolution.[44] In 1922 Koltsov authored the earliest cited article on blood group distributions and their potential eugenic and genetic applications. More effective in continuing this interest, however, was the work of Koltsov's protegé and fellow eugenicist Victor V. Bunak of the Anthropological Institute at Moscow University. Bunak's first article was published in 1924 describing the Hirszfelds' work and its significance for anthropology. The following year he conducted tests on 579 students at the Communist School for Eastern Peoples in Moscow, which gave him a sampling of 17 different ethnic groups. Most important, Bunak was editor of the *Russian Journal of Anthropology* (*Ruskii Antropologicheskii Zhurnal*) until 1932, which published more articles on blood group distribution between the wars than any other journal in the country except one.[45]

In addition to Koltsov and Bunak, there were eight other researchers who published articles on blood group distribution in the Soviet Union in 1924. Typically, these were doctors at remote locations who conducted research that was part of the early and strong interest in mapping the country serologically, but it also included an article by Boris N. Vishnevskii, the coordinator and proponent of the second center of research on blood group distribution at the Museum of Anthropology and Ethnography of the Soviet Academy of Sciences in Leningrad. Vishnevskii began conducting research on the anthropology of the Chuvash people, which utilized the new blood group discoveries.[46] In 1927 Vishnevskii established in Leningrad a "Bureau for Anthropological Investigations on Blood Groups of the Peoples of the U. S. S. R.," which produced numerous studies by him and his students, which were published in Soviet and foreign journals. Thus, both Moscow and Leningrad became centers of research on blood groups with a particular interest in anthropology.

There were other reasons besides anthropological ones for the interest in blood groups in the Soviet Union. Included among the articles published in 1924 were two on the blood groups of patients with malaria and one on patients with tuberculosis, which indicate the early and strong interest in possible links to disease. (Four articles followed in 1925.) In addition, an article also appeared that year in the most important Russian medical journal *Vrachebnoe Delo*, one of whose co-authors was V. I. Rubashkin, Professor of Histology and Cytology and director of the Institute for Protozoa Research at the University of Kharkiv.

Rubashkin was instrumental in founding the third and most important center of Soviet blood group research in the 1920s: the "Standing Committee for Blood Group Research" of the Medical Section of the Kharkiv Scientific Society of the Ukrainian Academy of Sciences.[47] Despite the seeming obscurity of this organization, Rubashkin's prestige helped the Ukrainian committee quickly succeed in its goal of coordinating, standardizing, and publishing the work of blood group researchers throughout the Soviet Union. The key element in this success was the creation of the *Ukrainisches Zentralblatt für Blutgruppenforschung*, a bilingual journal in German and Ukrainian edited by Rubashkin and V. N. Shamov, his colleague at Kharkiv. The choice of languages reflected a combination of

Ukrainian nationalism and scientific internationalism,[48] but its contributors included researchers from Leningrad, Moscow, Odessa, and all important centers of Soviet medical research. Finally, unlike the editors of the *Zeitschrift für Rassenphysiologie*, Rubashkin and Shamov successfully recruited the participation of the world leaders of blood group research such as Hirszfeld, Schiff, and Lattes plus Furuhata from Japan, Dujarric de la Rivière from France, and Thomsen from Denmark, not only as honorary members but as contributing authors. The result was that by the end of the 1920s, the *Ukrainisches Zentralblatt* provided its readers with the most comprehensive coverage of blood group research by any journal in the world.

Both Bunak and Vishnevskii worked closely with Rubashkin's committee in Kharkiv, and the result of all the activity was that the Soviet Union exceeded even Germany in the testing of its population for blood type.[49] From 1919 through 1930, Soviet authors published 108 articles of original research on blood group distribution, more than the 95 articles published by German researchers. In fact, together the articles by researchers in these two countries represented almost one-third of all such articles published worldwide. The breadth of the Soviet research is indicated by the fact that for the whole period between the two world wars 125 different authors in locations all over the country published articles on blood group distribution. The three centers made their findings available to national and even international audiences. For example, a large number of Soviet authors published in foreign journals, 23 such articles compared to only 5 German authors who published their findings in foreign journals during this period.

The Soviet affinity for publishing in German journals was the result of historical scientific ties rather than close cooperation between the German Society for Blood Group Research and the Kharkiv committee whose history it paralleled. Only five Soviet authors published original research on blood group distribution in the *Zeitschrift für Rassenphysiologie* (with most of these appearing after the Ukrainian journal ceased publication), and no German researchers did so in the Ukrainian journal. Nonetheless, the two publications did inform their readers about each other's work. Thus, Steffan authored a ten-page article on the work of the Deutsche Gesellschaft für Blutgruppenforschung in the first issue of the *Ukrainisches Zentralblatt*, and the German journal regularly gave abstracts of the contents of each issue of the Ukrainian journal. Although there was a regular bibliography of German blood group literature published by the Ukrainian journal, it was compiled by Schiff and only once were there abstracts of articles.

The *Ukrainisches Zentralblatt für Blutgruppenforschung* published increasing numbers of articles of original research on blood group distribution from 1927 through 1930, but Fig. 3.5 indicates that its share of all such Soviet articles was even smaller than that of the *Zeitschrift für Rassenphysiologie* for Germany.

Although in 1930 and 1931 the Ukrainian journal published over half the articles in the Soviet Union on blood group distribution, the main reason was the dramatic drop in articles by other journals. Thus, historically, the greatest significance of the *Ukrainisches Zentralblatt* was the bibliography of Soviet research it made available in a Western language for foreign countries as well as throughout the Soviet Union.

As the graph indicates, in most years (especially those with the largest number of articles), more Soviet researchers published their findings on

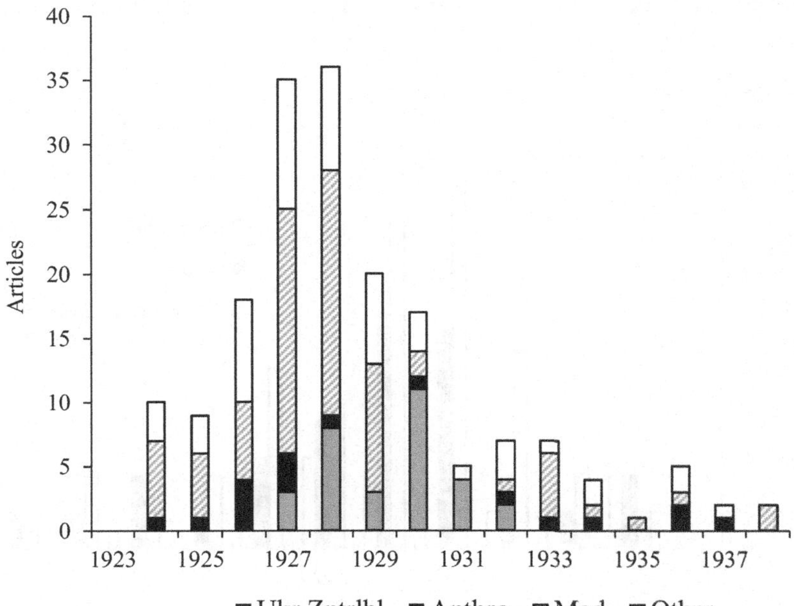

Fig. 3.5 Journals where articles appeared by Soviet researchers about blood group distribution, 1924–1938

blood group distribution in medical than any other type of journal. Only one or two articles appeared in anthropological publications (usually Bunak's *Russian Journal of Anthropology* and Vishnevskii's proceedings of the Academy of Sciences) albeit almost every year. Over one-third (34 percent) of medical journal articles appeared in national publications of general and clinical medicine (such as *Vrachebnoe Delo*), 22 percent were in regional publications and 44 percent appeared in journals of various medical specialties. Thus, the interest in blood group distribution could be found in all regions of the country and by a variety of medical specialists.

Despite the frequent appearance of articles in medical journals, as shown by Fig. 3.6 the link to disease was most often a close second to the subject of greatest interest to Soviet researchers from the start: the blood group distribution of the different peoples in different regions of the country.

In only one year between 1922 and 1938 (and late, after a dramatic decline in publications) did the number of articles about the blood groups and disease exceed those about distribution among the different peoples

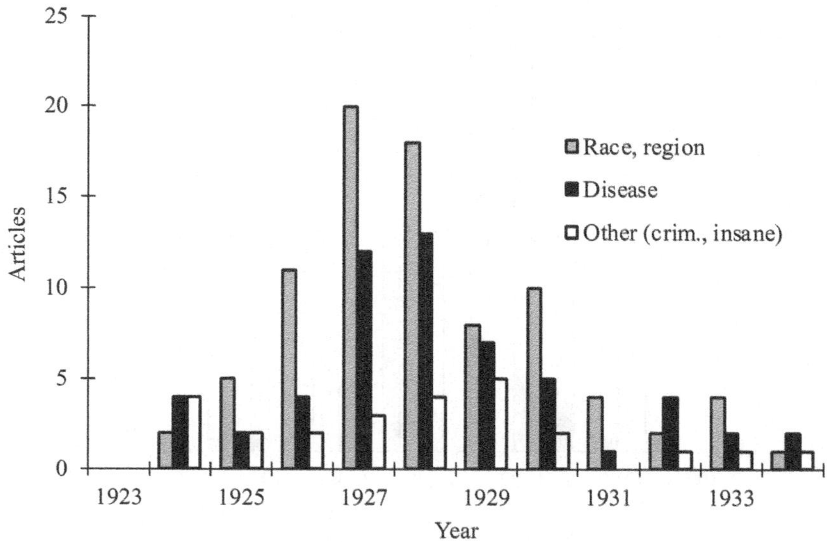

Fig. 3.6 Subjects of articles on blood group distribution by Soviet researchers, 1922–1938

of the Soviet Union. In total, over 60 percent of the articles published between the wars were on blood and race.

This anthropological interest in blood group distribution was evident as early as Koltsov's 1922 article which compared Russians and Jews, and it was quickly picked up by Bunak, whose tests of students from 17 different peoples of the Soviet Union mirrored the geographical pattern found by the Hirszfelds.[50] Vishnevskii's articles began appearing in 1925 and reported his findings from three trips to the Chuvash region of the Volga between 1924 and 1926.

An illustration of the interest in blood distribution of the Soviet nationalities is shown by the following list of different populations tested by researchers that were reported in articles published in 1926: Tatars, Udmuks, Wodjaks (Irkutsk), Ossetins (Caucasus), White Russians, and Bashkiri (Turks). Important sources of data were "Central Asian Anthropological Expeditions" sponsored by the Academy of Science beginning in the late 1920s and continuing through the early 1930s. The geographical extent of these efforts was so great that when the American serologist William Boyd compiled a summary list of all the literature published on blood group distribution through 1939, he found reports of testing at 257 locations in the Soviet Union, more than any other country in the world.[51]

In addition to the anthropologists Vishnevskii in Leningrad and Bunak in Moscow (and their students), medical researchers at Soviet facilities around the country were frequent authors of studies on their local populations. These included L. B. Vagner, a physiologist at Omsk, who published five articles between 1924 and 1926 on Siberian populations; B. W. Parin, who began studying local populations at the Bacteriological Institute of Perm before moving to Leningrad to work with Vishnevskii in 1929; and A. A. Melkikh at Irkutsk, who studied the local Buriat population and even created his own variation of the Hirszfeldss' biochemical index. Most often, however, one or two studies were done by local doctors who sent results to Bunak's or Rubashkin's journal, or else they published in their own local medical journal.

Other anthropological studies of ABO blood group distribution were done on more conveniently available subjects. Like the Kiel sailors, tested in 1926 by Steffan, Red Army soldiers and Great Russians were the subjects of a half dozen studies between 1927 and 1930. As in Germany, Jews were of interest in Koltsov's first report in 1922 and there were a dozen studies by 1928 with data on the blood groups of Jews plus varying conclusions about their difference or similarity compared to the local population.[52] Only a handful of studies were done by Soviet researchers through 1930 on foreign populations, usually residing in the country: two on Chinese, one on Arabs, and two on the descendants of German colonists in the Ukraine.[53]

The number of articles on blood groups and disease by Soviet researchers was overshadowed by those about anthropology, but compared to the rest of the world this disease research was formidable. In fact, through 1930, Soviet authors published more such articles (59) than researchers in any other country. Moreover, these were often the first attempts to test for correlation between blood groups and some diseases. For example, A. M. Liakhovetskii at the Tropical Institute of Moscow University was the first researcher in the world to test for a possible link between blood groups and malaria in 1924. Another disease which received early attention in the Soviet Union was tuberculosis. In fact, three different researchers in the country published studies in 1924 on the blood groups of patients with tuberculosis, which were the first such studies in the world.[54] Soviet researchers were also among the first to study links between blood groups and syphilis, although they were contemporary with studies published in Italy, Poland, and Germany. A Soviet researcher, Kaminskii, published the first results of blood group tests of patients with polio, although no other Soviet researchers followed. Curiously, one disease which received a great deal of attention for possible links to blood groups elsewhere but not in the Soviet Union was cancer. In fact, over 40 such articles were published on the subject between the wars but none by Soviet researchers.

Moscow, Leningrad, and Odessa, in addition to Kharkiv, were the most frequent places where this research was conducted, but authors from locations all over the Soviet Union reported their research on blood groups and disease. Moreover, the list of diseases studied by 1930 also included scarlet fever (among the earliest), epilepsy, goiter, leprosy, and typhus. More will be said about this line of research in a separate chapter on blood groups and disease, but for now it is worth noting that it reflects the early and strong interest by researchers in the Soviet Union in this possible link. There was also an unusual interest by researchers in the blood groups of the insane and criminals, especially the former which elicited several articles by Soviet authors in the late 1920s.

In hindsight at least, these Soviet researchers deserve priority credit for their pioneering work, but they rarely received it at the time. This is telling of the isolation of these researchers who, despite the efforts of the editors of the *Ukrainisches Zentralblatt* and the *Zeitschrift für Rassenphysiologie*, were rarely recognized or cited by researchers outside the country unless they published in Western journals. Thus, the three articles published by Soviet authors in 1924 on possible links between blood groups and tuberculosis, plus two others the following year, preceded any articles published in other countries. But these studies were never mentioned by subsequent researchers outside the Soviet Union. The earliest reference to Soviet research was a 1926 article by M. M. Alperin of the Institute for Tuberculosis Research in Odessa, because it was published in the *Beiträge zur Klinik der Tuberkulose*.[55] The oversight is even more glaring since Alperin's article cited the previous Soviet authors. The story was similar for studies of possible links between blood groups and malaria. Ljachovetskii published two articles on the subject in 1924, and it was the subject of papers at the second and third national congresses on malaria in 1924 and 1925.[56] None of this work, however, had an impact on Western medical research. Only when Austrian and German researchers reported results in 1927 did articles follow by Westerners (five in 1928). These later, independent studies show that the Soviets did not create the field of study, but ignorance of their pioneering work cost later researchers valuable and extensive comparative findings.

Two more general conclusions can be drawn from this research on blood groups and disease in the Soviet Union relative to the rest of the world. The first is that Soviet research (with some significant exceptions such as cancer) was quite extensive, reflecting the level of research in the country both in serology and the etiology of disease. The second conclusion is the isolation of the Soviet researchers. In 1924, for example, no Soviet journals were indexed by *Index Medicus*, which meant that Soviet researchers were aware of work elsewhere but had little impact outside the country. Thus, one can see the importance of a journal like the *Ukrainisches Zentralblatt*, not only to let Soviet researchers know about the work going on in their own country but also to bring their work into the mainstream of worldwide medical research. These efforts were not isolated nor in vain. By 1931 *Index Medicus* was indexing 31 Soviet journals, including 14 of which published articles on blood group distribution.

The Decline of German and Soviet Blood Group Research in the 1930s

If the most remarkable feature of blood group research in Germany and the Soviet Union was the extraordinary amount of interest in the 1920s, then as Fig. 3.1 shows, the decline of that interest in the following decade was equally striking. In both countries there were dramatic political changes in the early 1930s: Stalin's consolidation of power in the Soviet Union and Hitler's assumption of power in Germany. Yet only in the Soviet Union did the political change directly and dramatically affect the research on blood groups. In Germany the Nazi takeover was much less responsible for the decline of interest in the subject.

The decline of research on blood groups in Germany during the 1930s was all the more remarkable, because blood figured so prominently in Nazi rhetoric, at least as early as Hitler's *Mein Kampf.* Hence, one would expect that after taking power in January 1933, the Nazis would encourage blood group research, especially along the lines of the Steffan/Reche theories. Reche quickly tried to take advantage of this by renaming his Institute of Ethnology and Anthropology, the Institute of Racial Science and Ethnology in 1933.[57] But the only record of support mentioned by Geisenhainer was the purchase of 100 subscriptions of the *Zeitschrift für Rassenphysiologie* by the Ministry of the Interior for distribution to government offices, a courtesy also offered to the *Archiv für Rassen-und Gesellschaftsbiologie*. As Pauline Mazumdar has suggested, despite the fact that blood was primarily used as a metaphor for descent or inheritance, "this crossing over from symbolism to serology … gave a heightened significance to the work of the Deutsche Gesellschaft für Blutgruppenforschung."[58] The record shows, however, that this expected increase in interest never developed. In fact, rather than a rise, there was a decline in the number of articles published by German researchers on the distribution of blood groups during the 1930s.

As Fig. 3.1 shows, from 1926 through 1932 there was only one year in which less than 11 such articles were published, with an average of over 15 per year. Yet after 1933 in only one year were there as many as eight articles, with an average of less than five. The graph of articles shows that German publication on blood group distribution had been declining since the peak year of 25 articles in 1928. Only 4 articles were published in 1931, and although 18 were published in 1932, it was clearly the exception, as the number of articles never reached half that figure the rest of the decade.

Because publications on blood group began to drop before 1933 and did not revive once the Nazis were in power, one explanation of the decline of research may be simply that the initial subjects of possible blood testing were exhausted during the first rush of interest in the 1920s. Accordingly, the decline thereafter is partly the result of a maturation of research in the new field. Thus, the overwhelming number of early articles by German researchers were relatively simple tests of ABO blood type distribution of convenient subjects at hand: local populations not yet reported in the literature, pupils at schools with a cooperative administration, or visitors to medical clinics. The purpose of this research was typically to fill in a gap in the serological map or to see if an illness or other condition of those tested might be linked to a blood type that was above or below the frequency for the rest of the population.

This meant that for research to continue at the same pace, there had to be new populations to test or a reason to retest previous ones. Otherwise, the number of studies would decline. In fact, the overall record of German blood group research in the 1930s showed a decline with some minor exceptions. For example, in the late 1920s new blood groups were discovered that gave a new rationale for retesting. Some of these, such as the sub-groups of type A, were of little more than technical interest to researchers. Landsteiner and Levine's discovery of the MN system in 1928 was more significant, but it showed no pattern of geographical or ethnic distribution like the ABO system. The result was that its most immediate application was to legal questions of disputed paternity. This happened to be a subject of more interest in Germany than elsewhere because German courts were among the first to allow blood tests as evidence in legal cases.[59] Even with this additional interest, there was no rush to retest the population on the scale of the first ABO testing. Only eight articles published by German researchers between 1929 and 1937 included the MN distribution. The discovery of this new system, therefore, did not prompt a significant renewal of interest in blood groups, as was the case with the Rh discoveries of the 1940s.

The Nazi takeover had a similar, limited impact on the overall record of blood group research. In fact, one Nazi policy significantly (and ironically) hindered the work because it eliminated researchers of Jewish ancestry. There is a debate among scholars on the relative disruption or continuity of scientific research in Germany as a result of the Nazis coming to power.[60]

The disruption of blood group research was magnified beyond the actual numbers of Jews who left their laboratories, because of the importance of the positions they held and their potential for training and inspiring new researchers. For example, two of the most important Germans working on blood groups who emigrated were Bernstein and Schiff. Bernstein was in residence at Charles Davenport's laboratory at Cold Spring Harbor when Hitler took power, and he decided to stay in the U.S. Bernstein held a series of different positions in New York until the end of the war and returned to Göttingen with emeritus status in 1948.[61]

Schiff was able to stay at Friedrichshain (renamed Horst Wessel) Hospital until 1935 partly because he had served on the front lines during the First World War but also because of personal connections. He was, thus, able to continue the research which had made him the most important serologist in Germany. In addition to his work on the blood group distribution of the Berlin population, Schiff made contributions both to theoretical and applied research, which included the first testing for MN groups in Germany, establishment of serological evidence in the German courts, research on group factors in saliva, and a textbook on blood grouping techniques that went through three editions by 1932. The loss that Schiff's emigration meant to German serology can also be seen in a few examples of work he published while he continued to live in Germany under Nazi rule from 1933 to 1935: a significant monograph on blood groups and their applications, a second article on the blood groups of twins which he published with the eugenicist Otmar von Verschuer, and his fourth installment of research on the blood groups of the Berlin population.[62] The laws of 1935 removed Schiff from his civil service post, and the following year he took a position at Beth Israel Hospital in New York. Schiff was preparing the fourth edition in English of his textbook on blood grouping techniques in 1940 when he died suddenly at age 51. William Boyd completed the work on the book, for which Landsteiner wrote an introduction.[63]

The other potential source of additional subjects for blood group research by Germans was new populations to test. German researchers, however, had never shown much interest in studying people outside the country during the 1920s, and this continued into the 1930s with only a few exceptions, such as a study of some inhabitants of the South Pacific Loyalty Islands who visited Hamburg after the 1931 Colonial Exhibition in Paris.[64] The Nazis were responsible indirectly for one significant new source of subjects: testing of army personnel for possible use in blood transfusion beginning in 1936. Steffan had been one of the first to argue for such a policy, and in the late 1930s various techniques were reported by German researchers for blood typing the large numbers involved. Several articles collected and analyzed the results which were so extensive that, in effect, they completed the serological mapping which Steffan and Reche had called for over a decade earlier.[65]

Although blood group research in the Soviet Union showed a similar decline in the 1930s, the reasons were very different. If the revolutionary political circumstances of the 1920s made possible new approaches to medical and anthropological questions in the Soviet Union, the change in political climate of the 1930s brought the work to an abrupt end. Unlike German researchers, the Soviets had hardly exhausted the possible subjects of study, given the size of the country, diverse populations, and strong interest in possible links of blood groups to disease. Hence, there was a more abrupt change in blood group research in the Soviet Union, prompted not by a maturation of research but rather by political forces, usually referred to by Soviet historians as "the Great Break."[66]

This phrase is used to characterize the changes in Soviet society as a result of Stalin's consolidation of power after Lenin's death. The process of upheaval which emphasized replacement of "bourgeois" theoretical elements by proletarian and practical ones, began in 1928 and spread to various sectors of society at different times.[67] After Stalin's June 1, 1931 speech on "science as a weapon of class conflict," the impact reached those working in the anthropological and medical study of blood groups. Shortly thereafter the Ukrainian *Zentralblatt* added the word "Transfusion" to its title with an editorial announcement praising the value of "practical medicine," promising to conduct "further experimental and clinical research on hematological questions in the light of Marxist-Leninist methodology." The means would be "the linking of theoretical questions relative to the isoagglutination of the blood groups with the practice of blood transfusion."[68] M. S. Schindler published "Critical Remarks" on much of the research published in the *Zentralblatt* which he labelled "purely academic," and called for more "concrete, practical" research on applications like transfusion, the determination of paternity, etc.[69] In 1932 Bunak was replaced as editor of the *Russian Journal of Anthropology*. Of the early group of medical researchers only Shamov made the transition and took advantage of the new emphasis on practical applications. This was because of his early work on cadaver blood transfusion which became one of the most widely publicized of Soviet transfusion applications.[70]

Schindler's article was also critical of studies that suggested "the existence of good and bad blood." In fact, one of the articles he used as an example was on Stalin's home of Tiflis [Tblisi] in the Transcaucasus in which the author suggested that the region had seen an influx of Slavic peoples with a high percentage of type B blood.[71] That kind of conclusion may have been acceptable in the German *Zeitschrift für Rassenphysiologie* but not Stalin's Soviet Union. A more fundamental objection to such studies appeared in an article entitled "Race Theory -- Class Theory," in the *Russian Anthropological Journal* (renamed simply *Journal of Anthropology*) which appeared after the Nazis came to power in Germany and made specific reference to Nazi rule there.

> The fanning of nationalistic enmity and race hatred was for the ruling classes always a means of undermining and disorganizing the strength of their class enemies. Race theories in different forms have served the exploitation of man by man throughout the course of the history of class society, as a means of ideological foundation and justification of this exploitation.[72]

Conclusion

With the maturation of research and elimination of some key Jewish personnel, the field of blood group research in Germany shrank considerably in the 1930s, thus making it easier for Steffan and Reche to direct it. Rather than adding testing of new populations, Steffan and other contributors to the *Zeitschrift für Rassenphysiologie* attempted to devise new schemes for displaying all of the accumulated findings.[73] Meanwhile, elsewhere in Germany the publication of articles on blood group distribution almost disappeared from the national medical weeklies (only four articles appeared after 1932, none after 1935), and interest in potential links between blood groups and disease virtually ceased to be a subject of articles (only one appeared after 1936). Race and regional distribution of blood groups were left as the most frequent subjects of interest.

Given this greater importance, even if by default, of the Steffan/Reche agenda, it is surprising, as Mazumdar has shown, that there were few direct policy applications based on it. Geisenhainer provides analysis in depth that shows Reche played only a minor role after the war began in setting up the screening of populations for the German resettlement policy in the newly conquered eastern territories of Poland.[74] The idea was to select for consolidation of all German and potentially assimilable populations that were scattered in the lands of the east. Reche made numerous proposals to Nazi officials (including Rudolf Hess) for grander schemes to identify and remove Jewish and "Polish lice in our fur" in the newly conquered lands. But given his age (60) and the inflexibility of his schemes for implementation involving detailed screening, the Nazis chose more flexible and less costly approaches. Of note, given his extensive work on blood type as a definition of race, Reche did not push for its use in the screening. Mazumdar found that although there was a place for blood type on the form used by investigators who conducted the examinations, the blood testing was rarely done. Instead, the investigators used the more traditional physical anthropology measures of body form, hair, and eye color. The legacy of research on race and blood groups continued elsewhere, as shown by an article published in the *Zeitschrift für Rassenphysiologie* about tests and experiments conducted on non-Europeans in a prisoner of war camp. The *Zeitschrift* continued to be published through 1944.[75]

The *Ukrainisches Zentralblatt* ceased publication in 1932, with its last two articles on blood group distribution examining links to tuberculosis and the Ingush population of the Caucasus mountains. Without the journal's bibliographic record, it is difficult to know all Soviet articles on blood groups published thereafter, but from *Index Medicus* plus Boyd and Mourant's compilations, it appears that there were only a handful of articles on these subjects published by Soviet authors each year until the end of the 1930s. Anthropological articles appeared in the renamed *Journal of Anthropology* or local medical journals. Articles on blood groups and disease were published more frequently in local or foreign medical journals than national ones. Vishnevskii was the only leader of earlier anthropological research who survived the changes, remaining as director of the Anthropological Department of the Museum for Anthropology and Ethnography in Leningrad. An important source of subjects for his research were students at the Institute of the Peoples of the North, a school for about 500 students drawn from populations living in northern Russia and Siberia. As late as 1936 Vishnevskii published articles on his work in foreign journals.[76]

Only a few German blood group researchers were trained in the late 1930s and early 1940s who survived the war and became leaders of a new generation of serologists in the postwar period. Most important of these was Peter Dahr, who began his career in the early 1930s studying the blood groups of apes and anthropoids but changed to human studies in some articles for popular National Socialist journals in 1939–1940 on blood groups and race. During the war he was able to shift his research to the newly discovered Rh groups, thanks to his prewar work on anthropoids.[77] This coincided with the most important new line of blood group research after the war that was carried out by British and especially American researchers. Although very much behind German and Soviet serologists in the 1920s, Anglo-American researchers quite dramatically surpassed the Soviets who languished in the 1930s and the Germans who followed the dead-end path of racial research. A later chapter will describe this process in greater detail.

Notes

1. Soviet research has gone almost unnoticed by scholars. On the other hand, German blood group research has understandably received more attention, beginning with the work of Pauline Mazumdar cited below, and more recently Rachel E. Boaz, *In Search of "Aryan Blood": Serology in Interwar and National Socialist Germany* (Budapest: Central European University Press, 2012).
2. For example, see Allan Mitchell, *German Influences in France after 1870* (Chapel Hill: University of North Carolina, Press, 1979) and for French national science reform in late nineteenth century, see Harry Paul, *The Sorcerer's Apprentice: French Scientists' Image of German Science, 1840–1919* (Gainesville: University of Florida Press, 1972).
3. The classic study is Abraham Flexner, *Medical Education in Europe* (New York: Carnegie Foundation, 1912). A more recent assessment is Thomas N. Bonner, *American Doctors and German Universities: A Chapter in Intellectual Relations, 1870–1914* (Lincoln: University of Nebraska Press, 1963), and his subsequent, "German Model of Training Physicians in the United States, 1870–1914: How Closely Was It Followed?" *Bulletin of the History of Medicine* 64 (1990): 18–34, which became part of his more general book, *Becoming a physician: medical education in Britain, France, Germany, and the United States, 1750–1945* (New York: Oxford University Press, 1995).
4. W. Horsley Gantt, *Russian Medicine* (New York: Harper, 1937), pp. 78–9.
5. For background, see Nancy Frieden, *Russian Physicians in an Era of Reform and Revolution, 1865–1905* (Princeton: Princeton University Press, 1981), and on the standing of Russian and Soviet scientific research in the early decades of the twentieth century, see Loren R. Graham, "Formation of Soviet Research Institutes," *Social Studies of Science* 5 (1975): 303–29.

6. For a bibliography of this literature between 1900 and 1920, see articles by Hesch in *Zeitschrift für Rassenphysiologie* 1 (1928): 43–5; 101 and 2 (1929): 100–3.
7. Alan D. Beyerchen, "On the Stimulation of Excellence in Wilhelmina Science," in *Another Germany: A Reconsideration of the Imperial Era*, eds. Jack R. Dikes and Joachim Remak, (Boulder: Westview Press, 1988), 139–68.
8. Thomas Schlich, "'Welche Macht über Tod und Leben!' Die Etablierung der Bluttransfusion im Ersten Weltkrieg," in *Die Medizin und Der Erster Weltkrieg*, eds. Wolfgang U. Eckart and Christoph Gradmann (Pfaffenweiler: Centaurus-Verlagsgesellschaft, 1996), 109–30.
9. See Mark B. Adams, "Science, Ideology and Structure: The Koltsov Institute, 1900–1970," in *Social Context of Soviet Science*, eds. Linda L. Lubrano and Susan Gross Solomon. (Boulder: Westview Press, 1980), 173–209.
10. Brigitte Schroeder-Gudehaus, "Argument for the Self-government and Public Support of Science in Weimar Germany," *Minerva* 10 (1972): 537–70; and Paul Weindling, "Rockefeller Foundation and German Biomedical Science, 1920–1940," in *Science, Politics and the Public Good*, ed. Nicholaas A. Rupke (London: Macmillan, 1988), 119–40.
11. See, for example, a 1923 article which described to German readers the "American method" of agglutination testing: Gustav C. J. Scholten, "Unsere Bluttransfusionen und die amerikanische Methode zum Nachweis von Agglutininen," *Deutsche medizinische Wochenschrift* 49 (1923): 314–5.
12. Pauline M. H. Mazumdar, "Blood and Soil: The Serology of the Aryan Racial State," *Bulletin of the History of Medicine* 64 (1990): 187–219. For more on Steffan's mentor Reche, see Katja Geisenhainer, *"Rasse ist Schicksal:" Otto Reche (1879–1966) – Ein Leben als Anthropologe und Völkerkundler* (Leipzig: Evang. Verlagsanstalt, 2002).
13. Paul Schneider, "Untersuchung über den Isoagglutiningehalt im Menschenblut," *Zeitschrift für die gesamte experimentelle Medizin* 36 (1923): 153–63. The article by A. von Jeney, "Rassenbiologische Untersuchungen in Ungarn," *Deutsche medizinische Wochenschrift* 49 (1923): 546–7, was the third article on blood group distribution in Hungary to appear in a German journal since the war. The *Biochemische Zeitschrift* carried articles in 1920 and 1922 on tests by Verzar and Weszeczky. The ironic result was that when German researchers first reported their test results on the German population in 1924, they used as reference the blood group distribution results of Germans outside the country, such as the Hirszfelds' tests on German soldiers in Macedonia, Verzar's tests on German settlers in Transylvania, and even Liang's tests on

Germans in Shanghai. Such was the delay of German researchers' interest in the field.

14. The actual chronological sequence was as follows. Kirihara's article on Japan appeared March 24; Liang's on China in April; Schiff's original research on June 10; Hirszfeld on June 24, Bernstein in August and Schutz/Wohlisch on Sept. 2. Sucker in Leipzig also published an article probably in the fall of 1924. Only Schiff and Sucker mentioned Steffan's December 1923 article in the *Archiv*.
15. Personal correspondence with Frank Schiff, son of Fritz, who also furnished a "Curriculum vitae" and "Lebenslauf" from the personal papers of Fritz Schiff. The best published biographical account of Schiff is H. G. Moeller, "Friedrich Schiff - sein Wirken als Abteilungsdirektor am Krankenhaus im Friedrichshain, Berlin von 1922 bis 1935," *Deutsche Gesundheitswesen* 29 (1974): 1850–3.

    I am also grateful for a copy of a talk by Peter Voswinckel, "Fritz Schiff (1889–1940), His Life and Work," given at the ceremonial opening of the annual meeting of the German Blood Transfusion Society (Deutsche Gesellschaft für Transfusionsmedizin und immunhaematologie) in September 1993. The ceremony was to honor the work of Fritz Schiff in the presence of his son, on the occasion of the presentation of the society's Fritz Schiff prize which had been awarded since 1968.
16. Fritz Schiff and H. Ziegler, "Blutgruppenformel in der Berliner Bevölkerung," *Klinische Wochenschrift* 3 (1924): 1078.
17. Georg Schneider, "Weitere Beiträge zur Isohämagglutination," *Klinsche Wochenschrift* 4 (1925): 2383–7, and his article published somewhat later, "Ein Beitrag zur Blutgruppenforschung mit Untersuchungs-Ergebnissen der I. Internationalen Arbeiterolympiade," *Zeitschrift für Rassenphysiologie* 5 (1932): 140–3. See also Wilhelm Klein and H. Osthoff, "Haemagglutinine, Rasse- und anthropologische Merkmale," *Archiv für Rassen- und Gesellschafts-Biologie* 17 (1925): 371–8.
18. Max Gundel, "Rassenbiologische Untersuchungen an Strafangefangenen," *Klinische Wochenschrift* 5 (1926): 2165–6.
19. Hans Jacobsohn, "Uber die Blutgruppenzughörigkeit der Paralytiker," *Zeitschrift für die gesamte Neurologie und Psychologie* 105 (1926): 810–4.
20. For analysis of the völkisch link to blood group research, see Mazumdar, "Blood and Soil," 193–202. On the nationalist impact on medicine in the immediate postwar period, see Paul Weindling, *Health, Race and German Politics between National Unification and Nazism, 1870–1945* (Cambridge: Cambridge University Press, 1989), 305–25. For an individual case study of one doctor at this time, see Robert J. Lifton, *Nazi Doctors* (New York: Basic Books, 1986), 125–33.

21. Reche, "Zur ethnographie des abflusslosen Gebietes Deutsch-Ostafrikas," *Abhandlungen des hamburgisches Kolonialinstitut* 17 (1914): 1–129. For Reche's biographical background, see Geisenhainer, "'Rasse ist Schicksal'" and a more accessible summary, "'War in particular offers exceptionally favourable opportunities for surveying foreign racial material': The effects of World Wars on anthropologist Otto Reche's activities," *Anthropological Notebooks* 15 (2): 35–49. For a contemporary (and favorable) view that gives some indication of his stature at that time, see the festschrift in 1939 edited by Michael Hesch and Günther Spannaus, eds., *Kultur und Rasse* (Munich: Lehmanns Verlag, 1939). For his later role in the resettlement policy of the Nazis after the conquest of Poland, see Michael Burleigh, *Germany Turns Eastward* (Cambridge: Cambridge University Press, 1988), 166–76; and Karl Saller, *Rassenlehre des nationalsozialismus in Wissenschaft und Propagande* (Darmstadt: Progress Verlag, 1961), 48–9; 100–1.
22. No published or archival account has been found that indicates the first meeting of Reche and Steffan. There is, however, indirect evidence in addition to the coincidence of being in the same place at the same time. Reche joined the Nazi party late (in 1937) which meant certain privileges were not available to him. In the process of petitioning to back date his membership, a colleague attested that Reche had formed a "völkisch-soziale Partei" in 1919 in Hamburg with the motto, "Germany for the Germans." This would have given Reche the visibility to attract the attention of the returning war veteran Steffan. Letter dated Sept. 19, 1940, from Justizrat Willibald v. Zezschwitz to Reichsschatzminister Schwarz, Berlin Document Center, Partei Kanzlei Correspondence.
23. The article by Fritz Verzar and Oskar Weszeczky, "Rassenbiologische Untersuchungen mittels Isohamagglutinen," *Biochemische Zeitschrift* 133 (1922): 33–9, was one of those publications by foreigners appearing in German journals that informed German researchers about blood group distribution research in the early 1920s. Steffan's first article acknowledged the receipt of test sera from Verzar.

    Limited information was found about this stage of Steffan's career. He was born in 1885 near Heidelberg and received his medical degree from Freiburg i.B. with a thesis on "Operative Geburtshilfe." According to naval records, Steffan served on the small cruiser "Arcona" from May 1914 to July 1918, and then the "Bremse." In a 1921 article, "Beobachtungen über den Verlauf der künstlichen Infektion der Ratte mit Trypanosome," *Archiv für Schiffs-und Tropenhygiene* 25 (1921): 241–7, and also in a 1922 article in the same journal, Steffan listed himself as a naval medical officer at the Hamburg tropical medicine Institute. In a 1923 article, however, Steffan gave as his title, naval medical officer at the Ostsee Station, Kiel.

24. Paul Steffan, "Bedeutung der Bluntuntersuchung für die Bluttransfusion und die Rassenforschung," *Archiv für Rassen-und Gesellschafts-Biologie* 15 (1923): 148.
25. Steffan, "Bedeutung," p. 137. Even though the *Archiv* was the "official organ of the German Race Hygiene Society," and it was taken over by Lehmann in 1922 Peter Weingart, Jürgen Kroll and Kurt Bayertz *Rasse, Blut und Gene* (Frankfurt: Suhrkamp, 1988), p. 200 insist, "the *Archiv* remained until 1933 to a great extent free from taking one-sided political positions." Weindling, *Health, Race and German Politics*, 129–30, 314–5, shows that Ploetz was anti-völkisch and almost obsessed with asserting the scientific legitimacy of the journal.
26. Klein and Osthoff, "Haemagglutinine, Rasse- und anthropologische Merkmale." The *Archiv* was unusual among anthropological journals in the world to show such an early interest in the blood group research. As seen below, the only comparable journal was the *Ruskii Antropologicheskii Zhurnal.*
27. Steffan, "Weitere Ergebnisse der Rassenforschung mittels serologischer Methoden," *Mitteilungen der anthropologischen Gesellschaft in Wien* 56 (1926): 78–109; Steffan, "Rassenergebnisse der Blutforschung," *Die Sonne* 3 (1926): 49–64; Reche, "Fortschritte in der Anthropologie," *Mitteilungen der anthropologischen Gesellschaft in Wien* 57 (1927): 12–21; Reche, "Blutgruppenforschung und Anthropologie," *Volk und Rasse* 3 (1928): 1–13.
28. Reche, "Fortschritte in der Anthropologie," 18–9.
29. Mazumdar, "Blood and Soil," 191.
30. See, for example, Otto Reche, "Deutsche Gesellschaft für Blutgruppenforschung - Aufruf," *Artzliche Rundschau* 36 (1926): 347–8.
31. Carbon-copy of Schiff letter to Steffan, October 20, 1926; in Bernstein Archives, Niedersachsische Landes- und Universitätsbibliothek.
32. Hirszfeld letter to Bernstein, Nov. 18, 1927; in Bernstein Archives, Niedersächsische Landes-und Universitätsbibliothek.
33. "Mitteilungen des Vorstandes der Deutschen Gesellschaft für Blutgruppenforschung," *Zeitschrift für Rassenphysiologie* 1 (1928): 65; "Mitgliederverzeichnis," ibid. 2 (1930): 193–6.
34. Steffan, "Die Arbeitweise der Deutschen Gesellschaft für Blutgruppenforschung," *Zeitschrift für Rassenphysiologie* 1 (1928): 9.
35. Reche, "Die Deutsche Gesellschaft für Blutgruppenforschung - Aufruf," 447.
36. H. Schlossberger, K. Laubenheimer, et al., "Blutgruppenuntersuchungen an Schulkindern in der Umgebung von Frankfurt am Main," *Medizinische Klinik* 24 (1928): 851–2.

37. Paul Weindling, *Health, Race and German Politics*, 465–69. For published discussion of the Prussian Health Council, see Preußische Landesgesundheitsrat, "Ueber Blutgruppenuntersuchungen in den Schulen," *Veröffentlichungen aus dem Gebiete der Medizinalverwaltung* 25 (1927):278–306.
38. This was incorporated into Eugen Fischer's February 1928 proposal to the Emergency Fund for German Science (*Notgemeinschaft der Deutschen Wissenschaft*) to do a national anthropological survey that included blood group tests. Reche was one of seven anthropologists directing local research teams, and all but one of the directors was a member of the German Society for Blood Group Research. Eventually the Rockefeller Foundation gave 10,000 marks a year for five years beginning in 1930 for the project whose results were published as *Deutsche Rassenkunde*. Fischer excluded Jewish researchers from the entire venture.
39. As mentioned above, Lehmann also owned the *Archiv für Rassen-und Gesellschaftsbiologie* which published Steffan's first article, and he created the journal *Volk und Rasse* in 1926 which Reche edited. For more on Lehmann, see Mazumdar, "Blood and Soil," 199; and Klaus-Dieter Thomann, "Exkurs: Der medizinische Verlag J. F. Lehmann, Förderer und Finanzier von alldeutschem Verband und NSDAP," in *Medizin, Faschismus und Widerstand: Drei Beiträge*, eds. Barbara Bromberger, Hans Maustich and Klaus Dieter Thomann (Cologne: Paul Rugenstein, 1985), 97–110.

    An excellent account of neo-conservative publishers, of whom Lehmann combined the most extreme views and largest measure of success, see Gary D. Stark, *Entrepreneurs of Ideology: Neo-conservative Publishers in Germany, 1890–1933* (Chapel Hill: University of North Carolina Press, 1981). For an example of the heights to which the publisher rose during the Third Reich, see the 50th anniversary commemorative volume, Julius Friedrich Lehmann, *Fünfzig Jahre: J. F. Lehmanns Verlag, 1890–1940* (Munich: Lehmanns, 1940).
40. Reche, "Zum Geleit," *Zeitschrift für Rassenphysiologie* 1 (1928): 2–3; Reche, *Arztliche Rundschau* 36 (1926): 347.
41. On the importance of the *Münchener medizinische Wochenschrift* to Lehmann as a legitimate medical journal, see Stark, p. 20. On Springer and medical publications in Germany, see Heinz Sorkowski, *Springer Verlag* (Berlin: Springer, 1992), 1:280–2.
42. Geisenhainer, "'Rasse ist Schicksal,'" 130.
43. For an example of one effort at the time that combined anthropological and medical goals, see Susan Gross Solomon, "Soviet-German Syphilis Expedition to Buriat Mongolia, 1928: Scientific Research on National Minorities," *Slavic Review* 52 (1993): 204–32.

44. The phrase is Mark Adams, "Science, Ideology and Structure," 161. For more on Koltsov and the Institute, see also Adams, "Sergei Chetverikov, the Koltsov Institute, and the Evolutionary Synthesis," in *The Evolutionary Synthesis,* ed. Ernst Mayr and William B. Provine, 242–78 (Cambridge, Mass: Harvard University Press, 1980).

In a letter to Charles Davenport announcing he had organized a Russian eugenics society, Koltsov complained of the hardships of doing research. In particular, he asked for information about American work but also boasted of his own research on "the heredity of the chemical properties of blood." Koltsov kept up a correspondence through 1928. Koltsov letter to Davenport, June 25, 1921, APS Davenport Papers B:27.

45. Nikolai K. Koltsov, [the agglutination of human blood], *Uspechi Experimentalnoi Biologii*, (1922); Victor V. Bunak, [on agglutination reaction of human races], *Ruskii Antropologicheskii Zhurnal* [at this date it was also titled *Journal russe d'anthropologie*, with abstracts and some articles in French] 13 (1924): 115–9. Bunak, "Einige Daten uber die Isohamagglutination bei verschiedenen asiatischen Stammen," *Archiv für Rassen- und Gesellschaftsbiologie* 17 (1925): 316–8. For a brief biographical reference on Bunak, see Adams, 1990, p. 168.

46. Vishnevskii's article [New method for racial diagnosis with respect to the Chuvash] appeared in the Co*mptes rendus de l'Academie des Sciences de l'U.R.S.S.* (1924), as cited in G. I. Petrov, "Zur Frage der Isoagglutination des Blutes bei den Tadjiken," *Zeitschrift für Rassenphysiologie* 1 (1928): 90. The following year (1925) the Chuvash became an autonomous Soviet Socialist Republic.

47. *Ukrainisches Zentralblatt für Blutgruppenforschung*, 1 (1927), 1. For more on the Ukrainian Academy of Sciences which functioned autonomously in the 1920s, see Loren K. Graham, *The Soviet Academy of Sciences and the Communist Party*, 1927–32 (Princeton: Princeton University Press, 1967), 170–2. For background on Ukrainian nationalism during the period, see George Liber, *Soviet Nationality Policy, Urban Growth, and Identity Change in the Ukrainian SSR, 1923–1934* (New York: Cambridge University Press, 1992).

48. On the burst of publications in the Ukrainian language, see Liber, *Soviet Nationality Policy*, 110–2 and Liber, "Language, Literacy, and Book Publishing in Ukrainian SSR, 1923–1928," *Slavic Review* 41 (1982): 673–85.

49. Vishnevskii, "Anthropology in USSR in the Course of 17 Years (1917 to 1934)," *American Journal of Physical Anthropology* 21 (1936): 10–1; Vishnevskii, "Die Blutgruppenfrage aus dem IV Kongress der Zoologen, Anatomen und Histologen der U. d. S. S. R.," *Ukrainisches Zentralblatt für Blutgruppenforschung* 5 (1930): 47–55; G. I. Petrov, "Zur Frage des

Korrelativen zusammenhanges anthropometrischer Merkmale mit Blutgruppen," ibid., 73–88.

50. Viktor V. Bunak, "Einige Daten," 317. He stated, for example, "for the twelve Asian, Mongolian, and Turkish ethnic groups, the Hirszfeld Index varies within the rather narrow range between 0.55 and 1.80."
51. William C. Boyd, "Blood Groups," *Tabulae Biologicae* 17, no. 2 (1939): 189–98; 209–22. The next closest was Germany with 225. On other expeditions to Asia, see Solomon, "Soviet-German Syphilis Expedition," 208, n. 20.
52. See, for example, Avdeeva and Gritsevich, "[On the question of isohemagglutination in humans]," *Biulletin' Moskovskogo obshchestva ispytatelei prirody* 1 (1924): 108; and M. Dykhno, "[On the constitutional meaning of isoagglutination indices of human blood]," *Nauchnye izvestiia Smolenskogo Universiteta* 3 (1926): 93; W. J. Rubaschkin, "Der biologische Rassenindex der deutschen Koloniasten der Ukraine," *Ukrainische Zentralblatt für Blutgruppenforschung*, 1 (1927): 65–71; and Alexander Eisenberg, "Zur Frage nach den Isoagglutinationsgruppen des Blutes bei Menschen," *Folia Haematologica*, 36 (1928), 336. Their findings of biochemical race index are summarized as follows:

			Index	*Index for*
Author	*locale*	*date*	*for Jews*	*local popln*
Avdeeva, et al.	Moscow	1924	1.9	
Dychno	Smolensk	1926	1.7	
Eisenberg	Kharkiv	1928	1.81	1.53
Rubashkin	Ukraine	1927	1.6	1.44

53. There have been some suggestions of German colleagues inspiring the studies of these colonists, but Rubaschkin, "Der biologische Rassenindex," said he only undertook his study of German colonists in passing as part of a larger study in the Ukraine. To the extent he was prompted, it was by a similar study of German settlers in Hungary by Verzar and Weczecky in 1922.
54. A. M. Ljachovetskii, [The importance of hemo-agglutination in malaria] *Moskovskii meditsinskii zhurnal* 4 (1924): 25–36. On Tuberculosis, see Avdeeva and Gritsevich, [On the question], 108; Pantschenko and Agte, [Blood groups and Tuberculosis], *Archiv für klinische und experimentale Medizin* (1924); L. A. Barinstein, [Die Bluttransfusion im Lichte gegenwartiger Kenntnisse], *Sovremennye meditsina* 2 (1924): 39.

55. M. M. Alperin, "Ueber die Beziehungen zwischen Blutgruppen und Tubercule," *Beiträge zur Klinik der Tuberkulose* 64 (1926): 500. For example, in the same issue of the *Beiträge* an article by Julius Hollo and Wilhelm Léonard, "Gibt es einen Unterschied in der Häufigkeit der einzelnen Blutgruppen bei Lungentuberkulösen und bei gesunden Menschen?" 513–4, made no mention of the Soviet work. See also O. Connerth, "Uber Blutgruppen bei Tuberkulose," *Zeitschrift für Tuberkulose* 48 (1927): 140–2; or Zdislaw Swider and Natan Kon, "Badania nad grupami serologicznemi krwi u gruzlikow, I & II [Examination of groups of serum in tumors; Research on serological groups in the tuberculous; pigmentary syndromes, blood-groups and individual predisposition to tuberculosis]," *Polska Gazeta Lekarska* 6 (1927): 597–8; 972. And elsewhere, Rene Dujarric de la Rivière and Nicholas Kossovitch, "Au sujet des groups sanguins des tuberculeux et des cancereux," *Comptes rendus de la Société de biologie* 97 (1927): 137–9, did not cite Alperin, nor did American researchers Raphael et al. cite any Soviet references in a 1927 article, Theophile Raphael, Olive M. Searle, and William Scholten, "Blood Groups in Schizophrenic and Manic-depressive Psychosis," *American Journal of Psychiatry* 7 (1927): 153–61.
56. Ljachovetskii's article in *Moskovskii meditsinskii zhurnal* was, however, cited in the 1925 volume of *Index Medicus.* Communication was not much better in the Soviet Union. Neither Lisunova nor Minkevich's papers at the 1925 congress cited Ljachovetski's work. In fact, Lisunova credits Koltsov with suggesting her research on malaria and blood groups. A. Lisunova, "Gruppovaya gemoagglyutinatsiya i malyariya [Hemoagglutination Groups and Malaria]," Trudy 3-go vseross *Syezd malyar Moskva* (1925): 173.
57. Geisenhainer, "The effects of world wars," 40.
58. Mazumdar, "Blood and Soil," 195.
59. William H. Schneider, "Chance and Social Setting in the Application of the Discovery of Blood Groups," *Bulletin of the History of Medicine* 57 (1983): 553–4.
60. See Ute Deichmann and Benno Müller-Hill, "Biological Research at Universities and Kaiser Wilhelm Institutes in Nazi Germany," in *Science, Technology and National Socialism*, eds. Monika Renneburg and Mark Walker (Cambridge: Cambridge University Press, 1994), 160–1.
61. Bernstein made several requests for support to the Rockefeller Foundation while in the U.S. See Nov. 14, 1933, Note on Bernstein, RF 1.1 Ser. 100, Box 130, Folder 1603; background letter on Bernstein from Eric Ponder of Cold Spring Harbor Biological Laboratory to Raymond Fosdick October 30, 1939. One other of the Jewish researchers mentioned by

Schiff in his letter to Steffan also emigrated: Hans Sachs who directed the Cancer Institute at Heidelberg.

62. Fritz Schiff, *Blutgruppen und ihre Anwendungsgebiete* (Berlin: Springer, 1933); Fritz Schiff and Otto von Verscheurer, "Serologischer Untersuchungen an Zwillingen. II Mitteilung," *Zeitschrift für Morphologie und Anthropologie* 32 (1933): 244–9; Fritz Schiff and August Hien, "Zur Serologie der Berliner Bevölkerung. IV Mitteilung," *Klinische Wochenschrift* 13 (1934): 375–6.

    On Schiff's pioneer role in establishing the use of blood group findings in legal proceedings, see Herbert Patzak, "Ursprünge gerichtlich annerkannter Blutgruppenbefunde in deutschen Paternitätsgutachten" (Thesis: Marburg, 1990), pp. 32–3; 50–5. Lucie Adelsberger, one of his students, credits Schiff with "the first comprehensive studies on the group-specific substances in organs and secretions." See "In memory of Fritz Schiff," *Proceedings of the Virchow Medical Society* (New York) 9 (1950): 91–2.

63. See Landsteiner's introduction to Fritz Schiff and William C. Boyd, *Blood Grouping Technic* (New York: Interscience, 1940), p. iii.

64. Michael Hesch, "Papillarmuster bei Eingeborenen der Loyalty-Inseln. Beziehungen zwischen Papillarmustern und Blutgruppen," *Zeitschrift für Rassenphysiologie* 5 (1932): 163–8.

65. On techniques, see Paul Steffan, "Blutübertragung in der Kriegsmarine," *Veroffentlichungen aus dem Gebiete des Marine-Sanitätswesens*, 28 (1936): 5–40; Schreiber, "Zur Technik der Blutgruppenbestimmung bei Massenuntersuchungen," *Deutsche Militärarzt* 1 (1936): 97–9; G.W. Pontani, "Zur Frage der Technik der Blutgruppenbestimmung bei Massenuntersuchungen. Gleichzeitig ein Beitrag zur Blutgruppenverteilung in Schleswig-Holstein," *Deutsche Militärarzt* 2 (1937): 19–24; Hermann Eyer, "Ein einfaches Verfahren zur Steigerung der Sicherheit von Blutgruppenbestimmungen bei Massenuntersuchungen," *Deutsche Militärarzt* 4 (1939): 271–3.

    Reports of mass testing can be found in H. Hornung, "Uber die Beziehung der Blutgruppen zu rassischen Merkmalen," *Münchener Medizinische Wochenschrift* 87 (1940): 125–8; J. Mrugowsky, and H. Bernhart, "Die Ausführung von massen Untersuchungen auf Blutgruppenzugehörigkeit und das Eintätowaren der aufgefundenen Blutgruppen," *Münchener Medizinische Wochenschrift* 88 (1941): 669–72; Helmut Bernhart, "Beitrag zur Blutgruppengeographie Gross-Deutschlands," *Zeitschrift für Hygiene und Infektionskrankheiten* 123 (1942): 675–7.

    Of these researchers, Mrugowsky went on to achieve infamy because of his medical experiments on concentration camp inmates. These included tests of the safety of old blood plasma for transfusion, as well as experiments with typhus and malaria at Buchenwald. He was found guilty and hanged. See *Trials of War Criminals before the Nuernberg Military Tribunals* (Washington: Government Printing Office, 1949) 1:517–8; 598–606; 2:241–8.

66. For background, see Sheila Fitzpatrick, "Cultural Revolution as Class War," in *Cultural Revolution in Russia, 1928–1931*, ed. Sheila Fitzpatrick (Bloomington: Indiana University Press, 1978), 5–40. David Joravsky, *Soviet Marxism and Natural Science* (Columbia: Columbia University Press, 1961), pp. 233–49, calls the period from 1929 to 1932 "the Great Break."
67. For an example in one field, see David Joravsky, "Construction of Stalinist Psyche," in Fitzpatrick, *Cultural Revolution in Russia*, 105–28, which shows the relatively late impact on psychoneurological sciences. On the purge of the Academy of Sciences from September 1929 to March 1930 see Graham, *Soviet Academy of Sciences*, pp. 120–53.
68. *Ukrainisches Zentralblatt für Blutgruppenforschung und Transfusion* 1 (6) (1931): 5.
69. M. S. Schindler, "Der gegenwartige Stand der Lehre von Blutgruppen," ibid. 1 (6) (1932): 17.
70. Studies by Shamov and M. Kostiukov began in 1927 and were first published as, [Question of homoplasty from the cadaver. Blood transfusion from the cadaver], Trudi 3 *Ukrainskii siezda Khirurhiia* 18 (1929): 184–9. For an English summary, see Vladimir Nikolayevich Shamov, "Transfusion of Stored Cadaver Blood," *Lancet* (1937): 306–9.
71. The specific article was by L. M. Friedmann, "Die Blutgruppen grusinischer Kinder und der Zusammenhang des Gruppenmermals mit anderen erblichen Merkmale," Ukrainische*s Zentralblatt für Blutgruppenforschung* 4 (1930): 279–89.
72. M. S. Plissetzky and B. Smulevitsch, "Die Rassentheorie -- Klassentheorie,"*Journal d'anthropologie* 2 (1934): 23.
73. Mazumdar, "Blood and Soil," 202–9.
74. Geisenhainer, "The Effects of World Wars," 41–6; Mazumdar, "Blood and Soil," 211–16; and Burleigh, 166–76. For a description of the screening process, see Robert L. Koehl, *RKFDV: German Resettlement and Population Policy, 1939–1945* (Cambridge: Harvard University Press, 1957), 104–110.
75. Robert Stigler, "Rassenphysiologische Untersuchungen an farbigen Kriegsgefangenen in einem Kriegsgefangenlager," *Zeitschrift für Rassenphysiologie* 13 (1943): 26–57.
76. Vishnevskii, "Blood Groups of Tungus," *Human Biology* 8 (1936): 273–8. On the Leningrad Museum and Institute of the People of the North, see Tage Kemp, "Report of Visits to Various Institutes, Laboratories, etc. for

Human Genetics in Europe," July–October 1934, Rockefeller Archives, RG 1.2, 713, Box 2, Folder 16, pp. 37–38; and Vishnevskii, "Anthropology in the U.S.S.R.," 1–17.

77. Dahr published almost a dozen articles on the latest discoveries of ABO sub-groups and MN and P groups in apes, human families, and twins from 1936 to 1940. His popular articles were "Blutgruppenforschung und Rassenhygiene," *Ziel und Weg* 9 (1939): 98–108, which was the official organ of National Socialist doctors and in which Dahr listed himself as "komm. leiter des Amtes für Rassenpolitik im kreis der NSDAP Köln-sud." Another article was "Menschlichen Blutgruppen, -Untergruppen, und -Faktoren," *Volk und Rasse* 15 (1940): 13–20. Both articles were relatively restrained, considering the nature of the journals, about the claims of links between blood and race.

CHAPTER 4

Blood Group Research in Great Britain, France, and the U.S. Between the World Wars

Three countries where scientists ultimately developed strong interests in the new field of blood group research were Great Britain, France, and the U.S. Although initially their publication record on blood group distribution was greatly exceeded by that of researchers in Germany and the Soviet Union, a strong interest in the field developed in each of the three countries by the late 1930s. In fact, this became the basis for the explosion of research on blood groups in the years following the Second World War. The groundwork for this postwar work was laid in the 1930s, during which time researchers in Britain, France and the U.S. increased their publications from the 1920s, while in Germany and the Soviet Union there was a precipitous decline.

Of course, it should be no surprise that there was an interest in the new field of serology by American, French, and English researchers. At the beginning of the twentieth century, they, along with the Germans, had the best developed modern scientific traditions and medical research facilities in the world. Indeed, the most surprising feature of their research record was the relative lack of interest at first. Moreover, the timing, extent, and nature of their interest, as well as application of their findings, were very different, from each other as well as compared to researchers in other countries. Hence, a comparison of these developments offers another

W. H. Schneider, *Blood Groups and Human Heredity, 1900–1950*, Medicine and Biomedical Sciences in Modern History, https://doi.org/10.1007/978-3-031-69844-6_4

example of differences in the manner in which scientists came to the research. It also shows both similarities and differences in the workings of chance and local circumstances in their common pursuit of scientific truth.[1]

Background and Initial Interest

Although Landsteiner and other central Europeans such as Paul Ehrlich, Julius Morgenroth, Emil von Dungern, and Ludwik Hirszfeld are widely recognized for the initial discoveries about blood groups, there were many others working on the properties of blood at the time. For example, English and French contemporaries Samuel Shattock and Philippe Pagniez, as well as Jules Bordet in Belgium, worked simultaneously on the phenomenon.[2] In addition, researchers at hospitals and research institutes in the U.S., France, and Britain quickly followed up and added their own new discoveries to those coming out of central Europe prior to 1914. Reuben Ottenberg in New York who worked on blood typing before transfusion, made one of the first suggestions of Mendelian inheritance of immunologic properties.[3] Likewise, Ludwig Hektoen in Chicago and William Moss at Johns Hopkins are other notable researchers in the U.S. who quickly took up research and made key discoveries about blood groups.

The experience of the First World War only increased the interest in the properties of blood, especially as they related to transfusion needs. The simultaneous discovery of citrate as an anticoagulant (making blood storage possible) by researchers in Argentina, Britain, and Belgium demonstrates this widespread interest. The necessities of war increased the use and knowledge of transfusion on both sides of the trenches, giving a new generation of doctors experience with the handling of blood and its properties. Individual French, British, Canadian, and German researchers published some of the results of their experience with transfusion in 1915 and 1916, and the practice accelerated in 1917 with the arrival of the Americans on the Western front.[4]

Reports of transfusions grew independent of the war. *Index Medicus* cited an increasing number of articles well before the first publications on the war experience began appearing late in 1916. The war conditions, however, gave surgeons the opportunity to perform transfusions with enough frequency not only to perfect their techniques but also to produce a critical mass of data about the typing of donors when time permitted. In addition, the mass numbers of conscripts under medical surveillance made possible the first large-scale testing of blood types during and after the war, such as was done by the Hirszfelds in Macedonia.

In France one of the leading practitioners of blood transfusion was Emile Jeanbrau, a veteran of Verdun who first used citrated blood for an indirect transfusion in May 1917. He and his student Georges Giraud were among the most frequent authors of articles on transfusion and blood groups in the years coming out of the conflict.[5] British doctors preferred the indirect method of transfusion which first drained blood from the donor into a temporary storage container before giving it to the patient. They also learned other techniques from Canadian and American practitioners.[6] To a remarkable degree, doctors from the U.S. carried with them to France conditions of practice from home, as medical schools such as Harvard and Johns Hopkins set up their own hospital operations behind the front.[7]

In a sense this growing interest in blood and its properties was a common experience of the First World War, but the first testing of blood type distribution by researchers in the U.S., Britain, and France also showed some important differences. Of the three, it was the Americans who consistently showed the most interest in the distribution of blood groups. This is reflected in several isolated research reports that arose outside the immediate practical needs of wartime. For example, doctors at Ft. McPherson in Georgia reported testing in 1919 on a similar scale to what the Hirszfelds had done in Macedonia. The reason for their tests of over 1000 soldiers, however, did not go much beyond an interest in the techniques of blood typing, and although they reported the frequency of the four types, they made no attempt to compare it to other reports of distribution or break down their subjects into sub-groups for comparison. Another example of isolated interest was a 1919 article reporting tests on 131 newborns and children conducted by Johns Hopkins pediatrician William M. Happ, who looked at the appearance of blood types in newborns as well as their match to their mother's type.[8] Although the questions raised eventually led to a line of later research that produced the discovery of the Rh blood groups, Happ's results provided neither immediate inspiration for others nor any continuation of his own investigation of the phenomenon.

Another example of the numerous American researchers who became interested in blood group distribution at this time was Alson R. Kilgore, who went to work at the Red Cross Hospital of Shanghai in 1916 after finishing Harvard Medical School. Shortly after his arrival an emergency transfusion produced a hemolytic accident at the hospital, which gave Kilgore the opportunity to introduce some of the rapid agglutination tests developed recently in the U.S., that could test blood before transfusions even in an emergency. He took blood samples from an American doctor at Beijing whose blood type had been determined back home. Then following the transfusion, Kilgore and his Chinese colleague J. Hua Liu took the opportunity to crossmatch and determine the blood type of 100 Chinese subjects.[9] In their findings and indicative of the pervasive racism at the time, their most important conclusion was that Chinese blood could be grouped into the same four types as Europeans. Moreover, they went on, "Chinese bloods inter-agglutinate with European bloods just as they do with Chinese." Most noteworthy for purposes of the present study was that Kilgore and Liu found a significant difference between the distribution of blood types among the Chinese and Europeans. The fact that this article was published in 1918, meant that their discovery of differences in distribution appeared before the Hirszfelds' findings the following year. Of course, the small sample size and the limited circulation of the *China Medical Journal* severely limited the impact on Kilgore and Liu's research; hence, it is another example of isolated work, albeit telling of the general interest in the subject.

It was two years before another article was published on blood group distribution by American researchers, but the fact that there were four such articles in 1921 shows the continuing interest in the subject. One, by William L. Culpepper and Marjorie Abelson of the Parke Davis Laboratory in Detroit, was on another large group of 5000 subjects. Their interest was similar to the Ft. McPherson doctors mentioned above.[10] Results of a second large-scale testing project on blood groups and their relation to disease were also published that year by J. Arthur Buchanan and Edith T. Higley, who looked back at records for 3446 patients at the Mayo Clinic between 1917 and 1921.[11] Their research was inspired by an article published a few months earlier by the Scottish doctor William Alexander, who suggested a possible correlation between blood types and "malignant disease" based on 50 cases he had observed at hospitals in Dundee.[12] The third article published that year by American researchers was by Cristina Cabrera and Herbert W. Wade of the Department of Pathology at the Philippines General Hospital. Their research most closely resembled the Hirszfelds' in that they looked for differences in the distribution of blood groups in 204 Filipino subjects, male and compared them to other published tests of Chinese and American subjects. Although they cited the work of Kilgore in China, they were unaware of the work of the Hirszfelds.[13] The fourth article was by Ottenberg who tested 286 parents and children to confirm the Mendelian inheritance of blood types.[14]

One can already see in this initial research on blood group distribution by Americans some characteristics that would typify later work. This included the abundance of research subjects and a variety of settings and motivations for the research. For example, the existence of large numbers of army recruits, clinical patients, and exotic populations was an outgrowth of the American context that was defined by the great size and diversity of the populations and institutions in the country. From the start American research reflected these influences. In 1922 Julian Lewis and Deborah L. Henderson published the results of their tests of 270 blacks in Chicago, and the next year Arthur F. Coca and Olin Diebert published their landmark article describing the very high percentage of type O blood found in tests of a thousand native Americans.[15]

Despite the breadth of this interest by U.S. researchers, they also showed a relative isolation from the work of Europeans, especially those on the continent. The Hirszfelds' 1919 article, although published in *Lancet*, was not cited by American researchers until 1921. Coca's early interest in blood groups dates back to when Americans made efforts to keep up with the latest work of Europeans; in fact, he trained before the war with Hirszfeld at Heidelberg under Von Dungern. Another feature of American interest that will be examined in more detail below is the significant number of articles published in the U.S. with female co-authors.

There was some initial interest in the distribution of blood groups in Britain that was independent of the Hirszfelds' research as seen in Alexander's ground-breaking 1921 article which tested the association of disease and blood groups. He cited no other research in the article, and Alexander never published again on the subject. It was, however, an inspiration for later research on blood groups and disease, most immediately in a 1922 article by Buchanan and Higley which tested patients at the Mayo Clinic. Independent of Alexander but citing the Hirszfelds' 1919 article and some of the American work were two articles published that same year in *Lancet* and the *British Medical Journal* by S. C. Dyke of St. Thomas' Hospital in London.[16]

A second subject of interest by British researchers who tested large numbers for blood group distribution were the various populations in the far-flung reaches of the British empire. Among these early articles were those based on tests done in South Africa (1921), Australia (1922), and

Samoa (1924), which attempted to place the indigenous populations in the framework established by the Hirszfeld biochemical index.[17] Hence, the inspiration was similar to the line of research by Americans who looked at the different populations the U.S. had acquired through territorial expansion and immigration in the nineteenth and early twentieth centuries.

The publication pattern of British research on overseas populations differed significantly from that of researchers in the U.S. the next two decades. For example, from the start research on the blood group distribution among Australian aborigines appeared in the locally published *Australian Medical Journal*. Likewise, the first article published on subjects in South Africa appeared in a local journal. Although Cabrera's work in the then U.S.-occupied Philippines appeared in a locally published journal, that proved to be an exception, as almost all subsequent research on native Americans and overseas populations appeared in journals published in the U.S. Subsequent research on subjects in British colonial settings, on the other hand, was published in local journals.[18]

An obvious effect of this decentralized practice of British medical publication apparent at the outset was a limit on the audience reached back in the metropole. There is evidence, however, that it likely would not have mattered even if all the imperial and Commonwealth research had appeared in journals published in Britain. For example, the Hirszfelds' 1919 article appeared in *Lancet*, followed shortly by the Alexander and Dyke articles in other major medical journals (*British Journal of Experimental Pathology* and *British Medical Journal*) which reached a wide audience. Yet despite their suggestions of new medical as well as anthropological applications of the blood group distribution discoveries, a recent study concluded that interest in blood group research was "almost totally absent from Britain during the 1920s"; there were virtually no further articles published by English researchers during the remainder of the decade.[19]

French Research in the 1920s and 1930s

There is no immediate or obvious explanation for researchers in Britain not following up on the early interest but a possible clue comes from a comparison to what happened in France. To put the comparison in a broader context, the graph in Fig. 4.1 shows the frequency of articles published on blood group distribution testing by British, French, and American researchers between the two world wars.

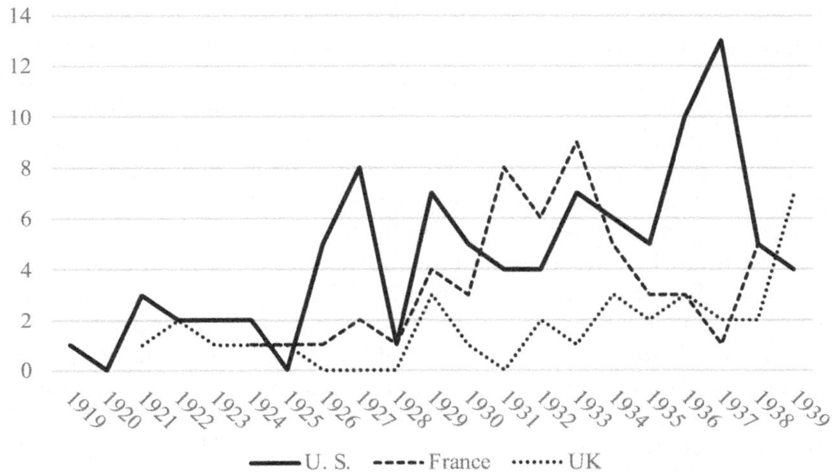

Fig. 4.1 Articles on blood group distribution by U.S., British, and French researchers, 1919–1939

There are several features of this data which beg explanation (and will be referred to later), but for now it is the initial pattern of the 1920s that is most instructive of why British interest remained low and the French steadily grew.

In France, as elsewhere interest in the blood groups was stimulated by the wartime practice of blood transfusion.[20] One of the most cited researchers was Emile Jeanbrau who, along with others, published articles on techniques of transfusion as well as various subjects related to the blood group discoveries. Typical was a January 1919 *Presse médicale* background article by a student of Jeanbrau's which, although ignoring Landsteiner and giving credit for discovery of the blood groups to the American Moss (misspelled Moos in the article), nevertheless provided a detailed description of how to test for blood types. It also described the importance of blood typing for anthropology and legal medicine as well as transfusion.[21]

Jeanbrau offers a good albeit dramatic example of how the war changed attitudes about the importance of blood groups for transfusion. Prior to and during the war, Jeanbrau like many surgeons rarely did blood compatibility testing, because he thought the urgency of the transfusions was greater than what his experience had shown was a low risk of compatibility problems. The end of the war (and wartime exigencies) plus the development of more rapid and simpler testing of blood type meant there was no longer an excuse for not testing. Moreover, transfusion accidents were more visible in civilian practice because they were less likely to be masked by other complications such as from war injuries, nor could they be accepted as unfortunate by-products of wartime conditions.

Despite these changes, surgeons in France at first continued to express their wartime view which minimized the dangers of hemolytic reactions. As late as 1923 in a presentation to the Congrès français de chirurgerie, Jeanbrau qualified a statement about the need to test in order to avoid hemolysis as follows, "But in the case of life-threatening hemorrhage, do not hesitate to give a transfusion without a prior test. The danger of fatal hemolysis from a donor chosen at random does not appear to exceed in effect 3 per cent."[22] Such statements by Jeanbrau and others were roundly criticized by fellow surgeons such as Georges Rosenthal, a former chef de service at Sainte-Antoine Hospital in Paris, who had also been one of the pioneers of blood transfusion in the French army during the war. In a 1925 article Rosenthal was adamant in his condemnation of these older attitudes toward testing. "*Never transfuse blindly; there is danger of death, and urgency is not an excuse for an inevitable error*"[23] [Italics are Rosenthal's]. These criticisms did their job. An article by Jeanbrau shortly thereafter made no reference to foregoing testing. He urged instead that if normal tests were impossible, then "indirect" or "biological" testing of compatibility be done, which entailed transfusing small amounts of the donor's blood (2–3 cc) at the beginning, then pausing every half minute to see if the patient showed any signs of hemolytic incompatibility before proceeding with the full transfusion.[24]

In the half dozen years following the war, publications about several features of the blood groups appeared in France with a frequency indicating interest comparable to other countries. This included original research on techniques of transfusion, studies of the blood groups of newborns and maternal-fetal incompatibility, as well as theoretical articles on medico-legal applications and summaries of the latest work in other countries.[25] Moreover, these postwar articles were published by researchers throughout France. Paul Michon in Nancy, for example, published several articles on blood groups and transfusion, while research done in such places as Strasbourg, Montpellier, and Alfort also appeared in the early 1920s.[26] The *Comptes rendus de la Société de biologie* was particularly important in allowing provincial researchers access to a national readership. The communications of the meetings of provincial societies as well as several foreign countries appeared in the journal.

There were, nevertheless, two noteworthy absences in this research in France during the period right after the war: participation by scientists at the Pasteur Institute and studies of the distribution of blood types from large samplings of the population.[27] In the mid-1920s, however, several new developments not only filled this gap but generally reshaped the interest in blood group research in France. One general change was the beginning of specialization as the amount of serological work grew, but by far the most important development which began work in France along the lines of the Hirszfelds' research was the arrival of Nicholas Kossovitch at the Pasteur Institute in 1924.

Kossovitch was from the former Austro-Hungarian Empire and his career involved much moving about. Details about his early life are limited, but most accounts indicate that he was born in Belgrade and studied medicine in Russia.[28] Accounts differ whether he studied with Landsteiner's in Vienna or came to Paris before the outbreak of the First World War, but better known and more important for his future career was that he was in the Serbian army during the First World War and was stationed in Salonica with Hirszfeld for most of the conflict. Kossovitch came to Paris following the war, and in 1924 he obtained a position at the Pasteur Institute in the laboratory of René Dujarric de la Rivière. Kossovitch quickly showed the value of his experience, publishing an article the following year in the *CRSB* on the blood group distribution of Czechs, using results from testing of soldiers at Salonica. Shortly thereafter he joined Dujarric at a new Centre d'études des groupes sanguins established at the Pasteur Institute, and they published a series of studies that not only set the standard for blood group research in France but also gave the center a worldwide reputation for research in the field.[29]

Thanks largely to Kossovitch's work, and the prestige of the Pasteur Institute, France took a prominent place internationally in blood group research much earlier than Britain. Because of his training with Hirszfeld, an important focus of Kossovitch's research was the anthropological implications of blood type distribution among different human populations. The subjects of his research (at first done in conjunction with Dujarric and later with junior assistants) included the French population as a whole (and Alsatians in particular), plus foreigners such as Armenian emigrés in Paris. The results were often published in the *CRSB*, although Kossovitch also held an appointment at the Ecole d'Anthropologie and published just as often in its *Revue Anthropologique*.[30]

Of note, Kossovitch's published only one article (jointly authored with Dujarric) in the *Annales de l'Institut Pasteur*, a lengthy 1930 article that included important details for the preparation of test sera and techniques for obtaining reliable agglutination results. Dujarric and Kossovitch did not focus solely on anthropological testing; they also published important work on other applications. For example, in the late 1920s they studied blood type frequency of patients with tuberculosis and cancer in France. They also published an early article in the *Annales de médecine legale* on blood groups in legal medicine.[31]

Despite the initial breadth of research topics, given Kossovitch's interests and the Pasteur's worldwide network of "*filiales*," it was not long before the French-directed blood group research became predominantly anthropological with important work done in French colonies and other countries. The pattern of the research was either for established doctors at a local Pasteur Institute, such as Indochina or Tunisia, to report the results of their blood group testing or individual doctors in far-off locales (the Congo, French West Africa, or Madagascar) to send back their findings to the *CRSB*. In virtually every article published in France until the mid-1930s, the Pasteur Institute supplied the test sera, and often Kossovitch or Dujarric presented the paper to the Société de biologie. In 1931 Kossovitch made his first field trip to Morocco where he did blood tests of various populations in conjunction with other anthropological observations.[32]

The result was that French research on the anthropology of blood groups overshadowed studies of correlations between blood groups and pathological conditions or other presumably inherited traits. More precisely, 11 such articles were published on the latter in the interwar years, whereas fully 50 articles reported the distribution among populations in France and a variety of other countries and colonies overseas. Thus, the research results in these 11 articles had less impact in France, whereas in other countries the study of links to disease and other characteristics led to major research programs. For example, early on Raymond Turpin was greatly impressed with the blood groups and their potential use in medical genetics, but he was disappointed by the negative results of his own attempt to correlate "Down syndrome" (Trisomy 21) with blood type. Although this was contemporary with similar research in the 1930s by Lionel Penrose in England, the two researchers apparently did not correspond. Thus, the matter was dropped until Turpin's student Lejeune took it up and contacted Penrose after the Second World War.[33] An earlier, similar example occurred when Edouard Toulouse published results of blood tests on 287 mental patients in 1926 at his psychiatric clinic in Ste. Anne Hospital. Finding no simple correlation between mental conditions and blood type, he dropped this line of research.[34]

Without much interest in medical or human genetics until the late 1930s, French researchers were noticeably less inclined than their foreign colleagues to draw conclusion from their work about grand evolutionary schemes or other biological theories. The French therefore did not participate in debates with foreign colleagues about the existence of primordial races, the origins of peoples such as the Amerindians or Roma, and whether blood groups might predate human evolution because they exist in anthropoids. An exception was research appearing in a number of articles by French researchers on the blood group distribution of Jews which they found frequently mirrored the population where they lived. This was an important contribution to the larger question of whether Jews were a distinct race.[35] This broad debate was unusual, and such speculation based on blood group studies was more often made by French eugenicists or extreme xenophobes such as René Martial who argued, for example, that blood tests should be given to prospective immigrants from the east to keep those with blood type B out of France.[36]

Revival of British Interest in Blood Group Research

The French experience indicates that the timely arrival of Kossovitch stimulated the early interest in the distribution of blood groups. In Britain, by contrast, despite an auspicious start, publications by researchers on blood group distribution did not lead to a sustained interest until the 1930s.[37] This included little or no immediate testing of the distribution of blood types of the population in the British Isles. For the whole decade of the twenties, *Lancet* and the *British Medical Journal* published the results of blood testing by only one researcher, and he was stationed in Syria. There was only one more isolated article in *Lancet*—a 1930 study by a doctor similarly stationed in a remote South American post—before Lionel Penrose's 1932 article on Down syndrome and blood groups among inmates at Colchester marked a new interest in such research inspired from a very different perspective.[38]

This record clearly shows that despite early initial publications there was little interest for several years in blood groups shown by medical or anthropological researchers in Great Britain. Nor was there much interest among British eugenicists who might potentially have been concerned about the subjects of race and the inheritance of blood type. The English Eugenics Society's *Eugenics Review* mentioned some reports on blood group research in other countries beginning in 1925, but it carried no articles of original research. The *Annals of Eugenics* said absolutely nothing about the new field until R. A. Fisher took over the journal in 1934 and made it into the most important research publication on blood groups in Britain.

When interest in blood group studies eventually revived in the late 1920s, it was British anthropologists who belatedly recognized the value of the Hirszfelds' discoveries. By itself this was not unusual, since anthropologists were often the first to show interest elsewhere. In the U.S. and other countries, it was also not until the late 1920s that anthropologists began to notice the potential value of blood group research. But in those countries medical researchers had been conducting studies for several years by the time the anthropologists recognized their importance. In Britain, however, because of the lack of medical interest, when articles on blood group distribution began appearing in anthropological journals in the late 1920s, they were the first to signal the importance of the new field.

The earliest, albeit brief, mention of the potential use of blood group studies in anthropology was by Reginald R. Gatesthe Canadian-born, University of Chicago-trained geneticist who became head of the Botany Department at King's College London after the First World War.[39] Hardly the reclusive bookworm, Gates' charming personality and wide range of interests won the hand of birth control radical Mary Stopes. His interest in human genetics and eugenics began in the 1920s, as a result of which he made reference to the blood groups in a 1925 article on "Mendelian Heredity and Racial Differences," that appeared in the *Journal of the Royal Anthropological Institute*.[40] It was, in fact, an isolated reference attached to a longer summary of the latest work in racial definition. Although Gates published an article of original blood group research in 1929, it was on Canadian Eskimos and was published in an American journal. Gates' greatest influence came later, in the 1930s when he conducted his own research and promoted blood group studies in India, Canada, and other overseas lands in the Commonwealth.

In the meantime, an extensive review of blood group research was done by Matthew Young for *Man*, another publication of the Royal

Anthropological Institute in 1928.[41] Although quite comprehensive, Young's article was neither the result of his own research nor even an appeal for British researchers to enter the new field. The intent and tone of the article was neutral and very circumspect. Young's conclusion was typical of most anthropologists' reactions in the 1920s.

> So far as can be seen at present, there would appear to be small warrant for the belief or claim that the evidence supplied by blood grouping will provide a complete and satisfactory basis for the classification of racial types ... The present indications are that blood grouping will not replace but may possibly supplement in some measure the racial criteria at present relied upon.[42]

Young's survey did prompt an article the following year in *Man* by the Australian doctor John B. Cleland, summarizing the research he had been conducting and publishing in Australia for eight years on blood group distributions among aborigines. But it was not until the mid-1930s that another article on the subject, let alone the results of original research, appeared in either *Man* or the *Journal of the Royal Anthropological Institute*. This represented the beginning of sustained interest in the subject that finally brought Britain into the worldwide mainstream of blood group research.

Most significant about the new interest in Britain was when and where it came from. It was neither medical nor anthropological researchers but rather a mathematician and a population geneticist who kindled the interest, and they were relatively late in recognizing the importance of the blood group studies—1931 to be exact. Despite this delay, these researchers in Britain made their greatest contribution by showing the importance of the blood group research for the new field of human genetics. The first to recognize the blood group research was John B.S. Haldane, the celebrated mathematician, physiologist, popularizer of science, and all-around polymath. His interest grew out of his work that helped create the field of population genetics in the 1920s along with colleagues Ronald Fisher and the American Sewall Wright.[43] To be sure, Haldane did not originate the idea that blood groups were a phenotype that could be analyzed by population genetics theory. As mentioned above, it was Felix Bernstein the German mathematician who did this when he worked out a three allele–two loci theory of inheritance in the early 1920s.[44] Haldane's interest in blood group studies came from their potential application to the anthropological question of human racial origins. His attempt at a new approach to an old question was similar to the Hirszfelds' research at Salonica, which was also outside their field of expertise.

One question about Haldane's rediscovery of the blood group studies is why he had not heard about them earlier. It was only at a talk he gave on February 20, 1931, at the Royal Institution on "Prehistory in the light of Genetics," that he first mentioned blood groups. Thus, over a decade of research and hundreds of articles had been done on seroanthropological research around the world. As mentioned, Haldane's talk focused on the study of race, specifically the problems of definition that resulted from the commonly used but environmentally modified traits of stature, skull shape, and skin color. He then announced, "Quite recently, however, a group of characters has been found which is not open to these objections. I refer to the human blood groups."[45] The "quite recent" discovery was Haldane's about the blood groups, but that was hardly the case for the rest of the world. As mentioned above, Hesch's book appearing the following year compiled a bibliography of almost 3000 articles published on blood group research since 1900.[46]

It is possible that Haldane might have missed the original article on the Hirszfelds' Salonica research published in a French journal or even the summary that appeared in *Lancet* in 1919. He might also be excused for missing the few articles on blood group research in British medical journals in the early 1920s or the brief paragraph in Gates' 1925 article in *Man*. More surprising is that he ignored Young's lengthy 1928 article in *Man* and all the other literature on the subject published on the continent. Even accounting for the difficulties of language, Haldane was also woefully ignorant of the steady publication of research on blood group distribution in American journals where almost 40 articles had appeared, including Gates' 1929 article on the blood groups of Canadian Indians and Eskimos in the *American Journal of Physical Anthropology*.[47] None were cited in his talk.

The source of Haldane's interest might have come from America, in a sense: the address given by Karl Landsteiner at the awarding of his Nobel Prize for medicine in December of 1930.[48] Unfortunately, we do not have Haldane's recorded words to verify the source of his inspiration. He cited only L. H. Snyder's 1929 book *Blood Grouping in Relation to Clinical and Legal Medicine* and Bernstein's earlier work in his first remarks on the "new evidence" of the blood groups at the February 1931 meeting of the Royal Institution. Another possibility is that his interest was kindled by the work of Charles Todd on the blood groups of chickens. In 1930 Haldane wrote to R. A. Fisher about Todd's research, which prompted a two-year correspondence between Todd and Fisher.[49]

Regardless of inspiration, 1931 was the turning point for the study of the blood groups in Britain. Although it would be wrong to overemphasize his influence, Haldane was a very well-known and influential public figure in the country. For example, when he gave another talk on blood groups and anthropology at a meeting of the Royal Anthropological Society the following year, it was reported in the two most important British medical journals: *Lancet* and the *British Medical Journal*.[50] This was the first time in four years that the *British Medical Journal* had mentioned blood group testing of human populations. Moreover, Haldane's talk was reported in the same *Lancet* issue as Penrose's landmark study on Down syndrome children, the first mention of a blood group study in *Lancet* in two years.

Equally significant were Haldane's personal contacts with leading British scientists and intellectuals. Attending the 1932 Royal Anthropological Institute meeting, for example, were Penrose, Gates, and Lancelot Hogben. The interest of Penrose and Gateshas already been mentioned, but there is some evidence that Hogben, the recently named Chair of Social Biology at the London School of Economics, may have been the first to rediscover the research on blood group distribution. Hogben, like Gates, was well connected with the inner circles of left-wing interwar British intellectuals. The several positions he held during his career, however, hindered his ability to develop an institutional base or build an ongoing group of collaborators from former students or colleagues. He came to the London School of Economics from South Africa, and when he left in 1938 it was for a post in Scotland. Hogben finished his career at the University of Birmingham. Nonetheless, Hogben's grasp of the statistical dimension of population genetics was first rate, and like Haldane he had a knack of writing for the general public which he learned from H.G. Wells.[51]

An example of Hogben's humor (and politics) is the following description of A.M. Carr-Saunders, noted statistician and President of the English Eugenics Society, which appears in Hogben's unpublished autobiography. "It used to puzzle me how anyone so facelessly devoid of charm and with so mediocre intellectual equipment attained such eminence." Carr-Saunders eventually became director of the London School of Economics and a Knight of the Realm. Hogben began his first appointment in 1919 as a lecturer in the Department of Imperial College headed by E. W. McBride, who was also head of the English Eugenics Society. According to Hogben, at the first meeting of the society he attended that year, McBride called for the mandatory sterilization of all males making less than £400 per year. Hogben noted that his beginning salary was £350.[52]

The best evidence of Hogben's recognition of the importance of the blood groups comes from an emergency meeting on January 31, 1931, of the governing council of the London School of Economics, prompted by a visitor from the Rockefeller Foundation. Hogben prepared a memorandum describing a "program of research" for his newly created chair which would study the genetic basis of social behavior. In it he stated, "Of such progress the most notable achievement is the recent work on the iso-agglutinins or 'blood-groups.'"[53] Hogben went on to co-sponsor, with R. A. E. Crew and C. C. Hurst another proposal on behalf of a "British Council for Research in Human Genetics" to the Rockefeller Foundation in September of 1931, which asked for £15,000 per year to support three research centers. It was unsuccessful, but Hogben published an article on human population genetics in November 1931 and devoted a whole chapter to blood group genetics in his book *Genetic Principles in Medicine and Social Science* published at about the same date.[54]

It is thus possible that Hogben learned of the blood group studies in January of 1931 and told his colleague Haldane who then prepared his talk for the Feb. 20 meeting of the Royal Institution. But the evidence suggests the flow of ideas more likely went the other way. In addition to the indirect testimony of Haldane's nephew, there is evidence to support the fact that Haldane was the senior in the relationship. Although Haldane was only 3 years older than Hogben, he had been interested in genetics far longer and was well established at Cambridge, thanks to family connections at Oxford. Before offering Hogben the appointment at LSE, the administration asked Haldane for his opinion of Hogben's qualifications, and before Hogben accepted the position, he wrote Haldane for advice.[55] The most important point, however, is not priority of rediscovery; it is the tight circle of colleagues that permitted the results of blood group research to spread immediately to Penrose and even more importantly to R. A. Fisher.

Although Hogben, Gates, and Penrose were already familiar, to a greater or lesser extent, with what Haldane announced, it was news for others in the audience, notably A. E. Mourant and C. G. Seligman.[56] Haldane can even be credited with stimulating the interest of one of the deans of American anthropology, Alfred Kroeber, about the importance of blood group research. Kroeber specifically cites Haldane as the inspiration for his 1934 article on blood groups and race which marked the entry into this research by a mainstream American anthropologist.[57] But the most important of those in Britain who followed up on Haldane's call for work on blood groups was his fellow population geneticist, R. A. Fisher.

Fisher's reputation, like that of Gates, has been somewhat tarnished by accusations of racism in his later years, but his importance to the development of population genetics remains unchallenged.[58] One clue to the role of blood group research in Fisher's work comes from his daughter who claims it dated back to as early as a 1926 article in the *Eugenics Review*. There is little evidence, however, to support this claim. No such article can be found, nor did Fisher mention blood groups in his monumental *Genetical Theory of Natural Selection*, which appeared in 1930. In fact, letters from some of the critics of Fisher's work such as Gates and the American William Boyd specifically mentioned the omission of references to blood group research. In response to their criticism Fisher later admitted that he "ought probably at least to have mentioned them [in *Genetical Theory of Natural Selection*]."[59] Fisher's ignorance notwithstanding, it suggests that even without Haldane's or Hogben's rediscovery, Fisher would have learned of the importance of blood group research sooner or later from others. Fisher's greatest importance is that like Hogben, he was soon in a position to do something about the lack of research in Britain, but whereas Hogben was unsuccessful, Fisher's efforts resulted in the creation of a laboratory specifically devoted to blood group research.

What gave Fisher the opportunity was the death in 1933 of Karl Pearson, who held the Galton Chair at University College in London. This position included the direction of the Galton Laboratory and the editorship of *Annals of Eugenics* which Pearson had created in the mid-1920s. Fisher was selected to replace Pearson and quickly took up genetic research, in general, and blood group research, in particular. This can be seen most immediately in the *Annals of Eugenics* which Pearson had started because of the lack of scientific rigor in the *Eugenics Review* which dated back to Galton himself and the establishment of the English Eugenics Society at the beginning of the century. Pearson's subtitle for his new journal minced no words, "a journal for the scientific study of race problems." One of Fisher's first actions was to go even further, expanding the editorial board to include such people as Haldane and Gates, but also reorganizing and changing the subtitle for the reorganized *Annals* to "a journal devoted to the genetic study of human populations."[60]

Another, even more concrete way that Fisher moved toward his new research goal came when D. P. O'Brien of the Rockefeller Foundation visited England in June of 1934 to talk with the Medical Research Council (MRC) about supporting new work in human genetics.[61] In response, as a member of the MRC's Council on Human Heredity, Fisher proposed establishing a serological genetics laboratory at the Galton Lab of University College. In April of 1935 Rockefeller offered funding of £1575 per year for five years. To avoid delay while equipment and staff were secured, Fisher hired a director for the new unit, George L. Taylor and arranged for him to spend a year of training with Oluf Thomsen at his research institute in Copenhagen. This was a frank admission of the lack of serological expertise in Britain at the time.

Taylor trained in Denmark from September 1936 to September 1937, and the first articles on the genetics of blood groups began appearing in the *Annals of Eugenics* in 1937 and 1938. Significantly, all were by foreigners, such as the 1937 Galton Lecture by Viggo Friedenreich of the Copenhagen Research Institute, and the Americans Alexander Wiener and William Boyd.[62] The initial results of Taylor's research finally began appearing in late 1938 and 1939. The opening of the first article admitted, "by comparison with other peoples, the numbers of English examined have been relatively few."[63]

Fisher changed the nature of the Galton Laboratory to engage significantly in blood group research. The dramatic events preceding the Second World War provided even greater opportunity to make up for lack of extensive blood group testing in the country. In the fall of 1938, the Munich Crisis began military mobilization throughout Europe. Accordingly, in anticipation of casualties from aerial bombardment of cities, plans were made for large-scale blood transfusions including the typing of potential donors which began in 1939. Very soon two brief letters appeared at the end of September in the *British Medical Journal* from directors of blood testing stations in Britain on the results of blood group distribution. One (September 30, 1939) pointed to the opportunity which testing presented for determining "the racial makeup of Britain" and speculated "perhaps some geneticist has undertaken the task."[64] Fisher and Taylor quickly published a letter in response on October 21, 1939, which urged test centers to send the results to the Galton Lab Serum Unit, which, they indicated, had been created for just such a purpose. Two months later a collection unit reported on 5000 tests.[65]

U.S. Research

Sustained British research on blood group distribution developed much later than the French, but in both countries the conduct of that research was shaped by relatively few individuals. In contrast, the Americans showed a broader and more varied interest that developed earlier and stronger; hence, it was shaped less by a few individuals and their circumstances. The beginning of this sustained research in the U.S. dated from the mid-1920s. Earlier articles were sporadic and isolated; hence, the timing was earlier than in Britain and roughly similar to France. But whereas French research was largely the result of the accidental establishment of one individual at the Pasteur Institute, American research grew out of much more widespread interest in a variety of applications of the blood group distribution discoveries as well as basic research on the nature of human isohemagglutinins. Indeed, this breadth of interest is probably the most distinguishing feature of blood group research in the U.S.

The beginning of coordinated efforts by U.S. researchers required first that they learn of the work of others and identify themselves as part of a common research field. This was a different process than one researcher or a small group starting a research laboratory as happened in France and Britain. After the appearance of the first articles reporting the results of blood group testing of large numbers of civilian and military personnel in the U.S. at the close of the First World War, there was a period of 3–4 years during which only sporadic and isolated articles appeared. Nonetheless, this research included some landmark studies and established lines of inquiry which were characteristic of later work in the U.S. First was the interest, following the lead of Moss at Johns Hopkins, in the basic nature of the ABO system which included such researchers as Huck and Guthrie who published four articles in 1923–1924 on the possible existence of sub-groups of blood type A. This was also the time when Landsteiner began his career at the Rockefeller Institute, which soon produced even more spectacular and influential results than his earlier research.[66]

Meanwhile, between 1921 and 1923 Reuben Ottenberg, one of the pioneers of blood transfusion before the war, wrote a series of articles on the inheritance of the blood groups which also publicized their "medico-legal" applications. The fact that they appeared in *JAMA* and the *Journal of Immunology* did much to spread word of the earlier work of Landsteiner, Lattes, and Hirszfeld. There were also a few articles in this period which examined the possible link between blood type and disease.[67] The most important work published at this time, however, was by Arthur Coca and Laurence Snyder.

Of the two, Coca's article on blood group distribution among native Americans was the more spectacular discovery.[68] In the course of studying allergic reactions, he tested almost 1000 students at Indian schools in Oklahoma, Kansas, and New Mexico, finding 78 percent were blood type O. This discovery had a great influence on the various race and blood group (not to mention anthropological) theories inspired by the Hirszfelds, even if the immediate appreciation of the discovery by U.S. researchers was limited. Yet, only three years later Ella Grove of Coca's lab followed up with a study of the Ainu of Japan, and in that same year Clara Nigg, a former assistant of Coca, tested 723 Kansas plains and Navajo Indians.[69] Both researchers were supported by money from the National Research Council's Committee on Scientific Problems of Human Migration, where Coca sat on a subcommittee (with Landsteiner and Ottenberg) that recommended funding.[70] The work they supported was strikingly similar to German proposals for systematic blood group testing.

These projects were approved at a conference called by the subcommittee on December 6, 1924, at New York Hospital, and it is clear from the conference report that the goal of participants was participation in a much broader plan for blood group testing around the world. The following details of agreement were reported from the meeting:

> (2) Systematic observation of isoagglutinative blood groupings should be continued and extended in order that reliable information about the percentages of blood groups in the different racial types may be secured.
>
> For this purpose, it was recommended that in all cases efforts be made to examine according to a standard method at least 500 persons if possible above the age of two years, about equally divided between the sexes, and so distributed as to be fair samplings of the population in question …
>
> (3) Careful determination of the blood groupage in special groups of persons subjected to anthropologic and psychologic study is urged with a view to correlation of the results with other characteristics …
>
> (5) The conference expressed itself in favor of giving careful consideration to any concrete projects for research in blood grouping that may be submitted through any of its members.

The subcommittee continued to meet throughout 1925, thus indicating the interest which the blood group discoveries elicited. It established contact with many of the most important blood group researchers throughout the world and made more specific plans for the systematic research proposed at the December conference. Although this work indirectly inspired much research—for example, that of Snyder in North Carolina and Oswald Streng in Norway—limited funds permitted only one other study besides those of Nigg and Grove that was supported by the council.

More important in the long run, Coca's discovery opened the pages of the *Journal of Immunology* which he edited to a series of articles on blood groups. Beginning in 1923, the journal published 33 articles in the next 16 years on the results of blood group testing which was more than all but two journals in the world. Among those who published in Coca's journal was Laurence H. Snyder, a graduate student of William Castle at Harvard who published an article in 1924 on agglutinins in rabbit sera. Shortly after he took up his first teaching position at North Carolina State College of Mining and Agriculture (now N. C. State University) in 1923, Snyder's attention turned from animal to human blood groups.[71] Two populations that attracted his attention were the large number of extended, inbred families in the mountains of western North Carolina and inhabitants of a Cherokee Indian reservation in the state. In 1924 Snyder published two articles giving preliminary results of this new research.[72]

As he studied the literature and established correspondence with such senior researchers as Hektoen of the National Research Council and Charles Davenport of the Eugenics Record Office, Snyder soon discovered how extensive this blood group research had become. In one effort to extend his own work, he proposed mailing blood samples from long distances. Hektoen encouraged Snyder to study black populations in North Carolina, and Davenport secured Snyder's participation in the study of race crossing in Jamaica.[73]

Snyder's most important early article, which marked the beginning of a cumulative and conscious study of blood groups in the U.S., appeared in the 1926 *American Journal of Physical Anthropology* and contained his own testing results plus an exhaustive survey of all blood group research in the world to date. This article immediately became the standard U.S. reference on the subject until Snyder's 1929 book superseded it.[74]

In the years immediately following publication of Snyder's *AJPA* article, American researchers published studies on a wide variety of topics including populations all over the world: Eskimos in Greenland, Yorubas in Nigeria, and Amerindians in Peru, as well as the first studies of Arabs in Lebanon and populations of Caribbean islands. In addition, blood group research was conducted by doctors in several medical institutions who published articles on possible genetic links between blood groups and disease.[75] This was also when Landsteiner and his assistant Philip Levine announced the existence of a new blood group system.

The discovery of the MNP groups in 1927 was dramatic evidence that U.S. researchers (led by the transplanted Landsteiner) were the equals of central Europeans and far ahead of their British and French counterparts in conducting fundamental serological research.[76] This was most clearly shown in 1939 when Landsteiner, Levine, and another of Landsteiner's protégés Alexander Wiener discovered the Rh blood group, which ushered in a new era in serological research after the Second World War. In the dozen years prior, there were 70 articles of original research on blood group distribution published by 42 different American authors. For the period 1931–1939, this was more such articles than were published by researchers from any other country.

The two most frequent subjects of interest in U.S. research were race and disease, with significantly more articles on the distribution of blood types among different peoples around the world. On average four to five articles appeared annually by U.S. researchers usually on populations in widely scattered overseas locales. For example, in 1927 a doctor with the Rockefeller Yellow Fever Commission in Lagos, Nigeria, published results of tests on Yorubas, and the same year two physicians who were part of an American Museum of Natural History expedition to Greenland authored an article on testing of Eskimos.[77] Shortly thereafter Moss and a colleague published findings in prior years from several research trips that tested populations in Peru, yaws patients in Santo Domingo, inhabitants in Yucatan, and prisoners at a detention farm in Texas. That same year (1929) Snyder reported the results of tests that accompanied Charles Davenport's study of "Race-crossing in Jamaica," and Leland Parr at the American University of Beirut authored the first of several studies on populations in the Middle East.[78] In 1931 Carleton Coon included blood group distribution testing that had been part of his anthropological fieldwork four years earlier for a monograph on populations in the Rif region of Morocco, and in 1933 William W. Howells did likewise for a study of Fiji Islanders.[79]

One of the most notable features of these studies was that they were done outside the U.S. In other words, they indicate the worldwide scope of U.S. medical and anthropological researchers who were stationed in hospitals or participated in expeditions funded by philanthropic and academic institutions, explaining why Kilgore was in China at the start of this research in 1918. In contrast, there were surprisingly few anthropological studies of populations within the U.S., and these were almost solely Native Americans. The first of these were by Coca in 1923, followed by Grove and Nigg in 1926. Seven years later Gustave Albin Matson of Washington University in St. Louis published an article announcing a very high percentage of blood type A among the Blackfeet Indians of Montana and Oregon. This touched off a new series of tests on American Indians to confirm and ultimately explain the phenomena of population "isolates" and genetic drift. Matson, along with William C. Boyd and P. B. Candela, was also the first to claim the possibility of conducting blood group tests on Indian burial remains and Egyptian mummies.[80]

Another feature of U.S. blood group research in the 1930s was strong interest in the possible relationship to disease. Beginning in 1927 articles regularly appeared which compared the distribution of blood types in "abnormal" populations (diseased, mentally ill, or criminal) with that of the population as a whole. Evidence of a blood type which occurred with significantly higher frequency in the abnormal individuals was taken as being linked genetically with the abnormality. This methodology was an oversimplification, but is basically similar to modern statistical human genetics methodology. In fact, relatively few of these studies found such a link; 18 of 20 articles published after 1927 found either no correlation or were inconclusive.

The persistence and extent of research on blood groups and disease, even in the face of negative results, was a notable feature of the American blood group research. This was far more interest than French or British publications. There were 7 articles on the subject by British and 11 by French researchers compared to 25 by Americans from 1919 through 1929. To be fair, as a proportion of all articles on blood group distribution there was surprising similarity: 24 percent of British, 21 percent of French, and 27 percent of American. Hence, the more accurate conclusion is that there was a widespread and consistent interest among researchers in all three countries in blood groups as genetic markers for disease. This fact is borne out by similar percentages mentioned earlier for other countries which were even higher, 36 percent of articles by Soviet researchers, 44 percent of German, and a remarkable 83 percent of Polish articles on blood groups and disease. The latter was the result of both the smaller overall number of articles and the special interest of Hirszfeld in constitutional serology.

Other features to this research on disease will be described in greater detail in a later chapter, but some can be noted briefly here for purposes of illustrating the U.S. research record. For example, there was the relative ease of testing institutionally confined subjects (e.g., in the case of mental patients) or those already under medical scrutiny (such as surgery patients or those taking the Wassermann test). Whether for the sake of convenience or other reasons, the most frequent subjects of interest at first were mental patients (six articles overall, three in 1927). Eventually, U.S. researchers tested the correlation of blood type with a variety of diseases such as polio (four articles), tuberculosis (three), syphilis (two), and allergy (two), with at least one study of malaria, scarlet fever, cancer, and even dental caries. As might be expected given the largely negative results, very few researchers published more than one article. Viewed in the light of all studies by U.S. researchers, these blood group distribution tests were almost the only ones done of the "white" population of the U.S., but they were "abnormal," hence like the exotic and foreign populations studied.

The lack of research on the rest of the population in the U.S. was not for want of subjects with potential racial or anthropological interest. There was much fertile ground for would-be racists or simply those interested in trans-Atlantic migrations of population. In fact, there were many examples of physical anthropologists using traditional morphological measures to bolster all sorts of racist stereotypes such as Ernest A. Hooten's 1939 attempt to connect crime with immigrant and other ethnic groups in the U.S.[81] There were also many examples of the new serological methods being used in central and eastern Europe where mixed populations lived in urban centers similar to the eastern U.S. Rumanian and Soviet researchers were greatly interested in former German colonists living in Transylvania and the southern Ukraine, but such studies were rarely done in the U.S.[82]

One exception that proves this rule was Landsteiner and Levine's tests of urban blacks and whites to confirm that their MNP discovery was a new blood group system. Their reasoning was that there would be different distributions according to race as was the case with ABO, and they did so again in 1942 with American Indians and the white population for the Rh discovery. The clear reason in each case was to test the properties of the new groups. They never showed an interest in a "biochemical" or any other blood group "index of race." In fact, the attempt to find a simple correlation between blood type distribution and race came under serious criticism earliest and strongest in the U.S. Among the most important of these critics was William C. Boyd.

Boyd went from a rural upbringing in Missouri to a Harvard undergraduate and master's degree in chemistry in 1926. He then pursued medical studies at Boston University, the institution with which he was affiliated the longest, albeit with several research leaves, until his retirement in 1969. His first interest in blood groups concerned their use in paternity exclusion, but beginning in 1934, and usually in conjunction with his wife Lyle G. Boyd, he became the most prolific and influential American author on blood group testing of diverse populations for the next 20 years. During that time Boyd was probably more responsible than any other U.S. researcher for moving blood group testing toward the study of population genetics.[83]

One final feature worth noting about American blood group researchers was the extent of participation by women. Over 20 percent of the almost 100 articles published by U.S. researchers on blood group distribution between the wars were authored or co-authored by women. One possible explanation is that since serology was new field there were fewer barriers to women participating than in long-established scientific specialties.[84] A few examples will illustrate, however, that participation by women was neither clear-cut nor simple. Many of the co-authorships were women with secondary or subservient appointments rather than true co-equal positions.

The careers of two important American women researchers, Ella Grove and Lyle Boyd, were greatly influenced by their husbands.[85] Ella Grove (1890–1966) who published an article on blood group distribution among populations in Japan and the Philippines in 1926, established a separate career first, albeit as a protégé of Arthur F. Coca. She studied with him at Cornell and like him trained overseas at Heidelberg. For her blood group field work, she took advantage of Coca's contacts in the Philippines where he had been stationed before the war, and he helped secure funding for her research from the National Academy of Science Committee on Scientific Problems of Human Migrations in 1925. Grove became an Instructor in Immunology at Cornell in 1925 and eventually married Coca (a second marriage for both) in 1930. They co-authored two articles in 1925 and gave a talk at the Galton Society of New York in 1926 on "the value of blood groups to the study of race," with Landsteiner in attendance. After publishing regularly on immunology since the mid-1920s, she gave up her research career shortly after the marriage. Her last publications appeared in 1932 based on research she had done while in Germany.[86]

Lyle Boyd's career was tied even closer to that of her husband. Details of her life are sketchy, but she had been the childhood sweetheart of William C. Boyd, and after their marriage she accompanied and assisted him on several studies beginning in the 1930s. Unlike her husband whose Ph.D. was in chemistry, Lyle Boyd eventually studied medicine and was listed as co-author of 14 articles published before the Second World War. A quite public example of William Boyd's close collaboration with his wife occurred when he insisted that she also participate in the 1949 UNESCO conference on race held at its headquarters in Geneva.[87]

Clara Nigg had been an assistant to Coca in the early 1920s before going to a bacteriology laboratory in Kansas. Her career was more independent. She was the sole author of an early article on Kansas plains Indians (also supported by the National Academy of Sciences) and another based on research in Hawaii. Her work caught the attention of no less a figure than Landsteiner who proposed her as an assistant in 1929. What followed illustrates some of the challenges faced by women doing scientific research at the time. Flexner who directed the Rockefeller Institute where Landsteiner worked opposed the appointment. He stated flatly in a letter to Landsteiner, "women do not have academic opportunities." Once appointed, he went on, they "proved an expensive embarrassment to us because when their period had expired, they had to be carried a long time before they could be let go. Indeed, it was always marriage and not other positions that relieved us of them."[88] Nonetheless, Landsteiner carried the day. Nigg was appointed in September of 1929 and remained an assistant at the Rockefeller Institute through the late 1930s, thus proving Flexner wrong in both the short and long run. During the Second World War she worked for the U.S. army and after the war at Squibb Biological Labs. Nigg ended her long career in the 1960s at the University of California Berkeley Naval Biological Labs.

A final example of an American woman who conducted independent research on blood group distribution was Eileen MacFarlane. She authored five articles from 1936 to 1938 on blood groups based on tests of various populations in India where she was a visiting professor of genetics. Later, she was listed as "Collaborator in Asiatic Research" at the University of Michigan, where she had received her Ph.D. in genetics. After the Second World War she developed a new research interest in cancer and also gave lectures to the public on her travels and research. She ended her career as a cancer researcher at Ohio State and died in 2002 at the age of 103.[89]

Women participated in blood group research elsewhere but less so than in the U.S. Although 15 percent of articles by French researchers were authored or co-authored by women, the number of articles were too limited (only nine) to draw any conclusions. There were, however, noteworthy individuals, such as Olga Grooten at Strasbourg who was sole or first author (with Kossovitch) on three articles in 1930 and 1931 on blood groups and polio. Likewise, three studies were published by Rina Younovitch of the Hadassah Municipal Hospital in Tel Aviv. Her work appeared in the *Comptes rendus de la Société de biologie* (1932–1933), reporting on blood tests of Jews from several different countries who resided in Palestine. In Britain there were even fewer articles (5) with female co-authors—three of which were by Elizabeth Ikin and one by Janet Vaughan of the Galton Lab—who became full equals if not leaders on their own of blood group research in Britain during and after the Second World War. There is insufficient information, other than name, about numerous women who participated in serological research elsewhere, including large numbers in the Soviet Union. A singularly important woman in Holland was Marianne van Herwerden who established herself as one of the most important geneticists in the country. As will be seen below, in the 1930s she directed the national survey of Dutch blood groups based at her laboratory at the University of Utrecht.[90]

Conclusion

Two important points for comparison about research on blood groups by British, French, and American researchers were the influence of individual scientists and the extent of studies in distant overseas locales. As the new field spread to different countries in the 1920s, often one or two scientists established a center that trained and directed a new generation of researchers. This was certainly the case with Kossovitch in France and Fisher in Britain,[91] but as in Germany and the Soviet Union, there was so much interest in the U.S. that several centers developed.

All three countries extended the geographical range of populations tested for blood type, but there were significant differences in the scope and extent of the testing, not to mention the motivation of researchers in each country. This can be seen in the different settings in which the French, British, and Americans conducted research in the distant settings. France, for example, had a large colonial empire, including a network of Pasteur Institute facilities provided access to subjects and medical personnel for the research. The French usually published their overseas results in France, in contrast to the British whose extensive empire had an even greater variety of subjects and extensive medical resources but where results of blood group studies were often published in overseas journals (South Africa, Australia, and India). The American researchers "informal" health empire offered many subjects for research but few opportunities for publication in the overseas lands of testing. Regardless of where published, the research done outside of the country was a large percentage of all articles by U.S. researchers (41 percent) and even more by French (28 of 60 or 47 percent). It will be seen below that this was also the case with Dutch researchers: 38 of 52 studies were done in the East Indies, although half of these articles appeared in journals published in the colony.

In France the development of new knowledge about blood groups followed a pattern similar to many other countries. This began with much general interest in the subject, then one individual became the center of a research program that included many studies of populations outside the country. One distinctively French feature of this research grew out of the peculiar Pasteur centralization and overseas connections. French interest in anthropological questions was not unusual, but the lack of work on disease increased the overall preponderance of French anthropological research on differences in blood group distribution in populations around the world. Although some French researchers like Martial were interested in proving racial hierarchy, the emphasis on the anthropology of blood groups in French publications was more the result of Kossovitch's interests that grew out of his experience with the Hirszfelds during the First World War. He continued this interest during the 1920s and 1930s even as his mentor Hirszfeld went on after 1919 to study links to disease and more fundamental questions of blood group biochemistry and physical constitution.

There were some changes in French blood group research by the end of the 1930s which reflected a move away from the model of centralized direction by the Pasteur Institute and primary concern with anthropological applications. Interest developed in practical applications of forensic medicine and paternity testing, and by 1939 a new research center was established at Lille. Moreover, as the chance of war increased, planning began for large-scale blood testing as part of establishing a national transfusion service in France.[92]

These changes late in the 1930s in France did not include interest in one of the most significant new fields related to the blood group discoveries: human population genetics. The major figures who picked up on the early work of German mathematician Felix Bernstein in the 1920s were primarily British geneticists Haldane, Hogben, and Fisher. Fisher's interest was especially important because he received funding from the Rockefeller Foundation in 1935 for a new Blood Group Research Center at the University of London. The researchers he assembled quickly established serious and sustained work which after the Second World War became one of the most important centers for study of blood group polymorphisms in the world.[93] Thus, the British who had initially shown so little interest in blood group distribution research eventually took the lead.

Perhaps the larger lesson from the record of the British research is not its eventual importance as the world center of blood group distribution studies. Rather, it is the delay in British interest, given its long-standing medical and anthropological traditions. Thus, the existence of well-established research facilities was not sufficient to guarantee that scientists in a given country would undertake research in human blood groups. Nor was research interest automatically sparked by the availability of information and the results obtained elsewhere. There is little doubt that British medical and anthropological researchers knew about the activity of others' work, but for over a decade they showed little interest.

Another lesson is more mixed: the importance of subjects available for research. It could be argued that in addition to its empire, the British had a mixed ethnic home population about which there was significant political debate, which thus offered a potential stimulus for blood group studies. To be fair, however, compared to countries in central and eastern Europe or the U.S., Great Britain had fewer recently arrived populations before and after the First World War. To put it another way, the mere existence of ethnic differences in the home population did not guarantee they would be studied serologically. As to populations overseas, the extent of the British empire did not automatically stimulate to interest in blood group research back in the home country. Perhaps Britain's empire was so well and long established that its decentralized nature had created local institutions which took up the interest in place medical researchers back in the metropole.

The American research on blood group distribution reflected some of the underlying features of scientific research in the U.S., which differed from those of Britain and France. One example is the breadth and resulting decentralization of interest. Although Snyder was similar to Kossovitch in publicizing new research on blood groups, there were other sources of inspiration to work in the field. Hence, it is likely that someone else would have written a defining reference work like Snyder's 1929 book. In fact, he moved on to other work, but about this same time William C. Boyd at Boston University Medical School began his research on human blood groups. By the end of the 1930s he had done eight studies on blood group distribution of peoples as varied as American Indians, the Irish, and Egyptians (both current residents and mummies). As a result, in 1939 Boyd published his 128-page summary article on all blood group distribution research to date that superseded Snyder's publication and became the new standard reference worldwide. In turn it was the basis for A. E. Mourant's postwar work.

The decentralized medical infrastructure of the U.S. also facilitated the breadth of American interest in the applications of blood group research to include links to disease and mental illness. For example, it was unlikely that any one American researcher announcing a negative finding could end a line of inquiry such as what happened for a time in France when Toulouse published his article finding no difference in blood group distribution among the mentally ill.

One final observation about the anthropological blood group studies by American researchers was the absence of their use in racial discrimination toward the black population. Filling the gap, however, was what might be called the "quasi-imperial" research of U.S. science and medicine in the years following the First World War. Opportunities grew in conjunction with research expeditions, Rockefeller projects (in Nigeria, Lebanon, and China), medical missionaries, and old-fashioned Yankee gunboat diplomacy that placed American medical researchers in positions around the world. It was these unforeseen opportunities that resulted in blood group testing of many different populations outside the U.S. This was possible, moreover, without the extensive and formal colonial structures that existed in the British and French empires.

Notes

1. Much of the research for part of this chapter was the basis for the following: William H. Schneider, "Blood Group Research in Great Britain, France, and the United States between the World Wars," *American Journal of Physical Anthropology* 38 supplement 21 (1995): 87–114.
2. Jules Bordet, "Le mécanisme de l'agglutination," *Annales de l'Institut Pasteur* 13 (1899): 225–50; Samuel George Shattock, "Chromocyte

Clumping in Acute Pneumonia and Certain Other Diseases and the Significance of the Buffy Coat in the Shed Blood," *Journal of Pathology and Bacteriology* 6 (1900), 303–14; and Jean Camus and Philippe Pagniez, "D'un pouvoir aggliutinant de certains serums humains pour les globules rouges de l'homme normal," *Comptes rendus de la Société de Biologie* [hereafter cited as CRSB], (1901) 242–4.

3. Reuben Ottenberg and Albert A. Epstein, "A Simple Method of Performing Serum Reactions," *Transactions of the New York Pathological Society* 8 (1908): 120–2.
4. See William H. Schneider, "Chance and Social Setting in the Application of the Discovery of Blood Groups," *Bulletin of the History of Medicine* 57 (1983): 550; and Schneider, "Blood Transfusion in Peace and War, 1900–1918," *Social History of Medicine* 10 (1997): 105–26.
5. Jean Juillard and Claude Raby, "La transfusion sanguin pendant la guerre 1914–1918," *Revue des corps de santé* 7 (1966): 835. For more on the experience of the early war years, see Maurice Guillot. Georges Dehelly, and Louis Morel, *La transfusion du sang* (Paris: A. Maloine, 1917). For Jeanbrau, see Emile Jeanbrau, "Une technique simple de transfusion," *Montpélier Médical* 39 (1917): 1142; Jeanbrau, "Technique simple de tranfusion du sang stabilisé par le citrate de soude," *Presse médicale* 26 (1918), 58–62; Jeanbrau and George Giroud, "Accidents de transfusion et moyens de les éviter," *Journal médicale française* 8 (1919), 203–9; and Giroud, "Groupes sanguins," *Presse médicale* 27 (1919), 21–2.
6. The Toronto surgeon L. Bruce Robertson published earliest and most frequently about transfusion in English journals. See, for example, "The Transfusion of Whole Blood: A Suggestion for Its More Frequent Employment in War Surgery," *British Medical Journal* 2 (1916): 38–40; or "A Contribution on Blood Transfusion in War Surgery," *Lancet* (1918): 759–62.
7. An example of an account by a member of the "Harvard Unit" is E.G. Crabtree, "Blood Transfusion in War Surgery in the British Army," *Boston medical and Surgical Journal* 181 (July 17, 1919): 60–3. For background and some observations on transfusion in the "official" government history, see "Collective Surgical Experiences at the Front and at the Base," in *The Medical Department of the United States Army in the World War*, vol. IX Surgery (Washington: Government Printing Office, 1927), 130–65.
8. William M. Happ, "Appearance of Iso-agglutinins in Infants and Children," *Journal of Experimental Medicine* 31 (1920):313–4. The article was received for publication in August 1919. George R. Moffitt, George F. Klugh and Chester E. Shepard, "Blood Type Classification, with a Slight Modification of Technic: Report of the Results of More than a Thousand

Tests," *JAMA* 73 (1919): 1821–2. Rather than give a breakdown of those tested, the authors boasted, "the sera used were from adults of all ages, from all classes of society, white and negro races."

9. Alson R. Kilgore and J. Hua Liu, "Iso-agglutination Tests of Chinese Bloods for Transfusion Compatibility," *China Medical Journal*, 32 (1918), 21–5. For more on the timing, see below.
10. William L. Culpepper and Marjorie Abelson, "Report of 5000 Bloods Typed Using Moss's Grouping," *Journal of Laboratory and Clinical Medicine*, 6 (1921): 276–83.
11. J. Arthur Buchanan and Edith T. Higley, "Relationship of Blood Groups to Disease," *British Journal of Experimental Pathology*, 2 (1921): 247–55.
12. William Alexander, "An Inquiry into the Distribution of Blood Groups of Patients Suffering from Malignant Diseases," *British Journal of Experimental Pathology*, 2 (1921): 66–9. Alexander cited no sources in his article.
13. Cristina Cabrera and Herbert W. Wade, "On Iso-agglutination Group Percentages in Filipino Blood," *Journal of the Philippine Islands Medical Association* 1 (1921): 100–2.
14. Reuben Ottenberg, "Heredity of Blood Qualities. Medico-legal Application of Human Blood Grouping," *Journal of Immunology*, 6 (1921): 363–85.
15. Julian Lewis and Deborah L. Henderson, "Racial Distribution of Isohemagglutinin Groups," *JAMA* 79 (1922): 1422–4; Arthur F. Coca and Olin Diebert, "A Study of the Occurrence of the Blood Groups among American Indians," *Journal of Immunology* 8 (1923): 487–91.
16. Sydney C. Dyke, "On Blood Grouping and Its Clinical Applications," *Lancet* 202 (1922): 579–82; "On the Medico-legal Importance of the Blood Groups," *Lancet* 203 (1922): 1271–3.
17. See, for example, James Hunter Harvey Pirie, "Blood Testing Preliminary to Transfusion: with a Note on the Group Distribution among South African Natives," *Medical Journal of South Africa* 16 (1921): 109–12; or Arthur H. Tebbutt and Sarah V. McConnel, "On Human Iso-haemagglutinins, with a Note on Their Distribution Amongst Some Australian Aborigines," *Medical Journal of Australia* 9 (1922): 201–9.
18. Out of 48 articles on blood groups published by all British and imperial researchers from 1928 to 1939, 22 articles appeared in journals published in Malaya, India, South Africa, Australia, and Canada. Of the 26 articles published in Britain, 15 appeared in journals outside the mainstream of medicine such as *Man*, *Journal of the Royal Anthropological Institute*, and the *Journal of Tropical Medicine*.
19. Jenny Bangham, *Blood Relations: Transfusion and the Making of Human Genetics* (University of Chicago Press, 2020), 42. There was one article

each in 1923 and 1924, then none on blood group distribution until 1932 except for 3 articles on work in Canada, India, and Malaya.

20. In addition to Guillot et al. and Juillard and Ruby cited above, for more detailed background on French blood group research, see William H. Schneider, "La recherche sur les groupes sanguins avant la deuxième guerre mondiale," in *Les sciences biologiques et médicales en France, 1920–1950*, eds. Claude Debru, Jean Gayon, and Jean-François Picard (Paris: CNRS-Editions, 1994), 311–27.
21. Georges Giraud, "Groupes sanguins," *Presse médicale*, 27 (1919): 21–2.
22. Emile Jeanbrau, "Transfusion Sanguine," *Congrès français de chirurgie. XXXII. Paris (8 octobre 1923) Procès-verbaux, mémoires et discussions* (Paris, 1923), 32:116.
23. Georges Rosenthal, "Transfusion sanguine," *Journal de médecine des praticiens* 96 (1925): 663.
24. Jeanbrau, "Comment, en dehors des cas d'extrême urgence, choisir un donneur pour la transfusion du sang?" *Clinique* 21 (1926): 141–4.
25. See, for example, J. Mouzon, "Recherches récentes sur les groupes sanguins," *Presse médicale* 31 (1923): 541–3; Roger Douris, "Applications médico-legales des groupes sanguins humains," *Bulletin des sciences pharmacologiques* 30 (1923): 90–107; M. Duvoir, "Le problème de la paternité," *La médecine* 5 (1924): 511–3; Prosper Emile-Weil and M. Lamy, "Sur une cause d'erreur dans la détermination des groupes sanguins due au vielleissement des sérums-étalons," *Bulletins et memoires de la société médicale des hôpitaux de Paris* 48 (1924): 859–61; or Amédée Laffont and Émile Gaujoux, "Recherches sur l'agglutination des globules sanguins avec les sérum maternal et foetal," *Comptes rendus de la Société de Biologie* 88 (1923): 730.
26. Michon's first article appeared in 1925, "Sur les variations quantitatives de l'isohemagglutination et les infractions aux schémas de Moss," *Comptes rendus de la Société de biologie* 92 (1925), 37–9. For a summary of his work, see his *Les groupes sanguins: Schémas d'application* (Paris: Masson, 1930). Others publishing similar articles included Meyer in Strasbourg, Falgarolle in Montpellier and Panniset and Verge in Alfort, all in *Comptes rendus de la Société de biologie.*
27. The latter is somewhat ironic because the first publication of the results (in full) of the Hirszfelds' research in Salonica was in a French journal, *Anthropologie*. Its appearance, however, was not in a medical journal, which meant it was little noticed by doctors. In fact, the source almost exclusively cited in later years was the 1919 *Lancet* article. It was only in 1927 that Prosper Emile-Weill and others founded a new journal *Sang*, which defined and focused attention on clinical aspects of serology. A few

years earlier, however, the new *Annales de médicine legale* offered a venue for work on blood groups and legal applications.

28. The best accounts are Pierre Lépine, "Necrologie: Nicholas Kossovitch (1884–1948)," *Annales de l'Institut Pasteur* 75 (1948): 62–4; and a preface by Henri Vallois to the posthumous volume of Kossovitch, *Anthropologie des groupes sanguins des populations au Maroc* (Paris: Mason, 1953), i-iii.
29. Letter from Dujarric de la Rivière to Director of Institut Pasteur, May 7, 1934, archives of Pasteur Institute. See also Dujarric de la Rivière and Kossovitch, "Dix années de fonctionnement d'un 'Centre d'études des groupes sanguins,'":*Bulletin de l'Academie de Médecine* 121 (1939): 487–94.
30. See Schneider, *Quality and Quantity: The Quest for Biological Regeneration in Twentieth Century France* (New York: Cambridge University Press, 1990), 301, for examples of Kossovitch's publications. Of 20 articles published between 1925 and 1935, 8 were in *CRSB* and 8 in the *Revue anthropologique.*
31. Raymond Dujarric de la Riviere and Nicholas Kossovitch, "Recherches sur les groupes sanguins," *Annales de l'Institut Pasteur*, 45 (1930): 107–53; "Au sujet des groups sanguins des tuberculeux et des cancereux," *Comptes rendus de la Société de biologie*, 97 (1927):137–9; "La question des groupes sanguins en médecine legale," *Annales de médecine legale*, 7 (1927): 390–400.
32. See Nicholas Kossovitch and Fernand Benoit, "Les groupes sanguins chez les Berberophones," *Comptes rendus de la Société de biologie*, 109 (1932): 198–200; or Kossovitch and Benoit, "Contribution à l'étude des indigènes du Maroc," *Revue anthropologique*, 43 (1933): 318–48.
33. Raymond Turpin and Armand Caratzali, "L'étude des groupes sanguins classiques chez les sujets atteints de mongolisme," *Revue critique de pathologie et de thérapeutique* 3 (1933): 789–97. For more on Turpin, see R. Laplane "Eloge de Raymond Turpin (1895–1988)," *Bulletin de l'Academir Nationize de la Medicine.* 173 (1989):535–43; and for broader context, see K. Codell Carter, "Early Conjectures That Down Syndrome Is Caused by Chromosomal Nondisjunction." *Bulletin of the History of Medicine* 76, no. 3 (2002): 528–63.
34. Edouard Toulouse, P. Schiff et R. Weismann-Netter, "Les groupes sanguins dans les maladies mentales et nerveuses," *Encephale* 21 (1926): 785–8.
35. See, for example, Nicholas Kossovitch and Fernand Benoit, "Contribution à l'étude anthropologique et sérologique des juifs modernes," *Revue anthropologique* 42 (1932): 99–125; Félix Regnault, "Il n'y a pas de race juive," *Revue anthropologique* 42 (1932): 390–3; and Rina Younovitch, "Les caractères sérologiques des juifs asiatiques," Comptes rendus de la Société de biologie 113 (1933): 1101–3.

36. For background, see Schneider, *Quality and Quantity*, 230–55; and Pierre-André Taguieff, "Immigrés, métis, Juifs: les raisons de l'inassimilabilité. Opinions et doctrines du Dr. Martial," in *Nationalismes, féminismes, exclusions: Mélanges en l'honneur de Rita Thalmann*, eds. Liliane Crips, et al. (Frankfurt: Peter Lang, 1993), 177–221.
37. On this point as well as the larger context of British research after 1945, see Bangham, *Blood Relations*.
38. Ernest H. R. Altounyan, "Blood Group Percentages for Arabs, Armenians and Jews," *British Medical* Journal (1928): 546; Lionel S. Penrose, "Blood Grouping of Mongolian Imbeciles," *Lancet* 222 (1932): 394–5 and Penrose, "Blood Group Distribution in the Eastern Counties of England," *British Journal of Experimental Pathology*, 14 (1933): 160–1.
39. On Gates see John A. Fraser-Roberts, "Reginald Ruggles Gates," *Biographical Memoirs of Fellows of the Royal Society* 10 (1964): 83–105.
40. Vol. 55 (1925): 468–82.
41. Matthew Young, "The Problem of Racial Significance of the Blood Groups," *Man* 28 (1928): 153–9; 171–6.
42. Young, 172.
43. On Haldane's new "fascination," see Bangham, *Blood Relations*, 43, and for background see Norman W. Pirie, "John Burton Sanderson Haldane," *Biographical Memoirs of the Royal Society* 12 (1966): 218–49 and Ronald W. Clark, *JBS: The Life and Work of J.B.S. Haldane* (New York: Coward McCann, 1969). For a more recent account of his later years, see Krishna R. Dronamraju, *Haldane: The Life and Work of J.B.S. Haldane with Special Reference to India* (Aberdeen: Aberdeen University Press, 1985).
44. Felix Bernstein, "Ergebnisse einer biostatistichen zusammenfassenden Betrachtung uber die erblichen Blutstrukturen des Menschen," *Klinische Wochenschrift* 3 (1924): 1495–7. On Bernstein, see Pauline M. H. Mazumdar in earlier chapters and, "Two models for human genetics: blood grouping and psychiatry in Germany between the World Wars." *Bulletin of the History Medicine* 70 (1996): 609–57; and Schneider, "Le rôle des groupes sanguins dans l'histoire de la génétique," in *Histoire de la génétique* (Paris: Editions Science en Situation, 1991), eds. Jean-Louis Fischer and William H. Schneider, 301–3.
45. J.B.S. Haldane, "Prehistory in the Light of Genetics." *Proceedings of the Royal Institution of Great Britain* 26 (1931): 356.
46. Hesch, "Die gesamte Schrifttum ..."
47. R. R. Gates, "Blood groups of Canadian Indians and Eskimos," *American Journal of Physical Anthropology* 12 (1929): 475–85. Thirty-three articles were published by U.S. researchers between 1921 and 1930.
48. I am grateful to Joan Austoker for this information, related to her by a nephew of Haldane.

49. As cited in Walter F. Bodmer, "Early British Discoveries in Human Genetics: Contributions of R. A. Fisher and J. B. S. Haldane to the Development of Blood Groups," *American Journal of Human Genetics* 50 (1992): 672–3.
50. "The Blood Groups in Genetics and Anthropology," *British Medical Journal*, (1932) 2: 26–7; "Blood Groups," *Lancet*, (1932) 1:1024–5. *Lancet* also showed a new interest in legal applications of blood group research prompted by a 1932 trial which culminated in 1937 legislation in Parliament to allow blood group tests as evidence in paternity cases. This was a whole decade after similar legislation had been passed in German state courts but approximately the same time as in the U.S. See William H. Schneider, "Chance and Social Setting": 553–5.
51. In fact, his income was supported considerably by royalties from a series of popular and frequently reprinted books, such as *Mathematics for the Million* (New York: Norton, 1937) and *Science for the Citizen* (New York: Knopf, 1938). Among the most useful items of Hogben's papers at Birmingham University is the manuscript of an unpublished autobiography, "Look Back with Laughter," L. T. Hogben Papers, A.3, University of Birmingham.
52. Hogben, "Look Back," 181–3.
53. "Memorandum by Professor L. T. Hogben concerning the scope and development of a science of Social Biology, together with a program of research and a statement of its financial requirements," LSE 6/15; Agenda, emergency CHee 3\0 Jan 1931, London School of Economics archives.
54. Hogben, *Genetic Principles in Medicine and Social Science* (London: 1931).
55. Hogben, "Look Back," 262. Haldane was also considered for the post.
56. "Blood groups," Lancet, (1932): 1025.
57. Alfred Kroeber, "Blood Group Classifications," *American Journal of Physical Anthropology* 18 (1934): 377–94. It is ironic that Kroeber heard about the work when he was at the University of California, some distance across the U.S. and the Atlantic.
58. To balance the informative but naturally slanted biography of Fisher by his daughter, Joan Fisher Box, *R. A. Fisher: The Life of a Scientist* (New York: John Wiley, 1978), see Bodmer, "Early British Discoveries in Human Genetics"; W. B. Provine, *The Origins of Theoretical Population Genetics* (Chicago: University of Chicago Press, 1971); and Provine, "The R.A. Fisher–Sewall Wright Controversy and its Influence Upon Modern Evolutionary Biology," in R. Dawkins and M. Ridley, eds., *Oxford Surveys in Evolutionary Biology, Vol. 2* (New York: Oxford University Press, 1985), 197–219.
59. "Fisher to W.C. Boyd, October 18, 1934, in *Natural Selection, Heredity and Eugenics: including Selected Correspondence of R.A. Fisher with Leonard*

Darwin and Others (Oxford: Clarendon Press, 1983), ed. J. H. Bennett, 183. See also 37 and 206–9.

60. Vol. 6. 1934–1935.
61. Fisher letter and proposal to O'Brien, July 18, 1934, Rockefeller Foundation archives, 401A; 1.1; Box 16, Folder 219. A running record of funding for the Galton blood group laboratory through Aug. 1940 is contained in folders 216–219. Corroborating records are in copies from MRC archives, courtesy of Joan Austoker. See also Joan Fisher Box, p. 344.
62. Alexander S. Wiener, J. Ziewe, and Joseph H. Fries, "On the Linkage Relations of the Genes for Allergic Disease and the Genes Determining the Blood Groups, MN-types, and Eye Colour in Man," *Annals of Eugenics* 7(1937): 163–78; Viggo Friedenreich, "Blood Groups and Genetics," *Annals of Eugenics* 8 (1937–1938): 152–65; and William C. Boyd, "Three Nomograms for Testing Agreement of Blood Grouping Data with Theories of Inheritance," *Annals of Eugenics* 8 (1937–1938): 337–42.
63. G. L. Taylor and Aileen M. Prior, "Blood Groups in England I. Examination of Family and Unrelated Material," *Annals of Eugenics* 8 (1937–1938): 343.
64. Edward Billing, "Racial Origins from Blood Grouping, *British Medical Journal* (Sept. 30, 1939): 712.
65. John C. Thomas, "Blood Group Distribution in England," *British Medical Journal* (1939): 1163. Fisher and Taylor letter of Oct. 21, 1939, "Blood Groups in Britain," *British Medical Journal*, 826. They also indicated they had already conducted 58,000 tests.
66. Charles G. Guthrie and John G. Huck, "On the Existence of More Than Four Isoagglutinin Groups in Human Blood," *Bulletin of Johns Hopkins Hospital* 34 (1923): 37–48; 80–8; 128–135. Landsteiner's first article after arriving at the Rockefeller Institute appeared in August 1923.
67. See, for example, George E. Pfahler and Bernard P. Widmann, "The Relation of Blood Groups to Malignant Disease and the Influence of Radiotherapy," *American Journal of Roentgenology and Radium therapy*, 12 (1924): 47–50.
68. Arthur F. Coca and Olin Diebert, "A Study of the Occurrence of the Blood Groups among American Indians," *Journal of Immunology* 8 (1923): 487–91.
69. Ella F. Grove, "On the Value of the Blood-group Relationship as a Means of Determining Racial Relationship," *Journal of Immunology* 12 (1926): 251–62; Clara Nigg, "A Study of the Blood Groups among the American Indians," *Journal of Immunology* 11 (1926): 319–22.
70. Ludvig Hektoen, "Report of Conference on Blood Grouping, Dec. 6, 1924," Archives of National Research Council, Anthropology and Psychology, 1924–1925, Committee on Scientific Problems of Human Migration: Projects.

71. Paul J. Schmidt, "Early Blood Grouping and Transfusion in North Carolina: Contributions of Laurence H. Snyder," *North Carolina Medical Journal* 47 (1986): 205–6. For more on Snyder, see "Historical Note: On the Role of Laurence H. Snyder in the Development of Human and Medical Genetics in the United States; an oral History Tape Interview," *American Journal of Medical Genetics* 8 (1981): 449–68; Daniel J. Kevles, *In the Name of Eugenics* (Cambridge: Harvard University Press, 1985), chapter 13; and Nathaniel Comfort, *The Science of Human Perfection* (New Haven: Yale University Press, 2014), 80–4.
72. Snyder, "Critical Tests of Blood Group Inheritance," *Southern Medicine and Surgery* 86, (1924):473–5; and "The Inheritance of Blood Groups," *Genetics* 9 (1924): 465–78. He also began a correspondence with Charles Davenport at the Eugenics Record office in Cold Spring Harbor.
73. Extensive correspondence by Snyder can be found in the Davenport Papers of the American Philosophical Society (Philadelphia) and the archives of the National Research Council, Anthropology and Psychology Division. See, for example, a letter of February 15, 1925, from Snyder to Hektoen, Chairman of the NRC Division of Medical Sciences.
74. Snyder, "Human Blood Groups: Their Inheritance and Racial Significance," *American Journal of Physical Anthropology* 9 (1926): 233–63; Snyder, *Blood Grouping in Relation to Clinical and Legal Medicine* (Baltimore: Williams and Wilkins, 1929).
75. Among the more exhaustive articles were Frederick Proescher and A. S. Arkush, "Blood Groups in Mental Diseases," *Journal of Nervous and Mental Diseases* 65 (1927): 569–84; Theophile Raphael, Olive M. Searle and William Scholten, "Blood Groups in Schizophrenic and Manic-depressive Psychosis," *American Journal of Psychiatry* 7 (1927):153–61.
76. Karl Landsteiner and Philip Levine, "A New Agglutinable Factor Differentiating Individual Human Bloods," *Proceedings of the Society for Experimental Biology and Medicine* 24 (1927): 600–2.
77. Henry R. Muller, "Blood Groups among the Yoruba Tribe of West African Negroes," *Proceedings of the Society for Experimental Biology and Medicine* 24 (1927): 437–8; Peter Heinbecker and Ruth Pauli, "Blood Groups of the Polar Eskimo," *Journal of Immunology* 13 (1927): 279–83.
78. William L. Moss and James A. Kennedy, "Blood Groups in Peru, Santo Domingo, Yucatan and Among the Mexicans at the Blue Ridge Prison Farm in Texas," *Journal of Immunology* 16 (1929): 159–74; Laurence H. Snyder, "Blood Groups of Jamaicans," *Race Crossing in Jamaica*, ed. by Charles Davenport (1929), 277–80; Leland W. Parr, "Studies in Isohemoglutination," *Journal of Immunology* 16 (1929): 99–107.
79. Carleton Stevens Coon, *Tribes of the Rif* (Cambridge: Harvard African Studies, 1931), vol. 9:393–402; William W. Howells, "Anthropometry

and Blood Types in Fiji and the Soloman Islands," *Anthropological Papers of the American Museum of Natural History* 33 (1933): 283–339.

80. Gustave Albin Matson, "Unexpected Differences in Distribution of Blood Groups among American Indians," *Proceedings of the Society for Experimental Biology and Medicine* 30 (1933): 1380–2. William C. Boyd and Lyle G. Boyd, "An Attempt to Determine the Blood Groups of Mummies," *Proceedings of the Society for Experimental Biology and Medicine* 31 (1934): 671–2; Gustave Albin Matson, "A Procedure for Determining Distribution of Blood Groups in Mummies," *Proceedings of the Society for Experimental Biology and Medicine*, 31 (1934): 964–8; P. B. Candela, "Blood-group Reactions in Ancient Human Skeletons," *American Journal of Physical Anthropology* 21 (1936): 429–32.
81. Ernest A. Hooten, *The American Criminal: An Anthropological Study* (Cambridge: Harvard University Press, 1939).
82. Use of blood groups to study "mixing" of populations in eastern Europe appeared as early as F. Verzar and Oskar Weszeczky, "Rassenbiologische Untersuchungen mittels Isohamagglutinen," *Biochemische Zeitschrift* 126 (1922): 33–9. On descendants of German colonists living in Transylvania and the southern Ukraine, see Sabin Manuila, "Recherches sero-anthropologiques sur les races en Roumanie par la methode de l'isohemagglutination," *Comptes rendus de la Société de biologie* 90 (1924), 1071–3, and W. J. Rubaschkin and S. Pauli, "Der biologische Rassenindex der deutschen Koloniasten der Ukraine," *Ukrainische Zentralblatt für Blutgruppenforschun*, 1–2 (1927): 65–71.
83. For a critical view of Boyd, see Rachel Silverman, "The Blood Group 'Fad' in Post-War Racial Anthropology," *Kroeber Anthropological Society Papers* 84 (2000): 11–27.
84. This was not just the case in the U.S. Hirszfeld, for example, collaborated with female researchers besides his wife. In an article aimed at encouraging American women to enter the medical field, Roscoe R. Spencer, "Opportunities for Women in War Medicine," *War Medicine*, 2 (1942): 574–79 found that there were 40 women in professional and scientific grades at the National Institute of Health (out of 289), with the top three specializations being bacteriology (13), statistics (9), and biochemistry (6).
85. Of course, Hirszfeld also collaborated with his wife. For historical perspective on the question of marital collaboration, see Marilyn B. Ogilvie, "Marital Collaboration: An Approach to Science," in Pnina G. Abir-Am and Dorinda Outram eds., *Uneasy Careers and Intimate Lives: Women in Science, 1789–1979* (New Brunswick: Rutgers University Press, 1987), 104–25.
86. Biographical details about her can be found in Sheldon G. Cohen, "Firsts in Allergy: The Contributions of Arthur F. Coca," *New England and*

Regional Allergy Proceedings 6 (1985): 287–92. Coca and Grove, "The Value of Blood Groups to the Study of Race," *Eugenical News* 11 (1926), 89–91. An obituary about her appeared in the *Bergen Record* (May 28, 1966).

87. See UNESCO letters. For an example of a newspaper account of the couple, see N. Gordon, "Dr. Boyd: Man of Many Talents" *Boston Sunday Herald* (Nov. 22, 1959) III:18.
88. Landsteiner to Flexner, April 18, 1929; Flexner to Landsteiner, April 18, 1929; Rockefeller Archive Center, RG450, L232, series 2, Box 3, folder 2.
89. As with most of the female researchers of the period, biographical information is sketchy. Much of the preceding on Macfarlane is based on materials, including a letter and attachment to Jack Schulz, Sept. 13, 1946, in the American Philosophical Society archives, Jack Schulz Papers, MS Collection 27. An obituary appeared in the *Cincinnati Enquirer* (February 19, 2002), https://www.legacy.com/us/obituaries/cincinnati/name/eileen-macfarlane-obituary?id=48013112.
90. CAB van Herwerden, *Marianne van Herwerden* (Rotterdam: W. L. & J. Brusse, 1948). M. Kirejczyk, "Vrouwen kozen exact; Studie en beroepsuitoefning rond de eeuwwisseling," *Gewina* 16 (1993): 234–47.
91. As will be seen in the next chapter, new centers that dominated research were established by Hirszfeld in Poland, Oluf Thomsen in Denmark, Leone Lattes in Italy, and Marianne van Herwerden in Holland.
92. Schneider, "La Recherche sur les Groupes Sanguins." 323–4.
93. Jenny Bangham, "Blood groups and human groups: Collecting and calibrating genetic data after World War Two," *Studies in History and Philosophy of Biological and Biomedical Sciences* 47 (2014): 74–86.

CHAPTER 5

Blood Group Research in Japan, Italy, and Elsewhere

The previous two chapters have examined the development of the new field of blood group research in the largest countries in Europe and U.S. The analysis has compared the role of specific biomedical institutions and the broader social and political influences as well as the peculiarities of individuals involved in shaping that research. There were some common themes and sharp differences in the amount and timing of interest, subjects studied, manner of communication, and organization of research.

As the overview chapter indicated, blood group research was a worldwide phenomenon with significant work conducted in many different countries. For example, Turda has shown the importance of seroanthropological research in Rumania and Hungary between the wars, and a recent article by Burton and Lefkatidou shows how Greek and Turkish researchers studied blood groups to justify their partition and movement of populations in the peace settlements between the two countries after the First World War.[1] A later chapter shows the acceleration of blood group studies by researchers from countries other than European and North America after the Second World War.

Because this research was so extensive, this book cannot be exhaustive in cataloging the record in every country. Neither space, time, nor linguistic ability permit a similar close analysis for the rest of blood group research in the world. That disclaimer notwithstanding, there are some features of research elsewhere that bear closer scrutiny either because of their

W. H. Schneider, *Blood Groups and Human Heredity, 1900-1950*, Medicine and Biomedical Sciences in Modern History,
https://doi.org/10.1007/978-3-031-69844-6_5

contribution to overall developments (e.g., Poland, Italy, and Japan) or for the sake of comparison (such as Holland, Finland, and Denmark). It is hoped these examples will stimulate further study, especially in the countries already examined.

Table 5.1 helps show where research in these additional countries fits into the overall record between the wars, at least as reflected by the amount of publication on blood group distribution.

Japanese and Italian authors conducted sufficient research (comparable to or exceeding that in countries previously examined) to warrant separate analysis in this chapter. Researchers in Holland, Denmark, Finland, and Poland were not quite as active, but their publications were significant enough for brief comparative analysis. The surprising amount of Dutch research was done mostly in the East Indies, and it will be more closely examined, along with research that was done in British and French colonies plus Latin America, in a separate section on blood group research outside Europe, Japan, and the U.S.

Table 5.1 Studies of blood group distribution by country of author, 1919–1939

Country or region	*Articles*	*Country or region*	*Articles*
With most research	819	Other Europe	83
USSR	183	Austria	26
Germany	149	Spain	18
Japan	143	Belgium	15
Italy	113	Switzerland	13
U.S.	99	Portugal	11
France	63		
Holland	44	Latin America	35
Britain	29	Brazil	17
		Argentina	10
Scandinavia	67	Lat. Amer (misc.)	8
Denmark	32		
Finland	24	Other	80
Norway, Sweden	11	Australia	23
		China	12
Eastern Europe	103	India	12
Poland	29	South Africa	11
Hungary	19	Unknown	22
Czechoslovakia	14		
Rumania	13	Total all articles	1106
Est, Latv, Lith	10		
E.Eur. (misc.)	18		

Blood Group Research in Japan

According to two basic criteria—amount of interest and peculiar differences—Japanese research on blood groups in the first half of the twentieth century warrants close and extensive analysis. Limitations of space and language, however, mean that this study can only indicate the overall pattern of that research along with some elements of that record which are instructive in comparison to other countries. Recent scholarship suggests that more extensive scrutiny of the history has already begun.[2]

At the beginning of the twentieth century Japan had just completed the first phase of Westernization that followed the Meiji Restoration.[3] In the field of scientific research and medical practice, the Western instructors who had arrived in the 1870s were being replaced at this time by their pupils and those Japanese returning from study abroad. Because Germany had been the foreign country to which the Japanese looked for medical instruction, this meant that the latest discoveries in immunology and serology were available in Japan, almost as they were being made. Kitasato's work with Koch and von Behring on serum therapy at the end of the 1880s was one of the most spectacular and best-known examples of how rapidly the Japanese became full participants in the dramatic advances in medical research after the turn of the century.[4]

Although it is not a sufficient explanation of why the Japanese showed such a strong interest in blood group research (England too had the scientific and medical infrastructure but developed much less interest until the 1930s), this rapid Westernization at least shows that the necessary medical research capabilities, such as training, research centers, plus medical journals, were in existence for the Japanese to participate in blood group research.[5] Whatever the reason, the earliest report of ABO blood group frequencies cited in the world literature was a 1916 article in the Japanese journal *Iji Shinbun* which reported tests of 350 inhabitants of Nagano.[6] Another isolated article appeared in 1920, but this was dwarfed by the publication of eight articles by Japanese researchers on blood group distribution in 1922 that signaled the beginning of a strong and sustained interest in the subject through the end of the 1930s.

A total of 136 articles on blood group distribution have been identified as published by Japanese researchers between 1922 and 1939, but this does not include a search of all Japanese-language medical journals. It is based on internal references from over 40 English-language articles plus Furuhata's efforts at compiling a bibliography of Japanese blood group research comparable to what was done in other countries.[7] So there is reason to believe that at least the articles from the 1920s are close to being complete. Some anecdotal evidence exists, however, to indicate the Japanese interest in blood groups went beyond the scientific literature to reach the popular imagination. For example, in 1933 Furuhata addressed the 5th Pan-Pacific Science Congress in Vancouver and sought to impress his audience with "how diligently young Japanese medical men are studying … blood groups." As a result of their work, he indicated, "there are no prefectures in Japan where the distribution of blood groups is not known." But the interest went further than that, Furuhata explained:

> There are some villages where the blood groups of all inhabitants in the village are tested and recorded in a list which is kept in the office. Every educated mother wishes to know the blood groups of her children. There are many schools where they tested the blood grouping of pupils in order to be ready to apply their knowledge in any case where it is necessary. In the Japanese Army and Navy they are testing the blood groups of soldiers and marines, which will be very useful in case of transfusion.[8]

Even if this search of articles on Japanese blood group distribution is not exhaustive, a greater number have been identified for the 1930s.[9] As a result, this body of research is useful for comparative purposes and gives an idea of the order of magnitude of Japanese work in the field as well as many of its more specific features over the period from 1920 through 1939. With that note of caution, Fig. 5.1 is offered to illustrate how Japanese research on blood group distribution rose and fell during this period compared to all research on the subject.

The unevenness of this graph of Japanese research on blood group distribution may very well be the result of incomplete references. Nonetheless, the number of articles which appeared in the 1920s (56) was high and increased significantly in the 1930s to 80 articles. In fact, it shows at least a steady or more probably an increase in interest while the number of articles published worldwide declined.

Many features of the research by Japanese authors were similar to those of blood group researchers in other countries. For example, studies were done by a variety of researchers in many different locations who published in a large number of different journals. Over 90 Japanese authors published articles on blood group distribution between 1922 and 1939. Of the 26 authors for whom institutional affiliation is known, only 5 were in

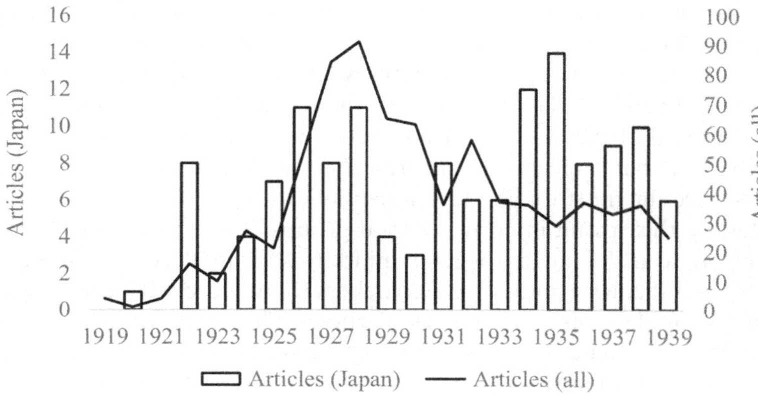

Fig. 5.1 Articles per year on blood group distribution by Japanese researchers, 1920–1939

Tokyo. Five others were in Taiwan, four in Kanazawa including Tanemoto Furuhata (about whom more will be said later), and the rest were in several other university and government positions around the country, including Sendai (two), Kyoto, Nagasaki, Jeijo, Nagoya (two), Hokkaido, Kumamoto, and Wakayama.

Despite the breadth of interest, in Japan as in most other countries there were few researchers who did extensive testing. In fact, only four individuals can be identified who published more than two articles on blood group distribution. Moreover, two locations, Taiwan and Kanazawa, stand out as centers of Japanese blood group research. Almost 20 articles were published by researchers in Taiwan, based at the Medical School of Taihoku University, where in 1931 Yoshito Maryuma began publishing a series of studies on the blood group distribution of the island's populations in the journal of the Taiwan Medical Association, ***Taiwan Igakkai Zasshi***. Although there had been a few earlier reports of testing on the island by Furuhata and Kirihara in 1925 and 1926, Maryuma and his associates conducted systematic tests of the Tayal, Paiwan, and other peoples indigenous to the island, the results of which were reported in nine articles that appeared in the 1930s.[10]

These were not all of the blood group studies done on the island. Some of the testing followed the pattern of what was done by researchers in other countries, such as the testing of school children and testing of the new MN blood groups. Others were more unusual tests of possible links between blood groups and other presumably inherited characteristics. Maryuma himself did a study of blood groups and dental caries, and in 1934 studies reported the blood types of groups as diverse as opium addicts and baseball players.[11] Because these researchers published mostly in the journal of the local medical society, the 18 articles on blood group distribution that appeared in *Taiwan Igakkai Zasshi* in the 1920s and 1930s were the most for any Japanese publication.

Despite this strong interest in blood groups, Taiwan was remote from the Japanese mainland both geographically and intellectually. Hence, it would be difficult to argue that researchers there exercised a great deal of influence on Japanese research as a whole. The other center of blood group study at Kanazawa was in a much better position to publicize and influence others in Japan. Moreover, it was directed by Tanemoto Furuhata who became the most important Japanese serologist and one of the country's leading human geneticists well into the post-Second World War era.

Furuhata followed the typical path of training for a budding Japanese researcher at the beginning of the twentieth century.[12] He graduated from the medical college of the Imperial University in Tokyo in 1916, and after the war he spent two years studying in Germany, England, France, and the U.S. In 1924 Furuhata received an appointment as Professor at the Kanazawa Medical College, where he established an Institute of Legal Medicine. The following year he was joined by K. Ichida and T. Kishi as assistants, and together they published many articles on blood group distribution and other subjects in forensic medicine. In 1936 Furuhata took a position at the Imperial University in Tokyo, where he became Dean of the Medical College after the Second World War.

Furuhata and his associates were well placed to influence Japanese serology during the 1920s and 1930s. They did this first by publication of a large number of articles on blood group distribution. Over 20 of the 136 articles identified by Japanese researchers were authored by Furuhata, his associates, or students at Kanazawa. Nor was this confined solely to their own journals. Only seven of their articles appeared in the journal of legal medicine published at Kanazawa, *Hanzaigaku Zasshi*. The rest were published in a variety of other Japanese as well as foreign medical journals. The foreign publications grew out of Furuhata's stature on the international scene. For example, he represented Japanese blood group researchers as early as the International Institute of Anthropology meeting in 1927 in Amsterdam, and meetings of the Pan-Pacific Science Congresses in Tokyo (1926), Java (1930), and Vancouver (1933). Furuhata was even more effective in making the results of Japanese research available to the rest of the world through his work with ***Japan Medical World***. He wrote articles and served on the editorial board of this English-language journal which was published in the 1920s to provide the wider world with original research as well as abstracts of articles from 50 Japanese-language medical publications. One of Furuhata's most important contributions was a bibliography of Japanese blood group research that appeared late in 1928.[13]

Furuhata is recognized for discovering a number of blood group agglutinogens (Q, E, T), but his greatest claim to theoretical discovery was an independent recognition of the error in Von Dungern and Hirszfeld's 2-gene 2-allele explanation of the inheritance of the ABO blood groups. Furuhata's suggestion of three genes was published shortly after Bernstein's 1924 and 1925 articles appeared, so his colleagues did not recognize his priority for the discovery.[14] In addition, he helped establish the legitimacy of using blood group testing in paternity exclusion cases in Japan.

There was no other blood group researcher of Furuhata's stature or influence in Japan during the 1920s and 1930s, but a large number of other researchers also published on the subject in a variety of journals. In fact, the numerous articles in the Taiwan Medical Society journal reflected the many other researchers publishing articles on blood group distribution in so many different publications. This included 20 articles in foreign journals with no single country or publication favored except the *Journal of Immunology*, where three articles between 1923 and 1926 gave early worldwide notice of Japanese serological research.[15] Otherwise, the majority of articles published in Japan appeared in journals of local medical societies (50) and medical specialty journals (37). Unlike other countries, there were relatively few articles on blood group distribution that appeared in national medical journals.

The subjects of interest to Japanese blood group researchers were similar to those in other countries: anthropology, disease, and other potentially inherited qualities. There was a difference, however, in emphasis. As Fig. 5.2 shows, only 21 of the 143 articles mentioned blood groups links to disease. With only a few articles each on such subjects as temperament, prostitution, criminals, and the Taiwanese studies of opium addicts and baseball players, this meant that the overwhelming majority of articles concerned race and anthropology.

These included the usual serological mapping of the Japanese population on the home islands, but there were also many studies of neighboring and subject peoples by Japanese researchers who took great pains to show

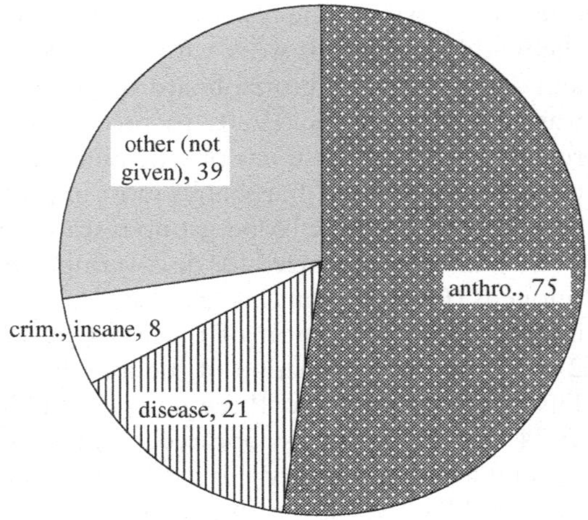

Fig. 5.2 Topics of Japanese articles on blood group distribution 1916–1939 (n = 143)

the differences between their blood type distribution and that of other people. The numerous articles in the 1930s on the indigenous population of Taiwan have already been mentioned. In addition, among the earliest subjects tested were Koreans, about whom three articles were published in 1922, and the Ainu whose testing was first reported in three articles in 1925, and who remained a subject of study well into the 1930s.[16]

Some of the first studies in 1922 were tests by Shinichi Kirihara and Rinsai Haku, two Japanese researchers residing in Korea who found a relatively higher percentage of blood type B in the north of the country than was found in Japan. Thus, in one article they noted "a marked difference between the serological constitution of these two peoples"; and in another article they found "quite distinct differences between the blood grouping percentages or biological indices of the Japanese and Koreans."[17] The authors, accordingly, placed the Koreans in the Hirszfelds' "Asio-African" group of races (percentage of blood type A lower than B), whereas the Japanese were classified in the "intermediate" group (blood type A between one and two times greater than B). Historian Hyun's reassessment of this blood group research argues that Furuhata's main goal was to establish the racial superiority of Japanese among Asian peoples.[18]

The Ainu people in Hokkaido, Japan's northernmost island, was the subject of great interest because they were presumed to be the indigenous population of the island.[19] There was less concern with the exact biochemical index of the Ainu than with the fact that their blood group distribution confirmed the obvious differences in physical appearance that anthropologists had already studied. Blood group testing of the Ainu served, therefore, not only to distinguish them from the Japanese but also to promise a possible new way of answering the long-standing question of the origins of the Ainu. This approach was hampered by some wide variations in the findings of different researchers, plus the fact that there was no population outside Japan with a blood group distribution that matched them.[20] The finding of large differences in blood group distribution among the seven aboriginal populations of Taiwan also did little to resolve a similar question as to their origins. Thus, Maryuma's testing in 1931 found the Tayal with a biochemical index comparable to the Russians, Spanish Jews, and the Chinese, while the Pawan matched the Philippine Islanders.

Confirming the conclusion of recent research by Hyun, the deeper-seated reason for the great interest in the anthropology of blood groups by the Japanese was to help confirm Japan's place in the world. The Hirszfelds' obviously Eurocentric classification scheme defined biochemical race indices of "European type" to be percentage of blood type A more than twice the percentage of type B, and "Asio-African type" to be percentage of A less than that of B, with all the rest in an "Intermediate type." From this perspective, one can understand the interest in the early Japanese findings of a distribution that fell in the intermediate as opposed to the Afro-Asian category where the Koreans, Indians, Chinese, and other Asian peoples were classified. As variations of the classification scheme became more complex, the response of Japanese researchers was to distinguish themselves from neighboring peoples. Furuhata, for example, found that the distribution of blood groups in Japan fit none of the Hirszfelds' categories; hence, he suggested that a new and distinct "Japanese type" was necessary in classification schemes.[21] In a later summary article, Matsui Akune, a Japanese collaborator of Schiff's in Berlin, echoed this same view.

> The whole of the truly Japanese populated area is clearly distinct serologically from neighboring areas. The characteristic combination for the Japanese is relatively higher A and lower B. A corresponding combination is found in no other population of the East.[22]

To conclude this section, the great concern with the anthropological standing of Japan's population helps explain the early and continuing interest in blood groups, which was one of the most striking features of

Japanese research on blood groups in the 1920s and 1930s. Even without assurance of a completely exhaustive search of articles, the research done was greater than that in almost any other country. For example, there were more articles by Japanese researchers on blood group distribution than by Americans in the 1920s and more than by Soviet or German researchers in the 1930s. Unlike the latter two, Japanese researchers found new populations to test outside the country and retested previously studied populations when the new MN system and other sub-groups were discovered in the 1930s. For example, the first tests in Japan using Landsteiner and Levine's MN discovery were done in 1933. In the next three years there were 19 studies published for 10 Japanese cities and prefectures as well as 2 in Taiwan. Hence, maturation of blood group research in Japan brought an increase rather than a decline in activity.

As in other countries, there was one researcher, Furuhata, who was clearly the most important in Japan, but he hardly controlled or dominated the work which was conducted in a variety of locations and was published in many different journals. Most of these were medical journals, but Japanese researchers were relatively less interested than their foreign counterparts in the relationship of blood groups and disease. Anthropological questions were the foremost subject of interest, despite the fact that Japanese anthropologists (and anthropological journals) were almost completely absent from the study of blood groups and race.

Blood Group Research in Italy

Research on blood groups in Italy between the wars was quite substantial. In fact, as reflected by articles on blood group distribution, there were only three countries where researchers published more such articles than the Italians. Unlike the Soviet Union or Germany where research declined abruptly or Japan where there was an increase during the 1930s, Fig. 5.3 shows that in Italy the blood group research mirrored closely the pattern of research worldwide, with a peak of interest in the late1920s, then a decline and levelling off in the1930s.

Generally following the worldwide pattern, this Italian interest in blood group research grew out of the peculiar nature of Italian science and medical practice as well as the geographical and political setting of the country between the wars. For example, the late unification of Italy meant that, like Germany, numerous intellectual and university centers had developed in the independent Italian polities that had existed since the Middle Ages.

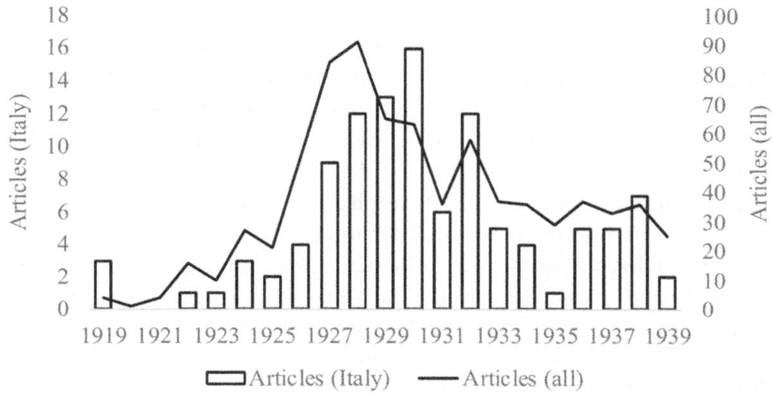

Fig. 5.3 Articles per year on blood group distribution by Italian researchers, 1919–1939

This meant the country had many centers of scientific and medical research by the end of the nineteenth century. Although newly independent Italy devoted fewer resources than Germany to medical research, as the twentieth century began, Italian researchers were certainly aware of new developments and had enough research centers and numerous medical and scientific publications to verify and spread the word of the blood group discoveries.

Beyond having the necessary research infrastructure, Italians interested in blood group studies were also influenced by at least two other circumstances that help explain the strong interest that eventually developed. One was the existence of historical, regional, and ethnic differences that reinforced the political and intellectual division in the country. After political unification in the 1860s these differences became the subject of extensive scholarly study, and blood groups provided an additional way for researchers to give scientific definition to the population differences in Italy, much as in the Soviet Union and Germany. A second reason for the interest in blood groups was the residual influence of Cesare Lombroso's work in criminal anthropology, especially its emphasis on hereditary or "constitutional" influences on behavior and physical condition.[23] More will be said about this in a later chapter, but the interest in "markers" of heredity that Lombroso popularized in the last third of the nineteenth century carried over into the twentieth century and provided very fertile ground in Italy for the growth of the idea that blood groups might be linked to all sorts of human conditions, especially diseases.

Mussolini's fascist rule began in 1922, but its influence on blood group research is difficult to gauge. Pressures on Jewish researchers were not comparable to those in Germany, at least until the end of the period, and the racial component of Mussolini's ideology was much less in evidence than in National Socialism. For example, Leone Lattes, the most famous Italian serologist who was Jewish, remained at his teaching post until the racial laws of 1939 forced him to flee Italy for Argentina. The one influence on blood group research that was an indirect consequence of Mussolini's policies was his interest in colonial empire. A significant number of articles (ten) were published on the blood groups of populations under colonial rule in Libya, Eritrea, and Ethiopia.

Lattes was the one Italian blood group researcher with a stature comparable to Schiff in Germany or Hirszfeld in Poland.[24] He was born in Turin in 1887 and completed his medical training there in 1909. He then studied in Frankfurt and returned to the Institute of Legal Medicine at the University of Turin in 1913. After war service, Lattes was appointed Professor of Legal Medicine at the University of Messina, then Modena, and finally the University of Pavia in 1933, where he remained, except for the break during the Second World War, until his death in 1954.

Lattes' work primarily concerned technical and theoretical questions about the role of blood groups in legal medicine. He did not author numerous or large studies of original research on blood group distribution. His most important influence, in addition to manuals and articles on applications of the latest blood group discoveries, was his attempt to summarize the work of the new field. For example, one of Lattes' first articles on blood groups appeared in 1915, entitled "Individuality of Human Blood," which summarized much of the prewar work as well as his own testing to confirm it. That title was used again for his most famous book, published first in 1923, but also translated into German, French, and English before a second Italian edition came out in 1934. Because of timing, *The Individuality of Human Blood* was probably the most important reference work on blood group testing results during the whole interwar period; moreso than Snyder's 1929 book and Steffan's 1933 handbook, neither of which were translated.

The first report of the blood group distribution among significant numbers of Italians (Lattes' 1915 article tested only 24 individuals) was the Hirszfelds' landmark 1919 article that included tests on 500 Italian soldiers in Macedonia. Despite a provocative breakdown in the longer version appearing in the French journal *Anthropologie* that showed differences between the ABO distribution in soldiers from northern (201 subjects), central (79), and southern Italy (220),[25] the Hirszfelds only inspired a handful of important regional studies by Italian researchers until the mid-1920s (see Table 5.2). This was followed shortly thereafter by two summaries of the whole country in 1928 by Ettore Cuboni in Milan and Domenico Viola in Pavia.[26]

This slow start in studying the anthropology of blood groups was partly a reflection of the generally delayed interest in blood group research in Italy. The first year that more than four articles appeared in Italy on any aspect of blood group testing was 1927, although during this time, researchers showed an interest in the possible relationship between blood groups and disease. In 1925, for example, articles appeared on the distribution of blood groups among cancer patients in Milan, and the following year there were reports of tests on patients with adenoids and children with diphtheria.[27] In 1927 there were two articles each on tuberculosis and cancer, as well as on syphilis and malaria.

Interest in anthropology and disease prompted the majority (75 percent) of articles in the late 1920s and early 1930s when research hit its peak. In fact, there was almost an equal number of both kinds of articles, as shown in Fig. 5.4.

Included in the anthropological articles were ten studies of overseas populations, most of which were inhabitants of the Italian colony of Libya.

Table 5.2 Early studies of blood group distribution in Italy, 1922–1927

Author	*Year*	*Location*	*No. of subj.*
Cavalieri	1922	Pavia	139
Mino	1923	Turin	734
Rizzatti	1924	Modena	559
Romanese	1926	Sardinia	947
Goldstein	1927	Trieste	1,488

Sources: Cavalieri, "Contributo allo studio dei gruppi sanguigni," *Archivio di patologia e clinica medica*, 1 (1922) ?; Prospero Mino, "La distribuzione dei gruppi sanguini in Italia," *Archivio di Antropologia Criminale*, 43 (1923): 438–45; E. Rizzatti, "Sulla Distribuzione dei Gruppi Sanguigni in Alcune Province DellaVal Padana," *Bolletino Della Societa Medica, Parma*, 3 (1924); Romanese, "Contributo Allo Studio Della Distribuzione dei Gruppi Sanguigni Nella Provincia di Cagliari," *Rassegna Internazionale di Clinica e Terapia*, 7 (1926): 272; Marco Goldstein, "I gruppi sanguigni degli abitanti de Trieste," *Policlinico*, 34 (1927), 523–6

Fig. 5.4 Subjects of Italian articles on blood group distribution, 1919–1939 (n = 114)

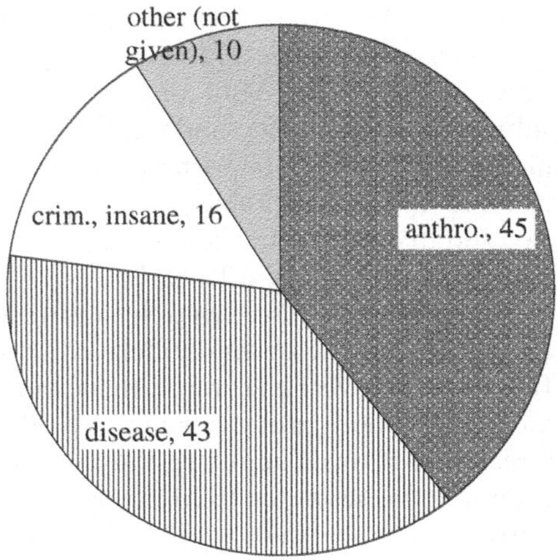

Carlo Tedeschi, director of a hospital at Derna, conducted or directed many of these studies.[28]

The diseases which were most often the subject of testing by Italian researchers were tuberculosis (ten articles), cancer (eight), and syphilis (nine) with malaria the subject of three articles. Hence, this pattern differed little from other countries. Peculiar to Italy was the strong interest of researchers in studies of blood groups among criminals and the insane. Sixteen articles on these subjects including constitutional predisposition to disease appeared between the wars. The assumption by researchers was that the blood groups were an easily tested phenotypic marker with a well-established genotype that was possibly linked to other presumably inherited conditions such as criminality and insanity, or more broadly, other diseases or body forms. Proponents of these "constitutional studies," as they were called in the 1920s and 1930s, were strongest in Italy and Germany and will be considered in greater detail in a later chapter.

There were a large number and variety of researchers who published articles on blood group distribution between the wars in Italy. In fact, much like the case in Japan, few researchers authored more than two such articles. The author with the most (eight articles) was Domenico Viola, who listed himself in articles as an army captain affiliated with the Institute for Legal Medicine at Pavia (before Lattes' appointment there). Viola's articles were on the anthropological significance of the blood groups, beginning in

1928 with one of the first articles to draw together all testing in Italy into an overall assessment of blood group distribution in the country. His work appeared primarily in anthropological journals and the bulletin of the medical society of Pavia, *Bollettino Della Societa Medico-Chirurgica di Pavia*. His articles often tested for correlation between blood type and such "constitutional factors" as head shape, hair and eye color, and height. His last blood group study was published in the *Giornale di medicina militare* in 1934 and examined the blood types of soldiers convicted of crimes, among whom he found a higher frequency of types B and AB which confirmed the controversial finding of Gundel in Germany.[29] Tedeschi, the head of the Derna Hospital in Libya, published three studies of the local population, and his colleagues published two more. Otherwise, besides Lattes, the only other frequent Italian author of blood group distribution studies was Ferdinando Nicoletti at the Institute for Legal Medicine of the University of Palermo who published four articles between 1928 and 1933 on the blood groups of the inhabitants of Sicily.

A composite picture of the Italian blood group researchers can be gleaned from their institutional affiliations, which are known in 63 cases. Of them 33 had positions at 13 different universities and 25 were at hospitals, clinics, or sanatoria. The majority of the university affiliations were with medical clinics and services in a variety of specialties, with pathology being the most common (six authors). Eight of the university researchers were at institutes of legal medicine. The non-university hospital affiliations were city and provincial as well as some independent clinics and sanatoria. There was even less of a discernable pattern to the specialties and services of these authors at the non-university institutions, although four were at psychiatric hospitals. The predominance of the medical affiliations explains why so many of the articles appeared in medical journals. It contradicts the fact, however, that a good percentage of articles were of anthropological interest.

Most striking about the geographical location of researchers was their wide range. The only cities where more than three researchers resided were Naples (eight researchers), Turin (six), and Milan (four). Only a handful of cities had 3 researchers (Cagliari, Palermo, Perugia, Sassari, and Parma), while 17 other cities had only 1 or 2 researchers, including Rome. The large number of researchers in Naples did not make it a research center, because only two of the authors were in the same practice (the ear, nose, and throat clinic of the university).

These two characteristics—the predominance of medical institutions and the broad geographical spread of researchers—are very evident in the journals where articles were published. The 114 articles on blood group distribution by Italian researchers appeared in 65 different publications. Forty of these journals carried only a single article, but none of the rest had more than six. The five journals with five or six articles were representative of the different kinds of publications. Thus, the *Archivio di Antropologia Criminale* and Lattes' *Bolletino della Sezione Italiana della Societa internazionale di Microbiologia* reflected the anthropological interests and the new field of microbiology. The three journals with five articles included a regional publication (*Bollettino Della Societa Medico-Chirurgica di Pavia*), one of a medical specialty (*Giornale italiano di dermatologia e sifiologia*) and the national medical journal *Policlinico*. As was shown in the overview chapter, Italy was unusual in having so much research on blood groups without a single journal carrying a significant number of blood group distribution articles. There was no new publication inspired by the discoveries, as was the case in Germany and the Soviet Union, nor did an established journal become the publication of choice for reporting the results of studies as happened in France and the U.S. The experience in Japan was probably the most comparable to Italy in that there was broad interest, but without the equivalent of a regional Japanese journal that published a large number of studies. Nor did Lattes establish a research center with students as Furuhata did.

The overall effect diminished the impact of the sum of Italian research since articles were spread over so many different publications. As Fig. 5.5 shows, the overwhelming number of articles appeared in medical journals (80 of 114 articles), with over half of them in medical specialty publications.

Only 13 articles appeared in more broadly read national medical publications such as *Policlinico* (five articles) or *Minerva Medica* (four articles). The most important anthropological journal was Lattes' *Archivio di Antropologia Criminale* (six articles). Interest in overseas populations was reflected in nine articles that appeared in journals of military and colonial medicine. Only three articles of original research on blood group distribution by Italian authors were published in foreign journals.

To summarize, the most notable features about the record of Italian blood group research between the wars were the large amount of interest and the importance of one researcher, Lattes. In addition, the subjects of interest to Italians were remarkably broad and balanced between anthropology, disease, and other conditions possibly linked to blood groups.

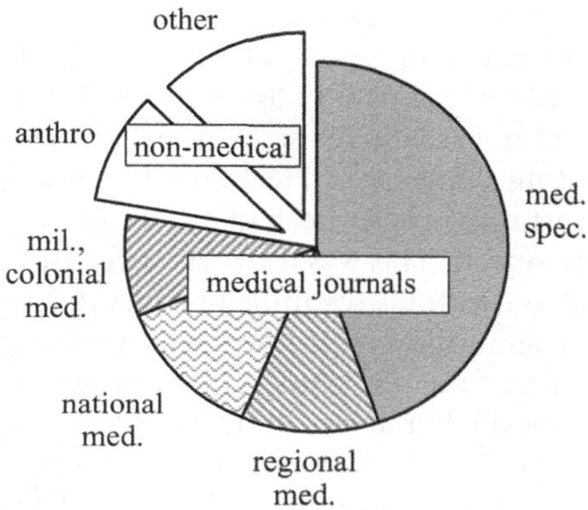

Fig. 5.5 Types of Italian journals where blood group distribution articles appeared, 1919–1939 (n = 114)

Despite the international recognition of Lattes as an expert in the new field, he failed to establish an important center that directed research on blood group distribution or gave it a focus.

Blood Group Research in Poland, Denmark, Finland, and Holland

Blood group research in Poland, Denmark, Finland, and Holland produced the next greatest number articles on blood group distribution between the wars (20–40 in each country). These countries were similar in some ways that help explain this level of interest. For example, their medical infrastructure was well enough developed to recognize the importance of and ability to extend the serological discoveries made in the first two decades of the twentieth century. They were also relatively small in size, or in the case of Finland and Poland, newly reestablished countries where the heightened nationalism following the First World War gave researchers a motive for using blood groups to help distinguish the population of their country from others. Moreover, the size and nature of the populations made national blood group surveys feasible. Finally, in each of these countries there was at least one center with a well-recognized expert in blood group research. Naturally, there were some features of history and geography, such as the existence of the Dutch colonial empire, which also explain some significant differences in the record of blood group research in these four countries.

The main research center in Poland was created by Ludwik Hirszfeld. Although in hindsight, it seems perfectly logical that Hirszfeld should settle in the new Polish state, he had not lived in Poland since he was18, and it was largely through the persuasion of his cousin Ludwik Rajchman of the Ministry of Health that he was appointed to run the State Hygiene Institute where he had the resources to create an Institute for Serum Research. This was fortunate because it gave him a practical purpose to go along with his scientific pursuits. Hirszfeld wasted no time training a new generation of researchers who were instrumental in advancing the discoveries of the war years. The institute soon became one of the leading serological laboratories in the world.[30]

One of the first and most important of these projects was the testing of new military recruits. In 1922 Jan Mydlarski of the Army Anthropological Service conducted the work in collaboration with Wanda Halber of Hirszfeld's Institute. In addition to more traditional anthropometric measurements, they recorded the blood types of over 12,000 recruits, using equipment as shown in Fig. 5.6.[31]

This immediately became the largest and most complete blood group study done anywhere in the world. Following the methods of the Hirszfelds' Macedonian research (and preceding Bernstein's new hypothesis), Mydlarski and Halber only reported the percentages of blood types A and B, confirming in the authors' words, "Poland occupies from the serological viewpoint, an intermediate place between European and Asian-African types." Their breakdown of regions in Poland showed the highest percentage of A in the West, and the researchers also suggested some correlation between blood type A, blond hair, and tall stature.

This interest in anthropological applications was the exception, however, in Polish blood group studies between the wars. The large majority of subsequent articles were on possible links between blood groups and disease or insanity. In fact, the only other anthropological study besides the Halber/Mydlarski study was a 1930 article by another of Hirszfeld's students who tested the recently discovered MN distribution in the Polish population.[32] There were two main reasons for this surprisingly strong emphasis on disease. The first was the comprehensive nature of the large army study which obtained results from all regions of Poland. Thus, after this testing was done, there was little need to repeat it locally. This was very different from Germany and the Soviet Union where because of the size of the countries even advocates of national surveys proposed

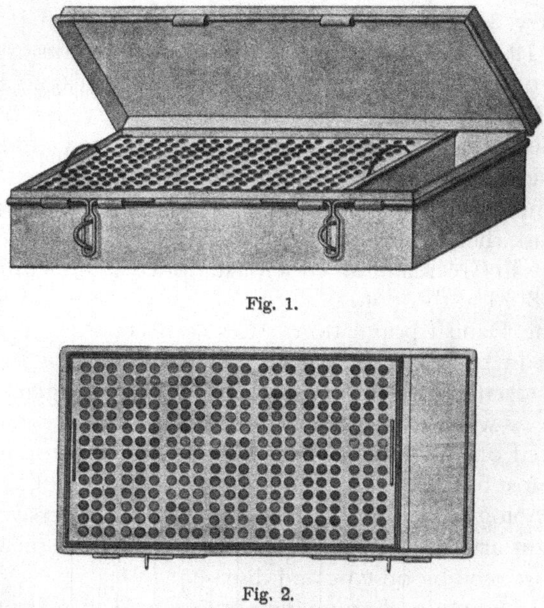

Fig. 5.6 Equipment of Halber and Mydlarski for testing military recruits. Source: Halber and Mydlarzki, 479

longer-term studies in stages. This Polish methodology was also the way that national testing was conducted in Finland, Denmark, and Holland.

Another reason for the great interest in disease was that Hirszfeld himself moved quickly in that direction following the war, beginning with his research on blood groups and the results of Schick tests for diphtheria. Added to this was the fact that in contrast to anthropological research there were no simple breakthrough discoveries either linking blood groups to disease or disproving a connection. Hence, the inconclusive and often contradictory findings prompted additional studies by Hirszfeld (and throughout the world) in the late 1920s and1930s.

In Finland a systematic study of the blood groups of the population was begun in 1925 and directed thereafter by Oswald Streng of the Helsinki University Sero-Bacteriology Institute. The primary interest of Streng and most of his students and co-workers was anthropological. They concentrated on distinguishing between the three main population groups in the country: Finnish-speakers, Swedish-speakers, and Lapps. Streng's first tests in 1925 were on a group of 1500 inhabitants, and it was followed in two years by a larger study with his colleague Elsa Ryuti of another 3500 subjects. By 1930 there had been 10 studies of over 25,000 people.[33] This anthropological research was conducted almost completely to the exclusion of any studies of blood groups and disease. The few studies of that kind were mostly done by Oluf Sievers of Streng's lab.[34]

In Denmark there were some early anthropological blood group studies of Eskimos in Greenland by a doctor stationed at a Julianhaab Hospital; then in 1928 an anthropological committee was created for systematic testing of the Danish population. After some confusion and questions about errors in testing, the project was taken over by Ib Freuchen of Thorvald Madsen's State Serum Institute in Copenhagen. Tests of over 20,000 subjects were done by 1935.[35] In the meantime extensive research was conducted on the possible links between blood groups and disease. One of the most frequent authors on the subject was Oluf Thomsen at the General Pathology Laboratory of Copenhagen University Clinic, who authored eight articles between 1927 and 1931, none of which showed correlation between blood type and disease.[36]

Most research on blood group distribution in Holland was done as part of a national survey officially sponsored by the Royal Academy of Sciences. In 1925 at the suggestion of the anatomist Louis Bolk, the academy created a "Committee for the Physical-anthropological Investigation of the Dutch Population." Its work was divided among five subcommittees which studied such features as the height and body-form indices.[37] The "Biochemical Committee" was to study blood group distribution, and the person whom Bolk chose to direct the research was Marianne van Herwerden of the Embryological and Histological Laboratory at the University of Utrecht. She quickly became the country's leading blood group serologist.

Van Herwerden (see Fig. 5.7), the daughter of a professor at Utrecht University, studied medicine and wrote a dissertation on the menstrual cycle of apes.[38] After receiving her medical degree, she worked in Vienna and contemplated establishing a private practice before her mentor C. A. Pekelharing, persuaded her to accept an appointment as an assistant at his physiology laboratory in Utrecht. Before her return in 1908, Van Herwerden worked at the Naples Zoological Station. In the next ten years she published on a variety of subjects in cytology and embryology, including the unusually large chromosomes in the salivary gland cells of flies (diptera) and the reproductive cycle of the water flea (daphnia). Van Herwerden's work in human genetics grew out of an interest in eugenics that followed a trip to the U.S. in 1920. The visit was arranged by

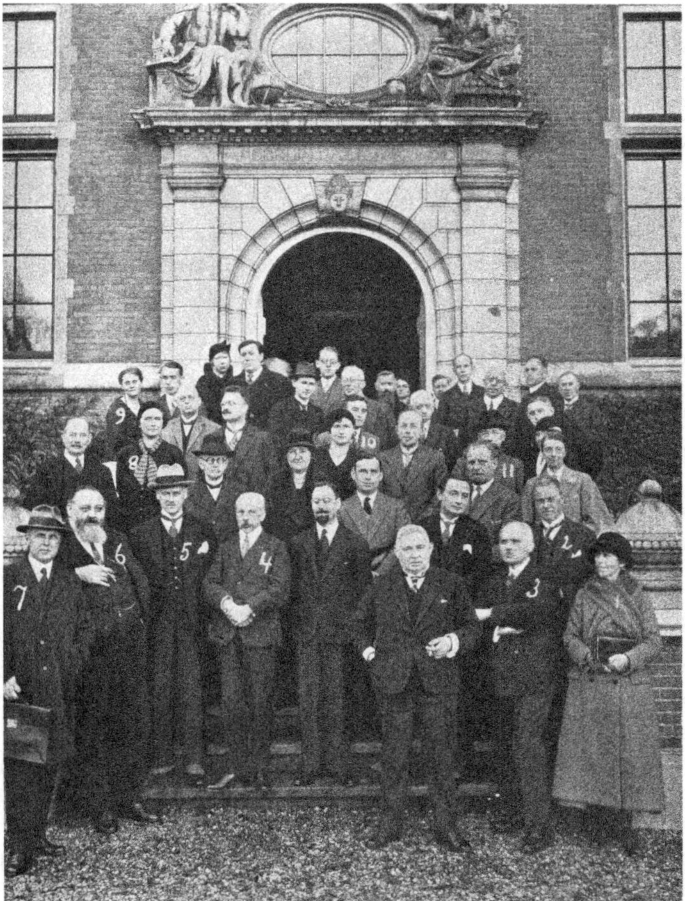

Fig. 5.7 "October 29, 1932 meeting of the Nederlandsch Nationaal Bureau voor Anthropology" (Van Herwerden is in the lower right corner). Source: Bork-Feltkamp, 1938, 132

Pekelharing when Van Herwerden was passed over as his replacement after his retirement in 1918. (The first female professor in Holland had only been appointed in 1917.) After her return she was named a lecturer at Utrecht.

During her three-month stay in America, Van Herwerden visited almost every major East coast biomedical research center between Johns Hopkins and Harvard, including Alexis Carrel's laboratory at the Rockefeller Institute and Morgan's at Columbia. Her interest in eugenics was stimulated by two visits to Charles Davenport's Eugenics Record Office at Cold Springs Harbor.[39] Two other significant features of Van Herwerden's American tour were her visits to the most important women's colleges (Goucher, Bryn Mawr, and Radcliffe) and the wide notoriety she received back in Holland as a result of her series of "Letters from America" which were published in the *Nederlandsch Tijdschrift voor Geneeskunde*.[40]

In the early 1920s Herwerden wrote occasional articles on eugenics for the *Tijdschrift* and was instrumental in founding the Genetics Committee which was the precursor of the Dutch Eugenics Society. Because of her American contacts, she was named the representative from Holland to the International Federation of Eugenics Organizations, and in 1926 Van Herwerden authored a book for the general public entitled, *Eugenics and Human Heredity*, which quickly went to a second printing.[41] When she was named to head the blood group survey, Herwerden had done no work on blood groups, although she had published some articles on serological techniques and trained one of the first Dutch researchers to publish on blood group distribution in 1924.[42] She, therefore, began the project with a background article on the blood groups in 1926 for the journal of the Dutch Anthropological Society, *Mensch en Maatschappij*, which also described plans for the survey project sponsored by the Academy of Sciences.[43]

Herwerden decided to do all testing for the survey, with a few exceptions, at her Utrecht laboratory. Her reasons were not only that the small size of the country made it possible but that methodologically it was desirable for uniformity. As she explained to the session on blood group research that she organized for the International Institute of Anthropology congress in Amsterdam in 1927, "It seems to me that a centralized investigation is absolutely necessary. Even if coordinated centrally, I have very little confidence in hemagglutination [tests] done hastily by various doctors in the middle of their daily practices without standardized procedures."[44] At that congress Herwerden reported the preliminary results of tests from several Dutch provinces, university students, a few remote villages, and Jews in Apeldoorn and Amsterdam.

The more detailed results of the national Dutch blood group survey were published in a series of articles in the proceedings of the Royal Academy of Sciences. The first was a 1930 article on tests of 3085 students at the universities of Leiden and Utrecht, plus 691 prisoners. This was followed by a 1932 article co-authored with C. P. J. Penning on 1074 inhabitants of the isolated region of "Over Velume." Both of these were reprinted in German periodicals. A third article appeared in 1933 co-authored with Floris Hers on 1591 inhabitants of another remote locale, "Hoeksche Waard."[45] Herwerden died in 1934, but a final report appeared in 1940 by Hendricus J. T. Bijlmer, a veteran of the Dutch East Indies blood group research team. In all the studies, which included over 20,000 tests, comparisons were done between blood groups and color of hair and eyes as well as head shape, but no correlations were found. As to other results, Bijlmer admitted "the whole is rather confusing." For example, the finding of highest percentage of type O and lowest of A in the northeast suggested no conclusions. On the other hand, the highest percentage of type B was found in the western provinces which indicated "the B factor may have reached the Netherlands from the side of the sea."[46]

Despite having conducted this large national study, not to mention all the research from the East Indies, the Dutch showed surprisingly little interest in the relationship between blood groups and disease or other potentially inherited characteristics. Herwerden included some tests of prisoners in her first study, and there were two articles in 1926 and 1928 on possible links to cancer and tuberculosis. Although these were early reports, there were no other studies done in Holland on blood groups and disease.

Before the decision to do a national survey, the only anthropological research on blood group distribution by Dutch researchers had been done in the East Indies.[47] This began a remarkable series of studies conducted at the same time as the research in Holland. The work was done largely by colonial health officers who published their results almost exclusively in the *Geneeskundig Tijdschrift voor Nederlandsch-Indië*. The results will be examined in more detail later, but the 30 articles reflected both the extent of the Dutch colonial medical service (over 500 European-trained doctors in 1927), as well as their interest in the complicated anthropology of the island's populations.[48]

Poland, Holland, Denmark, and Finland were similar in that they all possessed important serological research centers and conducted national blood group surveys between the wars. Their work was also similar in where researchers published their results. Most notable was a significant number of articles that appeared in foreign language journals, not surprising if researchers wished their findings to enter the mainstream of science. For early Polish blood group work when for a time there were limited numbers of Polish scientific publications, researchers used the proceedings of the Polish Biological Society which appeared in French as an annex of the *Comptes rendus de la Société de Biologie*. Ludwik Hirszfeld also often published in the *Klinische Wochenschrift*. Following this pattern, his two most important books were published in Berlin and Paris.[49] Later articles on blood groups and disease by Polish doctors from around the country appeared in Polish-language medical journals.

Danish, Finnish, and Dutch researchers had many well-established medical journals in their country where they published the results of blood group testing. To reach broader audiences, however, the Danes also published in German journals and occasionally in the *Journal of Immunology*. Finnish researchers published less often in foreign journals, but articles in *Acta Societatis Medicorum Fennicae Duodecim* were frequently in German, thus making them more accessible to a wider audience. Likewise, in Holland all the results of the Royal Academy of Sciences blood group studies were published in English. The Dutch East Indies research, however, was much less accessible to foreign readers. Even though the medical journal there had been published since the 1850s, it was entirely in Dutch and had a limited circulation. Researchers occasionally summarized the findings, however, in foreign journals.[50]

Other European Research

Blood group research in other European countries was not extensive enough to permit detailed analysis, but it was far from negligible. In fact, scholars in the remaining Scandinavian, east and central European countries plus Iberia, published over 160 articles on blood group distribution between the wars. The large amount of this work can be taken, at the least, as another indication of the widespread interest in blood groups. Beyond that, brief mention of some similarities and differences of timing, depth, and subjects of interest will round out the picture of research on the distribution of the blood groups before looking at research outside Europe, the U.S., and Japan.

Given the interest in Denmark and Finland, it is somewhat surprising that there was not more work in blood group research in the other Scandinavian countries of Sweden and Norway. In the latter, for example, only a handful of articles on blood group distribution were published before the end of the 1930s when a combination of anthropological interest in Eskimos and mass testing in preparation for wartime transfusion produced reports on the blood groups of tens of thousands of Norwegians.[51] There was even less interest in Sweden where only five articles were published on blood group distribution (three on the Lapps) during the whole interwar period. Given the state of medical research in the country and possible anthropological or race questions at the time, this lack of interest was surprising.

Such was not the case in eastern Europe where, as in Poland, researchers from most other countries showed an early and strong interest in the anthropology of blood groups. This began first in Hungary where articles on blood group distribution were published independently and shortly after the Hirszfelds' work in the First World War. The clear motivation of Oskar Weszeczky and Frigyes Verzar of the General Pathology Laboratory at the University of Debreczen, along with Andre Jeney who also published articles in the early 1920s, was the serological delineation of the mixed populations (German, Roma, Rumanian, as well as Hungarian) within the newly drawn boundaries of the Hungarian state. The early work of Sabin Manuila (trained in statistics) and Georges Popoviciu in Rumania showed a similar interest.[52] Rumanian authors published 13 articles on blood group distribution between the wars and Hungarians published19. Marius Turda has written in detail about the racial and political setting that produced much of this interest.[53] He shows how anthropologists and extreme nationalists used blood group testing which they thought more accurate than somatic measures (e.g., head shape), to support their claims, especially in contested regions like Transylvania. This anthropological interest in blood groups was also strong in Czechoslovakia (14 articles) and the Baltic states (10 articles).

Some Czech and Hungarian authors followed the lead of their German and Polish colleagues in studying the possible links between blood groups and disease. Almost half (15) of the 33 articles they published were on the blood group distribution of those with disease or the insane. This subject also received much attention by researchers in Austria and Switzerland (20 of the 39 articles on blood group distribution), which was not surprising given the strong influence of German medical research there. In fact, most of the Swiss articles were published in German-language journals, and the Austrian research, of course, had its own traditions that ran parallel if not precedent to work in Germany. The 26 articles on blood group distribution by Austrian researchers were an especially large number.

Researchers in Spain and Portugal published 29 articles on blood group distribution between the wars. In Portugal one reason for the interest was its colonial empire; in fact, 5 of 11 articles reported tests of inhabitants of Portuguese India and Africa. In Spain the first studies by Urra, Grifols y Roig, and Hoyos Sainz were anthropological in nature, focusing on possible differences between the blood group distribution of the inhabitants of Catalonia and Castille.[54] In 1932 the first tests were done of blood groups of the mentally ill in Spain, followed shortly by articles on blood groups and disease. By 1936 there had been 18 articles on blood group distribution published by Spanish authors, which reflect a broad interest in serology and partly explain why doctors there were able to make advances in blood transfusion during the Spanish Civil War.

This wide spread of interest indicates the level of medical research and degree to which researchers in these other European countries were part of the international community of scientific research. Another dimension of this is the number of articles that appeared in journals published in the researchers' own countries, which as Table 5.3 shows was almost half (75) of the 164 articles that appeared between the wars. Only Rumanian authors ignored their own journals, choosing instead to publish most often in the *Comptes Rrendus de la Société de Biologie*.

Table 5.3 Journals where authors from smaller European countries published blood group distribution articles

Author's Country	*Domestic Journal*	*Foreign Journal*
Austria	12	14
Czechoslovakia	9	5
Hungary	5	14
Scandinavia	9	4
Portugal	9	2
Rumania	1	12
Spain	13	5
Switzerland	5	8
Other	12	26
Total	**75**	**89**

Blood Group Research Conducted Outside of Europe, Japan, and the U.S.

The study of blood group distribution in Latin America, Africa, and Asia was of great importance to researchers who had talked from the start about mapping the world serologically. After first testing large numbers of Europeans, researchers increasingly turned to overseas lands for subjects to study. The conduct of this research took place during the "high noon" of Western colonialism between the wars, both in who was tested as well as how and by whom. Thus, for example, with the significant exception of Japan, only in Latin America and China was this research not conducted primarily by Europeans or colonial settlers. As Table 5.4 shows, Brazil (where 16 articles on blood group distribution were published between the wars) along with Argentina (14) and China (12) were independent countries outside Europe, North America, and Japan with sufficient numbers of trained medical personnel who had the knowledge and interest to conduct blood group research.[55]

In the remaining non-Western locations (the term here is used to describe locations other than Europe, North America, and Japan), the majority of testing was done by doctors of the settler community in the British Commonwealth lands (Australia, South Africa, and India), by French and Dutch medical personnel in their colonies, or American doctors overseas. As Fig. 5.8 indicates, the chronology of this research (excluding Japan and the USSR) shows a rather slow beginning in the 1920s,

Table 5.4 Articles on blood group distribution conducted in non-Western locations, 1918–1939

Independent		*British Commonwealth*		*Western Researchers in Colonial Setting*	
Country/region	*Articles*	*Country/region*	*Articles*	*Country/region*	*Articles*
Japan	139	Australia	23	U.S. abroad	39
China[a]	12	India	12	French overseas	29
Brazil	16	South Africa	11	Dutch East Indies	33
Argentina	14			Soviet Asia[a]	42
Other Lat. Amer.	8				

[a]Articles confirmed

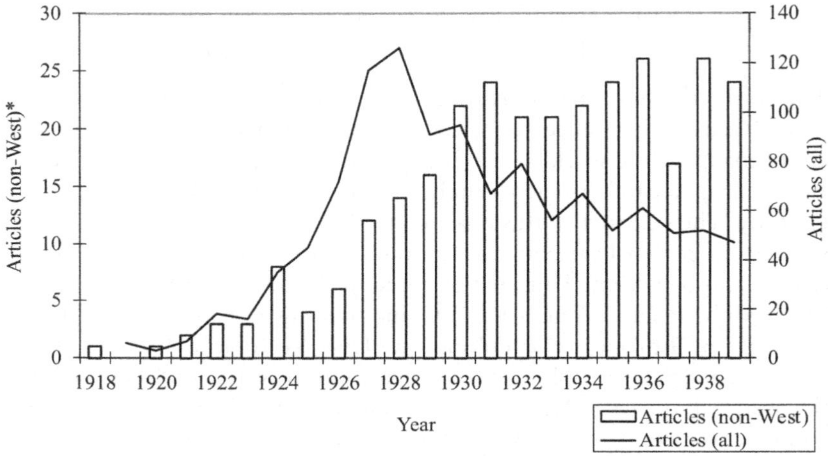

Fig. 5.8 Articles per year on blood group distribution research in non-Western locations, 1918–1939

then a rapid growth at the end of the decade to a level that was maintained throughout the 1930s.

The most striking feature about this record of research outside Europe, North America, and Japan is how it differed from the pattern of all blood group distribution articles which showed a decline of publications in the 1930s. The fact that non-Western research increased and remained strong while the overall number of articles declined, demonstrates dramatically the shift in focus of attention by researchers away from European and North American populations towards the rest of the world. This is further evidence of the maturing of blood group research which after the initial burst of activity in the 1920s, either sought new populations to test or new reasons (i.e., new blood groups) to restudy previously tested populations.

The first blood group testing in non-Western locations was done in China and Australia. The interest that developed in China was a reflection of the adoption of Western medical practice led largely by Europeans and Americans before and during the First World War. Most significant was the Rockefeller-funded Peking Union Medical College and hospitals jointly sponsored by missionaries and universities such as Harvard and Yale. Though small compared to the needs of so large a population, and late compared to Japan, efforts to introduce Western medicine in China resulted in 400 students in Western medical schools according to a 1914 Rockefeller Foundation China Medical Commission report. Of 17 such schools operating in China, 2 were run by the central government, 3 by provincial governments, 9 by missionaries, 2 by the Germans, 1 by the French, and 1 by the Japanese in Manchuria.[56] This is corroborated by other reports of 500–600 Western-trained physicians by 1915, and a 1920 survey reported 1700 medical school graduates of all kinds which rose to 2000 by 1925.[57]

Of the 24 studies of blood group distribution in China that were published by 1939, only 9 were by foreigners. Ten were by Chinese researchers alone and another five were co-authored by Chinese and foreigners.[58] In fact, as mentioned earlier one of the first articles in the world on the distribution of blood groups, antedating the Hirszfelds' work, was co-authored in 1918 by Alson R. Kilgore of Harvard and his co-worker at the Shanghai Red Cross Hospital J. Heng Liu, who had Harvard undergraduate and medical degrees and later became nominal Director of Peking Union Medical College and the first Vice-Minister of Health under the Nationalist government. Other articles on blood group testing soon appeared by Chinese doctors at Peking Union and Yale's Hunan Hospital in the early1920s. Subsequent research, however, appeared sporadically and in a variety of locations. With the exception of one article in 1931 by Dorothy Huie Wong and Foong Kong Chen of Peking Union on blood groups and syphilis, all Chinese research was anthropological. The most frequent publisher of Chinese articles was the *National Medical Journal of China*, although a few articles appeared in German medical journals.[59]

A similar, early interest in blood group research in Australia proved to be more persistent. Beginning with an article in 1922 on the blood groups of aborigines, Arthur H. Tebbutt of the Pathology Department of Prince Albert Hospital in Sydney published three more such articles in the next two years. This was followed in 1926 by the research of John B. Cleland, a Professor of Pathology at the University of Adelaide, who wrote the first of what was to be 11 articles on blood group distribution over the next 12 years.[60] These articles and those by other Australian researchers appeared most often in the *Medical Journal of Australia* (12 of the 23 Australian articles), the *Journal of Tropical Medicine and Hygiene* (7), or other Australian publications (3); hence, their audience was somewhat limited. All of these articles were on the anthropological significance of blood group distribution, principally the testing of aborigines.

The pattern of articles on blood group distribution published by South African researchers was similar, albeit later and less frequent than in Australia. In this case, with the exception of a very early article on testing before transfusion, all were written by only two researchers beginning in 1929: four by Adrianus Pijper at Pretoria and five articles by Ronald Elsdon-Dew, a pathologist at the South African Institute for Medical Research. Pijper conducted smaller studies, including one of South African Boers (descendants of seventeenth-century Dutch settlers) for Van Herwerden in Holland, whereas Elsdon-Dew conducted larger, more thorough studies. In fact, his first article was based on physical examinations given to almost 1500 black African miners.[61] All South African articles were anthropological in nature.

The other place in the British empire where there was significant interest in blood group research between the wars, was India. This was not only the result of anthropological interest in the peoples of India but also the level of medical training and research there. At the beginning of the twentieth century there were several Western medical colleges enrolling over 2000 students, plus five medical research centers, including the Haffkine Institute and two Pasteur Institute laboratories.[62] By the end of the 1920s enough Indians had received Western medical training that they, along with British expatriates and foreigners, undertook the study of blood group distribution which began to delineate the complexities of sub-continent populations. Of 18 articles on blood group distribution in India published through 1939, 11 were by Indian authors, 5 by foreigners, and 2 were co-authored by Indians and expatriate Englishmen.[63]

The first of these articles appeared late in 1928 presenting the work of a British army major and an Indian with support from the Indian Research Fund Association, both of whom went on to distinguished careers in medicine and microbiology. The article was quite sophisticated, pointing out the shortcomings of the Hirszfelds' tests of 500 Indian troops in the First World War, which had remained the only blood group study of Indians for almost a decade. The most obvious problem, according to the authors, was "it is impossible to say from the Hirschfields' [sic] paper which of India's many races and castes were examined."[64] Their article reported the results of over 3000 tests on troops in the Punjab as well as patients at the Pasteur Institute of Kasauli and Dravidians in central India. The challenge of this critique notwithstanding, it still took some time before other researchers in India responded to the challenge of serologically mapping the many different populations of the sub-continent. The next article appeared in 1931 and the first year of multiple articles was 1933.

In this research there were only three articles on blood groups and disease in India between the wars.[65] The anthropological focus of the rest of the research is not surprising, given the heterogeneous nature of the population. Another local influence on research was the existence of several scientific journals published in India, which provided many options for researchers to present their results. At the same time, however, the small circulation of these publications limited the impact of most research, although a number of articles appeared in journals back in Britain such as *Nature* and the *Journal of Tropical Medicine and Hygiene*, which gave the Indian results a much broader audience.[66] Finally, there were two foreigners whose involvement in this research is worth noting. One was the American Eileen MacFarlane who authored five articles between 1936 and 1938 on blood group distribution in places as diverse as South India, Tibet, and Bengal.[67] The other foreigner was Reginald Ruggles Gates, who had played an important role in stimulating interest in blood group research back in Britain. Gates was in touch with Indian researchers as well as MacFarlane beginning in 1935, offering test sera, advice, and information about the work of others in the field.[68]

The fact that Argentina and Brazil were the two Latin American countries where researchers showed extensive interest in blood groups is no surprise, given the development of medical research in the two countries. Researchers began their studies in the mid-1920s, and a steady flow of articles appeared through the end of the 1930s.[69] Indeed, five articles were published on blood group distribution by Argentinians in 1939. Another similarity was researchers' almost exclusive interest in the anthropology of the blood groups. In Brazil five articles compared the distribution of blood types among blacks, whites, and mulattos, while two studies were about isolated Indian populations. Only one Brazilian study departed from this anthropological interest: a 1938 article on criminals in Sao Paolo.[70] In Argentina there was even more research on the blood groups of Indians, thanks to the work of Salvador Mazza of the University of Buenos Aires Institute of Clinical Surgery. His five articles (four in 1927–1928) grew out of a study he directed on "Regional Pathology of the North." Also of note in Argentina was the publication of 5 articles (of a total of 14) on blood groups and disease or insanity.

This significant blood group research in the British Commonwealth and independent non-Western countries between the wars (96 articles) was matched by the extensive studies of French and Dutch researchers (62 articles) in their colonies and American researchers abroad (37 articles). With the exception of only two French studies and one by an American, all French and American overseas research was concerned with the anthropology of blood groups as mentioned in an earlier chapter. The steady report of American research began in the mid-1920s with Ella Grove's work in Japan and the Philippines. French overseas blood group research began at the end of the decade with articles on North and sub-Saharan African populations. Proof of the importance of this overseas testing to the overall record of publication by researchers in both countries can be seen in the percentage it represented of all blood group research conducted in the 1930s. Over half (28 of 52 or 54 percent) of articles by French researchers was done overseas, and the figures for U.S. researchers were 29 of 64 articles (45 percent).

The most frequent specific location of overseas French blood group testing was North Africa and the Middle East, where almost half (14 articles) of the research was done. Other locations were colonies in sub-Saharan Africa (six articles) and Southeast Asia (four). U.S. researchers also showed a surprising interest in North African and Middle East populations (14 articles), including Bedouins in Syria and Iraq, mummies in Egypt, and populations of the Rif in Morocco. The Asian research (12 articles) included MacFarlane's work in India as well as anthropological research in the South Pacific, Philippines, and China. The extent of this research around the world makes more surprising the relative lack of U.S. research conducted in Latin America (only seven articles).

The anthropological interest of U.S. researchers was also significant in that it reflected the entry of formally trained anthropologists into the field of blood group research, foreshadowing a change that greatly accelerated after the Second World War. For example, as was mentioned in an earlier chapter, this overseas research included the field work of Carleton Coon and William W. Howells. In addition, although William Boyd was trained and employed as an immunologist, already by the end of the 1930s, much of his work (notably three studies of blood types of mummies) was clearly written for anthropologists. A final reflection of the entry of the American blood group research into the formal domain of anthropology was the increasing publication of articles in the *American Journal of Physical Anthropology*. Ten of the twelve articles by U.S. researchers on blood group distribution that appeared in the journal between the wars were published after 1935, and seven of these ten articles were studies of overseas populations.

The series of articles by Dutch colonial officials in Indonesia was probably the most extensive testing of blood group distribution for a given non-European geographical location between the wars. Although there were a few early articles (notably by Bais and Verhoef[71]), the more intense study of the Indonesian population began in 1930 as a result of two developments. One was the holding of the Fourth Pan-Pacific Science Congress in Bandung (Java) in 1929, where reports were presented on blood group studies including the preliminary findings of Wilhemina M. van der Made, a government physician at the Mental Asylum at Sabang. She eventually tested over 10,000 subjects and incorporated her research into a medical dissertation at the University of Batavia published the following year.[72] Secondly, her work prompted J. P. Klieweg de Zwaan, a Professor of "Anthropology and Native Medicine" at the University of Amsterdam, to call for a standing committee to coordinate the investigation of blood groups in the East Indies. Little official record of the committee has been left and no formal report was published, but the results of the effort appeared in a number of articles published in the 1930s in the *Geneeskundig Tijdschrift voor Nederlandsch-Indië*.

Two examples of the conduct of this research explain why these investigations were possible. One was written by Hendricus J. T. Bijlmer, a frequent author of blood group articles (seven on Indonesian populations), who described a typical study he conducted in the Moluccas where he was stationed as a health officer in 1931. Before entering a village for testing, he obtained the cooperation of a "big man" who would provide an appropriate site, plus a table and chair. Often the subjects tested were school children. Van der Made prepared test kits ahead of time which permitted the testing of four subjects simultaneously. Bijlmer reported he could test 140 blood samples per hour.[73]

D. J. Buining gave another description of how research was conducted for his medical dissertation while he served as a naval health officer in East Java. His account is revealing because Buining required even more local cooperation for a study of the inheritance of blood groups. He not only needed to test for blood type, but he also required information about relationships in over 2300 families he tested. It was necessary, he said, to choose his subjects carefully. First, he determined "that all our regions were inhabited by a population which would lend itself without difficulty to the study of different family relations. This is indispensable for these studies of heredity." Then thanks to "collaboration of the government of East Java and the Public Health Service, which we liberally availed ourselves of," he acknowledged, "the collection of data was considerably facilitated."[74]

Both Bijlmer and Buining published early articles with detailed descriptions of blood testing techniques so that others might use them for their studies.[75] The combination of the official status of the researchers (the health service was largely in the hands of the military), their amateur interest in anthropology, and the ethnic diversity of the islands produced a very large study. Not counting Van der Made's research, there were 27 articles published by 15 different researchers on the blood group distribution of the Dutch East Indies between 1931 and 1940. They tested almost 47,000 inhabitants. Of note, because it was almost exclusively published in the *Geneeskundig Tijdschrift voor Nederlandsch-Indië*, this research only reached a limited audience. This was mitigated, to an extent, by occasional articles in more widely read journals that summarized the results for a larger audience.[76] This Indonesian research was duly noted by Boyd in his 1940 summary of anthropological testing of blood groups.

This completes the comparative analysis of blood group research as it was conducted in different countries. The final chapters will examine the applications of the blood group discoveries to two fields beyond anthropology: pathology and criminology. The use of blood groups for transfusion has been studied elsewhere,[77] and their application to forensic medicine, especially the question of individual identity, will be the subject of future study.

Notes

1. Marius Turda, "From Craniology to Serology: Racial Anthropology in Interwar Hungary and Romania," *Journal of the History of the Behavioral Sciences*, 43 (2007): 361–77; Marius Turda, "Entangled Traditions of Race: Physical Anthropology in Hungary and Romania, 1900–1940," *Focaal*, 58 (2010): 32–46; Elise K. Burton and Ageliki Lefkaditou. "Race in Circulation: Blood Banks and Forced Mobilities in the Eastern Mediterranean." *Bulletin of the History of Medicine* 96, no. 3 (2022): 375–402.
2. For example, see research by Jennifer Robertson, "Hemato-nationalism: The Past, Present, and Future of "Japanese Blood," *Medical Anthropology* 31 (2012): 93–112; and Jaehwan Hyun, "Blood Purity and Scientific

Independence: Blood Science and Postcolonial Struggles in Korea, 1926–1975" *Science in Context* 32 (2019): 239–60.

3. For general background, see Tuge Hideome, *Historical Development of Science and Technology in Japan* (Tokyo: Japan Cultural Society, 1968), 89–110; Nakayama Shigeru, et al., eds., *Science and Society in Modern Japan* (Cambridge: MIT Press, 1974); and James R. Bartholomew, *Formation of Science in Japan: Building a Research Tradition* (New Haven: Yale University Press, 1989).
4. On Japanese students abroad, see Minoru Watanabe, "Japanese Students Abroad and the Acquisition of Scientific and Technical Knowledge," *Cahiers d'études mondiales* 9 (1965): 254–93; and Bartholomew, *Formation of Science*, 68–82. Bartholomew's first work was on Kitasato, "Acculturation of Science in Japan: Kitasato Shibasaburo and the Japanese Bacteriological Community, 1885–1920," (Ph.D. dissertation, Stanford, 1972).

   Examples of background studies in English and French on this period in Japanese medicine include Pierre Huard, Zensetzou Ohya, and Ming Wong, *Médecine japonaise des origines à nos jours* (Paris: Roger Dacosta, 1974). John Z. Bowers gives some background on the adoption of German medicine in *Medical Education in Japan* (New York: Harper and Row, 1965), 32–41; and one of Bartholomew's earlier articles focuses on the creation of Japanese medical universities, "Japanese Culture and the Problem of Modern Science," in *Science and Values*, eds. Arnold Thackray and Everett Mendelsohn (New York: Humanities Press, 1974), 109–55.
5. Bartholomew, *Formation of Science*, 122, goes much further, claiming that on the eve of the First World War medical research was not only superior to the physical sciences in Japan but the equal of the best work being done at the Koch Institute in Berlin or the Pasteur Institute in Paris.
6. R. Hara, and S. Kobayashi, *Iji-Shinbun,* no. 954 (1916): 937, as cited in several subsequent articles, including Hozumi Fukamachi, "On the Biochemical Race Index of Koreans, Manchus and Japanese," *Journal of Immunology* 8 (1923): 291–4.
7. See, for example, Tanemoto Furuhata, "Japanese Literature on Isohemagglutination (1916–1928)," *Japan Medical World* 8 (1928): 321–4.
8. Tanemoto Furuhata, "On the Heredity of the Blood Group and its Application in Forensic Medicine," *Vancouver Medical Association Bulletin* 9 (1933): 204.
9. Evidence of even more research is the work of Takeo Satō, which has been analyzed in-depth by Hyun for comparison with Furuhata's research. Satō began publishing on the blood groups of Koreans in 1935 (which continued during and after the war), but that work did not turn up in the survey of literature used for this analysis. See, for example, Takeo Satō, Jiso

Kunifusa, Shoichi Nomura, and Hisashi Hagimori, [Blood Types of Koreans], *Japanese Journal of Legal Medicine* 9 (1935): 42–54.

10. Yoshito Maryuma's first article, co-authored with T. Wakeshima, was entitled, "Blood groups of Formosan savages," *Taiwan Igakkai Zasshi* 30 (1931): 35. An example of the earlier articles is T. Furuichi, "On the Heredity of Group Specific Characteristics of Human Blood," *Taiwan Igakkai Zasshi* 24 (1925): 581–90.

    For background on the medical school in Taiwan, see E. Patricia Tsurumi, *Japanese Colonial Education in Taiwan, 1895–1945* (Cambridge: Harvard University Press, 1977), 24–5; 122–4; 253. Medical training grew up around the Taihoku Hospital after 1907 and played a key role in producing sanitation personnel during Japanese rule. A formal medical school faculty of Taihoku Imperial University was not created until 1936.

11. T. Wakeshima, "Blood groups of Formosan-Chinese; Relation Between Blood Groups and Result of Study in Primary Schools," *Taiwan Igakkai Zasshi* 31(1932): 83; SeijiTerada, "Distribution of groups M and N among Japanese in the City of Taihoku and among Formosan Chinese and Formosan Savages," *Taiwan Igakkai Zasshi* 34 (1935): 1892; Yoshito Maruyama, "Blood Groups in Relation to Dental Caries," *Taiwan Igakkai Zasshi* 32 (1933): 88; Asho Ro, "On the Blood Types of Opium-addicts in Formosa," *Taiwan Igakkai Zasshi* 33 (1934): 33; and K. Amano, "On the Blood-types of Base-ball Players," *Taiwan Igakkai Zasshi* 33 (1934): 5–6.

12. The first part of Hyun, "Blood Purity" offers a recent assessment of Furuhata's role in blood group research. See also Robertson, "Hemato-nationalism," 98. For an assessment of his importance by one of the next generation of Japanese human geneticists, see E. Matsunaga, "History of Human Genetics and Eugenics in Japan," in *History and Development of Human Genetics: Progress in Different Countries*, ed. Krishna R. Dronamraju (Singapore: World Scientific, 1992), 130–2. There is no biography of Furuhata in English, only short obituary notices such as A. S. Wiener, "Tanemoto Furuhata," *Vox Sanguinis* 31 (1976): 77; and Jan Hirschfeld, "Tanemoto Furuhata (1891–1976)," *International Archives of Allergy and Applied Immunology* 54 (1977): 191–2.

    Just before his death, Furuhata published *Development of Haemotypology in Japan* (Tokyo: Matsumoto Institute, 1977), which unfortunately does not live up to the promise of its title and only presents minimal historical information. The following is also based on a "Personal History" dated Feb. 4, 1958, that accompanied a grant application by Furuhata to the Rockefeller Foundation, in the Rockefeller Archive Center, RG 1.2, series 609, box 15, folder 159.

13. Tanemoto Furuhata, "Japanese Literature on Isohemagglutination (1916–1928)."

14. His earliest publication was Tanemoto Furuhata, Kenkichi Ichida, and Takayoshi Kishi in *Nippon Gakujutsu Kyokai Hokoku*, 1 (1925): 314–25, which appeared in November of that year.
15. Fukamachi, "On the Biochemical Race Index"; Tanemoto Furuhata and Takayoshi Kishi, "On the Biological Racial-Index of the Japanese in the Hokiru District," *Journal of Immunology* 12 (1926): 83–9; and Kishi, "On the Biochemical Racial Index of the Ainu, Gilyak and Orokko in Karafu," *Journal of Immunology* 12(1926): 91–6.
16. On the early Korean articles see Hyun, "Blood Purity." Furuhata's first article was on the Ainu, [Japanese and Ainu Considered from the serological standpoint] *Nippon Gakujitsu Kyokwai Zasschi* (1925), 1. For one of the later studies, see Takehito Kobayasi, [On the blood groups of Korean schoolboys and schoolgirls] *Chiba Igakkai Zasshi* 16 (1938), 8–9.
17. Shinichi Kirihara and Rinsai Haku, [On the differences of the percentages of the blood groups between the Japanese and Koreans and on the heredity of blood group specificity] *Tokyo Iji-Shinshi* (1922), as abstracted in *Japan Medical World* 3 (1923):31; Kirihara and Haku, [On the differences of the percentages of the blood types of the Japanese and the Koreans and on the heredity of blood grouping specificity], *Chosen Igakkai Zasshi*, as abstracted in *Japan Medical World* 3 (1923): 59.
18. Hyun, "Blood Purity," 8–9.
19. For background, see Morris Low, "Physical Anthropology in Japan: The Ainu and the Search for the Origins of the Japanese" *Current Anthropology*, 53 suppl. (2012): 57–68; and Sakuzaemon Kodama, *Ainu: Historical and Anthropological Study* (Sapporo: Hokkaido University School of Medicine, 1970), especially 108–15 on blood group studies.
20. See Furuhata and Kishi, "Study of the Ainu Race from a Serological Standpoint," *Japan Medical World*, 8 (1928): 91–4.
21. Furuhata, "Study of the Geographical Distribution of Blood Groups of the Japanese," *Japan Medical World* 8 (1928): 119. Along similar lines, see Sen Nagai, "Die Körperkonstitution des Japaners. Der biochemische Rassenindex des Japaners," *Biologie der Person* 2 (1928): 437.
22. Matsui Akune, "Zur serologischen Anthropologie der Japaner," *Zeitschrift für Morphologie und Anthropologie* 30 (1932): 38.
23. See Daniel Pick, *Degeneration* (Cambridge: Cambridge University Press, 1989) on Lombroso and Italian unification.
24. For eulogies of uniformly high praise, see Ruggero Ceppellini, "In Memoriam: Leone Lattes, 1887–1954," *Bollettino dell instituto sieroterapico milanese*, 33 (1954): 649–50; Fernanda Domenici, "Leone Lattes (1887–1954)," *Minerva medicolegale*, 74 (1954): i-ii; and Giovanni Guglielmo, "Leone Lattes 1887–1954," *Haematologica*, 38 (1954): iii-vi.

25. L. and H. Hirschfeld [sic.], "Essai d'application des méthodes sérologiques au problème des races," *Anthropologie* 29 (1918–19): 522.
26. Ettore Cuboni, "Contributo Allo Studio Della Distribuzione dei Gruppi Sanguigni in Italia," *Bollettino dell'Instituto Sieroterapico Milanese* 7 (1928): 153–60; Domenico Viola, "I Gruppi Sanguigni Come Fattore Etno-Antropologico. Contributo Alla Distribuzione Regionale dei Gruppi Sanguigni in Italia," *Rivista di Antropologica* 28 (1928): 307–26.
27. Gaetano Dossena and Vincenzo Lancara, "L'Isoagglutinazione studiata nei riguardi dell'abito morfologico e delle neoplasie della sfera genitale muliebre," *Annali di ostetricia e ginecologia* 47 (1925):163–79; Francesco D'Onofrio, "Rapportio fra carattere ereditario gruppo sanguigno ed adenoidismo," *Archivio Italiana di Otologia, Rinologia e Laringologia* 37 (1926): 209–15; Filippo Ferraro, "[Studies Regarding Blood Groups in Infancy]," *Rivista di clinica pediatria* 24 (1926): 758.
28. Tedeschi's first article was "Osservazioni sul soma delle popolazioni indigene della Barra orientale secondo i concetti constituzionalistici," *Archivio Italiano di Scienze Mediche Coloniali* 10 (1929): 566–83.
29. Domenico Viola, "Contributo allo studio dei rapporti fra caratteri gruppo-specifici e caratteri psico-costituzionali," *Giornale di medicina militare* 82 (1934): 253–8.
30. These and other details are from Hirszfeld, *The Story of One Life*.
31. The first report was Wanda Halber and J. Mydlarski, "Recherches sero-anthropologiques en Pologne," *Comptes rendus de la Société de biologie*, 89 (1923): 1373–5. A lengthier analysis was published later by Wanda Halber and Jan Mydlarski, "Untersuchung uber die Blutgruppen in Polen," *Zeitschrift für Immunitätsforschung*, 43 (1925): 470–84.
32. Rose Amzel, "Distribution de l'élement M du sang dans la population polonaise," *Comptes rendus de la Société de biologie*, 104 (1930): 1083.
33. Eero Mustakallio, "Untersuchungen uber die Blutgruppen bei den Nordfinnen und Lappen," *Acta Societatis Medicorum Fennicae Duodecim* 20 (1938): 17, gives a good summary of work to date.
34. See, for example, Oluf Sievers, "Blodgruppsfördelningen bland friska och sjuka inom det i Finland samlade materialet [Blood group distribution of the sick and healthy as found in materials collected in Finland]," *Finska Lakaresallskapets Handlingar* 71 (1929): 836–48.
35. An example of early testing is ErikBay-Schmith, "Racebiologiske Undersogelser i Gronland [race biology research in Greenland]," *Ugeskrift for Laeger* 88 (1926): 880–2. On the larger study, see Soren Hansen, "Methodologisches uber Blutgruppenforschung durch Massenuntersuchungen," *Zeitschrift fur Rassenphysiologie* 2 (1929): 73–7; and Th. Madsen, E. T. Engle, Claus Jensen and I. B. Freuchen, "Blood Groups and Poliomyelitis: Report Based on 1118 Cases in the 1934

Epidemic in Denmark," *Journal of Immunology* 30 (1936): 213–9, which uses the national survey as a basis for comparison.

36. Oluf Thomsen, "Uber den Zusammenhang der Isoagglutinatorischen Bluttypen (Blutgruppen) mit Pathologischen Zustanden," *Acta Pathologica et Microbiologica Scandinavica* 4 (1927): 45–73; 163–4, was an early study; and for his most definitive study on cancer, see Thomsen, "Om mulighoben af forskellig Disposition til Cancerudviklung hos individer af forskelig "blodtype" [Possibilities of varying disposition to cancer development in individuals of various blood groups]," *Ugeskrift for Laeger* 93 (1931): 1008–15 which compiled the results from 1200 cases sent in from all over the country.
37. A. J. van Bork-Feltkamp, "Anthropological Research in the Netherlands. Historical Survey," *Verhandelingen der Koninklijke Nederlandsche Akademie van Wettenschappen. Amsterdam. Proceedings of the Section of Sciences* 37, no. 3 (1938): 1–166.
38. The most complete biography is by her sister C. A. B. van Herwerden, *Marianne van Herwerden 16 Februari 1874 - 26 Januari 1934* (Rotterdam: W. L. Brusse, 1948). For examples of her importance at her death, see G. C. Heringa, "Dr. M. A. van Herwerden," *Nederlandsch Tijdschrift voor Geneeskunde* 79 (1935): 4917–9, and Tina Tammes, "Bedeutung von Dr. Maria Anna van Herwerden für die Genetik und die Eugenik," *Genetica* 18 (1936), 3–9. Because she was one of the earliest female university researchers, Van Herwerden has also received attention from recent scholars. See, for example, Marta Kirejczyk, "Vrouwen kozen exact; Studie en beroepsuitoefning rond de eeuwwisseling," *Gewina* 16 (1993): 241–3. I am grateful to Ida Stamhuis for confirming the importance of Herwerden. See Stamhuis, "Female Contribution to Early Genetics: Tine Tammes and Mendel's Law for Continuous Character," *Journal of the History of Biology* 28 (1995): 495–6.
39. A fairly regular correspondence which followed between Davenport and Van Herwerden until her death in 1934 can be found in the Davenport Collection of the American Philosophical Society (Philadelphia).
40. Ten letters were published in volume 66 (1920). For an extensive account of her visit, see C. A. B. van Herwerden, pp. 67–138.
41. Herwerden, *Erfelijkheid bij den mensch en eugenetiek* (Amsterdam: Wereldbibliotheek, 1926). See Tammes, 3–4 on the influence of the book.
42. W. J. Bais and A. W. Verhoef, "Het verschijnsel der isohaemagglutinatie en de anthropologische Beteekenis Daarvan [anthropological blood studies of different races in Dutch East Indies]," *Geneeskundig Tijdschrift voor Nederlandsch-Indië* 68 (1924): 1212–31, which was translated and published as "On the Biochemical Racial Index of Various Races in the E. Indian Archipeligo," *Journal of Immunology* 9 (1924): 383–6.

43. Herwerden, "De Verdeeling der Menschheid in Bloedgroepen [subdivision of humanity according to blood groups]," *Mensch en Maatschappij* 2 (1926): 257–69.
44. Herwerden, "Groupes sanguins en Hollande," *Institut International d'Anthropologie, 3e Congrès, Amsterdam, Sept.1927*, (Paris: Noury, 1928): 456–60.
45. M. A. Van Herwerden and Th. Y. Boele-Nyland, "Investigation of Blood groups in Holland," *Koninklijke Akademie van Wettenschappen. Amsterdam. Proceedings of the Section of Sciences* 33 (1930): 659–73, reprinted in *Archiv für Rassen-und Gesellschafts-Biologie* 24 (1930): 198–207; C. P. J. Penning, M. A. van Herwerden, and Th. J. Boele-Nijland, "Bloodgroup-Investigation in the Over Veluwe (Harderwijk and Surrounding districts)," *Koninklijke Akademie van Wettenschappen. Amsterdam. Proceedings of the Section of Sciences* 35 (1932): 706–14; reprinted in *Zeitschrift fur Morphologie und Anthropologie* 31 (1932): 395–402; and Floris Hers, M. A. Van Herwerden, and Th. J. Boele-Nijland, "Bloodgroup Investigation in the 'Hoeksche Waard,'" *Koninklijke Akademie van Wettenschappen. Amsterdam. Proceedings of the Section of Sciences* 36 (1933): 849–61.
46. Hendricus J. T. Bijlmer, "Contribution to the Anthropology of the Netherlands, including the further elaboration of the Blood Group Research in Holland commenced in 1926 by the late M. A. Van Herweden," *Koninklijke Akademie van Wettenschappen. Amsterdam. Proceedings of the Section of Sciences* 43 (1940): 113–39.
47. Bais and Verhoef, "Het verschijnsel."
48. On medicine in the East Indies, see P. C. Flu, "Medical Science," in *Science in the Netherlands East Indies*, ed. L. M. R. Rutten (Amsterdam: Royal Academy of Sciences, 1927), 207–25.
49. *Konstitutionsserologie und Blutgruppenforschung* (Berlin: Springer Verlag, 1928); and *Groupes sanguins: leurs applications à la biologie, à la médecine et au droit* (Paris: Masson, 1938).
50. See, for example, D. J. Buining, "Recherches sur les groupes sanguin au Indes neerlandaises," *Anthropologie* 43 (1933): 289–312; or Hendricus J. T. Bijlmer, "Relation of Blood Groups to Race and Some Particulars of the SW Pacific," *Journal of the Royal Anthropological Institute*, 65 (1935): 123–31.
51. See, for example, Vibeke Fabricius-Hansen, "Blood Groups and MN-Types of Eskimos in East Greenland," *Journal of Immunology* 36 (1939): 523–30; and "Blood Type Determinations in the Southern Districts of Julianschaab, West Greenland (ABO and MN System)," *Journal of Immunology* 37 (1940): 497–9. On mass testing, see Otto Hartmann, Kare Hadland and Chr. Juel Bjerkelund, "Blood Group Distribution in Norway,"

Avhandlinger utgitt av Det Norske Videnskaps-Akademi i Oslo 5 (1940): 14–41.

52. Frigyes Verzar and Oskar Weszecky, "Rassenbiologische Untersuchungen mittels Isohamagglutinen," *Biochemische Zeitschrift,* 126 (1922): 33–9; Andre von Jeney, "Rassenbiologische Untersuchungen in Ungarn," *Deutsche medizinische Wochenschrift* 49 (1923): 546–7; Sabin Manuila, "Recherches sero-anthropologiques sur les races en Roumanie par la methode de l'isohemagglutination," *Comptes rendus de la Société de biologie* 90 (1924): 1071–3; Georges Popoviciu, "Differences dans la structure biologique en Roumanie d'après la situation géographique. Proprietés B et O," *Comptes rendus de la Société de biologie*, 90 (1924): 1069–71.
53. Marius Turda, "From Craniology to Serology: Racial Anthropology in Interwar Hungary and Romania," *Journal of the History of the Behavioral Sciences*, 43 (2007): 361–77; and Marius Turda, "Entangled Traditions of Race: Physical Anthropology in Hungary and Romania, 1900–1940," *Focaal* 58 (2010): 32–46.
54. See, for example, Juan Andreu Urra, "Los grupos sanguineos en Castilla," *Información medica* 5 (1928): 51–6; Luis de Hoyos Sainz, "Contribución al estudio seroanthopológico de Espana," *Institut International d'anthropologie, Lisbon, Sept. 1930* (1930): 553–60.
55. This was also the case in Soviet Asia under somewhat similar conditions.
56. See John Z. Bowers, *Western Medicine in a Chinese Palace, Peking Union Medical College, 1917–1951* (Philadelphia: Josiah Macy Foundation, 1972), 30–8. For more on Peking Union Medical College, see Mary Brown Bullock, *American Transplant: The Rockefeller Foundation and the Peking Union Medical College* (Berkeley: University of California Press, 1980). For more on the increasing literature on this topic, see also Peter Kong-Ming and Yuet-Wah Cheung, "Harvard Medical School of China, 1911–1916," *Social Science and Medicine* 16 (1982): 1207–15; and more recently, David Luesink, William H. Schneider, and Zhang Daqing, eds, *China and the Globalization of Biomedicine* (Rochester: University of Rochester Press, 2019).
57. Zhao Hongjun, "Chinese versus Western Medicine," *Chinese Science* 10 (1991): 21–37.
58. Most of the foreign articles were by H. M. Jettmar, an Austrian in the North Manchurian Plague Prevention Service whose work appeared primarily in Western language Chinese publications, such as "Biochemical Race Index of Mongols," *National Medical Journal of China* 14 (1928): 20–1. One exception was his article "Blutgruppenuntersuchungen in der Nordost Mongolei und der Mandschuriei," *Mitteilungen der anthropologischen Gesellschaft in Wien* 60 (1930): 39–47.

59. Dorothy Huie Wong and Foong Kong Chen, "Blood Groups in relation to syphilis and its Treatment," *National Medical Journal of China* 17 (1931): 354–9. See also Backiang Liang, "Blutgruppen in Kanton" *Münchener medizinische Wochenschrift* 76 (1929): 1466–7. For more on Liu, see Bowers, *Western Medicine in a Chinese Palace*, 86, 134; and Bullock, 58, 152–7.

    Note that this analysis only takes into account articles published in Western languages. Frank Dikötter who has written on racial and eugenic thought in Republican China, refers to other blood group articles in Chinese-language journals. Hence, there was greater interest among Chinese researchers than was found only by Western language publications. See Dikötter, "Discourse of Race and the Medicalization of Public and Private Space in Modern China (1895–1949)," *History of Science* 29 (1991): 416, 419; n. 12 and n. 13; and *Discourse of Race in Modern China* (Stanford: Stanford University Press, 1992), 134–5.
60. Tebbutt's first article was co-authored with Sarah V. McConnel, "On Human Iso-haemagglutinins, with a Note on Their Distribution Amongst Some Australian Aborigines," *Medical Journal of Australia* 9 (1922): 201–9. Cleland's first article was "Blood Grouping of Australian Aboriginals," *Australian Journal of Experimental Biology and Medical Science* 3 (1926): 33–5. For more on Cleland who was an important amateur anthropologist, see R. V. Southcott, "John Burton Cleland," *Medical Journal of Australia* 59 (1972):192–3.
61. Adrianus Pijper, "The Blood Groups of the South African Dutch," *Koninklijke Akademie van Wettenschappen. Amsterdam. Proceedings of the Section of Sciences* 32 (1929): 1159–63; Ronald Elsdon-Dew, "Serological Differences between Various Groups of the Bantu of Southern Africa," *Bantu Studies* 8 (1934): 361–6. Elsdon-Dew went on to write his medical dissertation on the blood group distribution of the Bantu, from which a very thorough study was extracted, "Blood Groups in Africa," *Publications of the South African Institute for Medical Research* 9 (1939): 29–94.
62. O. P. Jaggi, *History of Science, Technology and Medicine in India. vol. 13: Western Medicine in India* (Delhi: Atma Ram and Sons, 1979), 83–4; 179–87.
63. These do not include four articles on the Portuguese and one on the French possessions in India.
64. R. H. Malone and M. N. Lahiri, "Distribution of the Blood Groups in Certain Races and Castes of India," *Indian Journal of Medical Research*, 16 (1929): 963–4. Although the Hirszfelds could be excused for their ignorance of the details of Indian anthropology, especially considering the timing and circumstances of their research, Malone and Lahiri were even more critical of subsequent blood group researchers. "It is curious that this

lack of knowledge of the great diversity of races constituting the population of India has not been pointed out by writers who have supported or criticized the Hirszfelds' theory."

65. See, for example, A. Chaudhuri, "Blood groups and heredity," *Indian Medical Gazette* 66 (1931): 193–5; and P. N. Mitra, "Influence of Blood Group in Certain Pathological States," *Indian Journal of Medical Research* 20 (1933): 995–1004.
66. See A. J. Norohna and L. B. Kotbagi, "Some Anomalies Met With in Series of 300 Bloods Examined," *Journal of Tropical Medicine and Hygiene* 38 (1935): 295–6; and M. N. Basu, "Blood Groups of Noluas of Bengal," *Nature* 141 (1938): 649.
67. See, for example, Eileen W. Erlanson Macfarlane, "Eastern Himalayan Blood-Groups," *Man* 37 (1937):127–9; and Macfarlane, "Blood-group Distribution in India with Special Reference to Bengal," *Journal of Genetics* 36 (1938): 225–37.
68. Gates' letters can be found in the Gates Papers at Kings College (London) archives, 11/94. For example, see letter from A. Aiyappan, June 5, 1935; several MacFarlane letters to Gates, May 29, July 4, August 26, 1935; and June 18, 1936; and letter from P. K. Nandi, November 22, 1936.
69. The first study in Argentina was by Th. Furst, "Reactiones Differenciales Biologicas de la Sangre y su Empleo enla Biologia Racial y el Studio de la Constitucion," *Revista de Medicina* 12 (1924): 78; in Brazil it was Joao Montenegro, "Classifiaccao e Transfusaio do Sangue," *Brasil Medico* 1 (1925): 109–13.
70. Oscar Pereira Godoy, "Grupos sanguineos nos criminosos de Sao Paolo," *Archivos da sociedad de medecina legal e criminologia de Sao Paolo* 8 (1938): 185–91. On the state of medical research in Brazil during the first two decades of the twentieth century, see Nancy Stepan, *Beginnings of Brazilian Science: Oswaldo Cruz, Medical Research and Policy, 1890–1920* (New York: Science History Publications, 1976). She estimates that by the turn of the century there were 1500 medical students at Brazil's two medical schools. Stepan gives a broader view of science and medicine in Latin America in *Hour of Eugenics: Race, Gender and Nation in Latin America* (Ithaca: Cornell University Press, 1991), 39–43.
71. Their most important work was W. J. Bais and A. W. Verhoef, "Het verschijnsel."
72. For a summary, see Wilhemina M. van der Made, "Blood-groups of Sundanese Natives in West Java," *Fourth Pacific Science Congress, Java 1929*, 3 (1930):509–13.
73. Hendricus J. T. Bijlmer, "Bloedgroepenonderzoek in de Molukken," *Geneeskundig Tijdschrift voor Nederlandsch-Indië* 71 (1931): 1479–85.

For more on Biljmer and Klieweg de Zwaan, see G. A. Lindeboom, *Dutch Medical Biography* (Amsterdam: Rodopi, 1984), 145–6; 2239–40.

74. D. J. Buining, "Recherches sur les groupes sanguin au Indes neerlandaises," *Anthropologie* 43 (1933):301–2.
75. See, for example, Buining, "De techniek der bloedgroepdiagnostiek in Nederlandsch-Indië," *Geneeskundig Tijdschrift voor Nederlandsch-Indië* 71 (1931): 755–60. For background on the health service, see A. H. M. Kerkhoff, "Organization of the Military and Civil Medical Service in the Nineteenth and Twentieth Centuries," in *Dutch Medicine in the Malay Archipeligo, 1816–1942*, eds. G. M. van Heteren, et al. (Amsterdam: Rodopi, 1989), 9–24.
76. Bijlmer was the most active internationally. He presented a paper in 1934 on "The Relation of Blood Groups to Race, and Some Personal Enquiries in the South-west Pacific," at the International Congress of Anthropological and Ethnological Sciences, London, which was later published in the *Journal of the Royal Anthropological Institute* 65 (1935): 123–31.
77. See, for example, Schneider, "Blood Transfusion in Peace and War, 1900–1918," *Social History of Medicine* 10 (1997), 105–26; and Schneider, "Blood Transfusion Between the Wars," *Journal of the History of Medicine and Allied Sciences*, 58 (2003): 187–224.

CHAPTER 6

Blood Groups as Markers: Race and Disease

Previous chapters have shown the differences and similarities in research and findings about the different distributions of blood types around the world in the 1920s and 1930s. Striking as these may be, greatest interest in the Mendelian inheritance of blood types was their potential linkage with other conditions thought to be inherited. This is not surprising given the broad scientific and popular interest in heredity as manifested by the wide appeal of eugenics during this time. As to the traits or conditions that were of interest to blood group researchers, race and disease were clearly the most studied, and of the two, the concept of race was most changed by this new research. Initially, blood groups were taken as a new and more precise way to define race, as was shown in Chaps. 1 and 2 and will be briefly summarized below. By the end of the 1930s and especially after 1945, as will be shown in a later chapter, blood group genetics undermined the very concept of race and became the foundation of population genetics. The study of linkage to disease was extensive but less conclusive. It has received much less attention from scholars and will be examined in more detail below.

W. H. Schneider, *Blood Groups and Human Heredity, 1900–1950*, Medicine and Biomedical Sciences in Modern History,
https://doi.org/10.1007/978-3-031-69844-6_6

The Rise and Fall of Seroanthropology

From earliest times, humans have identified themselves as being different from others based on a variety of characteristics, cultural (e.g., language, customs, etc.) to be sure, but also including physical appearance. By the Middle Ages, in Europe, the Italian term *razza* was associated with ancestry and applied to plants and animals, and after the Scientific Revolution elaborate systems were adopted by Linnaeus, among others, to classify living things, including humans. Categories were based on appearance (as well as to a lesser extent function), and when applied to humans the obvious categories of skin, hair, and eye color, plus a variety of body measurements were used to search of a scientific basis for the delineation of the more or less widely used categories of human races, e.g., Caucasian, Negroid, Asiatic. Anthropometry was the name given to the measurement of various body parts, whose ratios were calculated to provide a measurable definition of the race categories. An example of one of the most widely used of these was the cephalic index, the ratio of the width to the length of the human head.[1]

There were serious problems with using these measurements, such as the changes in the human body over time, so that agreement on categories as well as range of measurement was impossible. The initial appeal of the Hirszfelds' discovery to the question of race was that blood type was a simple and more precisely defined characteristic to measure, and differences in distribution seemed to follow previously defined categories of race. In addition, blood type was clearly found to be inherited, unlike body parts, and it did not change over the course of a lifetime. Although they were not anthropologists, the Hirszfelds' conclusion from their discovery was that it offered a new way of defining and determining "biochemical" races, as they called them.

The venturing of medical researchers into anthropology was to be a pattern for decades to follow, but more important is that the link was made to race. As an aside, Ludwik Hirszfeld soon recognized the shortcomings of using only blood type as an indication of race, as shown by his research shifting to the broader concept of "constitutional serology."[2] At the same time, his interest shifted to possible links of blood groups to disease, such as diphtheria and maternal-fetal blood group incompatibility. The latter eventually led him close to the discovery of hemolytic disease and the new Rh blood group.[3]

Recently, Hirszfeld has come under criticism for his biochemical index in that it perpetuated racism.[4] Although in obvious ways this charge is warranted, Hirszfeld as well as his other colleagues of Jewish ancestry quickly saw the ways that racist ideologues in Germany made unwarranted claims and utilized blood group research to support their views of racial superiority. This regret can be found in Hirszfeld's correspondence (see Chap. 3) and more fully in his 1938 book, *Les groupes sanguins: leur application à la biologie, à la médecine et au droit*. Of course, it is most completely expressed in his autobiography written in hiding during the war after his escape from the Warsaw Ghetto.[5]

The 1919 article nonetheless set the pattern for subsequent research in the new field dubbed "seroanthropology." In addition to suggesting that there were two primordial races, the article questioned whether anatomical and biochemical races had different origins in time, and whether prehistoric distinctions might be determined by examining anthropoid apes. Much of the subsequent research attempted to verify or extend the results of the Hirszfelds by testing blood types among other peoples. As noted in previous chapters, these studies produced many surprises and problems. The first testing done in the early 1920s was on populations conveniently at hand in various place around the world: patients in hospitals in the U.S., China, South Africa, Rumania, Denmark, the Philippines, Australia, even Iceland. Most of these studies confirmed the Hirszfelds' general findings on geographical differences in blood type distribution. Then in 1923 Arthur F. Coca, a Cornell University immunologist who was studying the comparative susceptibility to allergies among American Indians and white Americans, found that more than 3/4 of native Americans he tested had type O blood, almost twice the frequency of any previously tested group.[6] Subsequent studies showed percentages as high as 90 to 95 percent for some isolated groups.

This began one of the major lines of inquiry in the 1920s and 1930s, including such questions as whether there was a third major center of racial definition, the timing of migration of humans to the New World, and the affinity of Amerindians to other groups such as Eskimos, Lapps, and Australian aborigines. For example, since Coca's findings suggested that there had existed a pre-Columbian native American race of entirely type O blood, some people tried to reconcile this hypothesis with the Hirszfelds' results by suggesting that the original (or aboriginal) human blood type was O and that subsequent new types A and B developed in western Europe and South Asia. The thesis did not hold up for very long, when it was realized that Australian aborigines, widely assumed to be one of the best examples of an earlier form of humanity, had a distribution of the ABO blood types identical to western Europeans: 45 percent A, 45 percent O, and 10 percent B. Then in 1925 Landsteiner and Miller found that anthropoid apes had blood types similar to A and B in humans, thereby suggesting that blood type differentiation pre-dated human evolution.[7]

In the 1930s a whole new dimension was added to the field of blood group anthropology when researchers began testing for blood type on the mummified archaeological remains of native American and Egyptians.[8] In a sense the methodology of the research was inspired by some of the early work of Landsteiner who found that dried blood stains could be accurately tested for blood type; in fact, criminological investigations had come to use the tests routinely by the 1930s. The additional discovery of blood type indicators in muscle tissue permitted the testing of mummified remains which sparked the imagination of anthropologists and archaeologists who saw a way of possibly testing the variation of blood types over a period of several thousand years, or at least testing the presumption of a pure type O pre-Columbian Indian population. It was apparent, however, by the end of the 1930s that the number of cases were too small and the possibility of contamination too great to produce reliable results.

Another major question which developed early in seroanthropology concerned the genetic determination of blood type. No one disputed the Mendelian inheritance of the ABO system, but as seen in Chap. 1, the exact number of allelomorphs was by no means settled, a fact which had important consequences in determining the Hirszfelds' Biochemical Index of Race. Initially, their simple ratio of type A to type B blood was modified to include the percentage of AB individuals in a given population. This was because they assumed the genetic basis of blood type to be the product of eight combinations of the two pairs of alleles (A and non-A, B and non-B), which could occupy two loci on the chromosome, with A and B dominant to both non-A and non-B but not each other.

In contrast, Bernstein, after some of his own testing and reviewing published statistics of blood type inheritance to date (1924), concluded the results could be explained better mathematically if only three possible alleles were assumed for the two loci of the chromosome determining ABO blood type. As Chap. 1 showed, he labelled these factors p (the A genotype), q (B genotype), and r (O genotype). With p and q dominant to r but not each other, only six combinations would result.

One immediate consequence of the new Bernstein theory was that it presumed a greater frequency of the O genotype (r factor) than was manifested in the phenotype of O blood, due to its being recessive. In two of his five non-O combinations, the O genotype was recessive. Thus, it magnified even more the frequency of the O gene in American Indian populations since half of those testing as A blood could be assumed to be heterozygous. But it was a long time before Bernstein's hypothesis was accepted, and in the meantime, all sorts of other proposals were made to resolve the problem, which produced a whole new area of seroanthropological debate.

Ultimately, as will be seen in a later chapter, the most important (albeit unintentional) result of research in seroanthropology was a dramatic change in the view of blood types from indicators of race to indicators of gene frequencies. The shift in emphasis was a crucial step for the beginning of the end of a scientific basis for the concept of race, especially when coupled with the fact that increasing numbers of studies had produced many contradictions to the simple patterns from which the Hirszfeldss first deduced their Biochemical Index of Race in 1919. The search for the genetic basis of blood types meant the ABO system eventually was seen primarily as a reflection of gene distribution. Thus, human population genetics with the concept of gene pools began replacing the categories of human races.

Blood Groups and Disease

In 1953 three researchers in London, Ian Aird, Hugh Henry Bentall, and J. A. Fraser Roberts, published a study entitled, "Relationship between Cancer of Stomach and the ABO Groups," which was a watershed in the study of possible links between blood groups and disease.[9] Reviving the line of inquiry begun by Alexander in 1921, this research studied almost 5700 patients at seven hospitals in England and Scotland, finding that people with blood type A were 5.8 percent more likely to have stomach cancer than those with blood type O. The article immediately prompted attention in a number of fields. Before this article was published, the standard text on blood groups by Race and Sanger (1st ed., 1950) devoted less than half a page to blood groups and disease, beginning with these words, "Excluding the effects of maternal-foetal differences there is as yet no evidence that any blood group is particularly susceptible to any disease." A dozen years after the article by Aird et al. the fifth edition of Race and Sanger's text (5th ed., 1962) included six pages on "Blood Groups and Susceptibility to Disease," citing references going back to Alexander's 1921 report, plus dozens of studies since 1953.[10]

The Aird et al. article and subsequent studies touched off a voluminous and sometimes strident debate about the validity of research linking blood groups and disease. In the process only a few authors took the time to review seriously the literature before 1953; both supporters and opponents dismissed this earlier work. Opponents such as A. S. Wiener (the most antagonistic), Alexander Manuila, and Otto Prokop, ridiculed the precursors, lumping them together with the most superficial and far-fetched tests of possible blood group links to such conditions as hangover, flat feet, homosexuality, and good teeth.[11]

Supporters, on the other hand, did not so much belittle the earlier work as point out its shortcomings in an attempt to magnify the differences in the "new" approach after 1953. In fact, Aird admitted that he was inspired from a completely different line of research, a 1950 article by Percy Stocks which reported a higher frequency of stomach cancer in the north of England as opposed to the south.[12] Aird did a quick literature search and found a few examples of earlier research which he described as "on very small series of cases without adequate controls." Race and Sanger echoed this criticism of earlier research for its use of "small numbers, disease groups which were too broad, and lack of control figures."[13]

A more careful examination of the research on blood groups and disease between the wars shows that although some of these characterizations were warranted, others were not. Most important, almost from the beginning researchers were remarkably thorough and penetrating in their criticisms and summary assessments of this line of research. In correcting the superficial picture painted by postwar researchers, the following analysis places the work of Aird and successors in a broader historical perspective. In the 1920s and 1930s over 300 studies were published on the association of specific blood types with a variety of illnesses. In fact, the strong interest makes this research a bellewether of experimental pathology (etiology) between the wars, giving some measure of which afflictions concerned medical research the most. In addition, this research reflects a method of "framing" disease which ran counter to the trend at the end of the nineteenth and beginning of the twentieth centuries which utilized environmental and contagion explanations. The search for predispositions marked by blood type shows that interest in hereditarian and constitutional explanations of disease was firmly rooted in the nineteenth century and, of course, has enjoyed an even stronger resurgence in recent years.[14]

Historical Interest in Inheritance and Disease

Several circumstances in the 1920s and 1930s helped produce this substantial interest in possible links between blood groups and disease, even in the face of inconclusive results. Most fundamental was the search for the causes of illness which had achieved such remarkable success at the end of the nineteenth and beginning of the twentieth centuries. Thanks to Pasteur, Koch, and their successors, the expectations from modern science to find the cause and prevention of disease were high not just among the general public but also the scientists themselves. Indeed, some historians have labelled this period as beginning the "Golden Age" of medicine.[15] After the first flush of discoveries made possible by the investigation of microbial organisms, however, there was a period of frustration in the early decades of the twentieth century, when results did not follow the inflated expectations.[16] As a result, medical researchers fell back on other modes of explanation for such illnesses as cancer and tuberculosis which proved to be more complicated to understand, let alone cure. In addition to environmental (miasmic) and microbial (germ) causes, many researchers returned to or continued to develop hereditarian explanations which had enjoyed a great vogue during the nineteenth century until their eclipse by the spectacular discoveries at the end of the century.[17]

Thus, by the 1920s there were two competing views of how disease was transmitted. Among the hereditarian explanations, the most widespread at the time were associated with the practice of "constitutional medicine." This was a very broad and sometimes amorphous view of health and healing which held that individuals' responses to the environment (including disease) were indirectly determined by hereditary features, usually manifested in body form.[18] Constitution was especially well suited to explain "predisposition," an explanation of disease that expanded to fill the growing gap between strict Mendelism and environmental or contagious explanations. Body type and personality were the most frequently studied manifestations of constitutional types which by 1940 had produced, according to a survey of the literature published in the *Quarterly Review of Biology*, over 300 articles which was hardly exhaustive.[19]

The historical roots of this view of humans, behavior, and disease went back to Hippocrates, Galen, and other classical theories of temperaments and humors. After a revival in the Renaissance (by Paracelsus, among others), there were attempts to give the idea logical underpinning in the Enlightenment under the name of diathesis which concentrated on predisposition. But with circular definitions of the term, such as "that state of the body which makes it acquire certain diseases," it is no wonder that researchers toward the end of the nineteenth century increased their efforts to use quantitative anthropometric measurements of the human body to define (and mark) basic human types with correlated diseases and temperaments. Perhaps the best known of these efforts were theories of phrenology and craniology which met with only limited success.[20] The research which was most often credited with inspiring twentieth-century constitutional medicine was done by Friedrich Wilhelm Beneke of Marburg, Germany, who published several studies in the late 1870s and early 1880s on measurements of various internal organs and their correlations with age, disease, and somatotype. Most important was his postulation of two main categories of humans: one of slight build with large lungs and a higher incidence of scrofula and phthisis (tuberculosis), and the other of large build with small lungs and a higher incidence of cancer in adults.[21]

Although some isolated researchers were inspired by these findings, two different schools of constitutional studies eventually developed in the twentieth century which exercised much wider influence. One was in Italy at the University of Padua, where Achille de Giovanni created what came to be known as a school of clinical anthropology. He and his students such as Giacinte Viola and Nicola Pende developed a system of classifying humans based largely on correlations of body type to disease.[22] The other school arose in central Europe (home of Jung and Rohrschach) where Emil Kraeplin and Ernst Kretschmer developed their theories which postulated a correlation between three somatotypes and temperament, specifically schizophrenia and manic-depression.[23] These two schools inspired hundreds of studies in the 1920s and 1930s, including those by George Draper who created a "constitutional clinic" affiliated with Columbia University in 1916.

In the meantime, there was another explanation of the inheritance of disease which had developed at the beginning of the twentieth century, inspired by the rediscovery of Mendel's work, and incorporated into the growing field of eugenics. Under the label of "morbid" or "familial" disease, this approach utilized, with varying success, the theoretical framework of dominant and recessive genes (or factors) plus the methodology of pedigree study in an effort to explain a wide variety of afflictions and conditions that were thought to be passed from one generation to another. In Bateson's 1909 book *Mendel's Principles of Heredity*, he listed alkaptonuria and brachydactyly as well as other abnormal conditions such as cataracts, hemophilia, and color blindness that seemed to follow a pattern of inheritance in humans similar to that found in peas by the Augustinian monk. By 1930 R. R. Gates' book *Heredity in Man* had added a considerable number of other traits, including many highly questionable or outright incorrect ones such as skin color, feeble-mindedness, and stature.[24] All were calculated and illustrated with the same Mendelian charts of crossing and breeding as if they were pea shapes or leaf colors.

First Studies of Blood Groups and Disease

Given this interest in the inheritance of disease, there was ample reason for researchers to examine possible links to blood groups soon after Von Dungern and Hirszfeld showed that blood type inheritance followed Mendelian{XE "Inheritance laws:Mendelian inheritance"} laws. Moreover, with only four possible ABO blood types which could be determined by simple tests after 1917, blood groups offered a highly promising alternative to the elaborate and varied anthropometric indices that had been devised to classify body types and forms for constitutional studies.

In fact, this advantage was a key part of the reason given for the first published study. As Alexander stated in the beginning of his 1921 article on blood groups and malignant disease, "we know that blood groups follow Mendelian laws." In addition, he added guardedly, "we do not know all the factors that determine the occurrence of malignant disease, but there is more than a suggestion that a hereditary factor, as distinct from inherited infection, plays some part in its causation."[25] Alexander admitted at the outset that "the number of cases so far dealt with - fifty - is not sufficiently large to justify any definitive conclusions being drawn." He ended the article, however, with the report that although malignant disease was found in people of all four blood types, "those in Group I (AB) and III (B) appear to be peculiarly susceptible." His reasoning and findings soon prompted an article by Buchanan and Higley at the end of 1921 on possible links between blood type and susceptibility to disease on a far larger number of patients (3446) at the Mayo Clinic.

Buchanan and Higley did not find any link between blood type and cancer, but equally as important for the subsequent pattern of research was that both of these studies found that people with all blood types had all the diseases; hence, there was no simple Mendelian link between blood type and disease.[26] Moreover, subsequent pedigree studies of possible links between blood types and other diseases, notably hemophilia and goiter, also showed no direct Mendelian link. The vast majority of subsequent research, therefore, shifted to the concept of predisposition and looked for evidence in the form of differences in frequency of blood types found in healthy and ill populations. The major point of debate thereafter was how much the distribution of blood types among patients with a given illness had to differ from that of the normal population to be significant.

Despite the different conclusions of these first two studies, there was no immediate rush by researchers to settle the matter. In 1922–1923 most blood group research concentrated on such matters as defining and explaining the phenomenon of agglutination and its inheritance, the possible existence of sub-groups, or confirmation of the Hirszfelds' discovery of a geographical pattern by a few scattered anthropological studies. Included among these were some articles comparing the blood types of mothers and newborns, a few of which pointed the way to the phenomenon of hemolytic disease of newborns that took more than 15 years to recognize.[27]

By far the strongest stimulus for the dramatic rise in research on blood groups and disease in the mid-1920s came from the work of the Hirszfelds: both the wider circulation of their First World War research as well as new studies that he and his students published at the Warsaw Serological Institute. In 1924 and 1925 several articles were published by a group of Polish researchers that included the Hirszfeldss, Henryk Brokman, Rose Amzel, Wanda Halber, and Adam Strazynski. They tested possible blood group links to syphilis and diphtheria. As might be expected from researchers as experienced and careful as the Hirszfelds, these were not hastily assembled or simplistic statistical comparisons. Instead, these researchers studied the existence of diphtheria antibodies as detected by the Schick test, which were found in individuals who had not been exposed to the disease. If both parents lacked the antibodies, such was also the case with their children. When both parents had the antibodies, almost all children did too. It was in the case where only one parent tested for the antibodies that the blood groups entered the picture. Specifically, when the child had the same blood type as the parent without antibodies, that child would not have the antibodies. In the opposite case, the child usually possessed the antibodies if it had the same blood type as the parent with them.

This diphtheria and Schick test research was more important in suggesting a possible mechanism for blood antigens to influence disease, as opposed to being a hereditary marker. There was no one blood type associated more or less frequently with the disease or antibodies. When the research was extended to Wassermann test results for syphilis, however, Amzel and Halber found that individuals with blood type O had a somewhat higher percentage of Wassermann-negative reactions (75.8 percent) than those of other blood type (66 to 64.1).[28] They even went so far as to link their findings to the questions raised by the Hirszfeldss' Macedonian research, which showed an uneven distribution of the blood types around the world.

> The study of the disease predisposition of different [blood] groups are of the greatest importance for considerations of an anthropological nature, because it concerns an answer to the question whether belonging to a particular group has an effect on selection.

This explicit mention of evolutionary implications was rare, however, among those testing blood groups and disease. The major effect of the Polish work was to give broader legitimacy to a whole new line of research.

There was one other independent beginning to the study of blood groups and disease inspired by early testing of blood groups in the Soviet Union by the biologist N. K. Koltsov. Beginning in 1924 with a study of malaria, and then tuberculosis, a number of Soviet researchers conducted studies on "how hemoagglutination properties of blood might affect the occurrence of disease."[29] In contrast to the Polish researchers who published in Western medical journals such as the *Zeitschrift für Immunitätsforschung*, the *Comptes rendus de la Société de Biologie*, and the *Journal of Immunology* which had wide circulation, this early Soviet research was published largely in local, Russian-language journals. Hence, it went unrecognized at first in the West. Only in 1926–1927 was it belatedly discovered, and thereafter at least part of the Soviet work was acknowledged in studies of blood groups and disease conducted around the world.

Overall Pattern of Research

The interest in potential links between blood groups and disease is evident in the large number of publications which appeared in the 1920s and 1930s. In fact, the overall pattern in Fig. 6.1 shows a remarkable similarity to that of all articles on blood group distribution between the wars.

The sharp rise of articles after 1925 was later and perhaps even more abrupt than for all articles, and the decline thereafter was more gradual,

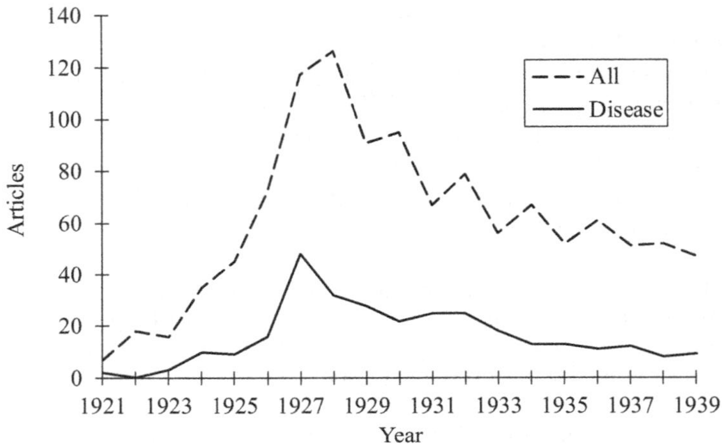

Fig. 6.1 Articles on blood groups and disease, 1921–1939

with eight to nine articles appearing by the end of the 1930s on the link between blood groups and disease. Thus, Aird and subsequent researchers can say with justification that interest had declined by 1939. Of course, the following year Landsteiner, Levine, and Wiener published their landmark findings on the Rh blood antigens which defined and explained hemolytic disease of the newborn, thus dramatically stimulating interest in the whole question of blood groups in general and disease in particular after the war. Thus, the commonly accepted characterization that "little emerged between 1921 and 1953" is wrong both generally as well as specifically with reference to the Rh discoveries.

The study of the link between blood groups and disease, like other blood group research, was widespread geographically. A chronology of the first articles to appear in 28 countries reveals the spread and speed with which this line of research was adopted.

Table 6.1 shows that there was a slight delay after the first articles appeared in the 1921 issues of the *British Journal of Experimental Pathology*. Then between 1924 and 1926 articles appeared by researchers from 11 countries in Europe and Japan. After 1927 the first articles were published by researchers in European countries with less medical research (Spain, Estonia, Greece) as well as overseas (Argentina, China, Egypt, and India). This pattern was, thus, very similar to that for all blood group

Table 6.1 First appearance of articles on blood group and disease by country of researcher, 1921–1938

Year	*Country*	*Researcher*	*Disease*
1921	Scotland (U.K.)	Alexander	Cancer
	U.S.	Higley & Buchanan	Various
1924	Poland	Hirszfeld, et al.	Diphtheria, syphilis
	USSR	Liakhovetzkii	Malaria
	USSR	Pantchenko	TB
1925	Denmark	Johanssen	Cancer
	Hungary	Weitzner	Cancer
	Italy	Dossena, et al.	Cancer
	Japan	Gondo	Cancer
1926	Austria	Hoche	Cancer
	Holland	Bendien	Cancer
	Romania	Mironescu	Infectious disease
	Switzerland	Niceforo	Cancer
1927	Finland	Sievers	Various
	France	Dujarric	TB, cancer
1928	Greece	Diamantopoulos	Various
	Spain	Urra	
1929	Estonia	Paldrok	Leprosy
1930	Argentina	Puente	Leprosy
1931	China	Wong	Syphilis
	Egypt	Ali	Leprosy
1933	India	Mitra	Various
1934	Belgium	Moureau	Various
1935	Czechoslovakia	Fiser	Cancer
	Yugoslavia	Kalic	Deaf-mutism
1937	Lithuania	Pautientis	Cancer
	Sweden	Lofgren	Haemophilia
1938	Canada	Erb	Polio

research, with the exception that researchers in some remote locations never developed an interest in blood groups and disease. For example, there was much more interest in the anthropological applications of blood group research in the East Indies, South Africa, Australia, and other Latin American countries, apparently to the exclusion of research on disease and blood groups.

As has been mentioned earlier in more detailed study of research in specific countries, there were differences in the extent of interest in links between blood groups and disease. Taken together, a comparison can be made by examining the proportion of all blood group articles with disease as a subject of interest published in countries where most research was done.

As shown in Table 6.2 the country where the greatest percentage of researchers were interested in disease was clearly Poland, thanks to the work of Hirszfeld and his associates. The rest of the countries fell into two groups. One was central and other eastern European countries (USSR, Germany, Italy, Austria, Demark) where a substantial percentage of all articles (34–42 percent) were on possible links between blood groups and disease. As the analysis of individual countries has revealed, these were also the countries where constitutional medicine had the strongest influence. The other group included the U.S., Britain, France, and Japan, where a significantly lower percentage of articles on disease (15–24 percent) reflected relatively less interest in the subject. In some countries, however, there was such a strong overall interest in blood group research that even a lower percentage of these articles represented a critical mass of work on blood groups and disease. Thus, in absolute numbers the most articles published between the wars were by authors in the Soviet Union, Germany, and Italy (43–56 articles), percentages (34–39 percent) well above the 25 percent average of articles on disease in all countries.

The most frequent criticisms of these studies by researchers after 1953 were their small subject size, the vagueness of disease or condition examined, and lack of control groups. Yet a close examination of the 300

Table 6.2 Percentage of articles on blood groups and disease by country of author

Country of author	*All Articles*	*Articles on disease*	*% of all*
Poland	30	23	77%
Denmark	33	14	42%
Austria	30	12	40%
Italy	111	43	39%
Germany	151	54	36%
USSR	166	56	34%
U.S.	94	23	24%
Britain	32	6	19%
France	57	11	19%
Japan	140	21	15%
Other & unknown	388	40	10%
Total	1232	303	25%

articles shows that the least valid criticism was lack of a control group. This may have originated from the fact that some of the initial studies simply reported the distribution of ABO blood types among disease populations, but they were generally the exceptions. In fact, the very first study by Alexander, although using small numbers, included tests of a control group of healthy individuals as well as blood types for patients with four diseases. Likewise, Buchanan and Higley's 1921 follow-up report on Mayo Clinic patients used the best available information on normal blood group distribution as a basis for comparison: the Hirszfelds' 1919 results. The authors even separated out the blood types of non-U.S. patients so as to account for the nationality differences which had been found among the different soldiers in Macedonia.

As blood group testing became more widespread in subsequent years, studies of possible links between blood groups and disease had larger and more specific control groups. For example, in 1924 two American researchers in Philadelphia who studied the blood group distribution of patients with cancer from radiation treatment exposure, compared their findings to the results reported by Ottenberg in 1921 for a study of blood group inheritance. By 1925 a researcher at Warsaw University Hospital reported the blood group distribution of 618 patients with skin diseases and used the recently completed study by Halber and Mydlarski of 12,000 Polish army recruits as a basis for comparison.[30]

In many other cases, the researchers tested their own control groups. For example, in 1926 J. Hollo and W. Lenard at Budapest Hospital compared the blood group distribution of 200 patients with pulmonary tuberculosis to 200 healthy patients. The largest studies done in this manner utilized the results of Wassermann tests for syphilis, a procedure that was widely used after its introduction in 1906. Testing for blood type soon became part of the procedure, and by the 1920s it was second only to testing for transfusion as a source of data for blood group distribution studies. Moreover, in the case of researchers interested in predisposition to disease, those with a negative Wassermann test provided an automatic control group for studying blood group links to syphilis. An example of such a study was done by Max Gundel in Kiel, who used the results of over 10,000 tests, comparing the blood type distribution of the 1710 who tested positive with those who tested negative. He found little difference.[31]

If the criticism is unwarranted about lack of control groups in studies of blood groups and disease, there is more of a basis for questions about the size of populations studied. In over 300 articles published between the wars on the blood group distribution of those with illnesses, accurate figures about the numbers tested were given for over 250 of the studies. They reported a total of 162,000 subjects tested, which meant an average of 635 for each study. The median number tested, however, was only 300, which indicates that most studies were on smaller populations. This can be shown more clearly by grouping the studies according to the numbers tested.

Table 6.3 indicates that over 160 articles (65 percent) reported tests on less than 500 subjects, a figure commonly mentioned as necessary for statistically meaningful results. Alexander Manuila, for example, reported that sampling errors ranging from 2 percent to 4 percent could arise in populations as large as 1000, with errors as high as 15 percent in samples less than 200.[32]

On the other hand, perhaps the most surprising thing about the numbers tested was that fully one-third of the articles included more than 500 subjects, and almost 40 had over 1000. To be sure, some of the large numbers are misleading, because they grouped together several different diseases. The Buchanan and Higley study, for example, compiled the results of blood group tests on 3400 patients at the Mayo Clinic for over four years. They included so many diseases (17) that only two, pernicious anemia (457 tests) and cancer (292), had more than 200 observations. In fact, because of the small numbers, the authors admitted that for half the diseases, the figures could be misleading. Some of the other large studies also simply offered tallies of hospital admissions, such as a 1933 study of 2000 patients at a hospital in India and another on a similar number of patients at a hospital in Udine, Italy.[33] The goal of the latter was simply to see if people with one blood type were more prone to illness than others, and the author reported that to be the case with blood type O.

Table 6.3 Size of blood groups and disease studies, 1921–1939

Numbers tested	*Number of studies*
0–199	86
200–499	77
500–999	52
1,000–1,999	28
Over 2,000	9

The disease that was most frequently tested for a link to blood groups was syphilis. Half of the dozen largest studies, utilizing the results of Wassermann and Schick tests, presented results of over 1000 subjects. The single largest study, by two researchers in northeast Japan, compared the blood group distribution of over 4000 sick people with 6400 healthy inhabitants. Among those who were sick, there were 2400 with syphilis, 895 with tuberculosis, and 713 with neurasthenia. When the results showed little difference in blood type distribution, the authors had enough syphilitic patients to divide them between those showing early and late-stage symptoms. They then found a lower percentage of those with blood type A in later-stage (30 percent compared to 39 percent in the control) and a higher percentage with type O (43 percent compared to 31 percent).[34]

Links to Specific Diseases

When the results of the early Polish and Soviet research on blood groups and disease reached central Europe, the home of constitutional studies, it stimulated a great deal of interest. The number of articles presenting research findings by German and Italian authors alone rose from 4 in 1926 to 17 in 1927. Table 6.4 indicates that the diseases of most interest were tuberculosis, cancer, and syphilis.

It is not difficult to understand why the three most studied diseases received so much attention. All were widespread, and the tuberculosis and syphilis bacilli had been identified in the last two decades of the nineteenth

Table 6.4 Articles on blood groups and most frequently studied diseases, 1921–1939

Disease	*1st study*	*1st author(s)*	*No. of studies*	*Notes*
Tuberculosis	1924	3 Soviets	66	
Cancer	1921	Alexander	47	Various cancers
Syphilis	1924	Amzel, Hirszfeld, et al.	41	1 art on gonorrhea
Malaria	1924	Liakhovetskii	22	
Scarlet fever	1927	3 Soviets	20	
Skin diseases	1924	Strazynski, Hirszfeld	14	Eczema, psoriasis
Leprosy	1930	Malinin	14	
Diphtheria	1924	Hirszfeld et al.	12	
Polio	1928	Kaminsky	12	

century. In addition, Ehrlich's treatment for syphilis raised hopes for similar "magic bullets" to cure other diseases. Syphilis and tuberculosis had a long history of being considered hereditary in origin, but the cause of cancer was more open to question. Like tuberculosis, cancer was discovered to present differences depending on where it was found in the body.

Besides the high incidence of these diseases, there were practical reasons that made it possible to do studies of potential linkage to blood type. As mentioned above, the large amount of research on blood groups and syphilis was possible because of the extensive Wassermann testing that was employed after the development of the procedure in the first decade of the twentieth century. One-third of the largest studies of links between blood groups and disease (each with over 1000 subjects) consisted partly or entirely of those who had been tested for syphilis. In fact, the most important early studies of syphilis and blood groups were by Polish researchers based on the results of almost 3000 Wassermann tests. They found a higher frequency of blood type O for positive Wassermann subjects than for those testing negative. Given the size of the Halber and Mydlarski army testing study (including the large control group) and the prestige of Hirszfeld, there was ample reason for follow-up testing by Italian, German, Russian, and Finnish researchers who did 16 studies in 1926–1927 alone. Some of these confirmed the lower frequency of blood type O among those testing negative or higher frequency of type A and AB among Wassermann positive tests, but more than half the studies found no difference in blood group frequencies between the ill and healthy population. Included among these was Gundel's large study (10,550 subjects) of the Schleswig-Holstein population.[35]

Whether from the lack of consistent results or the novelty of the problem wearing off, the number of these studies tapered off by the end of the decade. Through the 1930s, nonetheless, there were three to four studies published each year on blood groups and syphilis, including the first testing in Switzerland, Lebanon, the U.S., Romania, Hungary, China, and France. Only one study, by a researcher at the dermato-syphilis clinic of the University of Naples, found dramatic differences from the norm in the blood type distribution of patients.[36] He reported a much higher proportion of those with AB (27 percent) and B (17 percent) blood types among those with syphilis, and a low percentage of O (11 percent) compared to the normal population, thus confirming the first Polish results. But the numbers in the study were small (184 subjects), and there were other results based on far larger numbers which found a higher frequency of type O among those testing positive for syphilis. There were also additional large studies, such as Wong and Chen's at Peking Union Medical College, that found no difference in the blood group distribution of healthy and Wassermann positive individuals.[37]

The ambivalence of these results is illustrated by a simple tally of the studies reporting differences between the sick (or Wassermann positive) and healthy in their blood group distribution (14 articles) and those studies reporting no difference (16 articles). The impact of those finding a predisposition (or protection) according to blood type was further undercut by contradictory evidence of what blood type was associated with which condition. Thus, half the studies reporting differences confirmed the early Polish findings of a lower than normal incidence of blood type O and a higher AB among patients and those testing Wassermann positive, but almost the same number found a higher incidence of O or some different association.

Interest in studies of tuberculosis and blood groups also reflected the high prevalence of the disease in the first decades of the twentieth century when only pneumonia exceeded it as a cause of death in the U.S.[38] Even though a test for tuberculosis exposure was available after 1907, virtually all populations in Europe and North America tested positive; hence, there was no convenient control group of those testing negative as was the case with the tests for syphilis. On the other hand, the high prevalence of the disease and corresponding campaigns to identify and treat the afflicted especially at sanatoria, meant that there were large numbers of subjects available for blood testing.

Given this widespread concern with tuberculosis, coupled with the long-standing assumption that it was hereditary, it is surprising that the search for possible links between the disease and blood type did not occur sooner. For example, Alexander tested tuberculosis patients in his 1921 study, although Buchanan and Higley did not include them in their follow-up study later that year. The first studies to concentrate on tuberculosis patients were done in the Soviet Union in 1924, but only in late 1926 did these or other studies appear elsewhere in Europe. One of these was a study by Hungarian researchers ignorant of the Soviet work, but who attempted to extend the Polish work on diphtheria and syphilis. The other article in 1926 was a translation of Alperin's Russian work, which not only reported a higher percentage of blood group A among tubercular patients but also cited the previous work by other Soviet authors.[39]

Although late in appearance, publication of these studies about a possible link between blood groups and tuberculosis quickly prompted a flood of research. For example, in 1927 there were 17 tuberculosis studies by authors in 8 different countries and another 11 articles of original research in 1928. These studies involved significantly fewer individuals than the research on syphilis because no comparable body of data existed like the Wassermann testing. Nonetheless, although no tuberculosis study had more than 1000 patients, over half had more than 500, and these studies benefitted from the availability of control group comparisons from increasing anthropological blood group testing.

The tuberculosis results were no more conclusive about links to blood types than the research on syphilis. Some authors confirmed the higher incidence of tuberculosis among patients with blood type A and lower among those with type O, whereas others found no difference.[40] In an effort to find more conclusive results, some researchers refined the categories of patients. For example, all the early studies were of pulmonary tuberculosis, but Alperin introduced the distinction seen in the syphilis studies of dividing patients according to the three stages of the disease that was a common practice of diagnosis.[41] This approach was soon followed by others but with continuing mixed results. Alperin found a higher incidence of blood type A among those in the later, more severe cases of tuberculosis, but others did not.

As with the syphilis studies, the research on tuberculosis was almost evenly divided between those who found a difference between sick and healthy patients in the frequency of blood types. Of more than 60 articles, 24 reported differences and the same number did not. (About a dozen authors either made no comparisons or drew no conclusion.) As with syphilis, those who claimed to find differences were hampered by the fact that other research often produced contradictory results. Thus, nine of the researchers agreed with Alperin's initial finding of a higher percentage of blood type A and/or a lower O and B among tubercular patients, but seven articles reported the opposite: a lower percentage of type A and higher O.[42] Nor were the results much different among specialists in the disease. Of 18 studies published in journals specializing in tuberculosis, 7 found differences in blood type distribution between sick and healthy individuals and 8 found no difference.

The inconclusive nature of these results undoubtedly dampened the initial enthusiasm for the research. Indeed, if interest in blood groups and tuberculosis rose faster than with other diseases, it also dropped off more rapidly during the 1930s. There was an average of only two to three studies published per year from 1931 through 1939.

The large number of individuals tested for syphilis and tuberculosis was a main reason for so many blood group linkage studies, but that was not the case with cancer. Although it was not as frequently studied, cancer and its potential link to blood groups was the subject of the two most important landmark studies of all research on the subject: Alexander's 1921 article and Aird et al.'s 1953 work. In between, however, the results of testing were almost as inconclusive as the research on syphilis and tuberculosis in the 1920s and 1930s. For example, despite the short delay following the 1921 research, there were more studies earlier on cancer than the other diseases: five articles in 1925 and four in 1926. The rise in interest thereafter, however, was less abrupt for cancer than the other diseases: nine articles published in 1927 and only one in 1928.

There was no single research center or country that directed or led this work on blood groups and cancer. Of the handful of the earliest studies published by authors in Hungary, Denmark, Japan, and Italy, the article most often cited subsequently was by Geza Weitzner who compared the blood groups of 84 cancer patients at the Budapest Jewish Hospital to a healthy control group of one thousand.[43] The reason, however, was to refute his stunning finding of a fivefold higher frequency of blood type AB and half the percentage of type O among patients. One quick and unusually strong rebuke was by Fritz Schiff a few months after the article appeared, questioning Weitzner's testing methods. Another direct response was by Hirszfeld and Hittmair at the Berlin University Cancer Institute, who found little difference between the blood group distribution of 150 of their cancer patients and the healthy population.[44]

One reason for the failure to find the linkage between blood type and cancer was the smaller number of subjects in these early cancer studies. In fact, the only study with more than 500 patients was a national survey in Denmark. The most obvious reason for these smaller numbers was the lack of a screening test for cancer as existed for syphilis and tuberculosis. In addition, cancer did not have the same stigma as tuberculosis, and since its victims were generally far older, they were much more inclined to resignation and acceptance of their fate.[45] In fact, the main motivation of Aird and his colleagues to do a new study in 1953 was the availability of data from an unprecedented number of stomach cancer patients.

The national study in Denmark grew out of a 1926 doctoral dissertation by Erik W. Johannsen, who compared the blood group distribution of 512 healthy Danes with that of 263 patients with malignant tumors at the Institute of General Pathology of the University of Copenhagen. Johannsen sharpened his findings by comparing the frequency of type O with type A, which were approximately equal in the normal population but significantly different among the cancer patients (38 percent O vs. 49 percent A). Moreover, when he looked at only women with uterine cancer, the contrast was even sharper: 35 percent O to 54 percent A.[46] These results prompted the director of Johannsen's Institute, Oluf Thomsen, to conduct a series of studies that eventually included 1200 patients with malignant tumors. The research was supported by the Danish Cancer Committee and drew patients not just from Thomsen's own institute but from doctors at hospitals around the country. Thomsen's results, however, showed very little difference between the healthy population and cancer patients in their blood group distribution.[47]

There was similar disagreement in most findings on blood groups and cancer during the interwar period. A significant number of studies (12) found differences in the distribution among cancer patients compared to the norm, but there were almost twice as many studies (23) which found little difference. Of those finding a difference, there was somewhat more agreement on which blood types were associated with cancer. Thus, 8 of the 12 studies finding differences reported a lower percentage of blood type O and higher B and AB. Thus, buried in the results was a potential clue to the finding of a higher percentage of cancer with blood type A that Aird and his collaborators reported.

The only other country besides Denmark where researchers showed a strong interest in cancer and blood groups was Italy. In fact, researchers there actually published more articles (ten) than the Danes (nine), although it was not the result of a coordinated effort. Authors in each of these two countries published twice as many articles as their colleagues in France, Japan, or the U.S. Also of note was the fact that only two German studies were published on blood groups and cancer, and none were authored by Soviet researchers. This was in striking contrast to the 22 German and 17 Soviet articles on tuberculosis and syphilis, roughly equally divided. The Italian research included an early (1925) study by two gynecologists at the Obstetrics-Gynecology Institute of the University of Milan who tested 300 women, a large number for such an early study.[48] Their finding of little difference from the norm in the blood group distribution of their patients was corroborated by Marco Goldstein at the city hospital of Trieste. Goldstein, who was in the service of Adriano Sturli, a former assistant of Landsteiner (and a co-discoverer of the AB blood type), tested 218 cancer patients in an effort to verify the findings of Weitzner. In fact, he refuted them. A few years later, however, another researcher working under Sturli at Trieste found significant differences from normal blood group distributions in a study of 222 cancer patients.[49]

There were far fewer articles published on other diseases and their potential links to blood type. Of these the Soviets did the most studies on malaria (11 of the 22 articles found), perhaps because of the extent of the disease in the vast reaches of the country. Relatively few researchers followed up on Hirszfeld's initial research on diphtheria (he published four articles himself on the link). There were almost 30 other diseases receiving far less attention (five or fewer articles) for links to blood type, as indicated in Table 6.5.

As for diseases later found to be linked to blood type, although Buchanan and Higley's 1921 study of a number of diseases showed a marked increase in type O patients with duodenal ulcers (122 compared to 55 with blood type A), despite a few other articles testing correlations with several different diseases, it was not until a 1936 study of 244 patients in a Rome hospital that another article reported a higher incidence of patients with blood type O who had ulcers (52 vs. 37 percent).[50] No studies followed until the landmark 1954 article by Aird et al. Likewise, few

Table 6.5 Articles on blood groups and other disease, 1921–1939

Disease	*First study*	*No. of studies*	*Disease*	*First study*	*No. of studies*
Eclampsia	1923	4	Epilepsy	1930	1
Toxemia	1923	3	Alcoholism	1931	1
Adenoids	1926	1	Caries	1931	2
Leukemia	1926	2	Anemia	1932	2
Measles	1926	2	Hemophilia	1932	2
Hypertension	1927	1	Tonsillitis	1932	1
Infectious dis.	1927	3	Trachoma	1932	2
"Mongolism"	1927	5	Gallstones	1934	1
Eye diseases	1928	4	Herpes	1934	1
Typhus	1928	5	Friedrich's ataxia	1935	1
Diabetes	1929	1	Allergies	1936	3
Goiter	1929	3	Color blindness	1936	1
Hyperthyroid	1929	1	Ulcers	1936	1
Epilepsy	1930	1	Sickle cell	1937	1
Alcoholism	1931	1			

studies made distinctions between types of cancer, and none reported on a link to stomach cancer until Aird's article in 1953.[51] A final observation is that the goal of most researchers was at first to find a marker for disease: a direct link. This quickly shifted to "predisposition," the language of constitutional studies where heredity was broad and vague. Few except Snyder understood Mendelian heredity, and only late in the 1930s (Haldane, Fisher, Boyd) was there an appreciation of a link between disease and the overall distribution of blood groups around the world, through evolutionary selection.

Critics and Conclusion

In the introduction of William Boyd's 1939 article summarizing all research on blood group distribution in the previous two decades, the author included a brief paragraph on studies of the possible relationship between blood groups and disease. Despite his admission that it was an "incomplete survey," Boyd presented a table to support his own conclusion that "few of the studies have any value." Moreover, he went on to predict, "it may confidently be expected that if any differences in susceptibility of persons of different blood groups to different diseases do exist, they will be small, and not so easy to demonstrate conclusively."[52] A more complete survey (see Tables 6.6a and 6.6b) of these studies of blood groups and disease done in the 1920s and 1930s shows a remarkably consistent pattern of only one-third of researchers finding differences between sick and healthy patients in blood type distribution.

Although his survey was incomplete, Boyd's conclusions were supported by some of the most highly regarded researchers at the time. Some have been alluded to before, such as Schiff's early criticism of the findings of Geza Weitzner about Budapest cancer patients in 1926. That same year Philip Levine, then at the Cornell Department of Bacteriology and Immunology under the direction of Coca, tested Hirszfeld's theory of a link between blood type and inheritance of susceptibility to diphtheria. More specifically Levine was responding to a subsequent study by Th. Fürst of goiter in Bavarian families which he claimed supported Hirszfeld's theory. Levine pointed out, however, that the German study was only of four families, clearly "insufficient to warrant his conclusion." Levine did a larger study of 20 families including 74 parents and children, at least one of the parents and one of the children suffered from atopic allergy (hay fever and asthma).[53] His conclusion was that there was no evidence that

Table 6.6a William Boyd's table of links in Blood Group and Disease Studies (1939) compared to more exhaustive search (1921–1939)

Condition	*A increased and/or B decreased*	*A decreased and/or B increased*	*Some other change*	*No change*
Cancer	2	1	5	7
Syphilis	5	6	2	18
Tuberculosis	3		1	15

Table 6.6b (all authors' conclusions about blood groups and disease, 1921–1939)

Condition	*Difference found between sick & healthy individuals*	*No diff. found*	*No conclusion*
Cancer	12	22[a]	11
Syphilis	14[b]	16	10
Tuberculosis	24[c]	24	16

[a]Includes 5 followup studies by same authors

[b]Includes 2 followup studies by same authors

[c]Includes 6 followup studies by same authors

Source: William C. Boyd, "Blood Groups," *Tabulae Biologicae* 17 (1939): 144–5

atopic hypersensitivity is inherited conjointly with the serological group. As late as 1935 Schiff was still not persuaded that a single convincing case had been made that met Hirszfeld's own criteria as spelled out in his 1928 book *Konstitutionsserologie*.[54]

Another example of a well-regarded American critic of these studies linking blood groups and disease was Laurence Snyder. Shortly after these first reports appeared, he tested the blood group distribution of several hundred cases of epilepsy, insanity, and feeble-mindedness among both white and native American populations. Finding no difference in the distribution of blood types compared to the normal population, Snyder went on to criticize studies by Weitzner and Fürst for using such small numbers.[55] Three years later he was even more critical of "the wide range of speculation by many workers of late" which continued to be based on small studies. As one of the few people in the field trained in genetics, Snyder was especially frustrated by the "false claims or erroneous ideas of linkage." He, therefore, included a whole chapter on "Blood Groups and Pathology" in his 1929 book on blood groups, which began with a basic lecture on genetic linkage. Then surveying the literature which included many reports of differences from the norm of the blood group distribution of sick populations, Snyder concluded, "no abnormal distribution can as yet be accepted as final, and it seems likely that a normal distribution will eventually be demonstrated for these conditions."[56]

What accounts for this large literature and continuing research on blood groups and disease even in the face of such formidable opposition and at best mixed results? Why the persistence of studies, especially with so many negative findings? First, as in all blood group research was the Hirszfelds' (and Coca's) simple, spectacular success. This, combined with the relative ease of testing and availability of subjects to test, opened this research field to doctors in hospitals and testing laboratories around the world. Second was the fact that inconclusive results could act to some extent as an incentive to do more research. Then there was the variety of diseases and possibility of focusing on many subsets of illnesses. Finally, disease was a very practical concern much more so than race or any other application of blood group research.

The links between blood groups and disease were not the most questionable studies undertaken by researchers. The appeal of genetic determinism was also applied to other human traits, as seen in the wide spread of eugenics during the 1920s and 1930s. Much less studied but revealing of this appeal, as will be shown in the next chapter, were such traits as insanity, criminality, and related human conditions.

Notes

1. One of the more popular accounts of this history is Steven Jay Gould, *Mismeasure of Man* (New York: W.W. Norton, 1981).
2. Hirszfeld, *Konstitutionsserologie und Blutgruppenforschung* (Berlin: Springer, 1928).
3. Ludwik Hirszfeld, Hannah Hirszfeld, and Henryk Brokman, "On the Susceptibility to Diphtheria (Schick Test Positive) with Reference to the Inheritance of Blood Groups," *Journal of Immunology* 9 (1924): 571–91; Ludwik Hirszfeld and H. Zborowski, "Sur la permeabilité élective du placenta en rapport avec le groupe sanguin de la mère et la foetus," *Comptes rendus de la Société de Biologie* 92 (1925): 1253–5; Ludwik Hirszfeld and Roza Amzel, «Sur la presence des elements de groupe du foetus dans le sang retroplacentaire de la mere,» *Comptes rendus de la Société de Biologie* 109 (1932): 252–3.

4. For a summary of the controversial book by Myriam Spörri, *Reines und gemischtes Blut: Zur Kulturgeschichte der Blutgruppenforschung, 1900–1933* (Bielefeld: Transcript Verlag, 2013), see Frank Thadeusz, "Blood Purity: How a Bizarre Obsession Advanced Science," *Spiegel*, May 31, 2013. An attempt at a balanced assessment can be found in Katrin Steffen, and Maciej Górny, "Böses Blut. Die Blutgruppenforschung und der Serologe Ludwik Hirszfeld in Deutschland und in Polen," *JB historie*, 1 (2014): 97–119.
5. Hirszfeld, *The Story of One Life*, eds. Marta A. Balinska and William H. Schneider, (Rochester: University of Rochester Press, 2005).
6. Arthur F. Coca and Olin Diebert, "A Study of the Occurrence of the Blood Groups among American Indians," *Journal of Immunology* 8 (1923): 487–91.
7. Karl Landsteiner and C. P. Miller, "Serological Studies on the Blood of the Primates" *Journal of Experimental Medicine* 42 (1925): 841–52; 853–862; and 863–72.
8. William Boyd and Lyle G. Boyd, "An Attempt to Determine the Blood Groups of Mummies," *Proceedings of the Society for Experimental Biology* 31 (1934): 671–2; G. Albin Matson, "A procedure for Determining Distribution of Blood Groups in Mummies," *Proceedings of the Society for Experimental Biology and Medicine* 31 (1934): 964–8; P. B. Candela, "Blood Group Reactions in Ancient Human Skeletons," *American Journal of Physical Anthropology* 21 (1936): 429–32.
9. Ian Aird, H. H. Bentall and J. A. Fraser Roberts, "A Relationship between Cancer of Stomach and the ABO Blood Groups," *British Medical Journal* (1953) 1:799–801.
10. R. R. Race and Ruth Sanger, *Blood Groups in Man* (Oxford: Blackwell, 1950) 1st ed., 241; 5th ed. (1962), 393–9.
11. Otto Prokop and Gerhard Uhlenbruck, *Human Blood Serum and Serum Groups* (London: McLaren and Sons, 1969), 691; Alexander S. Wiener, "Modern Blood Group Mythology," *Journal of Forensic Medicine* 7 (1960):166–76; Wiener, "Blood-groups and Disease: a Critical Review," *Lancet* (1962) 1: 813–6; and Alexander Manuila, "Blood Groups and Disease -- Hard Facts and Delusions," *JAMA* 167 (1958): 2047–53.
12. Aird, "Discussion on the ABO Blood Groups and Disease," *Proceedings of the Royal Society of Medicine* 48 (1955): 139.
13. Race and Sanger (1962), 393–4. For another example, see the editorial "Blood Groups and Disease," *British Medical Journal* (Sept. 29, 1956), 757–8.
14. See Charles E. Rosenberg, "Disease and Social Order in America: Perceptions and Expectations," *Milbank Quarterly* 64, Suppl 1 (1986): 34–55; and Rosenberg, "Disease in History: Frames and Framers,"

Milbank Quarterly, 67 (1989): 1–15. On the interplay between heredity and infection, see Jean-Paul Gaudillière, "Le cancer entre infection et hérédité: gènes, virus et souris au National Cancer Institute (1937–1977)," *Revue d'histoire des sciences* 48 (1994): 57–89.

15. See, for example, Allan M. Brandt and Martha Gardner, "The Golden Age of Medicine?" in *Medicine in the Twentieth Century*, eds. Roger Cooter and John Pickstone (Netherlands: Harwood Academic Publishing, 2000), 21–37; and classic texts in the genre of Paul De Kruif, *Microbe Hunters* ((New York: Harcourt Brace, 1926).
16. See Paul De Kruif, *Sweeping Wind: A Memoir* (New York: Harcourt Brace, 1962), 13–22.
17. For the problem with explaining tuberculosis, see the chapter of "Contagion and Heredity," in Rene Dubos, *White Plague* (Boston: Little, Brown, 1952): 28–43. On conflicting views of cancer at the turn of the century, see James Patterson, *Dread Disease Cancer and Modern American Culture* (Cambridge: Harvard University Press, 1987), 21–8.
18. For an excellent overview, see Sarah W. Tracy, "George Draper and American Constitutional Medicine, 1916–1946: Reinventing the Sick Man," *Bulletin of the History of Medicine* 66 (1992): 53–89; and for the older notion of "diathesis" see Erwin H. Ackerknecht, "Diathesis: The Word and the Concept in Medical History," *Bulletin of the History of Medicine* 56 (1982): 317–25.
19. William B. Tucker and William A. Lessa, "Man: A Constitutional Investigation," *Quarterly Review of Biology* 15 (1940): 265–89; 411–55. This survey included only a handful of the many studies of blood groups and constitution.
20. For a contemporary introduction to the background of constitution studies, see Antonio Ciocco, "Historical Background of the Modern Study of Constitution," *Bulletin of the Institute of the History of Medicine* 4 (1936): 23–38. For more recent interpretations of phrenology, see Roger Cooter, *Cultural Meaning of Popular Science: Phrenology and the Organization of Consent in Nineteenth Century Britain* (Cambridge: Cambridge University Press, 1984).
21. Ciocco, "Historical Background," 30. Beneke's major works were, *Die anatomische Grundlagen der Constitutionsanomalien des Menschen* (Marburg: Elwert 1878) and *Constitution und constitutionelles Kranksein des Menschen* (Marburg: Elwert 1881).
22. See also Thorsten Sellin, "New Phase in Criminal Anthropology in Italy," *Annals of the American Academy of Political and Social Science* 125 (1926): 233–42; and Elio D. Monachesi "Trends in Criminological Research in Italy," *American Sociological Review* 1 (1936): 396–406 for the impact of the constitutional studies on criminology.

23. Kretschmer's most influential book translated into English was *Physique and Character* (New York: Harcourt, Brace, 1925).
24. See William Bateson, *Mendel's Principles of Heredity* (London: Constable & Co., 1929), 205–34; and R. R. Gates, *Heredity in Man* (London: Macmillan, 1930). The standard German reference work on human genetics by Erwin Baur, Eugen Fischer and Fritz Lenz, *Human Heredity* (New York: Macmillan, 1931), 213–494, devoted almost half the book to a section by Lenz entitled "Morbific Hereditary Factors." The most important French authority Eugène Apert, *Traité des maladies familiales et afflictions congénnitales and Hérédité morbide* (Paris: Flammarion, 1920), showed remarkable agreement with his foreign counterparts on the limited number of rare diseases that followed Mendelian inheritance. Their disagreement was on the workings of more complex illness such as tuberculosis and more vaguely defined conditions such as "feeble-mindedness."
25. William Alexander, "An Inquiry into the Distribution of Blood Groups in Patients Suffering from Malignant Diseases," *British Journal of Experimental Pathology* 2 (1921): 66–9.
26. J. Arthur Buchanan and Edith T. Higley, "Relationship of Blood Groups to Disease," *British Journal of Experimental Pathology* 2 (1921): 247–55.
27. In addition to Hirszfeld and Zborowski, "Sur la permeabilité élective du placenta," mentioned above, see Irvine McQuarrie, "Isoaaglutination in New-born Infants and Their Mothers: a Possible Relation Between Interagglutination and the Toxemia of Pregnancy," *Bulletin of Johns Hopkins Hospital* 34 (1923): 51–9; and Amédée Laffont and Émile Gaujoux, "Recherches sur l'agglutination des globules sanguins avec le sérum maternel et foetal," *Comptes rendus de la Société de Biologie* 88 (1923): 730–1.
28. Rose Amzel and Wanda Halber, "Ueber das Ergebnis der Wassermanschen Reaktion innerhalbe verschiedener Blutgruppen," *Zeitschrft für Immunitätsforschung* 42 (1925): 89–98.
29. A. Lisunova, "Gruppovaya gemoagglyutinatsiya i malyariya [Hemoagglutination Groups and Malaria]," *Trudy 3-go vseross Syezd malyar Moskva* (1925), 173–5.
30. G. E. Pfahler, and B. P. Widmann, "Relation of Blood Groups to Malignant Disease and the Influence of Radiotherapy," *American Journal of Roentgenology and Radiumtherapy* 12 (1924): 47–50; A. Straszynski, "Uber das Ergebnis der Wassermannschen Reaktion innerhalb verschiedener Blutgruppen bei behandelten Lues," *Klinische Wochenschrift* 4 (1925): 1962–3.
31. Julius Hollo and Wilhelm Lenard, "Gibt es einen Unterschied in der Häufigkeit der einzelnen Blutgruppen bei Lungentuberkulösen und bei gesunden Menschen?" *Beiträge zur Klinik der Tuberkulose*, 64 (1926): 513–4; Max Gundel, "Bestehen Zusammenhänge zwischen Blutgruppen

und Luesdisposition sowie zwischen Blutgruppe und Erfolg der Luestherapie?" *Klinische Wochenschrift* 6 (1927): 1703–5. For background on the history of the Wassermann test, see Ludwik Fleck, *Genesis and Development of a Scientific Fact* (Chicago: University of Chicago Press, 1979).

The first studies using this method had been done by the Hirszfelds and others in Poland. Beginning in 1924 they compared the blood groups of those with positive and negative Schick tests for diphtheria. Their finding of a difference, plus the prestige of the Hirszfelds, did much to inspire the whole line of research on blood groups and disease that developed in the 1920s and1930s. See below and Hannah Hirszfeld, Ludwik Hirszfeld, and Henryk Brokman, "Etude sur l'hérédité en rapport avec la sensibilité `a la diphtherie," *Comptes rendus de la Société de biologie* 90 (1924): 1198–1200, also published as, "On the Susceptibility to Diphtheria (Schick Test Positive) With Reference to the Inheritance of Blood Groups," *Journal of Immunology* 9 (1924): 571–91.

32. Alexandre Manuila, "Blood Groups and Disease," 1958. See also his *Quel est le nombre necessaire et suffisant d'examens dans les recherches biologiques?* Geneva: P.E. Grivet, 1945.
33. P. N. Mitra, "Influence of Blood Group in Certain Pathological States," *Indian Journal of Medical Research* 20 (1933): 995–1004; Sergio Pascoli, "Malattie e gruppi sanguigni," *Gazzetta degli ospedali* 61 (1940): 3–8.

    The belief in a general predisposition to disease was common among those studying constitutional medicine. Thus, Buchanan and Higley included a table for all sick patients at the Mayo Hospital. For more on these assumptions about heredity and disease, see below.
34. Yoshisada Ihara and Mototoshi Yanagihashi, "Ueber Krankheitsdisposition und Isohamagglutination," *Zeitschrift für Rassenphysiologie* 2 (1929): 32–8.
35. Max Gundel, "Bestehen Zusammenhänge zwischen Blutgruppen und Luesdisposition sowie zwischen Blutgruppe und Erfolg der Luestherapie?" *Klinische Wochenschrift* 6 (1927): 1703–5.
36. Candido Maderna, "Sifilide e gruppi sanguigni," *Riforma medica* 53 (1937): 527–9.
37. Dorothy Huie Wong and Foong Kong Chen, "Blood Groups in relation to syphilis and its Treatment," *National Medical Journal of China* 17 (1931): 354–9.
38. "CDC on Infectious Diseases in the United States: 1900–99," *Population and Development Review* 25 (1999): 636.
39. J. Hollo and W. Lenard, "Gibt es einen Unterschied in der Häufigkeit der einzelnen Blutgruppen bei Lungentuberkulösen und bei gesunden Menschen?" *Beitrage zur Klinik der Tuberkulose* 64 (1926): 513–14;

M. M. Alperin, "Ueber die Beziehungen zwischen Blutgruppen und Tubercule," *Beitrage zur Klinik der Tuberkulose* 64 (1926): 500.

40. Examples of those finding a link are Zdislaw Swider and Natan Kon, "Recherches sur les Groupes Sanguins Chez les Tuberculeux," *Comptes rendus de la Société de biologie* 98 (1928): 385–6 and Raymond Dujarric de la Riviere and Nicholas Kossovitch, "Au sujet des groups sanguins des tuberculeux et des cancereux," *Comptes rendus de la Société de biologie* 97 (1927): 137–9 found links.

    Those finding no link include O. Connerth, "Uber Blutgruppen bei Tuberkulose," *Zeitschrift fur Tuberkulose* 48 (1927): 140–2 and Theophile Raphael, Olive M. Searle, and Tom Horan, "Blood Groups in Tuberculosis," *Archives of Internal Medicine* 40 (1927): 328–31.
41. Alperin, "Ueber die Beziehungen zwischen Blutgruppen und Tubercule."
42. The latter were frequently found by Japanese and Italian authors. See, for example, Kaoru Miyamura, "Uber die Bedeutung der Blutgruppen im Gebiete der Dermatologie," *Japanese Journal of Dermatology and Urology* 30 (1930): 53; Paolo de Paoli, "Contributo allo Studio dei gruppi sanguigni nelle malattie tubercolari," *Lotta contro la tuberculosi* 3 (1932): 494–8; or Adolf Sylla, "Das Blutbild bei Lungentuberkulose, mit Berucksichtung der Blutkörperschensenkung (BKS) und der Blutgruppen," *Medizinische Klinik* 28 (1932): 686–8; 721–4.
43. Geza Weitzner, "Hämagglutiningehalt des Blutserums Karzinomkranker," *Medizinische Klinik* 21 (1925): 1960–1.
44. Hans Hirschfeld and Anton Hittmair, "Über Blutgruppenbestimmungen bei Krebskranken," *Medizinische Klinik*, 22 (1926): 1494–6. The Schiff note was in the same journal, 455.
45. James T. Patterson, *The Dread Disease*, 33–5.
46. Johannsen's first report appeared in "Classement de sujets affectés de tumeurs malignes selon les iso-agglutinines de leur sang," *Comptes rendus de la Société de biologie* 92 (1925): 112–15. For later results that eventually included 383 patients, see "Nogle studier over de menneskelige isohaemagglutininer med soerligt henblick paa forholdene ved kraeft," *Bibliotek for Laeger* 119 (1927): 42–7; and "Classification of Cancer Patients According to Their Blood Groups and Some Investigations Concerning Isohemagglutination," *Acta Pathologica et microbiologica Scandinavica* 4 (1927): 175–97.
47. Oluf Thomsen, "Om mulighoben af forskellig Disposition til Cancerudviklung hos individer af forskelig "blodtype" *Ugeskrift for Laeger* 93 (1931): 1008–15. In the process, Thomsen became a lively critic of Hirszfeld. See, for example, "Uber den Zusammenhang der Isoagglutinatorischen Bluttypen (Blutgruppen) mit Pathologischen Zustanden," *Acta Pathologica et Microbiologica Scandinavica* 4 (1927): 45–73; 163–4.

48. Gaetano Dossena, and Vincenzo Lancara, "L'Isoagglutinazione studiata nei riguardi dell'abito morfologico e delle neoplasie della sfera genitale muliebre," *Annali di ostetricia e ginecologia*, 47 (1925): 163–79.
49. Marco Goldstein, "La ripartizione dei gruppi sanguigni fra gli individui affetti da carcinoma," *Bollettino dell'Instituto Sieroterapico Milanese* 8 (1929), 293–6; Enrico Tagliaferro, "Gruppi sanguigni e carcinoma," *Minerva Medica* 28 (1937), 219–20.
50. Libero Ugelli, "Distribuzione dei gruppi sanguigni negli individui portatori di ulcere gastroduodenali," *Policlinico* (sezione pratica) 43 (1936): 1591–4.
51. Ian Aird, H.H. Bentall HH, and J.A. Mehigan JA, Roberts, "Blood Groups in Relation to Peptic Ulceration and Carcinoma of Colon, Rectum, Breast, and Bronchus; an Association between the ABO Groups and Peptic Ulceration," *British Medical Journal* 2 (1954): 315–21. Aird et al. (1953).
52. William C. Boyd, "Blood Groups," *Tabulae Biologicae* 17 (1939): 144–5.
53. Philip Levine, "Studies in Specific Hypersensitiveness," *Journal of Immunology* 11 (1926): 283–90.
54. Fritz Schiff, "Blutgruppen und Epidemiologie," *Klinische Wochenschrift* 14 (1935): 786–90.
55. Laurence H. Snyder, "Human Blood Groups: Their Inheritance and Racial Significance," *American Journal of Physical Anthropology* 9 (1926): 251. He was not entirely justified in his criticism since the numbers in his studies were as follows: 100 epileptics and 100 feeble-minded, although he did test 195 insane.
56. Snyder, *Blood Grouping and Its Relation to Clinical and Legal Medicine* (Baltimore: Williams and Wilkins, 1929), 106.

CHAPTER 7

Blood Groups and Behavioral Genetics: Crime, Insanity, and Temperament

The applications of the blood group discoveries which preoccupied researchers the most in the 1920s and 1930s were transfusion, race classification, and the genetics of disease. There is good reason for this given the obvious benefits in the case of transfusion and the potential for resolving questions about identifying differences in people around the world. In the case of links to disease, the blood group research was more ambivalent, but the promise of potential benefit was sufficient to produce substantial research in the interwar period.

Given the overall high level of interest in blood group research, there were surprisingly few studies done on blood types associated with human behavior. For example, only 18 of over 1200 articles published on blood group distribution from 1919 through 1939 had criminals as subjects. Despite this fact, these and other studies which sought to use blood types as genetic markers of behavior such as criminality or insanity were telling of some of the pitfalls of research in human biology in the twentieth century. These included pursuing research out of one's field, extrapolating from too little data, and of course, interpreting data to fit preconceived notions about human behavior.

W. H. Schneider, *Blood Groups and Human Heredity, 1900–1950*, Medicine and Biomedical Sciences in Modern History,
https://doi.org/10.1007/978-3-031-69844-6_7

The Search for "Criminal Man"

The study of the blood groups of criminals was the logical outgrowth of the "scientific" study of crime that began in the nineteenth century, although its roots can be found in the revolutionary proposal during the Enlightenment that punishment should fit the crime. This so-called Classical School of criminology had been a reaction to medieval practices of inquisition and torture. Cesare Beccaria and others argued that human nature being rational, criminal justice need only promise sure and sufficient punishment to make the cost of committing a crime exceed the potential benefits perceived by the criminal.[1]

The Enlightenment view assumed that criminal acts were rational choices which followed from calculating costs and benefits, an assumption which has remained a strong current in criminological thinking to the present day, since it is the basic premise of punishment as deterrence. One important effect at the time, however, was to focus attention on the crime and its punishment rather than the criminal. During the nineteenth century, however, a competing theory, self-proclaimed as "scientific," focused attention back on the criminal. Rather than being viewed as a rational actor, the criminal according to this theory was considered abnormal or at least not in control of his or her fate.[2]

At the risk of oversimplification, this new interest in the criminal was divided into two major lines of inquiry: one which examined environmental influences on criminals and the other examining the criminals themselves. In the first part of the nineteenth century, the emphasis was on the former, as grand social and economic theories emerged to explain the changing conditions of Europe's industrializing and urbanizing world. "Criminal and dangerous classes" to use the phrase of Louis Chevalier were produced in the process.[3] Then in the last half of the century, increasing attention was focused on the biological and psychological causes within the individual criminal.

The theorist who more than any other focused attention on the individual criminal by the end of the nineteenth century was the Italian physician Cesare Lombroso.[4] It was especially his notion of the "born criminal," recognizable by physical characteristics, which exercised the greatest influence on subsequent generations of criminologists in Europe and America. Although he had as many (if not more) critics as followers, virtually every history of criminology gives Lombroso major credit for shifting the focus of attention. As one early twentieth-century observer put it, "Whether

Lombroso was right or wrong is perhaps in the last analysis not so important as the unquestionable fact that his ideas proved so challenging that they gave an unprecedented impetus to the study of the offender."[5]

Lombroso's theories grew out of developments in physical anthropology during the middle nineteenth century. Popular observation had long used features of appearance such as skin color, size, hair, and eyes to distinguish between human groups. In Europe, as mentioned earlier, more systematic eighteenth-century systems of classifying humans developed along with other systems of classifying flora and fauna. Nineteenth-century racial classification claimed to be scientific by adding the element of measurement. A whole variety of body parts were measured or proportionally related to one another in an effort to find a quantifiable system of classification. For example, one of the best-known measurements was the cephalic index of skull shape that was widely used at the end of the century, but there were nasal indices, etc., that were also employed by physical anthropologists to categorize humans.[6]

Lombroso was trained as a physician, and while serving in the army of the new Italian state, he was struck by differences and similarities in the appearances of new recruits from the different regions of the peninsula. Ironically (or not so surprisingly according to some scholars such as Pick), in his search for a common Italian physical type, Lombroso began to recognize "abnormals," including those with a criminal background. This set him on his search for physical features marking criminals, such as ear lobes, toes, etc., which he described in his most influential work *Criminal Man* first published in 1876. This book defined the field of criminal anthropology and set the framework of criminology and its search for the causes of crime during the next several decades.

New scientific theories at the end of the nineteenth century and beginning of the twentieth century added—or to be more precise reinforced—one of the elements of Lombroso's criminal type. Inheritance had always been a part of Lombroso's theory, especially the idea of atavism or reversion to an earlier evolutionary stage. Hence, the influence of Darwin was one reason for the increased attention paid to the inheritance of criminality. Even more important after 1900, however, was the rediscovery of Mendel's research which found simple rules describing inherited traits. This linking of crime, genetics, and evolution not only gave eugenicists of the early twentieth century another item for their list of negative inherited traits to be eliminated, it also added a new dimension to the search for biological evidence of "born criminals." As a result, those manifesting the inherited criminal traits could be identified for differential punishment after the commission of a crime. Similarly, preventive measures might even be taken if they were recognized before a crime was committed. Naturally, Lombroso's findings of physical traits were to be the markers to watch for, although there were later refinements of general body type and morphology.

To summarize, Lombroso became the touchstone of hereditarian ideas about the causes of crime by the end of the nineteenth century. They took different form in different countries, but generally, they were viewed as "biological" (a term that encompassed inherited conditions as well as curable mental and physical illness) as opposed to "circumstantial" (including socio-economic as well as the individual's environment). Because Lombroso did not discover a simple marker for criminals, easily proven or disproven, the debate on the causes of crime became a shifting and complex one with sometimes whole countries identified with one "school" of thought, and at other times individuals who combined elements from each side.[7]

Blood Groups and Criminals

Such was the state of the scientific study of crime when the blood groups were discovered at the turn of the century. One can therefore appreciate the potential value they presented to some researchers. First, blood types were shown to be recognizable early in life and immutable. This prompted Landsteiner himself to suggest their use in individual criminal identification from blood stains. Within ten years the blood types were also recognized as being inherited according to simple Mendelian rules which prompted their use in cases of disputed paternity. Given the tradition and power of blood as a metaphor for heredity, the discovery of the differences and inheritance of blood types offered a cachet of scientific legitimacy to long-held popular ideas and descriptions of inheritance. This was similar to one of the driving forces behind the appeal of biological explanations for criminality. As an early history of Lombroso put it,

> The presence of a general popular superstition, which had existed for centuries, that the physical features of man somehow directly reflect his character and that criminals may be distinguished by obvious anatomical peculiarities was no doubt also an important factor in causing Lombrosian theories to receive considerable popular attention and publicity.[8]

The blood groups had the additional, intriguing quality of being hidden, that is internal so that someone who otherwise looked normal might have a telltale predisposition toward criminality that could only be revealed by testing of blood (which after 1915 was a simple enough test to determine blood type within a few minutes). Moreover, there were only a few mutually exclusive blood types, making their determination much less subjective or open to interpretation than deciding on features of body form.

Given these circumstances, it is perhaps surprising how long it took for the new blood group discoveries to be applied to the question of criminality. The first article devoted specifically to the blood type distribution among criminals appeared in 1926[9]; hence, it was relatively late compared to other studies. Moreover, although there had been some discussion in the legal medicine community about adding blood typing to the standard physical and mental exam given to those accused or convicted of crimes, this first published finding had a different origin. It was part of an attempt to test a very large segment of the population of the German province of Schleswig-Holstein. The researcher who conducted this essentially anthropological study was Max Gundel.

Although only 24 at the time, Gundel was an assistant at the Institute of Hygiene at the University of Kiel. He quickly published two articles based on his research in Schleswig-Holstein, and in the next few years he authored a total of nine articles on differences in blood group distribution among "abnormals," not only criminals but also patients with syphilis and the insane. Gundel remained in Kiel until 1928 when he became Privatdozent at the Hygiene Institute of Heidelberg University. Then in 1934 (at the age of 32) Gundel became a department head at the Robert Koch Institute in Berlin, where he did extensive work on streptococcus and pneumonia.[10]

Gundel's goal was to conduct the first large-scale blood group study of a relatively settled population in order to do tests of successive generations. It was no accident that such a study was attempted in Kiel, the home of the naval doctor Paul Steffan who in 1923, prompted by the Hirszfelds' 1919 *Lancet* article, published one of the first blood group studies in Germany, using tests of recruits stationed at the Kiel naval station. Steffan's fascination with the anthropological implications of the Hirszfelds' findings inspired several members of the local medical society at Kiel before he went on to be a co-founder of the German Society for Blood Group Research, and the journal *Zeitschrift für Rassenphysiologie* which proposed the serological mapping of the whole German-speaking world.[11]

Gundel published preliminary results of his research in June 1926 after testing over 3000 subjects, among whom he found some evidence of a higher percentage of blood type B among city dwellers compared to rural inhabitants.[12] Despite Gundel's primarily anthropological interest, his inclusion of 268 patients at the university psychiatric clinic had far more importance for subsequent research, because he found that 22 percent of them had blood type B compared to only 12 percent in the general population. (Subsequent testing of 134 more mental patients found 25.1 percent of over 400 tested had blood type B.) Following up on this finding, Gundel tested the blood types of 884 inmates at five prisons in Schleswig-Holstein to see, in his words, "whether perhaps similar proportions exist among prison inmates as among mental patients." The results were reported in a "Short Scientific Note" of the November 1926 issue of *Klinische Wochenschrift*.[13]

Even though by that time Gundel had tested over 8500 people in Schleswig-Holstein, this note focused only on the findings of prison tests which showed overall that 19 percent of prisoners had blood type B compared to 13.4 percent in the larger population of Schleswig-Holstein. To emphasize the potential of blood types as a marker for criminality (and despite the obvious risk of basing his conclusions on a small sampling), Gundel divided the 884 inmates by the types of crimes committed and found that of 110 serving sentences for serious crimes (murder, attempted murder, manslaughter), a higher percentage (33 percent) had blood type B. He also found that one-third of the 51 prisoners serving sentences longer than 9 years were type B, and that of 27 prisoners with previous offences that were serious crimes, 17 (or 63 percent) were blood type B.[14]

Dramatic as these numbers were, Gundel drew no conclusions from his findings, preferring to end his note with the promise of more detailed results once the whole study was completed. Nonetheless, the suggestion that blood groups (specifically blood type B) might be an indicator of a predisposition toward criminality, published in the widely read *Klinische Wochenschrift*, quickly prompted others to verify Gundel's results. One of the first was a study done by Kurt Böhmer of the Institute for Social and Legal Medicine at the University of Kiel. Böhmer was not just another junior colleague of Gundel's who was inspired by his and Steffan's work. He was an assistant at the prestigious Institute for Legal and Social Medicine headed by Ernst Ziemke, one of the founders of the *Deutsche Zeitschrift für die gesamte gerichtliche Medizin*, the leading journal of legal medicine in Germany.

In an initial report to the September 1926 meeting of the German Society for Legal and Social Medicine, which was published the following year in the society's journal, Böhmer confirmed Gundel's findings based on tests of 150 prisoners from the Kiel city jail (where Gundel had not conducted tests), of whom 20 percent were found to have blood type B.[15] Böhmer acknowledged that many of the prisoners he tested did not appear to be convicted of serious crimes, so like Gundel he divided them by the type of offense. Compared to the 13.4 percent blood type B found by Gundel in his large study of the overall population, Böhmer displayed his findings (see Table 7.1) next to Gundel's and concluded that it showed "a strong increase in group B among those with serious offenses against people and property."

Böhmer also followed Gundel's lead in distinguishing between what he called "casual criminality [*Gelegenheitsverbrechen*]" and "serious recidivism [*schwerer Rückfälligkeit*]" by examining those with previous criminal records. Although there was overall a high rate of recidivism among all prisoners, Böhmer found significant differences according to blood type. Thus, 73.3 percent of prisoners with blood type B were repeat offenders, compared to 63.3 percent for type O, 44.8 percent for type A, and 66.3 percent for type AB.[16] Böhmer also found what he called "an especially clear connection between recidivists and blood type B" when considering the seriousness of the previous crime. Of prisoners with previous convictions for murder, manslaughter, robbery, or bodily injury, he reported 44 percent with blood type B. The figure was 38 percent for those previously convicted of sex crimes and 18.7 percent for those previously convicted of lesser crimes of fraud and sale of stolen goods.

For the most part, Böhmer's method of analysis followed Gundel's very closely, but he went much further in describing the potential value of blood testing. For example, at the end of his 1927 article, Böhmer

Table 7.1 Percentage of prisoners with blood type B according to offense

Offense	*Findings of Böhmer*	*Gundel*
1. Murder, manslaughter, robbery bodily harm	17.4	30.0
2. Larceny, fraud	21.9	18.2
3. Arson	0	3.0

Source: Böhmer, "Blutgruppen und Verbrecher," *Deutsche Zeitschrift für die gesamte gerichtliche Medizin* 9 (1927), 426

described blood tests as a possible "new tool for the prison system to recognize recidivists and incorrigibles." In another article published that same year for a more general medical audience, Böhmer characterized the blood groups as "a means to separate the incorrigibles in prisons from those capable of rehabilitation."[17]

Such confidence in the value of blood groups to criminology was not shared by all criminologists and serologists. Among the critics was Fritz Schiff, the well-respected bacteriologist at the Berlin City Hospital, who had done a large study of the blood groups of the Berlin population in the early 1920s. At a meeting in late November 1926 of the German Society for Naturalists and Doctors (Gesellschaft deutscher Natursforscher und Ärtzte), Schiff suggested that Gundel's association of blood type B with criminality might be legitimate but only "parallel" to the real physiological or social causes of criminality. "As interesting as they may be," Schiff said,

> the meaning of these findings must not be overestimated. They are parallel to other correlations between bodily characteristics and social standing. Felix Bernstein pointed out a striking analogy to the observations of Lundborg in Sweden. There, it is not the blood type B but dark hair and eye color which is found in especially high frequency among prisoners. One explanation arises from the local variations (underlying social standing of the darker pigmented Lapp segment of the population).[18]

It is interesting that Schiff accepted Gundel's medical and statistical methods, choosing instead to question his causal explanation. This was despite the fact that Schiff was much better qualified as a serologist than a sociologist.

Böhmer's findings were also not long in being challenged on serological grounds. For example, in a December 1927 article of the *Deutsche Zeitschrift für die gesamte gerichtliche Medizin*, Augustin Foerster of the Institute for Legal and Social Medicine at Münster reported that his tests of 371 prisoners found only 12.7 percent with blood type B.[19] Moreover, he closely followed the procedure of Gundel and Böhmer by looking separately at serious offenders (136 subjects) of whom he found 14 percent had blood type B, which was very close to the percentage of the rest of the population. At the end of the article, Foerster stated his agreement with Schiff that the two earlier studies should not be overemphasized because blood group and criminality were parallel to "other correlations between bodily characteristics and social standing." He offered his own explanation of Gundel's and Böhmer's results based on the recent findings of German researchers who tested the blood groups of populations in certain regions of Germany (Oberhesse, Vogelberg, Giessen) where pockets of higher concentrations (17–25 percent) of blood type B were found.

The following year Gundel published the more detailed analysis of the blood groups of criminals he had promised in his preliminary report. Yet in this article of 20 pages, including 23 tables, he did not directly respond to or acknowledge any of his critics, nor did he add any additional tests to bolster his previous findings.[20] Instead, Gundel chose to elaborate in painstaking detail on the results of his original tests of prisoners in 1926.

A closer analysis of the main points of the article reveals that Gundel responded indirectly to at least some of his critics. For example, he noted that 98 percent of his prisoners came from Schleswig-Holstein, thus ruling out the explanation that they might be from regions with locally high proportions of the population with blood type B. But Gundel went even further, separating out prisoners by the birthplace of their parents, and for those whose parents were born elsewhere, he maintained that in each instance the percentage of blood type B was higher among the prisoners than the region of Germany from which their parents came.

Gundel went to similar lengths in ruling out such potential influences as the occupation of prisoners (no correlations were found). He also reinforced his earlier finding of a higher percentage of blood type B among recidivists, those convicted of more serious crimes, and those serving longer sentences. Yet, despite his evidence of links between criminality and blood type B, Gundel again refused to draw any further conclusions, preferring instead to end the article, "Understandably, I consider my research only a stimulus to further, more intensive research for which unfortunately there is insufficient material in the province of Schleswig-Holstein to enable us to draw final conclusions."[21] He and Böhmer had apparently tested all the prisoners in the region.

The discovery and initial reactions to the possible link between blood type and criminality show several features of research about the genetics of criminals, some of which have persisted to this day. First is the somewhat accidental way that a possible link was noted. It was a serologist looking at different populations who noticed in one of them an unexpected difference in distribution of blood types. Second, even if the discovery was inadvertent, there was sufficient understanding of the possible significance of blood types as a genetic marker to make Gundel's findings noticed quickly, both by supporters and skeptics. Also, because of the statistical nature of the proof, unlike what might have been the case had pedigree studies shown a simple direct link, there was a great deal of room for difference of opinion about the connection between blood groups and crime, including ambiguous references to predisposition, much as exists today. Finally, like today and by Gundel's own admission, it would be up to other scientists to do the additional research necessary to confirm his findings.

Of the dozen studies that appeared after 1928, some confirmed Gundel's link between blood type and criminality. For example, of two articles by Italians agreed with him, one by Vincent Palmieri on 98 mentally ill prisoners in Naples which reported 18 percent with blood type B, and another study by Giorgio Canuto at the University of Turin who concluded, "there is an evident correlation between having blood group B and the presence of constitutional somatic characteristics of the criminal type."[22]

Other studies, however, either found no confirmation of Gundel's findings or simply reported the results of testing prison populations. For example, two researchers in the Soviet Union and one in Yugoslavia found little difference between the distribution of blood types of criminals and the rest of the local populations.[23] Particularly ingenious was the study by Adam Schmidt, a researcher in Yugoslavia, who tested prisoners in the ethnically mixed region of Sombor, Yugoslavia. He broke down results by nationality and then tested several hundred school children of each nationality for normal control groups. Of 6 different nationalities studied, only the 60 Hungarian prisoners had a higher percentage of blood type B: 33.3 percent versus 20.1 percent in the control (student) population. Among the more surprising results was that, contrary to popular notions, about their criminality, "Gypsy" [Roma] prisoners were found by Schmidt to have only 13.8 percent blood type B among the 29 subjects he tested.

Given the mixed results, it is not surprising that the testing of criminals continued, albeit with diminished enthusiasm. This included some additional studies in Germany and Italy as well as one in Holland in the early 1930s. Then there was a revival of interest in the late 1930s in geographically widespread countries such as Cuba, Brazil, and Japan. The inspiration for the latter is similar to Gundel's initial interest: prisoners were a convenient, "captive" population for serologists to test in these new settings.

Beyond the lesson of how new discoveries about heredity were applied to old questions like the cause of crime, what impact did these results of blood group research have on the study of criminology? The simple (and unsurprising) answer is that the different sides in the debate between biological and circumstantial causes of crime used whichever findings of the blood group studies that supported their position. Thus, in Italy, the blood group studies not only fit quite naturally with the Lombrosian tradition, but they also were used to support a new line of research by endocrinologists who studied hormonal secretions (thought to be hereditarily determined) as a clue to the cause of criminality. In this context, blood type was viewed as another "internal" marker representing evidence, if not a cause, of criminality.[24] Palmieri who studied criminality, insanity, and constitutional body form at the Institute for Legal Medicine of the University of Naples, was eager to show the practical applications of his blood group research. His 1928 study which compared the blood types of 98 Italian criminals to the 500 Italian soldiers tested earlier by the Hirszfelds, explained the importance of the subject in his introduction as follows:

> The efforts to determine and study the relationship between psychological-constitutional characteristics and criminality, or even their specific forms, has not only a purely speculative and scientific purpose. If this research leads to positive and practical worthwhile conclusions, they would provide the necessary biological foundation for interested socio-legal applications, especially concerning the prevention of crime, as well as the form and extent of punishment.[25]

In Germany, the work of Gundel and Böhmer was offered as additional evidence by those seeking to show the biological differences between criminals and the normal population. The debate was surprisingly subtle and sophisticated, as shown by a 1930 article in the *Monatsschrift für Kriminalpsychologie* by Hans Brennecke, a prison doctor in Halle-Nietleben. Although the subject of the article was "the study of the personality of prisoners," two full pages were devoted to the blood group research of Gundel and Böhmer, whose findings Brennecke summarized as follows, "among prisoners in Schleswig-Holstein there has been found an increase of blood group B and an even higher amount among recidivists and incorrigibles." In fact, the results were so encouraging that Brennecke saw fit to caution as follows:

> As interesting as the findings of scientific researchers are up to now and as promising the insights for wider biological fields may be, one must warn against hasty conclusions. The increase in blood group B, for example,

> among the mentally ill and criminals generalized and interpreted as a pathological factor in the sense of an abnormal defect of the mental functions of criminals, would not only be a false conclusion, but also could produce dangerous criminal and penal consequences. Blood group or body build determination can never be decisive for the judgement between normal or pathological.[26]

Brennecke accepted the biological basis of certain criminal actions and even the practice of sterilization as a remedy for "incorrigible, recidivist, professional and habitual criminals." The longer quote above indicates, however, that he was not convinced that blood testing was a simple way to determine who fit this description. He did mention two other new approaches to the heredity of crime that he also thought promising: the general link to fingerprints and the twin studies of Johannes Lange.[27]

Outside of central Europe, the serological work attracted less attention from criminological researchers. For example, no study of a prison population was done between the wars in Britain, France, or the U.S. In part this was likely the result of differences in the way criminologists in these countries viewed the causes of crime. The French had been the strongest opponents of Lombroso from the start, and in Britain there was a well-established tradition of institutionally based administratively oriented medico-legal science that resisted the academic and theoretical search for "born criminals." In the U.S. the "circumstantial" causes of crime received a great deal of attention, especially from researchers of the new "Chicago School" that gained prominence in the 1920s. Their training, moreover, was in sociology and jurisprudence, as opposed to medicine which was most often the background of criminologists in Germany and Italy.[28]

This is not to say the hereditarian explanation of crime was absent from America between the wars. To be sure, one of the greatest dangers pointed out by eugenicists in the U.S. was the heredity of crime, but it was considered just one of the results of the broader problem of feeble-mindedness which was most easily measured by IQ tests.[29] Thus, it fell within the domain of psychology and intelligence rather than biology and crime. This was the case at least until the late 1930s when, as will be shown below, Sheldon and Hooten became interested in constitutional studies.

Even in central Europe and Italy much of the interest in the connection between blood groups and crime came not from criminologists but from serologists outside that field whose main interest was to demonstrate a practical value of their work. If prisoners offered a convenient, "captive" population to study, so much the better. If no obvious correlations appeared, however, or if disagreements emerged, there were other groups—races, the sick, or insane—that might show the value of serological testing. From this perspective, the best explanation of why serologists did not pursue more vigorously the hereditary link between blood group distribution and criminality, whether in central Europe or elsewhere, is that these researchers were serologists first and foremost. Hence, if they saw a more promising area of research or application—other behaviors or traits that might be genetically linked to blood groups—they would pursue it. Perhaps the best example was Gundel, clearly an outsider to criminology, and in fact, it would be more accurate to say that he stumbled upon his results in a search for the largest number of blood tests he could do. After conducting several studies, he left serology altogether and returned to his career in bacteriology.[30]

Blood Groups and Behavioral Genetics: The Insane

Looking at the wider context, one can see that a possible reason for lack of sustained interest in blood groups as a simple marker for criminality was not the result of researchers losing faith in the proposition that behavioral traits were inherited nor that blood groups could detect them. Rather, without conclusive proof of a blood group marker for criminality, researchers turned to other comparable traits that might be associated with criminals. Some of these additional behavioral traits with possible links to blood type were different from criminality which had a clearly defined population to study. Such conditions as insanity, character, temperament, or body build were complex and ambiguous, making it difficult to present simple confirmation or rejection of a link. At the same time, the wider choice of subjects gave serologists quite variable results and a much freer rein in interpreting or reinterpreting their findings.

One way to see this process is by examining the record of blood group studies of the mentally ill. The first feature of note is the significantly greater interest in the blood groups of the insane or mentally ill, as indicated by the publication of 51 studies on their blood group distribution from 1925 through 1939 compared to only 18 studies of blood types of criminals in that same period. On the other hand, similarly researchers in Germany (12 articles), the Soviet Union (8), and Italy (7) showed the most interest, although American, Czech, and English researchers each contributed three or four articles during this time period. Together, researchers in these countries accounted for about two-thirds of all articles on blood groups and the insane, but one or more articles were also published in eight other countries, revealing the wider geographical interest in blood groups as a marker for mental illness. Was this interest a result of a more commonly held assumption that insanity was hereditary, or did it follow from other reasons?

One clue comes from the way that early publications on the insane appeared, which was very different from the studies of criminals. Whereas Gundel's more or less accidental discovery in 1926 was the stimulus for subsequent work on the blood groups of criminals, many studies of the insane were conducted independently in the years from 1925 to 1927 by researchers before they realized that others were studying them as a separate population.[31] Almost without exception these researchers saw themselves as following the work of Alexander and Buchanan in England or Hirszfeld in Poland who took up the study of the relationship between blood groups and disease in the early twenties, albeit in this case mental illness.[32]

Similar to the studies of criminals, blood testing of the insane was also partly the result of research done for other purposes, such as serologists looking at another sub-group of patients to confirm the immutability of blood groups or a test for another link to disease. Even more important in making these studies possible was that the institutionalized insane, like prisoners, offered a conveniently sequestered hence easily tested population. This, after all, had been the case with Gundel's original research. In addition to these subjects being readily accessible, an important difference can be seen in one of the early articles published by doctors at the State Psychopathic Hospital of Michigan. They tested the blood groups of patients not to learn more about the nature of blood groups but rather the cause of disease: in this case to see if schizophrenia or manic-depression might be inherited.[33] Their search for biochemical determinants indicates that they found "nature" (i.e., heredity) a more viable explanation of insanity than the "nurture" (i.e., environment) of their patients. Another reason for a greater number of researchers with interest in the connection between blood groups and the insane was simply that institutions housing the insane were far more likely to be staffed with doctors than prisons were. In other words, although criminology (outside of central Europe) had passed largely into the hands of either sociologists or jurists, the study of mental illness was still firmly grounded in medical practice.[34]

The first studies of blood types among the mentally ill (after Jansky) were published in 1925 by Soviet researchers: Berstein who tested 87 patients and Feldman and Elmanovich who studied 815 subjects at Kharkiv in the Ukraine.[35] They were little noticed in the West, where at the same time studies were independently published on the topic beginning in France and Germany, then in Poland, Austria, and the U.S.[36] Of note is the fact that none of these studies made reference to any of the others. In the French and German cases, Toulouse et al. and Jacobsohn found little difference between the mentally ill tested and the general population, with the result in France being an end to this line of research for almost a decade.[37] Such was not the case in Germany, however, where Jacobsohn's 1926 study of patients at a Berlin asylum was soon noted by Ohnesorge and another German researcher in Breslau who reported the results of research on 800 patients at an asylum in Silesia.[38]

By 1928, when nine articles appeared, results had also been published by researchers, in Italy, the U.S., and Switzerland, who acknowledged the Soviet and German work as well as that done in Austria and Poland. This is a clear indication that these researchers had now developed a common interest in the link between blood groups and insanity, even if its inspiration had grown out of the general question of blood groups and predisposition to disease. Thereafter, an average of two to three articles appeared each year through the end of the 1930s on blood group distribution among the mentally ill, making it a distinct subfield of blood group research.

The problem posed and methodology used in these articles was similar to that of the studies of prisoners. Did the distribution of the blood types among the insane differ significantly from the overall population? Despite the lack of someone like Gundel who presented a provocative finding for verification, there eventually developed a lively debate on the relationship between the blood groups and mental illness. As mentioned above, early researchers examined mental patients primarily because of convenience in gathering as much data as possible for larger-scale studies.[39] The first researcher to find a difference in distribution was Eugenjusz Wilczowski, whose 1927 study found a higher percentage of type AB among mental patients in the late stages of syphilis (progressive paralysis) at a Warsaw hospital.[40] Equally significant (and indicative of subsequent methodology), however, was the fact that he had enough subjects (368) to give a breakdown by type of illness, in this case schizophrenia and progressive paralysis. In fact, only by this method did he notice that 14 of 78 subjects with progressive paralysis (17.9 percent) had a higher percentage of type AB than the normal 9 percent of the population. He found little difference in distribution among schizophrenics (8 percent AB). Ohnesorge's 1927 study also broke down subjects for analysis by sub-category and found over 70 percent of manic-depressives had type O blood (compared to 39 percent in the normal population). The number of patients in this category (21) was so small, however, that he could hardly draw any conclusions from the data.[41]

Far larger studies were reported at this same time by two groups of researchers in the U.S., but they differed in their conclusions. Two doctors at Agnew State Hospital in California found a higher percentage of type A among 2104 mental patients (52.7 percent vs. 43 percent in the normal population), a figure which varied little according to psychosis (from 51.4 percent for manic-depressives to 55.5 percent for general paralytics).[42] On the other hand, researchers at the Ann Arbor State Psychopathic Hospital found little difference in blood type distribution among 1100 patients tested with schizophrenia and manic-depression.[43]

In 1928 even more studies of blood groups among the insane were published, which reflected the growing debate in the literature on the subject. For example, as mentioned above, the German researcher Meyer published the results of tests at his provincial clinic in Silesia as a direct response to the work of Ohnesorge, while also citing the work of Wilczowski and Pilcz in Poland and Austria. Paul Würz in Basel also acknowledged the work of these earlier researchers as well as other Germans and the Americans before publishing his findings on tests of schizophrenics.[44] That same year (1928) Gundel published his findings on the blood groups of the insane that followed the pattern of his earlier work on prisoners, namely, that of 402 inmates tested at the Kiel mental asylum, 25.1 per cent were blood type B.[45] Despite the fact that most of these studies included enough tests that they could be broken down by the specific mental illness of the patients, researchers were still unable to reach agreement on the pattern of blood type distribution for the different sub-categories.

During the 1930s both these trends continued, with the addition of some new, if not always fruitful, lines of inquiry. Among the latter was the beginning of testing of MN blood groups of the insane. The first study published was by R. Hilgerman and his student Olga Hering on patients at the state mental hospital in Landsberg, Germany, in 1934.[46] In keeping with the methodology established in earlier studies, they tested enough patients (over 1300) to divide them into sub-categories by mental illness. The MN groups provided another set of variables, and their conclusions showed that some disorders, such as schizophrenia, showed little difference in blood group frequency compared to the normal population, whereas others such as progressive paralysis did.

Along this same line of research was Lionel Penrose's 1932 publication about his testing of blood types of "mongoloids" at the Colchester Asylum, which, as mentioned earlier, was a landmark in both the study of mental illness and the history of human genetics. This project was significant not only because it was an early study by one of the most important human geneticists of the mid-twentieth century but also because there had only been a handful of articles published in England on blood groups at all, let alone on their possible link to disease or insanity.[47] Penrose's failure to find any difference between the ABO distribution of "mongoloids" and the general population added to the conflicting opinions about whether blood groups were markers for "mental deficiency." It also was a crucial turning point in his career.

To summarize this comparison of the research on blood groups of criminals with research on the insane, the much greater amount of research done on the latter is not entirely explained by the ease of accessibility of subjects at insane asylums. Quite simply, there were even more potential subjects in prisons. Since both had "captive" populations at their disposal, this suggests that the better explanation for the greater interest in blood group testing of the insane might be that there were more physicians who staffed the mental institutions.

Another feature possibly influencing the amount of research on the mentally ill was the lack of clear definition of the subjects to be studied. Gundel's finding of a higher incidence of blood type B associated with criminals was relatively simple to test because prisoners and crime were legally determined. In contrast, there was no such clear definition of who was insane. The complexity, greater variety, and flexibility of defining mental illness differed from how the specific crimes of prisoners that were defined and adjudicated by the judicial system. Mental patients were not identified by such a clear-cut or externally defined process. The result was that the increased studies done on insanity included many more ways of defining subjects tested and interpreting results. No landmark study of the insane was published, such as Gundel's on criminals. In fact, the very search for such a breakthrough led to more blood group testing and a new classification of subjects: by human constitution.

Blood Groups, Temperament, and Human Constitution

A less focused but ultimately broader and more general attempt to use the blood groups as genetic markers with direct and indirect applications to human conditions such as criminology, insanity, and disease was research that correlated blood group distribution to findings in the fields of constitution/character/somatotype studies. Space only permits a brief look at this expansive and often amorphous field of inquiry, but it reveals the influence that Lombroso's "born criminal" had achieved by the mid-1900s. For example, by the late 1930s when studies began appearing by Americans Ernest A. Hooten and William H. Sheldon on body type and criminality,[48] they were part of a much larger international effort which for many years had looked at some of the same questions Lombroso proposed albeit from a different perspective. Whereas the Italian criminologist examined criminals in the hopes of finding telltale, abnormal anthropometric markers, these subsequent studies began with assumptions about general human somatotypes, then looked for association with criminality and signs of other differences from the norm. By 1940 the field of constitution and somatotype research was very broad. A survey of the literature published that year in the *Quarterly Review of Biology* listed over 300 articles, and it was hardly exhaustive.[49]

The historical roots of this view of humans goes back to Hippocrates, Galen, and other Classical theories of temperaments and humors. After a revival in the Renaissance (by Paracelsus, among others) and attempts to give logical underpinning in the Enlightenment, researchers in the nineteenth century increased their efforts to find experimental, quantitative anthropometric measurements of the human body which correlated with (and marked) basic human types. Perhaps the best known of these efforts were theories of phrenology and craniology which met with only limited success.[50] The research usually acknowledged as the inspiration of twentieth-century constitutional studies was done by a German contemporary of Lombroso, Friedrich Wilhelm Beneke of Marburg, who published several studies in the late 1870s and early 1880s on measurements of various internal organs and their correlations with age, disease, and somatotype. Most important was his postulation of two main categories of humans: one of slight build with large lungs and a higher incidence of scrofula and phthisis, and the other of large build with small lungs and a higher incidence of cancer in adults.[51]

Although some isolated researchers were inspired by these findings, two more influential schools of constitutional studies eventually developed in the twentieth century. One was in Lombroso's homeland at the University of Padua where Achille de Giovanni created what came to be known as a school of clinical anthropology. He and his students such as Domenico Viola and Nicola Pende developed a system of classifying humans based largely on correlations of body type to disease.[52] The other school arose in central Europe (home of Jung and Rohrschach) where first Emil Kraeplin and then Ernst Kretschmer published their theories which postulated a correlation between somatotypes and temperament, specifically schizophrenia and manic-depression.[53] These two schools inspired hundreds of studies in the 1920s and 1930s, including Hooten's and Sheldon's work. These findings were a logical body of research to test against the new discoveries about inheritance and blood group distribution in the 1920s.

Similar to the reaction of criminologists and alienists, the reception by the inner circle of constitutionalists to the new blood group discoveries was not overly enthusiastic. But serologists from far and wide (Japan, the Soviet Union, the U.S., and Germany) quickly tested the blood groups as markers for correlation with these typological systems. One can see the attraction that the blood group discoveries offered to this line of research, with its small number of mutually exclusive categories determined simply and quickly by laboratory testing. No less an authority than Ludwik Hirszfeld, who initially (1919) devised a "biochemical index" to measure race, became interested in more fundamental questions of immunology and correlation of blood type to disease and other human attributes during the mid-1920s. In a 1928 book entitled *Konstitutionsserologie*, he proposed that the normal blood group antibodies were "biochemically modeled entities whose phylogenetic creation and ontogenetic development follow rules similar to anatomical markers."[54] The majority of the book, however, was a summary of studies to date on the correlation between blood type distribution and such things as race, disease, mental illness, and criminality.

Hirszfeld's new concept of constitutional serology was adopted by a significant number of blood group researchers. Between 1924 and 1939 almost 30 articles used the term, but the majority of these studies simply tested for correlations between blood types and traditional morphological markers of physical anthropology, such as eye or hair color and head shape.[55] Among the articles that showed some awareness of the wider literature on constitution was a German study of 540 patients at Virchow Hospital in Berlin in 1928, which looked at the blood group distribution of the asthenic somatotype (tall and thin) and its association with tuberculosis.[56] Another example of a study at about the same time which drew on the wider constitutional literature was by a Soviet researcher who tested workers in a factory on the Dnieper River. Two years later, a more extensive study of 2400 Red Army soldiers in the Ukraine sought to correlate body type and blood type.[57]

Several important researchers attempted to correlate blood group distribution to the Kretschmer and other body types. One of the earliest of these was Böhmer's 1927 study, which, in addition to confirming Gundel's connection between blood type B and criminality, also looked at the body type of the prisoners tested. Because Böhmer also found a higher incidence of type B among prisoners with "asthenic-athletic" body forms that previous studies had associated with criminals, his study was often cited in subsequent literature on constitution and blood type.[58] It is not surprising that the greatest interest in the possible connection between blood types and constitution was in Italy, because of the work that Lombroso's successors had done in endocrinology and body-form studies. The largest effort to correlate blood groups, constitution, and criminality was a 1934 study by Viola of the Institute for Legal Medicine at the University of Pavia, who, while a captain in the military, tested 1500 soldiers who had been subjected to punishment for various forms of misconduct.[59]

Studies of temperament were another part of the broad field of constitutional research that used blood types to examine the genetics of crime. Although this approach originated in central Europe with the work of Kretschmer and others, Japanese researchers soon showed the most interest in this application of blood group research. The earliest and most influential of these studies was by Takeji Furukawa, a teacher at the Tokyo Higher Women's Normal School, who began publishing in 1927 and 1928.[60] Following the common practice of early blood group studies, he tested convenient populations at hand: 50 school teachers, 61 colleagues or visitors, and 248 school children. Although somatotype studies of Wundt and Kretschmer inspired him, Furukawa was most interested in devising a typology of temperament. He divided his subjects into "active," "passive," or "mixed" temperaments which he claimed to be correlated to blood types. Accordingly, people with O and B blood types were active, outgoing, intense, and bold, while those with A blood type he found were passive, timid, and indecisive.

Furukawa's real purpose, however, was revealed in a concluding section that characterized whole countries by temperament. Following the Hirszfelds' model, Furukawa devised a "National Temperament Index" which was the proportion of "active" to "passive" blood types in a country or (percent O + percent B)/(percent A + percent AB). This gave the Japanese the lowest, that is, most passive, index of 0.82 which was only rivalled by Swedes (0.82) and Norwegians (0.87). The highest, that is, most active, turned out to be Filipinos, American Indians, Gypsies, and Hindus (from 5.37 to 2.63), with most Europeans falling on the low end, from 1.08 for Austrians to 1.34 for Italians.[61]

Despite this questionable manipulation of numbers, Furukawa's research received surprisingly wide attention. He published an article in the respected *Zeitschrift für angewandte Psychologie und Charakterkunde*, and a refinement appeared in the first volume (1930) of the American John Dewey's *Journal of Social Psychology*.[62] As a result, his work was frequently cited in the literature thereafter. Among the articles it inspired in Japan was one in 1931 by a researcher in Okinawa who tested the correlation between the blood type and temperament of school children.[63] There is evidence, if somewhat anecdotal, that the link between blood type and temperament struck a responsive chord in wider Japanese society. A 1937 note in the *Journal of Heredity* cited an Associated Press report that a medical adviser to the Japanese Foreign Ministry recommended that diplomats be picked by blood type. Accordingly, there would be special preference given to those with blood type O who are "most suitable to represent Japan among the nations."[64]

In Germany, a more subtle study was done by Karl Goebbers at the Leipzig University Psychological Institute in 1937 that sought to correlate Rorschach results with blood type, but it described the work of Furukawa as "pioneering." A 1941 monograph published in Switzerland with the title *Character, Blood and Constitution* offered summary descriptions of individuals with the ABO blood types (type A were extroverts, etc.), much as Furukawa had done.[65] With the exception of a few racists in the late 1930s—notably just prior to and during Vichy France[66]—the attempts to use blood groups as a marker for temperament and other behavioral traits did not develop as extensively in western Europe and the U.S. as it did in central and eastern Europe or Japan.

Following the Second World War, however, there have been noticeable indications that the search for hereditary markers of complex behavior has persisted, including testing for correlation with blood groups. As will be seen in the final chapter, in 1973 *Nature* published an article which examined the relationship of ABO blood groups to IQ test results. Even more provocative was a 1983 article in the same journal claiming a higher percentage than normal of people with blood type A in higher socio-economic classes and a lower percentage of type O.[67] Meanwhile, in Japanese popular culture, blood types have approached the status of astrological signs for many people in making decisions about selection of mates and employment. Spinoffs have included a widely read book *You Are Your Blood Type*, which was translated into English in 1988 in the U.S., and a similar publication appeared in France under the title *Le secret de votre groupe sanguin*.[68]

Conclusion

It is not surprising that research on human heredity attempted to find a genetic marker for abnormal behavior. As seen in earlier chapters on race and disease, researchers sought evidence of the role of heredity in criminality and insanity, as proposed by many supporters of the widespread eugenics movement between the wars, and the test for blood groups offered a relatively simple way of identifying those whose behavior might otherwise appear to be normal. Even if there was no direct link between a specific blood type and insanity, blood testing might indicate a predisposition, to use today's language, that a prospective spouse, for example, might want to know about. This was like IQ testing that schools did for placing students or pedigree studies that were done for prospective spouses before marriage.

These studies demonstrate the workings of serendipity, chance, and presuppositions on the part of researchers, as well as honest retesting to confirm previous findings and verify results. The discovery of this new research "tool" (the Mendelian-inherited blood groups) was used, with some delay, to find statistical linkages to criminals or those determined to be insane, and this was clearly facilitated by easy access to populations for testing in prisons and insane asylums. When research produced negative or insufficient results, rather than leaving the search, there was a call to study more complex definitions of abnormal behavior.

Researchers who studied links of blood groups to abnormal behavior included practitioners of the new genetic techniques who were motivated by the desire to demonstrate the value of the discovery. But this was not necessarily shared by criminology and psychiatric professionals who had a vested interest in existing approaches to the problems. At the same time, others in the broader social setting (e.g., racists or politicians), with control and influence on funding and research, had their own interests that served neither the scientific, penal, nor mental health fields.

Notes

1. Most histories of criminology have followed the "great man" tradition, as indicated by titles from Hermann Mannheim, ed., *Pioneers in Criminology* (Chicago: Quadrangle, 1960) to Randy Martin et al., *Criminological Thought: Pioneers Past and Present* (New York: Macmillan, 1990). See below for recent, more broadly based approaches to criminology.
2. Michel Foucault's writings, especially *Discipline and Punish*, trans. Alan Sheridan (New York: Pantheon, 1977), are most responsible for turning contemporary scholars' attention to this development. For just two wide ranging examples from the literature, see Marie-Christine Leps, *Apprehending the Criminal: The Production of Deviance in Nineteenth-century Discourse* (Durham: Duke University Press, 1992) and John Tagg, "A Means of Surveillance; The Photograph as Evidence in Law," in John Tagg, *The Burden of Representation* (Amherst: University of Massachusetts Press, 1988): 66–102.
3. Louis Chevalier, *Dangerous Classes, Criminal Classes* (Princeton: Princeton University Press, 1981). For an overview of the philosophies that developed between the time of Beccaria and Lombroso, see Stephen Shafer, *Theories of Criminology* (New York: Random House, 1969), 111–22.
4. See Marvin Wolfgang's classic biographical account "Cesare Lombroso," in *Pioneers in Criminology*, ed. Hermann Mannheim (London: Stevens and Sons, 1960), 168–227, and more recently David G. Horn, *The Criminal Body: Lombroso and the Anatomy of Deviance* (New York: Routledge, 2003). For an updated bibliography, see Nicole Silvano Montaldo, "Lombroso: The Myth, The History." *Crime, Histoire & Sociétés / Crime, History & Societies* 22, no. 2 (2018): 31–61.
5. Thorsten Sellin, "The Lombrosian Myth in Criminology - Comment," *American Journal of Sociology* 42 (1937): 898–9.
6. See Ian Hacking, *The Taming of Chance* (Cambridge University Press, 1990). The title of Steven J. Gould's book is more critical of the process, *Mismeasure of Man* (New York: Norton, 1981).

7. For an excellent account of national differences, see Robert A. Nye, "Heredity or Milieu: The Foundation of Modern European Criminological Theory" *Isis* 67 (1976): 335–55. For a description of criminology in Britain at the turn of the century, see David Garland, "British Criminology Before 1935," *British Journal of Criminology* 28 (1988): 131–47. Lombroso's ideas became well-known late in Britain, after Havelock Ellis' 1890 writings. This lasted until Charles B. Goring's massive study, *The English Convict: A Statistical Study* (London: HMSO, 1913), was published which was widely interpreted as weakening the Lombrosian view because it failed to find criminal "types." Goring himself came to no such conclusion and in fact found notable differences between the height and weight of criminals and the normal population.

   In the U.S. Lombroso's ideas were also introduced in the 1890s, but it was not until 1909 that his or any other continental European criminologists' books were translated into English. For details, see Mark S. Gaylord and John F. Galliher, *The Criminology of Edwin Sutherland* (New Brunswick: Transaction Books, 1988), 53–8 and Mabel Elliott, *Crime in Modern Society* (New York: Harper, 1952).
8. Alfred Lindesmith and Yale Levin, "The Lombrosian Myth in Criminology," *American Journal of Sociology* 42 (1937): 668.
9. Max Gundel, "Rassenbiologische Untersuchungen an Strafangefangenen," *Klinische Wochenschrift* 5 (1926): 2165–6. A 1924 study by Frantz Schütz and Edgar Wöhlisch, "Bedeutung und Wesen von Haemagglutination und Blutgruppenbildung beim Menschcen," *Klinische Wochenschrift* 3 (1924): 1614–6, tested almost 1600 subjects which included 138 prisoners, but no difference in their blood group distribution was found.
10. E. Gotschlich, "Prof. Dr. Max Gundel zum Gedächtnis," *Zentralblatt für Bakteriologie* 153 (1949): 269–70.
11. In addition to Gundel's 1926 research, Steffan had inspired Frantz Schütz and Edgar Wohlisch's 1924 article, "Bedeutung und Wesen von Haemagglutination."For more on Steffan, see Pauline M. H. Mazumdar, "Blood and Soil: The Serology of the Aryan Racial State," *Bulletin of the History of Medicine* 64 (1990): 190–3.
12. Gundel, "Einige Beobachtungen bei der rassenbiologischen Durchforschung Schleswig-Holsteins," *Klinische Wochenschrift* 5 (1926): 1186. In a subsequent article, Gundel reported that of 310 subjects tested who said both parents had been born in the countryside, only 1.2 percent were blood type B, whereas of 112 who said both parents had been born in the city, 22.3 percent were blood type B. Gundel, "Blutgruppen bei Strafgefangenen," *Deutsche Zeitschrift für die gesamte gerichtliche Medizin* 11 (1928): 100.

13. Gundel, "Rassenbiologische Untersuchungen an Strafangefangenen," *Klinische Wochenschrift* 5 (1926), 2165–6.
14. Ibid.
15. Böhmer, "Blutgruppen und Verbrecher," *Deutsche Zeitschrift für die gesamte gerichtliche Medizin*, 9 (1927), 426.
16. The corresponding figures for Gundel were 79.8 percent B, 63.7 percent O, 63.6 percent A, and 38.8 percent AB.
17. Böhmer, "Blutruppen und Kriminalistik," *Forschungen und Fortschritte* 3 (1927): 142.
18. Fritz Schiff, "Die Blutgruppen und ihre Anwendung für Gericht," *Deutsche Zeitschrift für die gesamte gerichtliche Medizin* 9 (1927): 391.
19. Augustin Foerster, "Blutgruppen und Verbrecher," *Deutsche Zeitschrift für die gesamte gerichtliche Medizin* 11 (1928): 487–90.
20. Gundel, "Blutgruppen bei Strafgefangenen." The absence of additional testing was even more surprising because he had since moved to Heidelberg and presumably had a new prison population at his disposal.
21. Ibid., 119.
22. Canuto, "Distribuzione dei Gruppi Sanguigni nei Criminali Piemontesi," *Archivio di Antropologia Criminale* 48 (1928): 687–704; Palmieri, "Die Verteilung der Blutgruppen unter Geisteskranken Verbrechern," *Deutsche Zeitschrift für die gesamte gerichtliche Medizin* 12 (1928): 506–12. It should be noted that Palmieri used the Hirszfelds' First World War tests of Italian soldiers as a measure of the "normal" population, with 11 percent blood type B, whereas subsequent studies of Italians found a higher percentage of type B in the south of Italy: 14 percent in Naples, 17 percent in Sicily. See, for example, Raffaele Gaetano, "La distribuzione dei gruppi sanguigni nella provincia di Napoli," *Terapia* 21 (1931): 135–40.
23. G. A. Schusterov, "[Isohaemoagglutinierenden Eigenschaften des menschlichen Blutes nach den Ergebnissen einer Untersuchung an Straflingen des Reformatoriums (Arbeitshauses) zu Omsk]," *Moskovskii Meditsinskii Jurnal* 7 (1927): 1–6; W. Folomina, "Isohämagglutinationsgruppen bei Verbrechern," *Archiv Kriminologii i sudebnnoi meditsiny* 84 (1927): 145–8; and Adam Schmidt, "Blutgruppenbestimmungen an Strafgefangenen," *Deutsche Zeitschrift für die gesamte gerichtliche Medizin* 13 (1929): 373–6. Although Folomina did not know of Gundel's work, he reported a significantly higher percentage of type AB and O among thieves.
24. See, for example, Domenico Viola, "Contributo allo studio dei rapporti fra caratteri gruppo-specifici e caratteri psico-costituzionali," *Giornale di medicina militare* 82 (1934): 253–8. For more background on Italian criminology, see Thorsten Sellin, "A New Phase of Criminal Anthropology"; and Monachesi, "Trends in Criminological Research in Italy."

25. Palmieri, "Die Verteilung der Blutgruppen Unter Geisteskranken Verbrechern," 506. Palmieri claimed he only learned of Gundel's and Böhmer's research on blood groups and crime, well after he began his own study.
26. Hans Brennecke, "Die Erforschung der Personlichkeit des Gefangenen; ihre Methode und ihre Auswirkung im Strafvollzug," *Monatschrift für Kriminologie* 21 (1930):655–8.
27. Johannes Lange, *Verbrechen als Schicksal. Studien an kriminellen Zwillingen* (Leipzig 1929).
28. On the Chicago school, see Gaylord and Galliher, 135–41, who claim that Lombroso never had much influence on professional criminologists, which, when added to the early lack of interest in blood groups, explains why there were no studies of prisoners.
29. In addition to Gaylkord and Galliher on the Chicago School, see Lindesmith and Levin, "Lombrosian Myth," 669; and Cantor, 407. For Britain, see Paul Rock, *A History of British Criminology* (Oxford: Oxford University Press, 1988).
30. There is not time here to go into why a serologist in Germany tested prisoners while U.S. serologists did not. Suffice it to say that there was more research done overall on blood group distribution in Germany, while British, French, and American researchers had ample other subjects to test. A more thorough analysis of this question can be found in Schneider, "Science in National Context: Blood Group Research in Great Britain, France and the United States between the World Wars," *Yearbook of Physical Anthropology* 38 (1995): 87–114.
31. Some articles noted that the research of the Czech Jan Jansky in 1906, which discovered agglutination independently from Landsteiner, was based on mental patients in Prague. But the 20-year old study was not the stimulus for the new line of research in the mid-1920s. See Jan Jansky, "Haematologicke studie u psychotiku," *Sbornik Kliniky* 8 (1906–1907): 85–139. In any case Jansky found little difference between mental patients and the normal population.
32. See, for example, Eugenjusz Wilczowski, "Blutgruppenuntersuchungen bei Schizophrenie und progressiver Paralyse," *Klinische Wochenschrift* 6 (1927): 168; Viktor Ohnesorge, "Blutgruppenuntersuchungen Bei Nerven- und Geisteskrankheiten," *Archiv für Psychiatrie und Nervenkrankheiten* 81 (1927): 763–7; and Louis H. Snyder, "Human Blood Groups: Their Inheritance and Racial Significance," *American Journal of Physical Anthropology* 9 (1926): 233–63. The first work by Alexander was "An Inquiry into the Distribution of Blood Groups in Patients Suffering from Malignant Diseases," *British Journal of Experimental Pathology* 2 (1921): 66–9.

33. Theophile Raphael, Olive M. Searle and William Scholten, "Blood Groups in Schizophrenic and Manic-depressive Psychosis," *American Journal of Psychiatry* 7 (1927–1928): 153–61. As will be seen below, this had been proposed by Kretschmer and others who studied the connection between body form and temperament.
34. For more on doctors in English prisons, see Joe Sim, *Medical Power in Prisons: The Prison Medical Service in England, 1774–1989* (Buckingham: Open University Press, 1990).
35. G. Berstein, "Die Verteilung der Blutgruppen unter des Geisteskranken," Sovremnaj psycho-neurologica (1925) as cited in *Zentralblatt für die gesamte Neurologie und Psychiatrie* 41 (1925): 875; Feldman and Elmanovich, "Agglutinierende Eigenschaften des Blutes der Geisteskranken," *Mediko-biologicheskii zhurnal* 1 (1925): 125.
36. On France and Germany, see Edouard Toulouse, P. Schiff, and R. Weismann-Netter, "Les Groups Sanguins dans les Maladies Mentales et Nerveuses," *Encephale* 21 (1926): 785–8; Hans Jacobsohn, "Uber die Blutgruppenzugehörigkeit der Paralytiker," *Zeitschrift für die gesamte Neurologie und Psychologie* 105 (1926): 810–4. Elsewhere, see Wilczokowski, "Blutgruppenuntersuchungen bei Schizophrenie"; Raphael et al., "Blood Groups in Schizophrenic"; Alexander Pilcz, "Untersuchungen über die Blutgruppenzugehörigkeit bei Geisteskrankheiten," *Jahrbücher für Psychiatrie und Neurologie* 45 (1927): 120–31; and H.A. Bunker and S. Meyers, "Blood Groups in General Paralysis. A Study of Agglutinin-Agglutinogen Reactions in 91 Cases," *Journal of Laboratory and Clinical Medicine* 12 (1928): 415–26. The latter was in addition to Scholten and Searle mentioned above.
37. This was the result of a combination of Toulouse's prestige among psychiatrists, plus a general lack of interest in blood group studies at the time in France. This lasted until 1933 when Raymond Turpin reviewed the literature again on blood groups and mental illness. See Raymond Turpin and A. Caratzali, "Consideration sur la valeur constitutionnelle des groupes sanguins," *Revue française de puericulture* 1 (1933): 86–105.
38. Fr. Meyer, "Blutgruppenverteilung in der schlesichen Bevolkerung sowie die Beziehung der Blutgruppen zu Geisteskranken," *Deutsche medizinische Wochenschrift* 54 (1928): 1461; Ohnesorge, "Blutgruppenuntersuchungen bei Nerven- und Geisteskrankheiten," 763–7. Jacobsohn, 812; B. N. Chominskii and L. S. Schustova, "Zur Frage des Zusammenhangs zwischen Blutgruppe und psychischer Erkrankung," *Zeitschrift für die gesamte Neurologie und Psychiatrie* 115 (1928): 303–8. Jacobsohn acknowledged being in touch with two researchers in the Soviet Union who soon published some of their results in the West, but despite being at

Kiev, these Russians did not mention the earlier work of Feldman and Elmanovich at Kharkiv.

39. For example, Laurence H. Snyder included 395 patients and inmates who were epileptics, schizophrenics, and "feeble-minded" in his 1926 study of over 2200 subjects, "Human Blood Groups: Their Inheritance and Racial Significance," *American Journal of Physical Anthropology* 9 (1926): 233–63.
40. Wilczowski, "Blutgruppenuntersuchungen bei Schizophrenie."
41. Ohnesorge, 764.
42. Frederick Proescher and A. S. Arkush, "Blood Groups in Mental Diseases," *Journal of Nervous and Mental Diseases* 65 (1927): 578.
43. Theophile Raphael, Olive M. Searle, and William Scholten, "Blood Groups in Schizophrenic Disease."
44. Fr. Meyer, "Blutgruppenverteilung in der schlesichen Bevolkerung"; Paul Würz, "Uber die Blutgruppenverteilung bei Schizophrenen," *Schweizerische medizinische Wochenschrift* 58 (1928): 353–5.
45. Gundel, "Blutgruppen und Krankheiten," *Zeitschrift für Immunitätsforschung* 56 (1928): 60–76.
46. R. Hilgermann and H. Birnbaum, "Die Blutkörpercheneigenschaften M und N in Verbindung mit den 4 Blutgruppen in ihrer Beziehung zu Geisteskrankheiten," *Zeitschrift für die gesamte experimentelle Medizin* 94 (1934): 722–5; and Olga Hering, "Untersuchungen über Zusammenhänge zwischen den 4 klassischen Blutgruppenin. Verbindung mit den Blutkörpercheneigenschaften M und N und psychopathischer Veranlangung," *Zeitschrift für die gesamte experimentelle Medizin* 99 (1936): 547–56.
47. The results were published as Lionel S. Penrose, "Blood Grouping of Mongolian Imbeciles," *Lancet* (1932): 394–5; and M. Penrose and L. S. Penrose, "Blood Group Distribution in the Eastern Counties of England," *British Journal of Experimental Pathology* 14 (1933): 160–1.

    On Penrose, see Kevles, *In the Name of Eugenics.* On the lack of work in England, see above and Schneider "Blood Group Research in Great Britain, France and the United States between the World Wars."
48. Hooten's most notorious foray into the subject was *The American Criminal: An Anthropological Study* (Cambridge: Harvard University Press, 1939), which was supposed to be the first of three volumes, but subsequent ones on the "native and foreign-born white criminal" and "Negroes, Negroids, and Mexicans" were never completed. Hooten did publish a popular companion to the scientific study *Crime and the Man* (Cambridge: Harvard University Press, 1939), which boasted "not a single statistical table, practically no footnotes, and not even a bibliography."

    Sheldon began his research in the late 1920s with an article on "Morphological Types and Mental Ability," *Journal of Personnel Research*

5 (1927): 447–51, which developed into a more general prewar volume, *Varieties of Human Physique* (New York: Harper and Brothers, 1940), but only a brief section (pp. 254–9) on crime. Sheldon's postwar research, however, produced a ponderous volume devoted specifically to constitution and crime, *Varieties of Delinquent Youth* (New York: Harper and Brothers, 1949).

49. William B. Tucker and William A. Lessa, "Man: A Constitutional Investigation," *Quarterly Review of Biology* 15 (1940): 265–89; 411–55. For historical perspective, see Sarah W. Tracy, "George Draper and American Constitutional Medicine, 1916–1946: Reinventing the Sick Man," *Bulletin of the History of Medicine* 66 (1992): 53–89.
50. For a contemporary introduction to the background of constitution studies, see Antonio Ciocco, "Historical Background of the Modern Study of Constitution," *Bulletin of the Institute of the History of Medicine* 4 (1936): 23–38. For more recent interpretations of phrenology, see James Poskett, *Materials of the Mind: Phrenology, Race, and the Global History of Science, 1815–1920* (Chicago: University of Chicago Press, 2019).
51. Ciocco, 30. Beneke's major works were *Die anatomische Grundlagen der Constitutionsanomalien des Menschen* (Marburg: Eltwert, 1878) and *Constitution und constitutionelles Kranksein des Menschen* (Marburg: Elwert, 1881).
52. See Sellin, "New Phase in Criminal Anthropology in Italy," 236–42; and Monachesi "Trends in Criminological Research in Italy," for the impact of the constitutional studies on criminology.
53. Kretschmer's most influential book translated into English was *Physique and Character* (New York: Harcourt, Brace, 1925).
54. Ludwik Hirszfeld, *Konstitutionsserologie* (Berlin: Springer, 1928), 1.
55. See, for example, A. M. Gesselevic, "Zur Frage der Konstitution und der Hämagglutinationsgruppen des Blutes," *Ukrainische Zentralblatt für Blutgruppenforschung* 2 (1928): 5–23; a later version of which was published as "Die Korrelation zwischen den Körperbautypen und den Blutgruppen und ihre graphische Darstellung," *Zeitschrift für Konstitutionslehre* 17 (1932): 199–202.
56. Charlotte Lemke, "Kommen bei den Asthetikern und Tuberkulösen einzelne Blutgruppen besonders häufig vor?" *Zeitschrift für die gesamte Anatomie* 14 (1928): 333–46.
57. R. M. Fischmann, "[Isohemagglutination and constitution among workers in Petrovsky factory]," *Dnepro-Petrovsk. Med. Journ* (1929): 33; W. J. Rubaschkin and L. J. Leisermann, "Die Isohamagglutinationsgruppen und die Konstitutionsindexe bei den Ukrainegebürtigen Angehörigen der Roten Armée," *Ukrainische Zentralblatt für Blutgruppenforschung* 4 (1930): 145–55.

58. Brennecke, 665. For an example from the leading expert on body form and criminals, see Friedrich von Rohden, "Kriminalbiologische Untersuchungen an gesunden und geisteskranken Verbrechern," *Deutsche Zeitschrift für die gesamte gerichtliche Medizin* 10 (1927): 620–33; and "Methoden der Kriminalbiologie," *Handbuch der biologischen Arbeitsmethoden* 4:12/1 (1938), 643–7.
59. Viola, "Contributo allo studio."
60. Furukawa published a few articles in Japanese journals in 1927, but his most important work was published in Germany the following year. Takeji Furukawa, "Erforschung der Temperamente mittels der experimentellen Blutgruppenuntersuchung," *Zeitschrift für angewandte Psychologie und Charakterkunde,* 31 (1928), 271–99. For historical perspective, see Jennifer Robertson, "Hemato-nationalism: the past, present, and future of 'Japanese blood,'" *Medical Anthropology* 31 (2012): 98–9. Background on Furukawa is also provided by Isaac C.K. Tan, "The Scientific Appropriation of Blood-type Research in Interwar Japan," manuscript in preparation.
61. Furukawa, "Erforschung," 294.
62. Takeji Furukawa, "A Study of Temperament and Blood Groups," *Journal of Social Psychology* 1 (1930): 494–508. In this article, Furukawa simplified his characterization of blood types to the correlation of type O with "phlegmatic," type A with "melancholic" and type B with "sanguine" temperaments. His application of this to national temperament was even more simplistic, depending only on the percentage of blood type O. This, he said, meant the Japanese were the lowest and Europeans the highest, the latter proven by Europeans' "more phlegmatic temperament as shown in their study of science, in their diplomacy, military affairs, and other activities."
63. Kôzi Nisi, "[blood groups of inhabitants of Okinawa province and their temperament and talent from standpoint of blood group specificity]," *Bulletin of Legal Medicine Institute of Nagasaki* (1931): 42–9, abstracted in the *Deutsche Zeitschrift für die gesamte gerichtliche Medizin* 18 (1931–1932), 97. Another example is Kenichi Kushigemachi and Kengo Hamada, "[Blood groups of inhabitants of Kumamoto prefecture; relations to temperaments or some vocations]" *Kumamoto Igakkai Zasshi* [Journal of the Kumamoto Medical Society] 8 (1932) 5–6 (abstr).
64. "Blood Group of Diplomats," *Journal of Heredity*, 28 (1937): 221.
65. Karl H. Goebbers, "Blutgruppe und Typus," *Zeitschrift für angewandte Psychologie und Charakterkunde* 53 (1937): 19–47; K. Fritz Schaer, *Charakter, Blutgruppe und Konstitution* (Zürich and Leipzig: Rascher, 1941).

66. See Schneider, *Quality and Quantity: The Quest for Biological Regeneration in Twentieth Century France* (New York: Cambridge University Press, 1990), 227–9, 253–5.
67. John B. Gibson, G. A. Harrison, V.A. Clarke and R. W. Hiorns, "IQ and ABO Blood Groups," *Nature* 246 (1973): 498–500; J. A. Beardmore and F. Karimi-Booshehri, "ABO Genes are differentially distributed in socio-economic groups in England," *Nature* 303 (1983): 522–4 and "Blood group and socio-economic class," *Nature* 309 (1984): 395–9.
68. Toshitaka Nomi, *You Are Your Blood Type: The Biological Keys to Unlocking the Secrets of your Personality*, trans. Alexander Besher (New York: Pocket Books, 1988) and Jean-Louis Degaudenzi, *Le secret de votre groupe sanguin: Clé de la personnalité et du destin* (Paris: Filipucchi, 1991). For Japan, see Robertson, "Hemato-nationalism: the past, present, and future of 'Japanese blood,'" *Medical Anthropology* 31 (2012): 93–112.

CHAPTER 8

Conclusion: The Legacy of Blood Group Research After 1945

In a 1984 luncheon address to the 50th annual meeting of the American Association of Physical Anthropologists, the Oxford researcher G. Ainsworth Harrison presented "an outsider's view" of the development of physical anthropology since the founding of the association in 1930. He began with the observation, "Fifty years ago, the physical anthropology of recent populations was preoccupied, in North America as elsewhere in the world, with race and the reconstruction of racial phylogenetic affinities. Anthropometry was the main technique used." In ensuing years, he continued, the single most important change was the introduction of genetics to the field. "Fifty years ago, genetics was practically unheard of; today, it permeates all physical anthropological thinking."[1]

Although Harrison did not offer it, he could have presented proof of his observation from any current journal of physical anthropology. For example, at another session of the 50th anniversary meeting, William Pollitzer, a professor at the University of North Carolina, analyzed the growth of genetics and population studies as reflected in the pages of the *American Journal of Physical Anthropology*. His conclusion was, "The most important lesson from genetics, and its greatest influence upon our discipline, has been the shift from a static to a dynamic viewpoint. It sounded the death knell of typology and rang in the birth of populations."[2] The preceding study has shown that the line of research in human genetics that was best developed and most responsible for the changes in

W. H. Schneider, *Blood Groups and Human Heredity, 1900–1950*, Medicine and Biomedical Sciences in Modern History,
https://doi.org/10.1007/978-3-031-69844-6_8

the field of physical anthropology was the study of human blood groups that had flourished in the 1920s and 1930s. In 1951, Laurence H. Snyder, who began studying blood groups in the 1920s, said of their importance to the new field of human genetics which he pioneered, "the blood groups have been to human genetics what drosophila has been to classical genetics."[3]

These general observations notwithstanding, the history of blood group research, genetics, and race studies after the Second World Waris complicated and changed rapidly. Blood group testing was well established as an important tool of anthropology, genetics, and serology, and changes in these fields have been the subject of studies by historians since the 1990s. From that work it is possible to offer concluding remarks about the legacy of the interwar blood group research. There is space for only some examples of continuity and change, but to begin with the most obvious, the greatest changes were the result of wartime devastation in the countries most engaged in prewar research: Germany, the Soviet Union, and Japan.

Geography of Postwar Studies

As shown in an earlier chapter, Soviet research declined dramatically in the early 1930s as a result of Stalin's "Great Break." The new policy shut off anthropological and disease-related studies in favor of blood group research for practical uses like transfusion. Nor did Soviet research become part of the postwar worldwide shift to population genetics because of the political impact from the Lysenko affair which rejected Mendelian genetics.[4] Likewise, Eastern Bloc communist countries no longer had incentives to conduct racial studies, and genetics research there was similarly affected by Lysenkoism. There was an exception for a decade in Poland where Hirszfeld survived the war and helped create two Polish universities, including Wroclaw (former Breslau) which established an institute of immunology and experimental therapy.

Although even more devastated by the war, German blood group studies, in contrast, revived and became part of global biomedical genetics research after universities were reestablished in West Germany. In Japan the story is somewhat mixed, according to a recent study by Jaehwan Hyun. Furuhata, the leading figure in Japanese blood group research since the 1920s, survived the war and in 1952 established a center at Tokyo Dental and Medical University to study the distribution of the newly discovered blood groups as part of the field of "genetic distribution of human populations." Hyun concludes that this was similar to Furuhata's prewar serological racial anthropology, as his studies sought to differentiate the Japanese "ethnic nation" from neighboring East Asians.[5]

French researchers were late but soon began publishing articles on blood group distribution after the war, as many of them moved into the field of human genetics.[6] But as will be seen below, the interwar racial blood group claims of Réné Martial continued after 1945 with the work of one of his students Léone Bourdel. There was much more continuity of blood group research in the U.S. and Great Britain, but as will be seen, it quickly became involved in the postwar debate over the use of the term "race."

Despite the decline after 1945 in studies of the distribution of blood groups by researchers in many European countries, two lines of increased research can be identified overall. First was the rise in testing of populations outside Europe, North America, and Japan, and second was the summary, cumulative work of Arthur Mourant and his collaborators at Oxford on the worldwide distribution of blood groups. The latter was all the more necessary because of the dramatic growth of blood group testing in Latin America, the Middle East, Africa, and Asia in the second half of the twentieth century This was the result of both the relative neglect of such studies there during the interwar period and new generations of medical researchers in colonial and newly independent countries where schools and research centers were established after 1945. For example, Ana Barahona has shown how the development of medical genetics in Mexico began in the 1940s with the study of blood group distribution by Mario Salazar Mallén and Adolfo Karl. This made possible Rubén Lisker's landmark *Genetic Structure of the Mexican Population, Medical and Anthropological Aspects.*[7] Likewise, Projit Mukharji has published a study of the same time period in India when researchers such as Cambridge-educated D. N. Majumdar began the large-scale, systematic study of blood group distribution.[8] This work was added to anthropometric studies and became part of the debates about populations and castes in India until the 1960s when it provided the basis for the wider study of human genetics. A final example is blood group research in the Middle East (e.g., Israel and Iran) which also reflected Mourant's influence.[9] These are only a few examples of the extensive research on blood groups after 1945 conducted from Trinidad to Turkey, Chile to Pakistan, and by the late 2010s including Cameroun, Uganda, and Burkina Faso.[10]

The Work of Mourant

Arthur E. Mourant was a major figure in the postwar generation of serologists. First trained in geology, he entered medical school during the Second World War at age 34. Before he graduated in 1948 Mourant was co-discoverer of two new blood groups while working for the National Blood Transfusion Service, and in 1946 he took charge of the Blood Groups Reference Laboratory. Its purpose was to prepare reagents for blood testing in Britain and later was sanctioned by the World Health Organization to set standards for production. As such, the laboratory became the center of a much more coordinated worldwide network of postwar research on blood group distribution than existed before the war.[11]

Together with his colleagues, the brilliant statistician Ada Kopec and librarian Kasimiera Domaniewska-Sobczak, Mourant combined postwar research with previous interwar studies in the volume *The Distribution of Human Blood Groups* (1954), followed by *The Distribution of the Human Blood Groups and Other Biochemical Polymorphisms* (1976) and *Blood Groups and Diseases* (1978). Although Jenny Bangham raises questions about some subjective and undocumented procedures and methodology of Mourant,[12] at the time, the statement of his goal that appeared on the opening page of his 1954 *magnum opus* was widely accepted. "The study of the blood groups, besides having many purely scientific advantages over most other bases of classification has the merit of providing objective criteria far removed from the traditional marks of 'race'."

Blood Groups and Race

The quotation marks used by Mourant around race in 1954 are significant because the very concept of race was subject to painstaking scrutiny following the Second World War in reaction to the role it had played in fascist regimes since the 1930s. The revulsion against the Nazi racial atrocities produced numerous proposals in the scientific community for change, perhaps the most dramatic of which was the 1950 UNESCO Statement on Race which claimed that "race was less a biological fact than a social myth." This came close to the argument of UNESCO Director-General Julian Huxley that "ethnic" should replace the term "race."[13] Although pseudo-scientific racism was universally condemned, some prominent biologists and anthropologists objected to eliminating the concept altogether and complained there were no physical anthropologists or geneticists on the panel that issued the 1950 statement. This prompted UNESCO to convene a second panel with additional experts who in 1951 issued their own "Statement" which described their disagreement as follows:

> The concept of race is unanimously regarded by anthropologists as a classificatory device providing a zoological frame within which the various groups of mankind may be arranged and by means of which studies of evolutionary processes can be facilitated. In its anthropological sense, the word 'race' should be reserved for groups of mankind possessing well-developed and primarily heritable physical differences from other groups.[14]

Of course, not all anthropologists agreed with the 1951 statement, and blood group studies figured prominently in the ensuing debate among them about race after the war. Jonathan Marks and Rachel Silverman have shown that blood group data was used both by proponents and opponents of continuing the concept of race.[15] A major point of contention was whether and how scientists could define and distinguish differences between human groups. Through the interwar period the term race was used extensively, relying mostly on phenotypic, morphological features that had been the main way of defining the groups for over a century. The blood groups, as championed by proponents such as William Boyd, were a newly discovered feature that had a clear and simple genetic determinant.

Complicating their argument was that no one suggested any longer there were just four races defined by each ABO type. Rather it was the proportion of each (or the genes determining the types) in a given population which made those people distinct, i.e., a "race." The percentages, however, were just as subject to the criticism of being arbitrary as the shapes or measurements of the head used in defining earlier racial groups. While some die-hards like Carleton Coon argued to keep the old categories using blood groups to develop a more refined taxonomy, in the 1960s a movement developed following Huxley's argument to reject race altogether as distinct way of categorizing humans and replace it with the idea of gradually varying differences or clines. As found in the issues of *Current Anthropology* during the 1960s and in the writings of physical anthropologists such as Frank Livingstone and C. Loring Brace, those arguing against the concept of race claimed that blood types are an excellent example of genetically inherited traits that gradually vary in frequency depending on where populations had migrated and intermarried.[16] Richard Lewontin's "The Apportionment of Human Diversity," possibly the most often cited argument that "human racial classification is now seen to be of virtually no genetic or taxonomic significance," makes frequent use of the "embarrassment of riches" provided by blood group studies.[17]

Blood Groups and Disease

Contrary to debates about blood groups being markers for race, another interwar use of blood group studies was more widely recognized as valid in postwar research: the link between blood groups and disease. As mentioned in an earlier chapter, the 1953 research led by Aird is most widely cited as the first recognized proof of a link between blood type and stomach cancer.[18] It gave a great impetus for the continuation of such studies that had proliferated between the wars, but it did not eliminate all criticism. One of the best known and strongest critics of studies attempting to find links between blood type and diseases was Alexander Wiener, co-discoverer of the Rh system with Landsteiner. In a 1962 article Wiener argued that he found reliable investigators to have "failed to find any evidence of such a correlation and believe it unlikely that the blood-group of an individual does influence the occurrence or course of any disease in that individual."[19]

This criticism did little to stem the continuing research.[20] Mourant et al. found the subject worthy of another cumulative monograph in 1978 (*Blood Groups and Diseases*) which one reviewer described as providing "a huge amount of data," on "associations of the ABO blood groups with a wide variety of diseases including infectious, malignant, metabolic, mental, circulatory, respiratory, and digestive."[21] As to whether differences in blood type frequency were the result of random genetic drift or natural selection due to fitness in response to disease, Mourant et al. concluded, "Most workers now agree that both processes are operative, but their relative importance remains in question." Since then, although subsequent research still questions blood group links to cancer, the discovery of the molecular basis of the ABO blood group system has permitted a new line of research on the mechanisms of selection for infectious diseases, and statistical studies have continued to the present day.[22]

Blood Groups and Behavior

In his 1962 critique of blood group studies and disease, Alexander Wiener pointed to an even more questionable example "that blood group studies know no bounds." His example was a monograph on blood groups and temperament by French researcher Leone Bourdel. Her claims, he charged, were so far beyond the boundary of science that even "workers on blood-groups and disease have attempted to dissociate themselves from these claims."[23] The interwar work on blood types and temperament was not very extensive, but it survived in the research on constitution studies and body type, as well as the exceptional case of Bourdel. Although a student of the racist ideologue Rene Martial, Bourdel also conducted more widely accepted research on testing for professions and was employed by mainstream psychologists such as Henri Piéron of the École pratique des hautes études.[24] By the end of the 1930s and during the war, however, she followed the lead of Martial who argued for selection of immigrants according to blood types: rejecting B and accepting A and O. Her research focused on blood type, temperament, and race and concluded that type A indicated "harmonic" personality, type B "rhythmic," type O "melodic," and type AB "complex." After the war she published in respectable journals (e.g., *Journal de la société statistique de Paris*) and her 1946 book received a serious review in *Le Monde* (July 10, 1946)[25]

In one sense, perhaps confirming Wiener's view, there is little indication that Bourdel's work prompted much further study in France, although the subject of blood type and personality continues to the present day both in scholarly and popular publications.[26] For example, during a brief period beginning in the 1970s there was a flurry of interest in the association of ABO blood groups and intelligence as measured by IQ and other tests. This was sparked by a 1973 article in *Nature* published by researchers at Oxford and Cambridge who studied 534 people in 7 villages outside Oxford. They found "statistically significant" differences (higher IQ in A_1 blood type), although with the caution that the sample was small, and results might not be found in other populations. Nonetheless, given the recent interest at that time in genetics of intelligence prompted by the writings of Arthur Jensen and Richard Herrnstein, the article elicited several responses by colleagues at Oxford who suggested the differences were the result of local versus non-locally born subjects.[27]

Ten years later a much larger study was done by geneticists at Swansea examining blood groups as genetic markers of socio-economic status. They used records from all parts of England based on 400,000 blood donors from 1953 to 1963 (notably collected by Mourant), which included occupation as defined by the five official Registrar-General's Social Class categories: Professional, Managerial and Technical, Skilled (manual and non-manual), Partly skilled, and Unskilled. They found phenotype A was "highly significantly more" frequently found (15 percent more) in the higher socio-economic (professional and managerial) donors, while blood type O was less. They found no difference in Rh positive and negative blood types.[28]

The authors referenced the work of Jensen and Herrenstein on the genetic inheritance of intelligence that supported the view of a link to socio-economic status which once again generated, in the words of the journal, "a wealth of correspondence," some of which was published the following year with a reply from the original authors. The replies (from authors in the UK, as well as the U.S. and Chile) were all critical, some with analysis that replicated the study with different populations, while others criticized the methodologies.[29] At least one researcher in Chile has continued this line of study.[30]

Finally, there is the phenomenon in recent decades of the wider appeal of blood types as predictors of human behavior, similar to astrological signs and which can be found in popular writings and cultural practices around the world. For example, a book by Peter D'Adamo published in 1996 claimed that people with different ABO types processed food differently. As a result, he proposed different diets for each blood type. Translated into 60 languages, the book sold over 7 million copies and others soon attempted to cash in on the interest.[31]

These writings were widespread enough that they eventually prompted scientific studies, one of which was published in 2013 by staff at the Belgian Red Cross who received numerous inquiries from blood donors about diet and blood type. Their finding was, "No evidence currently exists to validate the purported health benefits of blood type diets."[32] The following year a laboratory study at the University of Toronto was published with the following conclusion by researchers, "Based on the data of 1,455 study participants, we found no evidence to support the 'blood-type' diet theory .... The way an individual responds to any one of these diets has absolutely nothing to do with their blood type and has everything to do with their ability to stick to a sensible vegetarian or low-carbohydrate diet."[33]

Japan is the country where blood type as genetic marker has enjoyed the most widespread popularity. The roots of this, as shown in a previous chapter, go back to the interwar period when blood type was considered in hiring for government service. Type O, for example, was seen as associated with a "universal" personality suitable for the diplomatic corps. Jennifer Robertson has recently summed up the legacy of interest in blood type after the war as follows, "For many Japanese today, blood is understood in terms of blood type, which, despite its controversial serological history, prevails as a popular mode of horoscopy, match-making, and personality analysis." The epitome of the pervasiveness of this attitude, she offers, are the blood donation mascots (kenketsu) which rival Hello-Kitty for cuteness and appeal, with each blood type characterized in cartoons, pendants, and songs as follows.

> Eitchi, the spirit of type A, is in charge of publicity, is very responsible, and organizes everyone. The spirit of type O, O^- tan, summons and attracts people, and is always an energetic mood maker. Bibi, the honest spirit of type B, is resolutely tenacious, while Ebirin, the spirit of type AB, is in charge of nursing, being of a kind and caring disposition.[34]

Although currently supported by and associated with blood collection in Japan, the broader association of blood type with personality which had lapsed after the war, was also revived in the 1970s by the popular publications of Masahiko Nomi and was carried on by his son Toshitaka after his father's death in 1981. According to a blogpost by Rachel Nuwer, despite numerous scientific studies refuting it, blood type categorization ["Ketsueki-gata"] is believed by 75 percent or more Japanese and influences many social interactions "from romance to work." Some kindergarten classrooms are reportedly divided into blood types so that teaching can be "tailored to blood group personalities" and "young Japanese commonly exchange blood types upon first meeting."[35]

Conclusion

The Japanese phenomenon has also been popularized in other countries, such as France and the U.S.[36] This leads to some final observations about the reasons for continuing studies of blood groups. From the start, the Hirszfelds' and others' initial discoveries (e.g., Coca's discovery of type O predominance among native Americans) were simple, spectacular, and easily understood.

Accordingly, they raised expectations of similar results while also promising that almost any findings would add to the accumulating knowledge of the new field. Moreover, as a new field, the testing of blood groups was open to researchers of many backgrounds. The technical expertise of the required methodology was not a major barrier for those interested in conducting research because the ease of doing blood typing, plus availability of populations to test, literally opened the whole world as a laboratory. The results could be presented by simple statistics which were less complicated to determine than conducting and interpreting pedigree studies.

To be sure, there were some problems with the new methodology. For example, trained statisticians challenged the size of populations studied as a source of potential for error. This was compounded by the need to have representative samples to account for differences of ethnic makeup in the population studied. One could argue that the Hirszfelds were lucky (although perhaps it was inevitable) to stumble upon the first and most important discovery about blood groups and inheritance: differences in distribution according to ethnic makeup. But the dramatic nature of this finding which inspired the search for other revelations, tempted others to forego the care and painstaking attention to detail that the Hirszfelds actually followed: testing very large sample sizes with some use of controls.

Another source of errors was the application of results to several areas of study (i.e., anthropology, medicine, criminology, psychology) by researchers with little or no expertise in the fields. On the other hand, the problem of inconclusiveness invited further research, and the vagueness of some definitions (e.g., insanity, predisposition, etc.) gave proponents much leeway to adjust their claims and respond to criticisms. Finally, the possibility of a link between blood groups and a subject of such widespread concern as disease meant that there was great incentive for blood group testing that might have quite practical value. As shown, despite lack of conclusive results, this line of research continued after 1945, and there is evidence that if Aird et al. had not done their study, others would have soon published similar results. For example, the same month that the Aird collaborators published their article, another article appeared in a 1954 issue of the *AMA Archives of Surgery* by two surgeons at the Mayo Clinic reporting results of ABO and Rh frequencies in over 1400 patients with several diseases. Likewise, at an October 1954 meeting of the International Union against Cancer in London, two Sheffield University researchers gave a preliminary report on a five-year study of blood groups and cancer, although prompted by the publication of Aird and his colleagues.[37]

Returning to the overall appeal of blood group research, genetic determinism has been a siren song for the general populace and scientists especially after Mendel's modern formulation of the concept at the end of the nineteenth century. The discoveries about the human blood groups and their Mendelian inheritance after 1900 made them the first widely studied genetic markers that stimulated great interest in whether this inheritances from past ancestors could predict the traits of present and future generations. This long-standing quest is perhaps the most important underlying reason for the beginning of blood group studies by the Hirszfelds and their continuation afterward despite the exaggerated expectations and limited practical applications between the wars and after.

Notes

1. G. Ainsworth Harrison, "The Last Fifty Years of Human Population Biology," in *History of Physical Anthropology*, Frank Spencer, ed. (New York: Academic Press, 1982), 467.
2. William Pollitzer, "The Development of Genetics and Population Studies," *American Journal of Physical Anthropology* 56 (1981): 488.
3. Louis H. Snyder, "Old and New Pathways in Human Genetics," in *Genetics in the Twentieth Century*, ed. by L.C. Dunn (N.Y.: Macmillan, 1951), 371. See also C. Loring Brace, "The Roots of the Race Concept in American Physical Anthropology," in Spencer, 11–29 and Jonathan Marks, "The Legacy of Serological Studies in American Physical Anthropology," *History and Philosophy of the Life Sciences*, 18 (1995): 345–62.
4. The classic study of this challenge to Mendelism is David Joravsky, *The Lysenko Affair* (Chicago: University of Chicago Press, 1970). For a more recent assessment, see W. DeJong-Lambert, *The Cold War Politics of Genetic Research: An Introduction to the Lysenko Affair* (New York: Springer, 2012).
5. Jaehwan Hyun, "Blood Purity and Scientific Independence: Blood Science and Postcolonial Struggles in Korea, 1926–1975" *Science in Context* 32 (2019): 246–7.
6. Henri-V. Vallois and Paulette Marquer, "La distribution des groupes sanguins en France," *Comptes rendus hebdomadaires des seances de l'Academie des sciences 258 (1964): 2179–82.* French Nobel laureate Jean Dausset began his career giving blood transfusions in North Africa during the Second World War. See "Jean Dausset: Biographical," Accessed February 13, 2024, https://www.nobelprize.org/prizes/medicine/1980/dausset/biographical/.

7. Rubén Lisker, *Estructura genética de la población mexicana. Aspectos médicos y antropológicos* (Mexico City: Salvat Mexicana de Ediciones, S.A. de C. V., 1981). Salazar Mallen's first study was Marion Salazar Mallén and R. Hernández de la Portilla, "Existencia del aglutinógeno Rh en los hematíes de 250 individuos Mexicanos." *Revista de la Sociedad Mexicana de Historia Natural* 5 (1944): 183–5.
8. Projit B Mukharji, "From Serosocial to Sanguinary Identities: Caste, Transnational Race Science and the Shifting Metonymies of Blood Group B, India c. 1918–1960," *Indian Economic and Social History Review* 51 (2014): 143–76. For early work of Majumdar, see D. N. Majumdar, "Blood Groups of the Doms," *Current Science* 11 (1942): 153–4; and D.N. Majumdar and Kunwar Kishen. "Blood Groups Distribution in the United Provinces: Report on the Serological Survey of the UP," *The Eastern Anthropologist* 1(1947) 8–15.
9. Elise K Burton, "'Essential Collaborators': Locating Middle Eastern Geneticists in the Global Scientific Infrastructure, 1950s–1970s." *Comparative Studies in Society and History* 60, no. 1 (2018): 119–49.
10. J. D. Arneaud and O. Young, "A Preliminary Survey of the Distribution of A B O and Rh Blood Groups in Trinidad, B.W.I.," *Documenta de medicina geographica et tropica* 7 (1955): 375–8; B. Sevgen and N. Mizan, "[Blood groups and the Rh factor in Turkey]," *Tip Fakültesi mecmuasi* [Bulletin de la Faculté de medecine d'Istanbul] 23 (1960): 560–3; S. Sandoval, C. Henckel, and L. Givovich, "The Blood Groups, Subgroups, and Rh Factor of the Mapuche Indians of the Province of Cautin, Chile," *Blood* 1 (1946):555–9; M. Afzal, Ziaur-Rehman, F. Hussain, R. Siddiqi, "A Survey of Blood Groups," *Journal of the Pakistan Medical Association* 27 (1977): 426–8.

    For contemporary Africa, see ST Ndoula, JJ Noubiap, JR Nansseu, and A Wonkam, "Phenotypic and Allelic Distribution of the ABO and Rhesus (D) Blood Groups in the Cameroonian Population," *International Journal of Immunogenetics* 41 (2014): 206–10; RO Apecu, EM Mulogo, F Bagenda, et al., "ABO and Rhesus (D) Blood Group Distribution Among Blood Donors in Rural Southwestern Uganda: A Retrospective Study." *Biomed Central Research Notes* 9 (2016): 513; S Worlledge, SE Ogiemudia, CO Thomas, BN Ikoku, and L Luzzatto, "Blood Group Antigens and Antibodies in Nigeria," *Annals of Tropical Medicine and Parasitology* 68 (1974): 249–64; and S Sawadogo, K Nebie, T Millogo, et l., "Distribution of ABO and RHD Blood Group Antigens in Blood Donors in Burkina Faso," *International Journal of Immunogenetics* 46 (2019): 1–6.
11. Mourant's autobiography *Blood and Stones: An Autobiography* (La Haule, Jersey: La Haule Books, 1995) has not been widely distributed, but more accessible is Gary P. Misson, A. Clive Bishop, and Winifred M Watkins,

"Arthur Ernest Mourant. 11 April 1904–29 August 1994," *Biographical Memoirs of Fellows of the Royal Society. Royal Society* 45 (1999): 329–48. For background and a recent assessment of his work, see Jennifer Bangham, *Blood Relations: Transfusion and the Making of Human Genetics* (University of Chicago Press, 2020), 135–74.

12. Jenny Bangham, "Blood Groups and Human Groups: Collecting and Calibrating Genetic Data after World War Two." *Studies in history and philosophy of biological and biomedical sciences* 47 Pt A (2014): 74–86.
13. Huxley was a co-author with Hogben and Haldane of the popular 1935 book *We Europeans* which presented one of the earliest arguments that blood group distribution was evidence against pseudo-scientific racial biology. See Jenny Bangham, *Blood Relations*, 53–5 and Marianne Sommer, "Biology as a Technology of Social Justice in Interwar Britain: Arguments from Evolutionary History, Heredity, and Human Diversity," *Science, Technology, & Human Values* 39, no. 4 (2014): 561–86.
14. "Statement on the Nature of Race and Race Differences by Physical Anthropologists and Geneticists--June 1951," in *The Race Concept: Results of an Inquiry* (Paris: UNESCO, 1952), 11. See also Brattain, 1401–2.
15. Marks, "The Legacy of Serological Studies"; Rachel Silverman, "The Blood Group 'Fad' in Post-War Racial Anthropology," *Kroeber Anthropological Society Papers* 84 (2000): 11–27.
16. Frank R. Livingstone, "On the Non-Existence of Human Races," *Current Anthropology* 3 (1962): 279; C. Loring Brace, "On the Race Concept," *Current Anthropology* 5 (1964): 313.
17. Richard C. Lewontin, "The Apportionment of Human Diversity," in *Evolutionary Biology*, eds. William C. Steere, Theodosius Dobzhansky, and Max K. Hecht (New York: Springer; 1972), 381–98. On Lewontin's significance, see Michael D. Edge, Sohini Ramachandran, and Noah A. Rosenberg, "Celebrating 50 Years Since Lewontin's Apportionment of Human Diversity," *Philosophical Transactions of the Royal Society of London. Series B, Biological Sciences*, 377 (June 2022), https://doi.org/10.1098/rstb.2020.0405.
18. Ian Aird, H. H. Bentall and J. A. Fraser Roberts, "A Relationship between Cancer of Stomach and the ABO Blood Groups," *British Medical Journal* (1953) 1:799–801.
19. Alexander S. Wiener, "Blood-groups and Disease. A critical review," *Lancet*. 21 (1962):813–6.
20. See Alexander S. Wiener, "Controversy in Human Genetics. Blood groups and Disease," *American Journal of Human Genetics* 22 (1970):476–83.
21. Frank B. Livingstone, "Review of *Blood Groups and Disease: A Study of Associations of Diseases with Blood Groups and Other Polymorphisms*. A. E. Mourant, A. C. Kopec, and K. Domaniewska-Sobczak," *Human Biology* 51:600–1.

22. Massimo Franchini, Giancarlo M. Liumbruno, and Giuseppe Lippi, "The Prognostic Value of ABO Blood Group in Cancer Patients," *Blood Transfusion*, 14 (2016):434–40; on molecular mechanisms, see David. J. Anstee, "The Relationship between Blood Groups and Disease," *Blood* 115 (2010): 4635–43; Laura Cooling, "Groups in Infection and Host Susceptibility," *Clin Microbiol Rev.* 28 (2015):801–70. For an example of COVID-19 correlation studies (mostly negative), see Nicholas Mielke, Rebecca Gorz, Amit Bahl, Lili Zhao, and David A. Berger, "Association between ABO Blood Type and Coronavirus Disease. 2019 Severe Outcomes Across Dominant Variant Strains." *Journal of the American College of Emergency Physicians open*, 5 (2024), https://doi.org/10.1002/emp2.13115.
23. Even more critical was Wiener's, "Blood Groups and Personality Traits," *American Journal of Human Genetics* 17 (1965): 369–70.
24. Annick Ohayon, "Ce qui énervait Henri Piéron," *Bulletin de psychologie* 533 (2014): 409–14.
25. Léone Bourdel, "Sang - Tempéraments - Travail – Races," *Journal de la société statistique de Paris* 87 (1946): 162–78; Jacques Genevay and Léone Bourdel, *Sang, Tempéraments, Travail et Races* (Paris: Maloine, 1946).
26. Rihab Alsadi, "Personality Traits and Their Relationship with Blood Groups among of Palestinian University Students," *International Journal of Psychology and Behavioral Sciences* (2020) 10(2): 34–42.
27. John B. Gibson, G. A. Harrison, V.A. Clarke, and R. W. Hiorns, "IQ and ABO Blood Groups," *Nature* 246 (1973): 498–500; Glenys Thomson and Walter F. Bodmer, "Letter: Population stratification as an explanation of IQ and ABO association." *Nature* 254 (1975): 363–4.
28. J. A. Beardmore and F. Karimi-Booshehri, "ABO Genes are Differentially Distributed in Socio-economic Groups in England," *Nature*, 303 (1983): 522–4.
29. J. A. Beardmore and F. Karimi-Booshehri, "Blood Group and Socio-economic Class," *Nature* 309 (1984): 395–9 (6 replies); G. C. Ashton, "Blood Polymorphisms and Cognitive Abilities," *Behavior Genetics* 16 (1986): 517–29.
30. Carlos Y. Valenzuela, Carolina Pastene, and Cynthia M. Pérez. "Intelligence and Genetic Markers in Chilean Children," *Biological Research* 31 (1998): 81–92; Carlos Y. Valenzuela, "Human Sociogenetics," *Biological Research* 44 (2011): 393–404.
31. Peter J. Adamo, *Eat Right 4 Your Life: The Individualized Blood Type Diet Solution* (New York: G.P. Putnam, 1996). For imitators, see Dina Khader, *The Food Combining/Blood Type Diet Solution: a Personalized Diet Plan and Cookbook for Each Blood Type* (New York: McGraw Hill: 2000); Joseph

Christiano, *Joseph Christiano's Blood Type Diet O: a Custom Eating Plan for Losing Weight, Fighting Disease, and Staying Healthy for People with Type O Blood* (Lake Mary, FL: Siloam, 2010).

32. Leila Cusack, Emmy De Buck, Veerle Compernolle, and Philippe Vandekerckhove, "Blood Type Diets Lack Supporting Evidence: a Systematic Review," *American Journal of Clinical Nutrition* 98, (2013): 99–104.
33. Jingzhou Wang, Bibiana García-Bailo, Daiva E. Nielsen, and Ahmed El-Sohemy, "ABO Genotype, 'Blood-Type' Diet and Cardiometabolic Risk Factors," *PLoS ONE*, 9 (2014): 1–9.
34. Jennifer Robertson, "Hemato-nationalism: The Past, Present, and Future of "Japanese Blood," *Medical Anthropology* 2012;31(2): 93–5.
35. Rachel Nuwer, "You are what you bleed: In Japan and other east Asian countries some believe blood type dictates personality," *Scientific American* Guest Blog (February 15, 2011) https://blogs.scientificamerican.com/guest-blog/you-are-what-you-bleed-in-japan-and-other-east-asian-countries-some-believe-blood-type-dictates-personality/
36. Jean-Louis Degaudenzi, *Le secret de votre groupe sanguin: Clé de la personnalité et du destin* (Paris: Filipucchi, 1991); Toshitaka Nomi and Alexander Besher, *You Are Your Blood Type* (New York: Pocket Books; 1988).
37. Harry N. Green and Ivor Dunsford, "Relationship of Blood groups to Cancer," *Acat – Unio Internationalis contra cancrum*, 10 (1954): 125–7; Charles W. Mayo and James O. Ferguson, "Are Certain Diseases Associated with Specific Blood Groups or Rh Antigens?" *AMA Archives of Surgery* 66 (1953): 406–9.

Selected Bibliography

Note on Sources

References to archives are found in notation of individual chapters. In addition, materials consulted for this book can be found in "William H. Schneider History of Blood Groups Research Collection" (RLML-016), History of Medicine Collection, Ruth Lilly Medical Library, Indiana University School of Medicine. These include copies of research articles, archival and other unpublished materials, and a spreadsheet database with entries for over 1000 research articles published before 1939.

Research Publications Before 1945

Akune, Matsui. "Zur serologischen Anthropologie der Japaner." *Zeitschrift für Morphologie und Anthropologie* 30 (1932): 38.

Alexander, William. "An Inquiry into the Distribution of Blood Groups of Patients Suffering from Malignant Diseases." *British Journal of Experimental Pathology* 2 (1921): 66–9.

Alperin, M. "Ueber die Beziehungen zwischen Blutgruppen und Tubercule." *Beiträge zur Klinik der Tuberkulose* 64 (1926): 500.

Altounyan, Ernest H. R. "Blood Group Percentages for Arabs, Armenians and Jews." *British Medical* Journal (1928): 546.

Amano, K. "On the Blood-types of base-ball players." *Taiwan Igakkai Zasshi* 33 (1934): 5–6.

W. H. Schneider, *Blood Groups and Human Heredity, 1900–1950*, Medicine and Biomedical Sciences in Modern History, https://doi.org/10.1007/978-3-031-69844-6

Amzel, Rose and Wanda Halber. "Ueber das Ergebnis der Wassermanschen Reaktion innerhalbe verschiedener Blutgruppen." *Zeitschrft für Immunitätsforschung* 42 (1925): 89–98.

Amzel, Rose. "Distribution de l'élement M du sang dans la population polonaise." *Comptes rendus de la Société de biologie*, 104 (1930): 1083.

Apert, Eugène. *Traité des maladies familiales et afflictions congénnitales and Hérédité morbide*. Paris: Flammarion, 1920.

Avdeeva and Gritsevich. "[On the question of isohemagglutination in humans]," *Biulletin' Moskovskogo obshchestva ispytatelei prirody* 1 (1924): 108.

Bais W. J. and A. W. Verhoef. "Het verschijnsel der isohaemagglutinatie en de anthropologische Beteekenis Daarvan [anthropological blood studies of different races in Dutch East Indies]." *Geneeskundig Tijdschrift voor Nederlandsch-Indië* 68 (1924a): 1212–31.

Bais W. J. and A. W. Verhoef. "On the Biochemical Racial Index of Various Races in the E. Indian Archipeligo." *Journal of Immunology* 9 (1924b): 383–6.

Barinstein, L. A. [Die Bluttransfusion im Lichte gegenwartiger Kenntnisse]. *Sovremennye meditsina* 2 (1924): 39.

Basu, M. N. "Blood groups of Noluas of Bengal." *Nature* 141 (1938): 649.

Bateson, William. *Mendel's Principles of Heredity*. London: Constable & Co., 1929.

Baur, Erwin, Eugen Fischer, and Fritz Lenz. *Human Heredity*. New York: Macmillan, 1931.

Bay-Schmith, Erik. "Racebiologiske Undersogelser i Gronland [race biology research in Greenland]." *Ugeskrift for Laeger* 88 (1926): 880–2.

Beneke, Wilhelm. *Die anatomische Grundlagen der Constitutionsanomalien des Menschen*. Marburg: Elwert 1878.

Beneke, Wilhelm. *Constitution und constitutionelles Kranksein des Menschen*. Marburg: Elwert 1881.

Bernhart, Helmut. "Beitrag zur Blutgruppengeographie Gross-Deutschlands." *Zeitschrift für Hygiene und Infektionskrankheiten* 123 (1942): 675–7.

Bernstein, Felix. "Ergebnisse einem biostatistischen zusammenfassenden Betrachtung über die erblichen Blutstrukturen des Menschen." *Klinische Wochenschrift* 3 (1924):1495–7.

Bernstein, Felix. "Zusammenfassende Betrachtungen über die erblichen Blutstrukturen des Menschen." *Zeitschrift für induktive- Abstammungs und Vererbungslehre* 37 (1925): 237–70.

Bijlmer, Hendricus J. T. "Bloedgroepenonderzoek in de Molukken." *Geneeskundig Tijdschrift voor Nederlandsch-Indië* 71 (1931): 1479–85.

Bijlmer, Hendricus J. T. "Contribution to the Anthropology of the Netherlands, including the further elaboration of the Blood Group Research in Holland commenced in 1926 by the late M. A. Van Herweden." *Koninklijke Akademie van Wettenschappen. Amsterdam. Proceedings of the Section of Sciences* 43 (1940): 113–39.

Bijlmer, Hendricus J. T. "Relation of Blood Groups to race and Some Particulars of the SW Pacific." *Journal of the Royal Anthropological Institute*, 65 (1935): 123–31.

Billing, Edward. "Racial Origins from Blood Grouping, *British Medical Journal* (Sept. 30, 1939): 712.

"Blood Group of Diplomats." *Journal of Heredity*, 28 (1937): 221.

Böhmer, Kurt. "Blutruppen und Kriminalistik." *Forschungen und Fortschritte* 3 (1927a): 142.

Böhmer, Kurt. "Blutgruppen und Verbrecher." *Deutsche Zeitschrift für die gesamte gerichtliche Medizin*, 9 (1927b), 426–30.

Bordet, Jules "Le mécanisme de l'agglutination." *Annales de l'Institut Pasteur* 13 (1899): 225–50.

Borgman, Christine L. ed. *Scholarly Communication and Bibliometrics*. Newbury Park, CA: Sage, 1990.

Bouchet, Nadia du. "Interagglutination positive malgré l'identité des groupes entre le sang de la mére et du nouveau-né." *Comptes-rendus de la Société de Biologie* 94 (1926): 16–17.

Boyd, William C. "Blood Groups." *Tabulae Biologicae* 17, no. 2 (1939): 113–240.

Boyd, William C. "Three Nomograms for Testing Agreement of Blood Grouping Data with Theories of Inheritance." *Annals of Eugenics* 8 (1937–1938): 337–42.

Boyd, William C. and Lyle G. Boyd. "An Attempt to Determine the Blood Groups of Mummies." *Proceedings of the Society for Experimental Biology* 31 (1934): 671–2.

Boyd William C. and Lyle G. Boyd. "Blood Grouping by Means of Preserved Muscle." *Science* 78 (1933): 578.

Brennecke, Hans. "Die Erforschung der Personlichkeit des Gefangenen; ihre Methode und ihre Auswirkung im Strafvollzug." *Monatschrift für Kriminologie* 21 (1930):655–8.

Buchanan, J. Arthur and Edith T. Higley. "Relationship of Blood Groups to Disease." *British Journal of Experimental Pathology* 2 (1921): 247–55.

Buining, D. J. "Recherches sur les groupes sanguin au Indes neerlandaises." *Anthropologie* 43 (1933):289–312.

Buining, D. J. "De techniek der bloedgroepdiagnostiek in Nederlandsch-Indië." *Geneeskundig Tijdschrift voor Nederlandsch-Indië* 71 (1931): 755–60.

Bunak, Victor V. [on agglutination reaction of human races]. *Ruskii Antropologicheskii Zhurnal* 13 (1924): 115–9.

Bunak, Victor V. "Einige Daten uber die Isohamagglutination bei verschiedenen asiatischen Stammen." *Archiv für Rassen- und Gesellschaftsbiologie* 17 (1925): 316–8.

Bunker, H.A. and S. Meyers. "Blood Groups in General Paralysis. A Study of Agglutinin-Agglutinogen Reactions in 91 Cases." *Journal of Laboratory and Clinical Medicine* 12 (1928): 415–26.

Cabrera, Cristina and Herbert W. Wade. "On Iso-agglutination Group Percentages in Filipino Blood." *Journal of the Philippine Islands Medical Association* 1 (1921): 100–2.

Camus, Jean and Philippe Pagniez. "D'un pouvoir aggliutinant de certains serums humains pour les globules rouges de l'homme normal." *Comptes rendus de la Société de Biologie* [hereafter cited as *Comptes rendus de la Société de biologie* (1901) 242–4.

Candela, P. B. "Blood Group Reactions in Ancient Human Skeletons." *American Journal of Physical Anthropology* 21 (1936): 429–32.

Canuto, Giorgio. "Distribuzione dei Gruppi Sanguigni nei Criminali Piemontesi." *Archivio di Antropologia Criminale* 48 (1928): 687–704.

Chaudhuri, A. "Blood groups and heredity." *Indian Medical Gazette* 66 (1931): 193–5.

Cleland, John B. "Blood Grouping of Australian Aboriginals." *Australian Journal of Experimental Biology and Medical Science* 3 (1926): 33–5.

Coca Arthur F. and Olin Diebert. "A Study of the Occurrence of the Blood Groups among American Indians." *Journal of Immunology* 8 (1923): 487–91.

Coca Arthur F. and Ella Grove. "The Value of Blood Groups to the Study of Race." *Eugenical News* 11 (1926), 89–91.

Chominskii B. N. and L. S. Schustova. "Zur Frage des Zusammenhangs zwischen Blutgruppe und psychischer Erkrankung." *Zeitschrift für die gesamte Neurologie und Psychiatrie* 115 (1928): 303–8.

"Collective Surgical Experiences at the Front and at the Base." In *The Medical Department of the United States Army in the World War*, vol. IX Surgery, 130–65. Washington: Government Printing Office, 1927.

Connerth, O. "Uber Blutgruppen bei Tuberkulose." *Zeitschrift für Tuberkulose* 48 (1927): 140–2.

Coon, Carleton Stevens. *Tribes of the Rif.* Cambridge: Harvard African Studies, 1931.

Crabtree, E.G. "Blood Transfusion in War Surgery in the British Army." *Boston medical and Surgical Journal* 181 (July 17, 1919): 60–3.

Culpepper William L. and Marjorie Ableson. "Report on Five Thousand Bloods Typed using Moss's Grouping." *Journal of Laboratory and Clinical M*edicine 6 (1921), 276–83.

Cuboni, Ettore. "Contributo Allo Studio Della Distribuzione dei Gruppi Sanguigni in Italia." *Bollettino dell'Instituto Sieroterapico Milanese* 7 (1928): 153–60.

Dahr, Peter. "Blutgruppenforschung und Rassenhygiene." *Ziel und Weg* 9 (1939): 98–108.

Dahr, Peter. "Menschlichen Blutgruppen, -Untergruppen, und -Faktoren." *Volk und Rasse* 15 (1940): 13–20.

Decastello, Alfred von and Adriano Sturli. "Ueber die Isoagglutinine im Serum gesunder und kranker Menschen." *Münchener medizinische Wochenschrift* 49 (1902): 1990–5.

Diamond, Louis K., Kenneth D. Blackfan, and James M. Baty. "Erythroblastosis fetalis and its association with universal edema of the fetus, icterus gravis neonatorum and anemia of the newborn." *Journal of Pediatrics* 1 (1932): 269–309.

D'Onofrio, Francesco. "Rapportio fra carattere ereditario gruppo sanguigno ed adenoidismo." *Archivio Italiana di Otologia, Rinologia e Laringologia* 37 (1926): 209–15.

Dossena, Gaetano and Vincenzo Lancara. "L'Isoagglutinazione studiata nei riguardi dell'abito morfologico e delle neoplasie della sfera genitale muliebre." *Annali di ostetricia e ginecologia* 47 (1925):163–79.

Douris, Roger. "Applications médico-legales des groupes sanguins humains. *Bulletin des sciences pharmacologiques* 30 (1923): 90–107.

Dujarric de la Rivière, Rene and Nicholas Kossovitch. "Dix années de fonctionnement d'un 'Centre d'études des groupes sanguins.'" *Bulletin de l'Academie de Médecine* 121 (1939): 487–94.

Dujarric de la Rivière, Rene and Nicholas Kossovitch. "La question des groupes sanguins en médecine legale." *Annales de médecine legale*, 7 (1927a): 390–400.

Dujarric de la Rivière, Rene and Nicholas Kossovitch "Recherches sur les groupes sanguins." *Annales de l'Institut Pasteur*, 45 (1930): 107–53.

Dujarric de la Rivière, Rene and Nicholas Kossovitch "Au sujet des groups sanguins des tuberculeux et des cancereux." *Comptes rendus de la Société de biologie*, 97 (1927b):137–9.

Dungern, Emil Von and Ludwik Hirszfeld. "Uber Nachweis und Vererbung biochemischer Strukturen. I," "Uber Vererbung gruppenspezifischer Strukturen des Blutes. II," "Uber gruppenspezifische Strukturen des Blutes. III." *Zeitschrift für Immunitätsforschung* 4 (1910): 531–46; 6(1910): 284–92; and 8 (1911): 526–62.

Duvoir, M. "Le problème de la paternité." *La médecine* 5 (1924): 511–3.

Dyke, Sydney C. "On Blood Grouping and Its Clinical Applications." *Lancet* 202 (1922a): 579–82.

Dyke, Sydney C. "On the Medico-legal Importance of the Blood Groups." *Lancet* 203 (1922b): 1271–3.

Dykhno, M. "[On the constitutional meaning of isoagglutination indices of human blood]." *Nauchnye izvestiia Smolenskogo Universiteta* 3 (1926): 93.

Eisenberg, Alexander. "Zur Frage nach den Isoagglutinationsgruppen des Blutes bei Menschen." *Folia Haematologica*, 36 (1928), 336.

Elsdon-Dew, Ronald. "Blood Groups in Africa." *Publications of the South African Institute for Medical Research* 9 (1939): 29–94.

Elsdon-Dew, Ronald. "Serological Differences between Various Groups of the Bantu of Southern Africa." *Bantu Studies* 8 (1934): 361–6.

Emile-Weil, Prosper and M. Lamy. "Sur une cause d'erreur dans la détermination des groupes sanguins due au vielleissement des sérums-étalons." *Bulletins et memoires de la société médicale des hôpitaux de Paris* 48 (1924): 859–61.

Epstein, Reuben and Albert E. Ottenberg. "A Simple Method of Performing Serum Reactions." *Transactions of the New York Pathological Society* 8(1908): 117–23.

Macfarlane, Eileen W. Erlanson. "Eastern Himalayan Blood-Groups." *Man* 37 (1937):127–9.

Eyer, Hermann. "Ein einfaches Verfahren zur Steigerung der Sicherheit von Blutgruppenbestimmungen bei Massenuntersuchungen." *Deutsche Militärarzt* 4 (1939): 271–3.

Fabricius-Hansen, Vibeke. "Blood Groups and MN-Types of Eskimos in East Greenland." *Journal of Immunology* 36 (1939): 523–30.

Fabricius-Hansen, Vibeke. "Blood Type Determinations in the Southern Districts of Julianschaab, West Greenland (ABO and MN System)." *Journal of Immunology* 37 (1940): 497–9.

Feldman and Elmanovich. "Agglutinierende Eigenschaften des Blutes der Geisteskranken." *Mediko-biologicheskii zhurnal* 1 (1925): 125.

Ferraro, Filippo. "[Studies Regarding Blood Groups in Infancy]." *Rivista di clinica pediatria* 24 (1926): 758.

Fischmann, R. M. "[Isohemagglutination and constitution among workers in Petrovsky factory]." *Dnepro-Petrovsk. Med. Journ* (1929): 33.

Fisher R. A. and G. L. Taylor. "Blood Groups in Britain." *British Medical Journal* (Oct. 21, 1939): 826.

Flexner, Abraham. *Medical Education in Europe*. New York: Carnegie Foundation, 1912.

Flu, P. C. "Medical Science." In *Science in the Netherlands East Indies*, edited by L. M. R. Rutten, 207–25. Amsterdam: Royal Academy of Sciences, 1927.

Foerster, Augustin. "Blutgruppen und Verbrecher." *Deutsche Zeitschrift für die gesamte gerichtliche Medizin* 11 (1928): 487–90.

Folomina, W. "Isohämagglutinationsgruppen bei Verbrechern." *Archiv Kriminologii i sudebnnoi meditsiny* 84 (1927): 145–8.

Friedenreich, Viggo. "Blood Groups and Genetics." *Annals of Eugenics* 8 (1937–1938): 152–65.

Friedenreich, Viggo and A. Zacho. "Die Differentialdiagnose zwischen den 'Unter'- Gruppen A1 und A2." *Zeitschrift für Rassenphysiologie* 4 (1931):164–91.

Friedmann, L. M. "Die Blutgruppen grusinischer Kinder und der Zusammenhang des Gruppenmermals mit anderen erblichen Merkmale." Ukrainisches *Zentralblatt für Blutgruppenforschung* 4 (1930): 279–89.

Fukamachi, Hozumi, "On the Biochemical Race Index of Koreans, Manchus and Japanese." *Journal of Immunology* 8 (1923): 291–4.

Furuhata, Tanemoto. "On the Heredity of the Blood Group and its Application in Forensic Medicine." *Vancouver Medical Association Bulletin* 9 (1933): 203–13.
Furuhata, Tanemoto. [Japanese and Ainu considered from the serological standpoint]. *Nippon Gakujitsu Kyokwai Zasschi* (1925), 1.
Furuhata, Tanemoto. "Japanese Literature on Isohemagglutination." *Japan Medical World* 8 (1928a): 321–4.
Furuhata, Tanemoto. "Study of the Geographical Distribution of Blood Groups of the Japanese." *Japan Medical World* 8 (1928b): 119.
Furuhata, Tanemoto, Kenkichi Ichida, and Takayoshi Kishi. [no title] *Nippon Gakujutsu Kyokai Hokoku*, 1 (1925): 314–25.
Furuhata, Tanemoto and Takayoshi Kishi. "On the Biological Racial-Index of the Japanese in the Hokiru District." *Journal of Immunology* 12 (1926): 83–9.
Furuhata, Tanemoto and Takayoshi Kishi. "Study of the Ainu Race from a Serological Standpoint." *Japan Medical World*, 8 (1928): 91–4.
Furuichi, T. "On the Heredity of Group Specific Characteristics of Human Blood." *Taiwan Igakkai Zasshi* 24 (1925): 581–90.
Furukawa, Takeji. "Erforschung der Temperamente mittels der experimentellen Blutgruppenuntersuchung." *Zeitschrift für angewandte Psychologie und Charakterkunde,* 31 (1928), 271–99.
Furukawa, Takeji. "A Study of Temperament and Blood Groups." *Journal of Social Psychology* 1 (1930): 494–508.
Furst, Th. "Reactiones Differenciales Biologicas de la Sangre y su Empleo enla Biologia Racial y el Studio de la Constitucion." *Revista de Medicina* 12 (1924): 78.
Gaetano, Raffaele. "La distribuzione dei gruppi sanguigni nella provincia di Napoli." *Terapia* 21 (1931): 135–40.
Galton, Francis. *Natural Inheritance.* London: Macmillan, 1889.
Gates, R. R. "Blood groups of Canadian Indians and Eskimos." *American Journal of Physical Anthropology* 12 (1929): 475–85.
Gates, R. R. *Heredity in Man.* London: Macmillan, 1930.
Gesselevic, A. M. "Zur Frage der Konstitution und der Hämagglutinationsgruppen des Blutes." *Ukrainische Zentralblatt für Blutgruppenforschung* 2 (1928): 5–23.
Gesselevic, A. M. "Die Korrelation zwischen den Körperbautypen und den Blutgruppen und ihre graphische Darstellung." *Zeitschrift für Konstitutionslehre* 17 (1932): 199–202.
Giroud, Georges. "Groupes sanguins." *Presse médicale* 27 (1919), 21–2.
Godoy, Oscar Pereira. "Grupos sanguineos nos criminosos de Sao Paolo." *Archivos da sociedad de medecina legal e criminologia de Sao Paolo* 8 (1938): 185–91.
Goebbers, Karl H. "Blutgruppe und Typus." *Zeitschrift für angewandte Psychologie und Charakterkunde* 53 (1937): 19–47.
Goldstein, Marco. "La ripartizione dei gruppi sanguigni fra gli individui affetti da carcinoma." *Bollettino dell'Instituto Sieroterapico Milanese* 8 (1929), 293–6.

Goring, Charles B. *The English Convict: A Statistical Study* London: HMSO, 1913.

Grove, Ella F. "On the Value of the Blood-group Relationship as a Means of Determining Racial Relationship." *Journal of Immunology* 12 (1926): 251–62.

Guillot, Maurice, Georges Dehelly, and Louis Morel. *La transfusion du sang*. Paris: A. Maloine, 1917.

Gundel, Max. "Einige Beobachtungen bei der rassenbiologischen Durchforschung Schleswig-Holsteins." *Klinische* Wochenschrift, 5 (1926a): 1186.

Gundel, Max. "Bestehen Zusammenhänge zwischen Blutgruppen und Luesdisposition sowie zwischen Blutgruppe und Erfolg der Luestherapie?" *Klinische Wochenschrift* 6 (1927): 1703–5.

Gundel, Max. "Blutgruppen bei Strafgefangenen." *Deutsche Zeitschrift für die gesamte gerichtliche Medizin* 11 (1928): 100.

Gundel, Max. "Rassenbiologische Untersuchungen an Strafangefangenen. *Klinische Wochenschrift* 5 (1926b): 2165–66.

Guthrie, Charles G. and John G. Huck. "On the Existence of More than Four Isoagglutinin Groups in Human Blood." *Bulletin of the Johns Hopkins Hospital*, 34 (1923): 37–48.

Halber, Wanda and J. Mydlarski. "Recherches sero-anthropologiques en Pologne." *Comptes rendus de la Société de biologie*, 89 (1923): 1373–5.

Halber, Wanda and Jan Mydlarski. "Untersuchung uber die Blutgruppen in Polen." *Zeitschrift für Immunitätsforschung*, 43 (1925): 470–84.

Haldane, J.B.S. "Prehistory in the Light of Genetics." *Proceedings of the Royal Institution of Great Britain* 26 (1931): 355–71.

Hansen, Soren. "Methodologisches uber Blutgruppenforschung durch Massenuntersuchungen." *Zeitschrift fur Rassenphysiologie* 2 (1929): 73–7.

Happ, William M. "Appearance of Isoagglutinins in infants and Children." *Journal of Experimental Medicine* 31 (1920): 313–34.

Hara, R. and S. Kobayashi. [no title]. *Iji-Shinbun*, no. 954 (1916): 937.

Hartmann, Otto, Kare Hadland, and Chr. Juel Bjerkelund. "Blood Group Distribution in Norway." *Avhandlinger utgitt av Det Norske Videnskaps-Akademi i Oslo* 5 (1940): 14–41.

Heinbecker, Peter and Ruth Pauli. "Blood Groups of the Polar Eskimo." *Journal of Immunology* 13 (1927): 279–83.

Hering, Olga. "Untersuchungen über Zusammenhänge zwischen den 4 klassischen Blutgruppenin. Verbindung mit den Blutkörpercheneigenschaften M und N und psychopathischer Veranlangung." *Zeitschrift für die gesamte experimentelle Medizin* 99 (1936): 547–56.

Hers, Floris, Marianne Van Herwerden, and Th. J. Boele-Nijland. "Bloodgroup Investigation in the 'Hoeksche Waard.'" *Koninklijke Akademie van Wettenschappen. Amsterdam. Proceedings of the Section of Sciences* 36 (1933): 849–61.

Herwerden, Marianne van. *Erfelijkheid bij den mensch en eugenetiek.* Amsterdam: Wereldbibliotheek, 1926a.

Herwerden, Marianne van. "Groupes sanguins en Hollande." In *Institut International d'Anthropologie, 3e Congrès, Amsterdam, Sept.1927,* 456–60. Paris: Noury, 1928.

Herwerden, Marianne van. "De Verdeeling der Menschheid in Bloedgroepen [subdivision of humanity according to blood groups]." *Mensch en Maatschappij* 2 (1926b): 257–69.

Herwerden, Marianne Van and Th. Y. Boele-Nyland. "Investigation of Blood groups in Holland." *Koninklijke Akademie van Wettenschappen. Amsterdam. Proceedings of the Section of Sciences* 33 (1930): 659–73, reprinted in *Archiv für Rassen- und Gesellschafts-Biologie* 24 (1930): 198–207.

Hesch, Michael. "Die gesamte Schrifttum der Blutgruppenforschung in der drei ersten Jahrzehnten ihrer Entwicklung, 1901–1931. In *Handbuch der Blutgruppenkunde,* edited by Paul Steffan, 539–645. Munich: Lehmans Verlag, 1932a.

Hesch, Michael. "Papillarmuster bei Eingeborenen der Loyalty-Inseln. Beziehungen zwischen Papillarmustern und Blutgruppen." *Zeitschrift für Rassenphysiologie* 5 (1932b): 163–8.

Hesch, Michael and Günther Spannaus, eds. *Kultur und Rasse.* Munich: Lehmanns Verlag, 1939.

Hilgermann, R. and H. Birnbaum, "Die Blutkörpercheneigenschaften M und N in Verbindung mit den 4 Blutgruppen in ihrer Beziehung zu Geisteskrankheiten." *Zeitschrift für die gesamte experimentelle Medizin* 94 (1934): 722–5.

Hirschfeld, Hans and Anton Hittmair. "Über Blutgruppenbestimmungen bei Krebskranken." *Medizinische Klinik,* 22 (1926): 1494–6.

Hirszfeld, Hannah, Ludwik Hirszfeld, and Henryk Brokman. "Etude sur l'hérédité en rapport avec la sensibilité `a la diphtherie." *Comptes rendus de la Société de biologie* 90 (1924a): 1198–1200.

Hirszfeld, Ludwik, *Les groupes sanguins: leurs applications à la biologie, à la medicine et au droit,* trans. by Hanna Hirszfeld (Paris: Masson, 1938).

Hirszfeld, Ludwik. *Konstitutionsserologie und Blutgruppenforschung.* Berlin: Springer Verlag, 1928.

Hirszfeld, Ludwik and Roza Amzel. « Sur la presence des elements de groupe du foetus dans le sang retroplacentaire de la mere,.» *Comptes rendus de la Société de Biologie* 109 (1932): 252–3.

Hirszfeld, Ludwik and Hannah Hirszfeld. " Serological Differences Between the Blood of Different Races." *Lancet* 194 (1919): 675–9.

Hirszfeld, Ludwik, Hannah Hirszfeld, and Henryk Brokman. "On the Susceptibility to Diphtheria (Schick Test Positive) with Reference to the Inheritance of Blood Groups." *Journal of Immunology* 9 (1924b): 571–91.

Hirszfeld, Ludwik and H. Zborowski. "Sur la permeabilité elective du placenta en rapport avec le groupe sanguin de la mére et la foetus." *Comptes rendus de la Société de biologie* 92 (1925): 1253–5.

Hogben, Lancelot. *Genetic Principles in Medicine and Social Science*. London: 1931.

Hollo, Julius and Wilhelm Léonard. "Gibt es einen Unterschied in der Häufigkeit der einzelnen Blutgruppen bei Lungentuberkulösen und bei gesunden Menschen?" *Beiträge zur Klinik der Tuberkulose* 64 (1926): 513–4.

Hooten, Ernest A. *The American Criminal: An Anthropological Study*. Cambridge: Harvard University Press, 1939a.

Hooten, Ernest A. *Crime and the Man*. Cambridge: Harvard University Press, 1939b.

Hornung, H. "Uber die Beziehung der Blutgruppen zu rassischen Merkmalen." *Münchener Medizinische Wochenschrift* 87 (1940): 125–8.

Howells, William W. "Anthropometry and Blood Types in Fiji and the Soloman Islands." *Anthropological Papers of the American Museum of Natural History* 33 (1933): 283–339.

Hoyos Sainz, Luis de. "Contribución al estudio seroanthopológico de Espana." *Institut International d'anthropologie, Lisbon, Sept. 1930* (1930): 553–60.

Ihara, Yoshisada and Mototoshi Yanagihashi. "Ueber Krankheitsdisposition und Isohamagglutination." *Zeitschrift für Rassenphysiologie* 2 (1929): 32–8.

"Isoagglutination. Recommendation that the Jansky Classification be Adopted for Universal use." *JAMA* 76 (1921): 130.

Jacobsohn, Hans. "Uber die Blutgruppenzughörigkeit der Paralytiker." *Zeitschrift für die gesamte Neurologie und Psychologie* 105 (1926): 810–4.

Jansky, Jan. "Haematologicke studie u. psychotiku." *Sbornik Klinicky* 8 (1907): 85–139.

Jeanbrau, Emile. "Comment, en dehors des cas d'extrême urgence, choisir un donneur pour la transfusion du sang?" *Clinique* 21 (1926): 141–4.

Jeanbrau, Emile. "Une technique simple de transfusion." *Montpélier Médical* 39 (1917): 1142.

Jeanbrau, Emile. "Technique simple de tranfusion du sang stabilisé par le citrate de soude." *Presse médicale* 26 (1918), 58–62.

Jeanbrau, Emile. "Transfusion Sanguine." *Congrès français de chirurgie. XXXII. Paris (8 octobre 1923) Procès-verbaux, mémoires et discussions* (Paris, 1923), 32:116.

Jeanbrau, Emile and George Giroud. "Accidents de transfusion et moyens de les éviter." *Journal médicale française* 8 (1919), 203–9.

Jeney, A. von. "Rassenbiologische Untersuchungen in Ungarn." *Deutsche medizinische Wochenschrift* 49 (1923): 546–7.

Jettmar, H. M. "Biochemical Race Index of Mongols." *National Medical Journal of China* 14 (1928): 20–1.

Jettmar, H. M. "Blutgruppenuntersuchungen in der NordostMongolei und der Mandschuriei." *Mitteilungen der anthropologischen Gesellschaft in Wien* 60 (1930): 39–47.

Johannsen, Erik W. "Classement de sujets affectés de tumeurs malignes selon les iso-agglutinines de leur sang." *Comptes rendus de la Société de biologie* 92 (1925): 112–15.

Johannsen, Erik W.. "Classification of Cancer Patients according to their blood groups and some Investigations concerning Isohemagglutination." *Acta Pathologica et microbiologica Scandinavica* 4 (1927a): 175–97.

Johannsen, Erik W. "Nogle studier over de menneskelige isohaemagglutininer med soerligt henblick paa forholdene ved kraeft." *Bibliotek for Laeger* 119 (1927b): 42–7.

Karsner, Howard T. "Transfusion with Tested Bloods." *JAMA* 70 (1918): 769–71.

Kennedy, James A. "Blood Group Classifications Used in Hospitals in the United States and Canada." *JAMA* 92 (1929): 614–5.

Kilgore, Alson R. and J. Heng Liu. "Iso-agglutination Tests of Chinese Bloods for Transfusion Compatibility." *China Medical Journal* 32 (1918): 21.

Kirihara, Shinichi. "Uber die Isohämagglutination beim menschlichen Blute." *Zeitschrift für klinische Medizin* 99 (1924): 530.

Kirihara, Shinichi and Rinsai Haku. [On the differences of the percentages of the blood types of the Japanese and the Koreans and on the heredity of blood grouping specificity], Chosen Igakkai Zasshi [as abstracted in *Japan Medical World* 3 (1923): 59].

Kishi, Takayoshi. "On the Biochemical Racial index of the Ainu, Gilyak and Orokko in Karafu." *Journal of Immunology* 12(1926): 91–6.

Klein, Wilhelm and H. Osthoff. "Haemagglutinine, Rasse- und anthropologische Merkmale." *Archiv für Rassen- und Gesellschafts-Biologie* 17 (1925): 371–8.

Kobayasi, Takehito. [On the blood groups of Korean schoolboys and schoolgirls]. *Chiba Igakkai Zasshi* 16 (1938), 8–9.

Koenig, E. *Bibliography on Blood Transfusion.* Leningrad: Vestnik Chirurguii and Research Institute of Blood Transfusion in Leningrad, 1935.

Koltsov, Nikolai K. [the agglutination of human blood]. *Uspechi Experimentalnoi Biologii*, (1922).

Kossovitch, Nicholas and Fernand Benoit. "Contribution à l'étude anthropologique et sérologique des juifs modernes." *Revue anthropologique* 42 (1932a): 99–125.

Kossovitch, Nicholas and Fernand Benoit. "Contribution à l'étude des indigènes du Maroc." *Revue anthropologique*, 43 (1933): 318–48.

Kossovitch, Nicholas and Fernand Benoit. "Les groupes sanguins chez les Berberophones." *Comptes rendus de la Société de biologie* 109 (1932b): 198–200.

Kretschmer, Ernst. *Physique and Character.* New York: Harcourt, Brace, 1925.

Kroeber, Alfred. "Blood Group Classifications." *American Journal of Physical Anthropology* 18 (1934): 377–94.

Kushigemachi, Kenichi and Kengo Hamada. "Blood Groups of inhabitants of Kumamoto prefecture; relations to temperaments or some vocations." *Kumamoto Igakkai Zasshi* [Journal of the Kumamoto Medical Society] 8 (1932) 5–6.

Laffont, Amédée and Émile Gaujoux. "Recherches sur l'agglutination des globules sanguins avec le sérum maternal et foetal." *Comptes rendus de la Société de biologie* 88 (1923): 730–1.

Landsteiner, Karl. "Zur Kenntnis der antifermentativen lytischen und aglutinierenden Wirkungen des Blutsera und der Lympho." *Centrallblatt für Bakteriologie* 27 (1900): 361.

Landsteiner, Karl. "Ueber Agglutinationserscheinungen normalen menschlichen Blutes." *Wiener klinische Wochenschrift* 14 (1901): 1134.

Landsteiner, Karl and Philip Levine. "A New Agglutinable Factor Differentiating Individual Human Bloods." *Proceedings of the Society for Experimental Biology and Medicine* 24 (1927a): 600–02.

Landsteiner, Karl and Philip Levine. "Further Observations on Individual Differences of Human Blood." *Proceedings of the Society for Experimental Biology and Medicine 24 (1927b):* 941–2.

Landsteiner, Karl and Philip Levine. "On the Racial Distribution of Some Agglutinable Structures of Human Blood." *Journal of Immunology* 16 (1929): 123–31.

Landsteiner, Karl and C. P. Miller. "Serological Studies on the Blood of the Primates." *Journal of Experimental Medicine* 42 (1925): 841–52; 853–72.

Landsteiner, Karl and Max Richter. "Ueber die Verwertbarkeit individueller Blutdifferenzen für die forenzische Praxis." *Zeitschrift für Medizinbeamten* 16 (1903): 85–9.

Landsteiner, Karl and Alexander S. Wiener. "Studies on an Agglutinogen (Rh) in Human Blood Reacting with Anti-Rhesus Sera and with Human Isoantibodies." *Journal of Experimental Medicine* 74 (1941): 309–20.

Lange, Johannes. *Verbrechen als Schicksal. Studien an kriminellen Zwillingen.* Leipzig 1929.

League of Nations. Permanent Commission on Biological Standardisation, *Report of the Permanent Commission on Standardisation of Sera, Serological Reactions, and Biological Products (Frankfurt, April 25–28, 1928)* (Geneva, 1928).

Lee, Roger I. "A Simple and Rapid Method for the Selection of Donors." *British Medical Journal* (1917): 683–84.

Lehmann, Julius Friedrich. *Fünfzig Jahre: J. F. Lehmanns Verlag, 1890–1940.* Munich: Lehmanns, 1940.

Lemke, Charlotte. "Kommen bei den Asthetikern und Tuberkulösen einzelne Blutgruppen besonders häufig vor?" *Zeitschrift für die gesamte Anatomie* 14 (1928): 333–46.

Levine, Philip. "Studies in Specific Hypersensitiveness." *Journal of Immunology* 11 (1926): 283–90.

Levine, Philip L. Burnham, E.M. Katzin, and P. Vogel. "The Role of Isoimmunization in the Pathogenesis of Erythroblastosis Fetalis." *American Journal of Obstetrics and Gynecology* 42 (1941): 925–37.

Levine, Philip and Rufus E. Stetson. "An Unusual Case of Intra-Group Agglutination." *JAMA* 113 (1939): 126–7.

Lewis, Julian and Deborah L. Henderson. "Racial Distribution of Isohemagglutinin Groups." *JAMA* 79 (1922): 1422–4.

Liang, Backiang. "Blutgruppen in Kanton." *Münchener medizinische Wochenschrift* 76 (1929): 1466–7.

Lisunova, A. "Gruppovaya gemoagglyutinatsiya i malyariya [Hemoagglutination groups and malaria]." Trudy 3-go vseross *Syezd malyar Moskva* (1925): 173.

Ljachovetskii, A. M. [The importance of hemo-agglutination in malaria]. *Moskovskii meditsinskii zhurnal* 4 (1924): 25–36.

Macfarlane, Eileen. "Blood-group Distribution in India with Special Reference to Bengal." *Journal of Genetics* 36 (1938): 225–37.

Maderna, Candido. "Sifilide e gruppi sanguigni." *Riforma medica* 53 (1937): 527–9.

Madsen, Th., E. T. Engle, Claus Jensen, and I. B. Freuchen. "Blood Groups and Poliomyelitis: Report based on 1118 Cases in the 1934 Epidemic in Denmark." *Journal of Immunology* 30 (1936): 213–9.

Majumdar, D. N. "Blood Groups of the Doms." *Current Science* 11 (1942): 153–4.

Malone R. H. and M. N. Lahiri. "Distribution of the Blood Groups in Certain Races and Castes of India." *Indian Journal of Medical Research*, 16 (1929): 963–4.

Manuila, Sabin. "Recherches sero-anthropologiques sur les races en Roumanie par la methode de l'isohemagglutination." *Comptes rendus de la Société de biologie* 90 (1924), 1071–3.

Maryuma, Yoshito and T. Wakeshima. "Blood groups of Formosan savages." *Taiwan Igakkai Zasshi* 30 (1931): 35.

Maruyama, Yoshito. "Blood Groups in relation to dental caries." *Taiwan Igakkai Zasshi* 32 (1933): 88.

Matson, Gustave Albin. "A procedure for Determining Distribution of Blood Groups in Mummies." *Proceedings of the Society for Experimental Biology and Medicine* 31 (1934): 964–8.

Matson, Gustave Albin. "Unexpected Differences in Distribution of Blood Groups among American Indians." *Proceedings of the Society for Experimental Biology and Medicine* 30 (1933): 1380–2.

McQuarrie, Irvine. "Isoaaglutination in new-born infants and their mothers: a possible relation between interagglutination and the toxemia of pregnancy." *Bulletin of Johns Hopkins Hosptial* 34 (1923): 51–9.
Meyer, Fr. "Blutgruppenverteilung in der schlesichen Bevolkerung sowie die Beziehung der Blutgruppen zu Geisteskranken." *Deutsche medizinische Wochenschrift* 54 (1928): 1461.
Michon, Paul. *Les groupes sanguins: Schémas d'application*. Paris: Masson, 1930.
Michon, Paul. "Sur les variations quantitatives de l'isohemagglutination et les infractions aux schémas de Moss." *Comptes rendus de la Société de biologie* 92 (1925), 37–9.
Mitra, P. N. "Influence of Blood group in certain pathological states." *Indian Journal of Medical Research* 20 (1933): 995–1004.
"Mitgliederverzeichnis." *Zeitschrift für Rassenphysiologie* 2 (1930): 193–6.
"Mitteilungen des Vorstandes der Deutschen Gesellschaft für Blutgruppenforschung." *Zeitschrift für Rassenphysiologie* 1 (1928): 65
Miyamura, Kaoru. "Uber die Bedeutung der Blutgruppen im Gebiete der Dermatologie." *Japanese Journal of Dermatology and Urology* 30 (1930): 53.
Moffitt, George R., George F. Klugh, and Chester E. Shepard. "Blood Type Classification, with a Slight Modification of Technic: Report of the Results of More than a Thousand Tests." *JAMA* 73 (1919): 1821–2.
Montenegro, Joao. "Classifiaccao e transfusaio do sangue." *Brasil Medico* 1 (1925): 109–13.
Moss, William L. "A Simplified Method for Determining the Isoagglutinin in Group in the Selection of Donors for Blood Transfusion." *JAMA* 68 (1917):1905–6.
Moss, William L. "Studies in Isoagglutinins and Isohemolysis." *Bulletin of the Johns Hopkins Hospital* 21 (1910): 63–70.
Moss, William L. and James A. Kennedy. "Blood Groups in Peru, Santo Domingo, Yucatan and Among the Mexicans at the Blue Ridge Prison Farm in Texas." *Journal of Immunology* 16 (1929): 159–74.
Mouzon, J. "Recherches récentes sur les groupes sanguins." *Presse médicale* 31 (1923): 541–3.
Mrugowsky, J. and H. Bernhart. "Die Ausführung von massen Untersuchungen auf Blutgruppenzugehörigkeit und das Eintätowaren der aufgefundenen Blutgruppen." *Münchener Medizinische Wochenschrift* 88 (1941): 669–72.
Muller, Henry R. "Blood Groups among the Yoruba Tribe of West African Negroes." *Proceedings of the Society for Experimental Biology and Medicine* 24 (1927): 437–8.
Mustakallio, Eero. "Untersuchungen uber die Blutgruppen bei den Nordfinnen und Lappen." *Acta Societatis Medicorum Fennicae Duodecim* 20 (1938): 17.
Nagai, Sen. "Die Körperkonstitution des Japaners. Der biochemische Rassenindex des Japaners." *Biologie der Person* 2 (1928): 437.

"New Designation for Blood groups According to Iso-agglutinins." *JAMA* 88 (1927): 1421.

Nigg, Clara. "A Study of the Blood Groups among the American Indians." *Journal of Immunology* 11 (1926): 319–22.

Nisi, Kôzi. "[blood groups of inhabitants of Okinawa province and their temperament and talent from standpoint of blood group specificity]." *Bulletin of Legal Medicine Institute of Nagasaki* (1931): 42–9.

Norohna, A. J. and L. B. Kotbagi. "Some anomalies met with in series of 300 bloods examined." *Journal of Tropical Medicine and Hygiene* 38 (1935): 295–6.

Ohnesorge, Viktor. "Blutgruppenuntersuchungen Bei Nerven- und Geisteskrankheiten." *Archiv für Psychiatrie und Nervenkrankheiten* 81 (1927): 763–7.

Ottenberg, Reuben. "Heredity of Blood Qualities. Medico-legal Application of Human Blood Grouping." *Journal of Immunology*, 6 (1921): 363–85.

Ottenberg, Reuben and Albert A. Epstein. "A Simple Method of Performing Serum Reactions." *Transactions of the New York Pathological Society* 8 (1908): 120–2.

Palmieri, Vincent. "Die Verteilung der Blutgruppen unter Geisteskranken Verbrechern." *Deutsche Zeitschrift für die gesamte gerichtliche Medizin* 12 (1928): 506–12.

Pantschenko and Agte, [Blood groups and tuberculosis], *Archiv für klinische und experimentale Medizin* (1924), as cited in S. Birkenfeld. [Tuberculosis and blood groups]. *Polska Gazeta Lekarska* 18 (1939): 485–7.

Paoli, Paolo de. "Contributo allo Studio dei gruppi sanguigni nelle malattie tubercolari." Lotta contro la tuberculosi 3 (1932): 494–8.

Parr, Leland W. "Studies in Isohemoglutination." *Journal of Immunology* 16 (1929): 99–107.

Pascoli, Sergio. "Malattie e gruppi sanguigni." *Gazzetta degli ospedali* 61 (1940): 3–8.

Penning, C. P. J., Marianne van Herwerden, and Th. J. Boele-Nijland. "Bloodgroup-Investigation in the Over Veluwe (Harderwijk and Surrounding districts)." *Koninklijke Akademie van Wettenschappen. Amsterdam. Proceedings of the Section of Sciences* 35 (1932): 706–14; reprinted in *Zeitschrift fur Morphologie und Anthropologie* 31 (1932): 395–402.

Penrose, Lionel S. "Blood Group Distribution in the Eastern Counties of England." *British Journal of Experimental Patholog*, 14 (1933): 160–1.

Penrose, Lionel S. "Blood Grouping of Mongolian Imbeciles." *Lancet* 222 (1932): 394–5.

Petrov, G. I. "Zur Frage der Isoagglutination des Blutes bei den Tadjiken." *Zeitschrift für Rassenphysiologie* 1 (1928): 90.

Petrov, G. I. "Zur Frage des Korrelativen zusammenhanges anthropometrischer Merkmale mit Blutgruppen." *Ukrainisches Zentralblatt für Blutgruppenforschung* 5 (1930): 73–88.

Pfahler, George E. and Bernard P. Widmann. "The Relation of Blood Groups to Malignant Disease and the Influence of Radiotherapy." *American Journal of Roentgenology and Radium therapy*, 12 (1924): 47–50.

Pijper, Adrianus. "The Blood Groups of the South African Dutch." *Koninklijke Akademie van Wettenschappen. Amsterdam. Proceedings of the Section of Sciences* 32 (1929): 1159–63.

Pilcz, Alexander. "Untersuchungen über die Blutgruppenzugehörigkeit bei Geisteskrankheiten." *Jahrbücher für Psychiatrie und Neurologie* 45 (1927): 120–31.

Pirie, James Hunter Harvey. "Blood Testing Preliminary to Transfusion: with a Note on the Group Distribution among South African Natives." *Medical Journal of South Africa* 16 (1921): 109–12.

Plissetzky M. S. and B. Smulevitsch. "Die Rassentheorie – Klassentheorie." *Journal d'anthropologie* 2 (1934): 23.

Pontani, G. W. "Zur Frage der Technik der Blutgruppenbestimmung bei Massenuntersuchungen. Gleichzeitig ein Beitrag zur Blutgruppenverteilung in Schleswig-Holstein." *Deutsche Militärarzt* 2 (1937): 19–24.

Popoviciu, Georges. "Differences dans la structure biologique en Roumanie d'après la situation géographique. Proprietés B et O." *Comptes rendus de la Société de biologie*, 90 (1924): 1069–71.

Preußische Landesgesundheitsrat. "Ueber Blutgruppenuntersuchungen in den Schulen." *Veröffentlichungen aus dem Gebiete der Medizinalverwaltung* 25 (1927):278–306.

Proescher, Frederick and A. S. Arkush. "Blood Groups in Mental Diseases." *Journal of Nervous and Mental Diseases* 65 (1927): 569–84.

Raphael, Theophile, Olive M. Searle, and William Scholten. "Blood Groups in Schizophrenic and Manic-depressive Psychosis." *American Journal of Psychiatry* 7 (1927): 153–61.

Rautmann, H. "Über Blutbildung bei fötaler allgemeiner Wassersucht." Bei*träge zur pathologischen Anatomie* 54 (1912): 332–49.

Reche, Otto. "Blutgruppenforschung und Anthropologie." *Volk und Rasse* 3 (1928): 1–13.

Reche, Otto. "Deutsche Gesellschaft für Blutgruppenforschung – Aufruf." *Artzliche Rundschau* 36 (1926): 347–8.

Reche, Otto. "Fortschritte in der Anthropologie." *Mitteilungen der anthropologischen Gesellschaft in Wien* 57 (1927): 12–21.

Reche, Otto. "Zur ethnographie des abflusslosen Gebietes Deutsch-Ostafrikas." *Abhandlungen des hamburgisches Kolonialinstitut* 17 (1914): 1–129.

Regnault, Félix. "Il n'y a pas de race juive." *Revue anthropologique* 42 (1932): 390–3.

Ro, Asho. "On the Blood types of opium-addicts in Formosa." *Taiwan Igakkai Zasshi* 33 (1934): 33.

Robertson, L. Bruce. "The Transfusion of Whole Blood: A Suggestion for its more Frequent Employment in War Surgery." *British Medical Journal* 2 (1916): 38–40.

Robertson, L. Bruce. "A Contribution on Blood Transfusion in War Surgery," *Lancet* (1918): 759–6.

Rohden, Friedrich von. "Kriminalbiologische Untersuchungen an gesunden und geisteskranken Verbrechern." *Deutsche Zeitschrift für die gesamte gerichtliche Medizin* 10 (1927): 620–33.

Rohden, Friedrich von. "Methoden der Kriminalbiologie." *Handbuch der biologischen Arbeitsmethoden* 4:12/1 (1938), 643–7.

Rosenthal, Georges. "Transfusion sanguine." *Journal de médecine des praticiens* 96 (1925): 663.

Rous, Peyton and Joseph R. Turner. "A Rapid and Simple Method of Testing Donors for Transfusion." *JAMA* 64 (1915): 1980–2.

Rubaschkin, W. J. and L. J. Leisermann. "Die Isohamagglutinationsgruppen und die Konstitutionsindexe bei den Ukrainegebürtigen Angehörigen der Roten Armée." *Ukrainische Zentralblatt für Blutgruppenforschung* 4 (1930): 145–55.

Rubaschkin W. J. and S. Pauli. "Der biologische Rassenindex der deutschen Koloniasten der Ukraine." *Ukrainische Zentralblatt für Blutgruppenforschung*, 1 (1927): 65–71.

Salazar Mallén, Marion and R. Hernández de la Portilla. "Existencia del aglutinógeno Rh en los hematíes de 250 individuos Mexicanos." *Revista de la Sociedad Mexicana de Historia Natural* 5 (1944): 183–5.

Satō, Takeo, Jiso Kunifusa, Shoichi Nomura, and Hisashi Hagimori. [Blood Types of Koreans]. *Japanese Journal of Legal Medicine* 9 (1935): 42–54.

Schaer, K. Fritz. *Charakter, Blutgruppe und* Konstitution. Zürich and Leipzig: Rascher, 1941.

Schiff, Fritz. "Die Blutgruppen und ihre Anwendung für Gericht." *Deutsche Zeitschrift für die gesamte gerichtliche Medizin* 9 (1927): 369–401.

Schiff, Fritz. *Blutgruppen und ihre Anwendungsgebiete*. Berlin: Springer, 1933.

Schiff, Fritz. "Blutgruppen und Epidemiologie," *Klinische Wochenschrift* 14 (1935): 786–90.

Schiff, Fritz and William C. Boyd. *Blood Grouping Technic*. New York: Interscience, 1940.

Schiff, Fritz and August Hien. "Zur Serologie der Berliner Bevölkerung. IV Mitteilung." *Klinische Wochenschrift* 13 (1934): 375–6.

Schiff, Fritz and Otto von Verscheurer. "Serologischer Untersuchungen an Zwillingen. II Mitteilung." *Zeitschrift für Morphologie und Anthropologie* 32 (1933): 244–9.

Schiff, Fritz and H. Ziegler. "Blutgruppenformel in der Berliner Bevölkerung." *Klinische Wochenschrift* 3 (1924): 1078.

Schindler, M. S. "Der gegenwartige Stand der Lehre von Blutgruppen." *Ukrainisches Zentralblatt für Blutgruppenforschung und Transfusion* 1 (6) (1932): 17.

Schlossberger, Hans, K. Laubenheimer, W. Fischer, and F.W. Wichmann. "Blutgruppenuntersuchungen an Schulkindern in der Umgebung von Frankfurt am Main." *Medizinische* Klinik 24 (1928): 851–2.

Schmidt, Adam. "Blutgruppenbestimmungen an Strafgefangenen." *Deutsche Zeitschrift für die gesamte gerichtliche Medizin* 13 (1929): 373–6.

Schneider, Georg. "Weitere Beiträge zur Isohämagglutination." *Klinsche Wochenschrift* 4 (1925): 2383–7.

Schneider, Georg. "Ein Beitrag zur Blutgruppenforschung mit Untersuchungs-Ergebnissen der I. Internationalen Arbeiterolympiade." *Zeitschrift für Rassenphysiologie* 5 (1932): 140–3.

Paul Schneider, "Untersuchung über den Isoagglutiningehalt im Menschenblut," *Zeitschrift für die gesamte experimentelle Medizin* 36 (1923): 153–63.

Scholten, Gustav C. J. "Unsere Bluttransfusionen und die amerikanische Methode zum Nachweis von Agglutininen." *Deutsche medizinische Wochenschrift* 49 (1923): 314–5.

Schreiber, "Zur Technik der Blutgruppenbestimmung bei Massenuntersuchungen," *Deutsche Militärarzt* 1 (1936): 97–9.

Schusterov, G.A. "[Isohaemoagglutinierenden Eigenschaften des menschlichen Blutes nach den Ergebnissen einer Untersuchung an Straflingen des Reformatoriums (Arbeitshauses) zu Omsk]." *Moskovskii Meditsinskii Jurnal* 7 (1927): 1–6.

Schütz, Frantz and Edgar Wöhlisch. "Bedeutung und Wesen von Haemagglutination und Blutgruppenbildung beim Menschcen." *Klinische Wochenschrift* 3 (1924): 1614–6.

Sellin, Thorsten. "New Phase in Criminal Anthropology in Italy." *Annals of the American Academy of Political and Social Science* 125 (1926): 233–42.

Shamov, Vladimir Nikolayevich and M. Kostiukov. [Question of homoplasty from the cadaver. Blood transfusion from the cadaver]. Trudi 3 *Ukrainskii siezda Khirurhiia* 18 (1929): 184–9.

Shamov, Vladimir Nikolayevich. "Transfusion of Stored Cadaver Blood." *Lancet* (1937): 306–9.

Shattock, Samuel George. "Chromocyte Clumping in Acute Pneumonia and Certain Other Diseases and the Significance of the Buffy Coat in the Shed Blood." *Journal of Pathology and Bacteriology* 6 (1900), 303–14.

Sheldon, William H. "Morphological Types and Mental Ability." *Journal of Personnel Research* 5 (1927): 447–51.
Sheldon, William H. *Varieties of Human Physique*. New York: Harper and Brothers, 1940.
Sievers, Oluf. "Blodgruppsfördelningen bland friska och sjuka inom det i Finland samlade materialet [Blood group distribution of the sick and healthy as found in materials collected in Finland]." *Finska Lakaresallskapets Handlingar* 71 (1929): 836–48.
Snyder, Louis H. *Blood Grouping in Relation to Clinical and Legal Medicine*. Baltimore: Williams and Wilkins, 1929.
Snyder, Louis H. "Blood Groups of Jamaicans." In *Race Crossing in Jamaica*, edited by Charles Davenport, 277–80. Washington: Carnegie Institution of America, 1929b.
Snyder, Louis H. "Critical Tests of Blood Group Inheritance." *Southern Medicine and Surgery* 86, (1924a):473–5.
Snyder, Louis H. "Human blood groups: Their inheritance and racial significance." *American Journal of Physical Anthropology* 9 (1926), 233–63.
Snyder, Louis H. "The Inheritance of Blood Groups," *Genetics* 9 (1924b): 465–78.
Spencer, Roscoe R. "Opportunities for Women in War Medicine." *War Medicine*, 2 (1942): 574–9.
Steffan, Paul. "Die Arbeitweise der Deutschen Gesellschaft für Blutgruppenforschung." *Zeitschrift für Rassenphysiologie* 1 (1928): 9.
Steffan, Paul. "Bedeutung der Blutuntersuchung für die Bluttransfusion und die Rassenforschung." *Archiv für Rassen- und Gesellschafts-Biologie* 15 (1923): 148.
Steffan, Paul. "Beobachtungen über den Verlauf der künstlichen Infektion der Ratte mit Trypanosome." *Archiv für Schiffs-und Tropenhygiene* 25 (1921): 241–7.
Steffan, Paul. "Blutübertragung in der Kriegsmarine." *Veröffentlichungen aus dem Gebiete des Marine-Sanitätswesens*, 28 (1936): 5–40.
Steffan, Paul. "Rassenergebnisse der Blutforschung." *Die Sonne* 3 (1926a): 49–64.
Steffan, Paul. "Weitere Ergebnisse der Rassenforschung mittels serologischer Methoden." *Mitteilungen der anthropologischen Gesellschaft in Wien* 56 (1926b): 78–109.
Stigler, Robert. "Rassenphysiologische Untersuchungen an farbigen Kriegsgefangenen in einem Kriegsgefangenlager." *Zeitschrift für Rassenphysiologie* 13 (1943): 26–57.
Straszynski, A. "Uber das Ergebnis der Wassermannschen Reaktion innerhalb verschiedener Blutgruppen bei behandelten Lues." *Klinische Wochenschrift* 4 (1925): 1962–3.
Swider, Zdislaw and Natan Kon. "Badania nad grupami serologicznemi krwi u gruzlikow, I & II [Examination of groups of serum in tumors; Research on serological groups in the tuberculous; pigmentary syndromes, blood-groups

and individual predisposition to tuberculosis]." *Polska Gazeta Lekarska* 6 (1927): 597–8; 972.

Swider, Zdislaw and Natan Kon. "Recherches sur les Groupes Sanguins Chez les Tuberculeux." *Comptes rendus de la Société de biologie* 98 (1928): 385–6.

Sylla, Adolf. "Das Blutbild bei Lungentuberkulose, mit Berucksichtung der Blutkörperschensenkung (BKS) und der Blutgruppen." *Medizinische Klinik* 28 (1932): 686–8; 721–4.

Tagliaferro, Enrico. "Gruppi sanguigni e carcinoma." *Minerva Medica* 28 (1937), 219–20.

Tammes, Tina. "Bedeutung von Dr. Maria Anna van Herwerden für die Genetik und die Eugenik." *Genetica* 18 (1936), 3–9.

Taylor, G. L. and Aileen M. Prior. "Blood Groups in England I. Examination of Family and Unrelated Material." *Annals of Eugenics* 8 (1937–1938): 343–55.

Tebbutt, Arthur H. and Sarah V. McConnel. "On Human Iso-haemagglutinins, with a note on their Distribution amongst some Australian Aborigines." *Medical Journal of Australia* 9 (1922): 201–9.

Tedeschi, Carlo. "Osservazioni sul soma delle popolazioni indigene della Barra orientale secondo i concetti constituzionalistici." *Archivio Italiano di Scienze Mediche Coloniali* 10 (1929): 566–83.

Terada, Seiji. "Distribution of groups M and N among Japanese in the city of Taihoku and among Formosan Chinese and Formosan savages." *Taiwan Igakkai Zasshi* 34 (1935): 1892.

Thomas, John C. "Blood Group Distribution in England." *British Medical Journal* (1939): 1163.

Thomsen, Oluf. "Om mulighoben af forskellig Disposition til Cancerudviklung hos individer af forskelig "blodtype" [Possibilities of varying disposition to cancer development in individuals of various blood groups]." *Ugeskrift for Laeger* 93 (1931): 1008–15.

Thomsen, Oluf. "Uber den Zusammenhang der Isoagglutinatorischen Bluttypen (Blutgruppen) mit Pathologischen Zustanden." *Acta Pathologica et Microbiologica Scandinavica* 4 (1927): 45–73; 163–4.

Toulouse, Edouard, P. Schiff, and R. Weismann-Netter. "Les groupes sanguins dans les maladies mentales et nerveuses." *Encephale* 21 (1926): 785–8.

Tucker, William B. and William A. Lessa. "Man: A Constitutional Investigation." *Quarterly Review of Biology* 15 (1940): 265–89; 411–55.

Turpin, Raymond and A. Caratzali. "Consideration sur là valeur constitutionnelle des groupes sanguins." *Revue française de puericulture* 1 (1933a): 86–105.

Turpin, Raymond and Armand Caratzali. "L'étude des groupes sanguins classiques chez les sujets atteints de mongolisme." *Revue critique de pathologie et de thérapeutique* 3 (1933b): 789–97.

Ugelli, Libero. "Distribuzione dei gruppi sanguigni negli individui portatori di ulcere gastroduodenali." *Policlinico* (sezione pratica) 43 (1936): 1591–4.

Urra, Juan Andreu. "Los grupos sanguineos en Castilla." *Información medica* 5 (1928): 51–6.

Van der Made, Wilhemina M. "Blood-groups of Sundanese Natives in West Java." *Fourth Pacific Science Congress, Java 1929* 3 (1930): 509–13.

Verzar, Fritz and Oskar Weszeczky. "Rassenbiologische Untersusuchungen mittels Isohamagglutininen." *Biochemische Zeitschrift 126* (1921):33–9.

Vincent, Beth. "A Rapid Macroscopic Agglutination Test for Blood Groups, and Its Value inn Testing Donors for Transfusion." *JAMA* 70 (1918): 1219–20.

Viola, Domenico. "Contributo allo studio dei rapporti fra caratteri gruppo-specifici e caratteri psico-costituzionali." *Giornale di medicina militare* 82 (1934): 253–8.

Viola, Domenico. "I Gruppi Sanguigni Come Fattore Etno-Antropologico. Contributo Alla Distribuzione Regionale dei Gruppi Sanguigni in Italia." *Rivista di Antropologica* 28 (1928): 307–26.

Vishnevskii, Boris N. "Anthropology in USSR in the Course of 17 Years (1917 to 1934)." *American Journal of Physical Anthropology* 21 (1936a): 1–17.

Vishnevskii, Boris N. "Blood Groups of Tungus." *Human Biology* 8 (1936b): 273–8.

Vishnevskii, Boris N. "Die Blutgruppenfrage aus dem IV Kongress der Zoologen, Anatomen und Histologen der U. d. S. S. R." *Ukrainisches Zentralblatt für Blutgruppenforschung* 5 (1930): 47–55.

Vishnevskii, Boris N. "Professor Dr. W. J. Rubaschkin und seine Arbeiten auf dem Gebiete der Blutgruppenforschung." *Zeitschrift für Rassenphysiologie* 6 (1933).

Vishnevskii, Boris N., [New method for racial diagnosis with respect to the Chuvash]. Appeared in the *Comptes rendus de l'Academie des Sciences de l'U.R.S.S.,* (1924).

"Von der medizinischen Sektion der Charkower Wissentschaftlichen Gesellchaft." *Ukrainische Zentralblatt für Blutgruppenforschung* 1 (1927): 5–7.

Wakeshima, T. "Blood groups of Formosan-Chinese; relation between blood groups and result of study in primary schools." *Taiwan Igakkai Zasshi* 31(1932): 83.

Weitzner, Geza. "Hämagglutiningehalt des Blutserums Karzinomkranker." *Medizinische Klinik* 21 (1925): 1960–1.

Weszeczky, Oskar. "Untersuchungen über die gruppenweise Hämagglutination beim Menschen." *Biochemische Zeitschrift* 107 (1920): 160.

Wiener, Alexander S. J. Ziewe, and Joseph H. Fries. "On the Linkage Relations of the Genes for Allergic Disease and the Genes Determining the Blood Groups, MN-types, and Eye Colour in Man." *Annals of Eugenics* 7(1937): 163–78.

Wilczowski, Eugenjusz. "Blutgruppenuntersuchungen bei Schizophrenie und progressiver Paralyse." *Klinische Wochenschrift* 6 (1927): 168.

Wong, Dorothy Huie and Foong Kong Chen. "Blood Groups in relation to syphilis and its Treatment." *National Medical Journal of China* 17 (1931): 354–9.

Würz, Paul. "Uber die Blutgruppenverteilung bei Schizophrenen." *Schweizerische medizinische Wochenschrift* 58 (1928): 353–5.

Young, Matthew. "The Problem of Racial Significance of the Blood Groups." *Man* 28 (1928): 153–9; 171–6.

Rina Younovitch, "Les caractères sérologiques des juifs asiatiques," *Comptes rendus de la Société de biologie* 113 (1933): 1101–3.

Research Publications After 1945

Adamo, Peter J. *Eat Right 4 Your Life: The Individualized Blood Type Diet Solution.* New York: G.P. Putnam, 1996.

Afzal, M., F. Ziaur-Rehman, F. Hussain, R. Siddiqi. "A Survey of Blood Groups. *Journal of the Pakistan Medical Association* 27 (1977): 426–8.

Aird, Ian. "Discussion on the ABO Blood Groups and Disease." *Proceedings of the Royal Society of Medicine* 48 (1955): 139.

Aird, Ian, H. H. Bentall, and J. A. Fraser Roberts. "A Relationship between Cancer of Stomach and the ABO Blood Groups." *British Medical Journal* (1953) 1:799–801.

Aird, Ian, H.H. Bentall, J.A. Mehigan, and J. A. Roberts. "Blood groups in relation to peptic ulceration and carcinoma of colon, rectum, breast, and bronchus; an association between the ABO groups and peptic ulceration." *British Medical Journal* 2 (1954): 315–21.

Alsadi, Rihab. "Personality Traits and Their Relationship with Blood Groups among of Palestinian University Students." *International Journal of Psychology and Behavioral Sciences* (2020) 10(2): 34–42.

Anstee, David J. "The relationship between blood groups and disease." *Blood* 115 (2010): 4635–43.

Apecu, R. O., E. M. Mulogo, F. Bagenda, et al. "ABO and Rhesus (D) blood group distribution among blood donors in rural southwestern Uganda: a retrospective study." *Biomed Central Research Notes* 9 (2016): 513.

Arneaud JD, and O. Young. "A preliminary survey of the distribution of A B O and Rh blood groups in Trinidad, B.W.I." *Documenta de medicina geographica et tropica* 7 (1955): 375–8.

Ashton, G. C. "Blood polymorphisms and cognitive abilities." *Behavior Genetics* 16 (1986): 517–29.

Bangham, Jenny. "Blood groups and human groups: Collecting and calibrating genetic data after World War Two." *Studies in History and Philosophy of Biological and Biomedical Sciences* 47 (2014): 74–86.

Beardmore, J. A. and F. Karimi-Booshehri. "ABO Genes are Differentially Distributed in Socio-economic Groups in England." *Nature* 303 (1983): 522–4.

Beardmore, J. A. and F. Karimi-Booshehri "Blood Group and Socio-economic Class." *Nature* 309 (1984): 395–9.

"Blood Groups and Disease." *British Medical Journal* (Sept. 29, 1956): 757–8.

Bourdel, Léone. "Sang - Tempéraments - Travail – Races." *Journal de la société statistique de Paris* 87 (1946): 162–78.

Cavalli-Sforza, Luigi, Luca Paolo Menozzi, and Alberto Piazza. *History and Geography of Human Genes*. Princeton: Princeton University Press, 1994.

"CDC on Infectious Diseases in the United States: 1900–99." *Population and Development Review* 25 (1999): 635–40.

Christiano, Joseph. *Joseph Christiano's blood type diet O: a custom eating plan for losing weight, fighting disease, and staying healthy for people with type O blood*. Lake Mary, FL: Siloam, 2010.

Cooling, Laura. "Groups in Infection and Host Susceptibility." *Clin Microbiol Rev.* 28 (2015):801–70.

Cusack, Leila, Emmy De Buck, Veerle Compernolle, and Philippe Vandekerckhove. "Blood type diets lack supporting evidence: a systematic review." *American Journal of Clinical Nutrition* 98, (2013): 99–104.

Degaudenzi, Jean-Louis. *Le secret de votre groupe sanguin: Clé de la personnalité et du destin*. Paris: Filipucchi, 1991.

Edge, Michael D., Sohini Ramachandran, and Noah A. Rosenberg. "Celebrating 50 years since Lewontin's apportionment of human diversity." *Philosophical transactions of the Royal Society of London. Series B, Biological sciences*, 377 (June 2022), https://doi.org/10.1098/rstb.2020.0405.

Fisher, R.A. "The Rhesus Factor: A Study in Scientific Method." *American Scientist* 35 (1947): 95–102.

Franchini, Massimo, Giancarlo M. Liumbruno, and Giuseppe Lippi. "The prognostic value of ABO blood group in cancer patients." *Blood Transfusion*, 14 (2016):434–40.

Furuhata, Tanemoto. *Development of Haemotypology in Japan*. Tokyo: Matsumoto Institute, 1977.

Genevay, Jacques and Léone Bourdel. *Sang, Tempéraments, Travail et Races*. Paris: Maloine, 1946.

Gibson, John B., G. A. Harrison, V.A. Clarke, and R. W. Hiorns. "IQ and ABO Blood Groups." *Nature* 246 (1973): 498–500.

Green, Harry N. and Ivor Dunsford. "Relationship of Blood groups to Cancer." *Acat – Unio Internationalis contra cancrum*, 10 (1954): 125–7.

Khader, Dina *The food combining/blood type diet solution: a personalized diet plan and cookbook for each blood type*. New York: McGraw Hill: 2000.

Kodama, Sakuzaemon. *Ainu: Historical and Anthropological Study*. Sapporo: Hokkaido University School of Medicine, 1970.

Kossovitch, Nicholas. *Anthropologie des groupes sanguins des populations au Maroc*. Paris: Mason, 1953.

Lewontin, Richard C. "The apportionment of human diversity." In *Evolutionary Biology*, edited by William C. Steere, Theodosius Dobzhansky, and Max K. Hecht, 381–98. New York: Springer; 1972.

Lisker, Rubén. *Estructura genética de la población mexicana. Aspectos médicos y antropológicos.* Mexico City: Salvat Mexicana de Ediciones, S.A. de C. V., 1981.

Livingstone, Frank R. "On the Non-Existence of Human Races." *Current Anthropology* 3 (1962): 279.

Livingstone, Frank B. "Review of *Blood Groups and Disease: A Study of Associations of Diseases with Blood Groups and Other Polymorphisms.* A. E. Mourant, A. C. Kopec, and K. Domaniewska-Sobczak." *Human Biology* 51:600–1.

Majumdar, D.N. and Kunwar Kishen. "Blood Groups Distribution in the United Provinces: Report on the Serological Survey of the UP." *The Eastern Anthropologist* 1(1947) 8–15.

Manuila, Alexandre. "Blood Groups and Disease -- Hard Facts and Delusions." *JAMA* 167 (1958): 2047–53.

Manuila, Alexandre. *Quel est le nombre necessaire et suffisant d'examens dans les recherches biologiques?* Geneva: P.E. Grivet, 1945.

Mayo, Charles W. and James O. Ferguson. "Are Certain Diseases Associated with Specific Blood Groups or Rh Antigens?" *AMA Archives of Surgery* 66 (1953): 406–9.

Mielke, Nicholas, Rebecca Gorz, Amit Bahl, Lili Zhao, and David A. Berger. "Association between ABO blood type and coronavirus disease 2019 severe outcomes across dominant variant strains." *Journal of the American College of Emergency Physicians open*, 5 (2024) https://doi.org/10.1002/emp2.13115.

Mourant, A. E. *The ABO Blood Groups* Oxford: Blackwell, 1958.

Mourant, A. E., A. C. Kopec, and K. Domaniewska-Sobczak. *Blood Groups and* Diseases. Oxford: Oxford University Press, 1978.

Mourant, A. E. *Blood and Stones: An autobiography.* La Haule, Jersey: La Haule Books, 1995.

Mourant, A. E. *The Distribution of the Human Blood Groups.* Oxford: Blackwell, 1954, updated 1976.

Ndoula, S.T., J. J. Noubiap, J. R. Nansseu, and A Wonkam. "Phenotypic and allelic distribution of the ABO and Rhesus (D) blood groups in the Cameroonian population." *International Journal of Immunogenetics* 41 (2014): 206–10.

Nomi, Toshitaka. *You Are Your Blood Type: The Biological Keys to Unlocking the Secrets of your Personality.* Translated by Alexander Besher. New York: Pocket Books, 1988.

Prokop, Otto and Gerhard Uhlenbruck. *Human Blood Serum and Serum Groups.* London: McLaren and Sons, 1969.

Provine, William A. *Origins of Population Genetics.* Chicago: University of Chicago Press, 1971.

Provine, William A. "The R.A. Fisher–Sewall Wright Controversy and its Influence Upon Modern Evolutionary Biology." In *Oxford Surveys in Evolutionary Biology*, Vol. 2, edited by R. Dawkins and M. Ridley, 197–219. New York: Oxford University Press, 1985.

Race R. R. and Ruth Sanger. *Blood Groups in Man*. Oxford: Blackwell, 1950.

Sandoval, S., C. Henckel, and L. Givovich. "The blood groups, subgroups, and Rh factor of the Mapuche Indians of the Province of Cautin, Chile." *Blood* 1 (1946): 555–9.

Sapha Shibeeb, S. and Aisha Khan. "ABO blood group association and COVID-19. COVID-19 susceptibility and severity: A review." *Hematology, Transfusion and Cell Therapy* 44 (2022): 70–5.

Sawadogo, S. K Nebie, T. Millogo, et al. "Distribution of ABO and RHD blood group antigens in blood donors in Burkina Faso." *International Journal of Immunogenetics* 46 (2019): 1–6.

Sevgen, B. and N. Mizan. "[Blood groups and the Rh factor in Turkey]." *Tip Fakültesi mecmuasi* [Bulletin de la Faculté de medecine d'Istanbul]. 23 (1960): 560–3.

Sheldon, William H. *Varieties of Deliquent Youth*. New York: Harper and Brothers, 1949.

Snyder, Louis H. "Old and New Pathways in Human Genetics." In *Genetics in the Twentieth Century*, edited by L.C. Dunn, 369–92. N.Y.: Macmillan, 1951.

"Statement on the Nature of Race and Race Differences by Physical Anthropologists and Geneticists--June 1951." In *The Race Concept: Results of an Inquiry*. Paris: UNESCO, 1952.

Trials of War Criminals before the Nuernberg Military Tribunals. Washington: Government Printing Office, 1949.

Valenzuela, Carlos Y. "Human sociogenetics," *Biological Research* 44 (2011): 393–404.

Valenzuela, Carlos Y., Carolina Pastene, and Cynthia M. Pérez. "Intelligence and genetic markers in Chilean children," *Biological Research* 31 (1998): 81–92.

Vallois, Henri-V. and Paulette Marquer. "La distribution des groupes sanguins en France." *Comptes rendus hebdomadaires des seances de l'Academie des sciences 258 (1964): 2179–82.*

Wang, Jingzhou, Bibiana García-Bailo, Daiva E. Nielsen, and Ahmed El-Sohemy. "ABO Genotype, 'Blood-Type' Diet and Cardiometabolic Risk Factors." *PLoS ONE*, 9 (2014): 1–9.

Wiener, Alexander S. "Blood-groups and disease: a critical review." *Lancet* (1962) 1: 813–6.

Wiener, Alexander S. "Blood Groups and Personality Traits." *American Journal of Human Genetics* 17 (1965): 369–370.

Wiener, Alexander S. "Controversy in human genetics. Blood groups and disease." *American Journal of Human Genetics* 22 (1970):476–483.

Wiener, Alexander S. “Modern Blood Group Mythology.” *Journal of Forensic Medicine* 7 (1960):166–76.

Wiener, Alexander S. “Tanemoto Furuhata.” *Vox Sanguinis* 31 (1976): 77.

Wintrobe, Maxwell M., ed. *Blood Pure and Eloquent.* N.Y: McGraw-Hill, 1980.

Wolfgang, Marvin. “Cesare Lombroso.” In *Pioneers in Criminology, edited by* Hermann Mannheim, 168–227. London: Stevens and Sons, 1960.

Worlledge, S., S. E. Ogiemudia, C. O. Thomas, B. N. Ikoku, and L. Luzzatto. “Blood group antigens and antibodies in Nigeria.” *Annals of Tropical Medicine and Parasitology* 68 (1974): 249–64.

Zallen, Doris T., Daphne Christie, and Elizabeth M. Tansey. *The Rhesus Factor and Disease Prevention: Wellcome Trust Centre Witness Seminar.* London: Wellcome Trust Centre for the History of Medicine, 2004.

Zwaan, Klieweg de. See G. A. Lindeboom, *Dutch Medical Biography* (Amsterdam: Rodopi, 1984), 145–6; 2239–40.

Secondary Sources

Ackerknecht, Erwin H. “Diasthesis: The Word and the Concept in Medical History.” *Bulletin of the History of Medicine* 56 (1982): 317–25.

Adams, Mark B. “Science, Ideology and Structure: The Koltsov Institute, 1900–1970.” In Social Context of Soviet Science, edited by Linda L. Lubrano and Susan Gross Solomon, 173–209. Boulder: Westview Press, 1980a.

Adams, Mark B. “Sergei Chetverikov, the Kol’tsov Institute, and the Evolutionary Synthesis.” In *The Evolutionary Synthesis,* edited by Ernst Mayr and William B. Provine, 242–78. Cambridge, Mass: Harvard University Press, 1980b.

Adelsberger, Lucie. “In memory of Fritz Schiff.” *Proceedings of the Virchow Medical Society* (New York) 9 (1950): 91–2.

Bangham, Jenny. *Blood Relations: Transfusion and the Making of Human Genetics.* University of Chicago Press, 2020.

Bartholomew, James R. “Acculturation of Science in Japan: Kitasato Shibasaburo and the Japanese Bacteriological Community, 1885–1920.” Ph.D. diss., Stanford University, 1972.

Bartholomew, James R. *Formation of Science in Japan: Building a Research Tradition.* New Haven: Yale University Press, 1989.

Bartholomew, James R. “Japanese Culture and the Problem of Modern Science.” In *Science and Values,* edited by Arnold Thackray and Everett Mendelsohn, 109–55. New York: Humanities Press, 1974.

Bartrip, P. W. J. *Mirror of medicine: The British Medical Journal.* Oxford: Clarendon Press, 1995.

J.H. Bennett, ed. *Natural Selection, Heredity and Eugenics: including Selected Correspondence of R.A. Fisher with Leonard Darwin and Others.* Oxford: Clarendon Press, 1983.

Beyerchen, Alan D. "On the Stimulation of Excellence in Wilhelmina Science." In *Another Germany: A Reconsideration of the Imperial Era*, edited by Jack R. Dikes and Joachim Remak, 139–68. Boulder: Westview Press, 1988.

Boaz, Rachel E. *In Search of "Aryan Blood": Serology in Interwar and National Socialist Germany.* Budapest: Central European University Press, 2012.

Bodmer, Walter F. "Early British Discoveries in Human Genetics: Contributions of R.A. Fisher and J.B.S. Haldane to the Development of Blood Groups." *American Journal of Human Genetics* 50 (1992): 671–6.

Bonner, Thomas N. *American Doctors and German Universities: A Chapter in Intellectual Relations, 1870–1914.* Lincoln: University of Nebraska Press, 1963.

Bonner, Thomas N. *Becoming a physician: medical education in Britain, France, Germany, and the United States. 1750–1945* (New York: Oxford University Press, 1995.

Bonner, Thomas N. "German Model of Training Physicians in the United States, 1870–1914: How Closely Was It Followed?" *Bulletin of the History of Medicine* 64 (1990): 18–34.

Bork-Feltkamp, A. J. van. "Anthropological Research in the Netherlands. Historical Survey." *Verhandelingen der Koninklijke Nederlandsche Akademie van Wettenschappen. Amsterdam. Proceedings of the Section of Sciences* 37, no. 3 (1938): 1–166.

Bowers, John Z. *Medical Education in Japan.* New York: Harper and Row, 1965.

Box, Joan Fisher *R. A. Fisher: The Life of a Scientist.* New York: John Wiley, 1978.

Brace, C. Loring. "On the Race Concept." *Current Anthropology* 5 (1964): 313.

Brace, C. Loring. The Roots of the Race Concept in American Physical Anthropology." In *History of Physical Anthropology, edited by* Frank Spencer, 11–29. New York: Academic Press, 1982.

Brandt, Allan M. and Martha Gardner. "The Golden Age of Medicine?" In *Medicine in the Twentieth Century*, edited by Roger Cooter and John Pickstone, 21–37. Amsterdam: Harwood Academic Publishing, 2000.

Bullock, Mary Brown. *American Transplant: The Rockefeller Foundation and the Peking Union Medical College.* Berkeley: University of California Press, 1980.

Burnham, John C. "The British Medical Journal in America." In *Medical Journals and Medical Knowledge*, edited by Stephen Lock and Roy Porter, 165–87. London: Routledge, 1992.

Burleigh, Michael. *Germany Turns Eastward.* Cambridge: Cambridge University Press, 1988.

Burton, Elise K. "'Essential Collaborators': Locating Middle Eastern Geneticists in the Global Scientific Infrastructure, 1950s–1970s." *Comparative Studies in Society and History* 60, no. 1 (2018): 119–49.

Burton, Elise K. and Ageliki Lefkaditou. "Race in Circulation: Blood Banks and Forced Mobilities in the Eastern Mediterranean." *Bulletin of the History of Medicine* 96, no. 3 (2022): 375–402.

Ceppellini, Ruggero. "In Memoriam: Leone Lattes, 1887–1954." *Bollettino dell instituto sieroterapico milanese*, 33 (1954): 649–50.

Chevalier, Louis. *Dangerous Classes, Criminal Classes.* Princeton: Princeton University Press, 1981.

Ciocco, Antonio. "Historical Background of the Modern Study of Constitution." *Bulletin of the Institute of the History of Medicine* 4 (1936): 23–38.

Clark, Ronald W. *JBS: The Life and Work of J.B.S. Haldane.* New York: Coward McCann, 1969.

Carter, K. Codell. "Early Conjectures That Down Syndrome Is Caused by Chromosomal Nondisjunction." *Bulletin of the History of Medicine* 76, no. 3 (2002): 528–63.

Cohen, Sheldon G. "Firsts in Allergy: The Contributions of Arthur F. Coca." *New England and Regional Allergy Proceedings* 6 (1985): 287–92.

Comfort, Nathaniel. *The Science of Human Perfection* New Haven: Yale University Press, 2014.

Cooter, Roger. *Cultural Meaning of Popular Science: Phrenology and the Organization of Consent in Nineteenth Century Britain.* Cambridge: Cambridge University Press, 1984.

"Jean Dausset: Biographical." Accessed February 13, 2024 https://www.nobelprize.org/prizes/medicine/1980/dausset/biographical/.

DeJong-Lambert, W. *The Cold War Politics of Genetic Research: An Introduction to the Lysenko Affair.* New York: Springer, 2012.

Deichmann, Ute and Benno Müller-Hill. "Biological Research at Universities and Kaiser Wilhelm Institutes in Nazi Germany." In *Science, Technology and National Socialism*, edited by Monika Renneburg and Mark Walker, 160–83. Cambridge: Cambridge University Press, 1994.

de Solla Price, Derek J. "Citation Measures of Hard Science, Soft Science, Technology, and Nonscience." In *Communication among Scientists and Engineers*, edited by Carnot E. Nelson and Donald K. Pollock, 3–22. Lexington, Ma: D.C. Heath, 1970.

Diamond, Louis K. "The Rh Problem: A Personalized History." *Turkish Journal of Pediatrics* 24 (1982): 35–47.

Dikötter, Frank. *Discourse of Race in Modern China.* Stanford: Stanford University Press, 1992.

Dikötter, Frank. "Discourse of Race and the Medicalization of Public and Private Space in Modern China (1895–1949)." *History of Science* 29 (1991): 411–20.

Domenici, Fernanda. "Leone Lattes (1887–1954)." *Minerva medicolegale*, 74 (1954): i–ii.

Dronamraju, Krishna R. *Haldane: The Life and Work of J.B.S. Haldane with Special Reference to India.* Aberdeen: Aberdeen University Press, 1985.

Dubos, Rene. *White Plague.* Boston: Little, Brown, 1952.

Elliott, Mabel. *Crime in Modern Society.* New York: Harper, 1952.

Farr, Andrew D. "Blood Group Serology -- The First Four Decades (1900–1939)." *Medical History* 23 (1973): 215–26.
Fitzpatrick, Sheila. "Cultural Revolution as Class War." In *Cultural Revolution in Russia, 1928–1931*, edited by Sheila Fitzpatrick, 115–48. Bloomington: Indiana University Press, 1978.
Fleck, Ludwik. *Genesis and Development of a Scientific Fact.* Chicago: University of Chicago Press, 1979.
Foucault, Michel. *Discipline and Punish.* Translated by Alan Sheridan. New York: Pantheon, 1977.
Fraser-Roberts, John A. "Reginald Ruggles Gates." *Biographical Memoirs of Fellows of the Royal Society* 10 (1964): 83–105.
Frewer, Magdalene. "Das wissentschaftliche Werk Felix Bernsteins." Ph.D. diss., University of Göttingen, 1977.
Garland, David. "British Criminology Before 1935." *British Journal of Criminology* 28 (1988): 131–47.
Gantt, W. Horsley. *Russian Medicine.* New York: Harper, 1937.
Gaudillière, Jean-Paul. "Le cancer entre infection et hérédité: gènes, virus et souris au National Cancer Institute (1937–1977)." *Revue d'histoire des sciences* 48 (1994): 57–89.
Gaylord, Mark S. and John F. Galliher. *The Criminology of Edwin Sutherland.* New Brunswick: Transaction Books, 1988.
Geisenhainer, Katja. *Rasse ist Schicksal: "Otto Reche (1879–1966) – Ein Leben als Anthropologe und Völkerkundler.* Leipzig: Evang. Verlagsanstalt, 2002.
Geisenhainer, Katja. "'War in particular offers exceptionally favourable opportunities for surveying foreign racial material': The effects of World Wars on anthropologist Otto Reche's activities." *Anthropological Notebooks* 15 (2): 35–49.
Frieden, Nancy. *Russian Physicians in an Era of Reform and Revolution, 1865–1905.* Princeton: Princeton University Press, 1981.
Fruton, Joseph S. *Contrasts in Scientific Style: Research Groups in the Chemical and Biochemical Sciences.* Philadelphia: American Philosophical Society, 1990.
Gotschlich, E. "Prof. Dr. Max Gundel zum Gedächtnis." *Zentralblatt für Bakteriologie* 153 (1949): 269–70.
Gould, Steven Jay. *Mismeasure of Man.* New York: W.W. Norton, 1981.
Graham, Loren R. "Formation of Soviet Research Institutes." *Social Studies of Science* 5 (1975): 303–29.
Graham, Loren K. *The Soviet Academy of Sciences and the Communist Party,* 1927–32. Princeton: Princeton University Press, 1967.
Guglielmo, Giovanni. "Leone Lattes 1887–1954." *Haematologica*, 38 (1954): iii–vi.
Hacking, Ian. *The Taming of Chance.* Cambridge University Press, 1990.

Harrison, G. Ainsworth. "The Last Fifty Years of Human Population Biology." In *History of Physical Anthropology*, edited by Frank Spencer, 467–72. New York: Academic Press, 1982.

Harwood, Jonathan. *Styles of Scientific Thought: The German Genetics Community, 1900–1933*. Chicago: University of Chicago Press, 1993.

Heringa, C. "Dr. M. A. van Herwerden." *Nederlandsch Tijdschrift voor Geneeskunde* 79 (1935): 4917–19.

Herwerden, C. A. B. van. *Marianne van Herwerden*. Rotterdam: W. L. & J. Brusse, 1948.

Hideome, Tuge. *Historical Development of Science and Technology in Japan*. Tokyo: Japan Cultural Society, 1968.

Hirschfeld, Hans. "Tanemoto Furuhata (1891–1976)." *International Archives of Allergy and Applied Immunology* 54 (1977): 191–2.

Hirszfeld, Ludwik. *The Story of One Life*. Translated and edited by Marta A. Balinska and William H. Schneider. Rochester: University of Rochester Press, 2005.

Hogben, Lancelot. *Mathematics for the Million*. New York: Norton, 1937.

Hogben, Lancelot. *Science for the Citizen*. New York: Knopf, 1938.

Hongjun, Zhao. "Chinese versus Western Medicine." *Chinese Science* 10 (1991): 21–37.

Horn, David G. *The Criminal Body: Lombroso and the Anatomy of Deviance*. New York: Routledge, 2003.

Huard, Pierre, Zensetzou Ohya, and Ming Wong. *Médecine japonaise des origines à nos jours*. Paris: Roger Dacosta, 1974.

Hyun, Jaehwan. "Blood purity and scientific independence: blood science and postcolonial struggles in Korea, 1926–1975." *Science in Context* 32 (2019): 239–60.

Jaggi, O. P. *History of Science, Technology and Medicine in India. vol. 13: Western Medicine in India*. Delhi: Atma Ram and Sons, 1979.

Joravsky, David. "Construction of Stalinist Psyche." In *Cultural Revolution in Russia, 1928–1931*, edited by Sheila Fitzpatrick, 105–28. Bloomington: Indiana University Press, 1978.

Joravsky, David. *The Lysenko Affair*. Chicago: University of Chicago Press, 1970.

Joravsky, David. *Soviet Marxism and Natural Science*. Columbia: Columbia University Press, 1961.

Juillard Jean and Claude Raby. "La transfusion sanguin pendant la guerre 1914–1918." *Revue des corps de santé* 7 (1966): 821–38.

Karel, Leonard. "Selection of Journals for *Index Medicus*. A Historical Review." *Medical Literature Association Bulletin*, 55 (1967), 259–78.

Kerkhoff, A. H. M. "Organization of the Military and Civil Medical Service in the Nineteenth and Twentieth Centuries." In *Dutch Medicine in the Malay Archipeligo, 1816–1942*, edited by G. M. van Heteren, 9–24. Amsterdam: Rodopi, 1989.

Kevles, Daniel J. *In the Name of Eugenics.* Cambridge: Harvard University Press, 1985.

Kirejczyk, Marta. "Vrouwen kozen exact; Studie en beroepsuitoefning rond de eeuwwisseling." *Gewina* 16 (1993): 234–47.

Koehl, Robert L. *RKFDV: German Resettlement and Population Policy, 1939–1945.* Cambridge: Harvard University Press, 1957.

Kohler, Robert E. *Lords of the Fly.* Chicago: University of Chicago Press, 1994.

Kong-Ming Peter and Yuet-Wah Cheung. "Harvard Medical School of China, 1911–1916." *Social Science and Medicine* 16 (1982): 1207–15.

Kruif, Paul de. *Microbe Hunters.* (New York: Harcourt Brace, 1926.

Kruif, Paul de. *Sweeping Wind: A Memoir.* New York: Harcourt Brace, 1962.

Laplane R. "Eloge de Raymond Turpin (1895–1988)." *Bulletin de l'Académie nationale de médecine* 173 (1989):535–43.

Leon, George B. *Greece and the Allied Powers, 1914–1917.* Thessaloniki: Institute for Balkan Studies, 1974.

Lépine, Pierre "Necrologie: Nicholas Kossovitch (1884–1948)." *Annales de l'Institut Pasteur* 75 (1948): 62–4.

Leps, Marie-Christine. *Apprehending the Criminal: The Production of Deviance in Nineteenth-century Discourse.* Durham: Duke University Press, 1992.

Liber, George. "Language, Literacy, and Book Publishing in Ukrainian SSR, 1923–1928." *Slavic Review* 41 (1982): 673–85.

Liber, George *Soviet Nationality Policy, Urban Growth, and Identity Change in the Ukrainian SSR, 1923–1934.* New York: Cambridge University Press, 1992.

Lifton, Robert J. *Nazi Doctors.* New York: Basic Books, 1986.

Lindesmith, Alfred and Yale Levin. "The Lombrosian Myth in Criminology." *American Journal of Sociology* 42 (1937): 653–71.

Low, Morris. "Physical Anthropology in Japan: The Ainu and the Search for the Origins of the Japanese." *Current Anthropology,* 53 suppl. (2012): 57–68.

Luesink, David, William H. Schneider, and Zhang Daqing, eds. *China and the Globalization of Biomedicine.* Rochester: University of Rochester Press, 2019.

Mannheim, Hermann, ed. *Pioneers in Criminology.* Chicago: Quadrangle, 1960.

Marks, Jonathan. "The Legacy of Serological Studies in American Physical Anthropology." *History and Philosophy of the Life Sciences,* 18 (1995): 345–62.

Martin, Randy, Robert J. Mutchnick, and W. Timothy Austin. *Criminological Thought: Pioneers Past and Present.* New York: Macmillan. 1990.

Matsunaga, Ei. "History of Human Genetics and Eugenics in Japan." in *History and Development of Human Genetics: Progress in Different Countries,* edited by Krishna R. Dronamraju, 128–44. Singapore: World Scientific, 1992.

Mazumdar, Pauline M. H. "Blood and Soil: The Serology of the Aryan Racial State." *Bulletin of the History of Medicine* 64 (1990): 187–219.

Mazumdar, Pauline M.H. *Species and Specificity: An Interpretation of the History of Immunology through the Work of Karl Landsteiner.* Cambridge: Cambridge University Press, 1995.

Mazumdar, Pauline M. H. "Two Models for Human Genetics: Blood Grouping and Psychiatry in Germany between the Wars." *Bulletin of the History of Medicine* 70 (1996), 609–57.

McCain, Katherine W. "Mapping Authors in Intellectual Space: Population Genetics in the 1980s." In *Scholarly Communications and Bibliometrics,* edited by Christine L. Borgman, 194–216. Newbury Park, CA: Sage Publications, 1990.

McCain, Katherine W. "The Paper Trails of Scholarship: Mapping the Literature of Genetics." *Library Quarterly* 56 (1986), 258–71.

Misson, Gary P., A. Clive Bishop, and Winifred M Watkins. "Arthur Ernest Mourant. 11 April 1904 — 29 August 1994." *Biographical memoirs of fellows of the Royal Society. Royal Society.* 45 (1999): 329–48.

Mitchell, Allan. *German Influences in France after 1870.* Chapel Hill: University of North Carolina, Press, 1979.

Monachesi, Elio D. "Trends in Criminological Research in Italy." *American Sociological Review* 1 (1936): 396–406.

Montaldo, Nicole Silvano. "Lombroso: The Myth, The History." *Crime, Histoire & Sociétés / Crime, History & Societies* 22, no. 2 (2018): 31–61.

Mukharji, Projit B. "From Serosocial to Sanguinary Identities: Caste, Transnational Race Science and the Shifting Metonymies of Blood Group B, India c. 1918–1960." *Indian Economic and Social History Review* 51 (2014): 143–76.

Moeller, H. G. "Friedrich Schiff - sein Wirken als Abteilungsdirektor am Krankenhaus im Friedrichshain, Berlin von 1922 bis 1935." *Deutsche Gesundheitswesen* 29 (1974): 1850–3.

Moulin, Anne-Marie. *Le dernier langage de la médecine: Histoire de l'immunologie de: Pasteur au Sida.* Paris: Presses Universitaires de France, 1991.

Nuwer, Rachel. "You are what you bleed: In Japan and other east Asian countries some believe blood type dictates personality." *Scientific American* Guest Blog (February 15, 2011). Accessed February 13, 2024. https://blogs.scientificamerican.com/guest-blog/you-are-what-you-bleed-in-japan-and-other-east-asian-countries-some-believe-blood-type-dictates-personality/.

Nye, Robert A. "Heredity or Milieu: The Foundation of Modern European Criminological Theory." *Isis* 67 (1976): 335–55.

Ogilvie, Marilyn B. "Marital Collaboration: An Approach to Science." In *Uneasy Careers and Intimate Lives: Women in Science, 1789–1979*, edited by Pnina G. Abir-Am and Dorinda Outram, 104–25. New Brunswick: Rutgers University Press, 1987.

Ohayon, Annick. "Ce qui énervait Henri Piéron." *Bulletin de psychologie* 533 (2014): 409–14.

Patterson, James. *Dread Disease Cancer and Modern American Culture.* Cambridge: Harvard University Press, 1987.

Patzak, Herbert. "Ursprünge gerichtlich annerkannter Blutgruppenbefunde in deutschen Paternitätsgutachten." Ph.D. diss., Marburg, 1990.

Paul, Harry. *The Sorcerer's Apprentice: French Scientists' Image of German Science, 1840–1919.* Gainesville: University of Florida Press, 1972.

Pick, Daniel. *Degeneration.* Cambridge: Cambridge University Press, 1989.

Pirie, Norman W. "John Burton Sanderson Haldane." *Biographical Memoirs of the Royal Society* 12 (1966): 218–49.

Pollitzer, William. "The Development of Genetics and Population Studies." *American Journal of Physical Anthropology* 56 (1981): 488.

Poskett, James. *Materials of the Mind: Phrenology, Race, and the Global History of Science, 1815–1920.* Chicago: University of Chicago Press, 2019.

Reingold, Nathan. *Science, American Style: Selected Writings of Nathan Reingold.* New Brunswick: Rutgers University Press, 1991.

Robertson, Jennifer. "Hemato-nationalism: The Past, Present, and Future of 'Japanese Blood.'" *Medical Anthropology: Cross-Cultural Studies in Health and Illness* 31 (2012): 93–112.

Rock, Paul. *A History of British Criminology.* Oxford: Oxford University Press, 1988.

Rogers, Frank B. "Index Medicus in the Twentieth Century." In *Centenary of Index Medicus*, edited by John B. Blake, 53–61. Bethesda: U.S. Department of Health and Human Services, 1980.

Rosenberg, Charles E. "Disease and Social Order in America: Perceptions and Expectations." *Milbank Quarterly* 64, Suppl 1 (1986): 34–55.

Rosenberg, Charles E. "Disease in History: Frames and Framers." *Milbank Quarterly*, 67 (1989): 1–15.

Rous, Peyton. "Karl Landsteiner." *Obituary Notices of Fellows of the Royal Society* 5 (1947): 295–324.

Saller, Karl. *Rassenlehre des nationalsozialismus in Wissenschaft und Propagande.* Darmstadt: Progress Verlag, 1961.

Schlich, Thomas "'Welche Macht über Tod und Leben!' Die Etablierung der Bluttransfusion im Ersten Weltkrieg." In *Die Medizin und Der Erster Weltkrieg*, edited by Wolfgang U. Eckart and Christoph Gradmann, 109–30 Pfaffenweiler: Centaurus-Verlagsgesellschaft, 1996.

Schmidt, Paul J. "Early Blood Grouping and Transfusion in North Carolina: Contributions of Laurence H. Snyder." *North Carolina Medical Journal* 47 (1986): 205–8.

Schneider, William H. "Blood Group Research in Great Britain, France, and the United States Between the World Wars." *American Journal of Physical Anthropology* 38 supplement 21 (1995): 87–114.

Schneider, William H. "Blood Transfusion in Peace and War, 1900–1918." *Social History of Medicine* 10 (1997): 105–26.

Schneider, William H., "Chance and Social Setting in the Application of the Discovery of Blood Groups." Bulletin of the History of Medicine 57 (1983): 545–62.

Schneider, William H. "La Recherche sur les Groupes Sanguins avant la Deuxième Guerre Mondiale." In *Les sciences biologiques et médicales en France, 1920–50*, edited by Claude Debru, Jean Gayon, and Jean-François Picard, 311–27. Paris: CNRS-Editions, 1994.

Schneider, William H. "Le rôle des groupes sanguins dans l'histoire de la génétique," in *Histoire de la génétique* (Paris: ARPEM, 1990a), eds. Jean-Louis Fischer and William H. Schneider, 293–308.

Schneider, William H. *Quality and Quantity: The Quest for Biological Regeneration in Twentieth Century France*. New York: Cambridge University Press, 1990.

Schroeder-Gudehaus, Brigitte. "Argument for the Self-government and Public Support of Science in Weimar Germany." *Minerva* 10 (1972): 537–70.

Sellin, Thorsten. "The Lombrosian Myth in Criminology – Comment." *American Journal of Sociology* 42 (1937): 898–9.

Shafer Stephen, *Theories of Criminology*. New York: Random House, 1969.

Shigeru, Nakayama, David L. Swain, and Yagi Eri eds. *Science and Society in Modern Japan*. Cambridge: MIT Press, 1974.

Silverman, Rachel. "The Blood Group 'Fad' in Post-War Racial Anthropology." *Kroeber Anthropological Society Papers* 84 (2000): 11–27.

Silverstein, Arthur M. *History of Immunology*. New York: Academic Press, 1989.

Sim, Joe. *Medical Power in Prisons: The Prison Medical Service in England, 1774–1989*. Buckingham: Open University Press, 1990.

Snyder, Louis H. "Human and Medical Genetics in the United States; an oral History Tape Interview." *American Journal of Medical Genetics* 8 (1981): 449–68.

Solomon, Susan Gross. "Soviet-German Syphilis Expedition to Buriat Mongolia, 1928: Scientific Research on National Minorities." *Slavic Review* 52 (1993): 204–32.

Sommer, Marianne. "Biology as a Technology of Social Justice in Interwar Britain: Arguments from Evolutionary History, Heredity, and Human Diversity." *Science, Technology, & Human Values* 39, no. 4 (2014): 561–86.

Sorkowski, Heinz. *Springer Verlag*. Berlin: Springer, 1992.

Southcott, R. V. "John Burton Cleland." *Medical Journal of Australia* 59 (1972):192–3.

Speiser, Paul. *Karl Landsteiner, Entdecker der Blutgruppen*. Vienna: Hollinek, 1961.

Spörri, Myriam. *Reines und gemischtes Blut: Zur Kulturgeschichte der Blutgruppenforschung, 1900–1933*. Bielefeld: Transcript Verlag, 2013.

Stamhuis, Ida. "Female Contribution to Early Genetics: Tine Tammes and Mendel's Law for Continuous Character." *Journal of the History of Biology* 28 (1995): 495–531.

Stark, Gary D. *Entrepreneurs of Ideology: Neo-conservative Publishers in Germany, 1890–1933*. Chapel Hill: University of North Carolina Press, 1981.

Steffen, Katrin and Maciej Górny. "Böses Blut. Die Blutgruppenforschung und der Serologe Ludwik Hirszfeld in Deutschland und in Polen." *JB historie* 1 (2014): 97–119.

Stepan, Nancy. *Beginnings of Brazilian Science: Oswaldo Cruz, Medical Research and Policy, 1890–1920*. New York: Science History Publications, 1976.

Stepan, Nancy. Hour of Eugenics: Race, Gender, and Nation in Latin America. Ithaca: Cornell University Press, 1991.

Storm van Leeuwen, Willem. *Indrukten van een statieris naar America*. Groningen: J.B. Wolters, 1920.

Tagg, John. "A Means of Surveillance; The Photograph as Evidence in Law." In *The Burden of Representation*, edited by John Tagg, 66–102. Amherst: University of Massachusetts Press, 1988.

Taguieff, Pierre-André. "Immigrés, métis, Juifs: les raisons de l'inassimilabilité. Opinions et doctrines du Dr. Martial." In *Nationalismes, féminismes, exclusions: Mélanges en l'honneur de Rita Thalmann*, edited by Liliane Crips, Michel Cullin, Nicole Gabriel, and Fritz Taubert, 177–221. Frankfurt: Peter Lang, 1993.

Thackray, Arnold. "Measurement in the Historiography of Science." In *Toward a Metric of Science*, edited by Yehuda Elkana, Joshua Lederberg, Robert K Merton, Arnold Thackray, and Harriet Zuckerman, 11–30. N.Y.: John Wiley, 1978.

Thadeusz, Frank. "Blood Purity: How a Bizarre Obsession Advanced Science." *Spiegel*, May 31, 2013.

Thomann, Klaus-Dieter. "Exkurs: Der medizinische Verlag J. F. Lehmann, Förderer und Finanzier von alldeutschem Verband und NSDAP." In *Medizin, Faschismus und Widerstand: Drei Beiträge*, edited by Barbara Bromberger, Hans Maustich and Klaus Dieter Thomann, 97–110. Cologne: Paul Rugenstein, 1985

Tracy, Sarah W. "George Draper and American Constitutional Medicine, 1916–1946: Reinventing the Sick Man." *Bulletin of the History of Medicine* 66 (1992): 53–89.

Tsurumi, Patricia. *Japanese Colonial Education in Taiwan, 1895–1945*. Cambridge: Harvard University Press, 1977.

Turda, Marius. "Entangled Traditions of Race: Physical Anthropology in Hungary and Romania, 1900–1940." *Focaal*, 58 (2010): 32–46.

Turda, Marius. "From Craniology to Serology: Racial Anthropology in Interwar Hungary and Romania." *Journal of the History of the Behavioral Sciences*, 43 (2007): 361–77.

Watanabe, Minoru. "Japanese Students Abroad and the Acquisition of Scientific and Technical Knowledge." *Cahiers d'études mondiales* 9 (1965): 254–93.

Weindling, Paul. *Health, Race and German Politics between National Unification and Nazism, 1870–1945*. Cambridge: Cambridge University Press, 1989.

Weindling, Paul. "Rockefeller Foundation and German Biomedical Science, 1920–1940." In *Science, Politics and the Public Good*, edited by Nicholas A. Rupke, 119–40. London: Macmillan, 1988.

Weingart, Peter, Jürgen Kroll, and Kurt Bayertz. *Rasse, Blut und Gene*. Frankfurt: Suhrkamp, 1988.

Index[1]

[1] Note: Page numbers followed by 'n' refer to notes.

W. H. Schneider, *Blood Groups and Human Heredity, 1900–1950*, Medicine and Biomedical Sciences in Modern History, https://doi.org/10.1007/978-3-031-69844-6

D

E

F

G